ASHP's
PharmPrep

Interactive Case-Based Board Review

Third Edition

Diane B. Ginsburg, M.S., R.Ph., FASHP
  Clinical Professor
  Assistant Dean for Student Affairs
  Regional Director, Internship Program
  The University of Texas at Austin
  College of Pharmacy
  Austin, Texas

American Society of Health-System Pharmacists®
Bethesda, Maryland

Any correspondence regarding this publication should be sent to the publisher, American Society of Health-System Pharmacists, 7272 Wisconsin Avenue, Bethesda, MD 20814, attention: Special Publishing.

The information presented herein reflects the opinions of the contributors and advisors. It should not be interpreted as an official policy of ASHP or as an endorsement of any product. The information contained in this program, and the companion workbook, are to be used as guidance.

Because of ongoing research and improvements in technology, the information and its applications contained in this text are constantly evolving and are subject to the professional judgment and interpretation of the practitioner. The editors, contributors, and ASHP have made reasonable efforts to ensure the accuracy and appropriateness of the information presented in this document. However, any user of this information is advised that the editors, contributors, advisors, and ASHP are not responsible for the continued currency of the information, for any errors or omissions, and/or for any consequences arising from the use of the information in the document in any and all practice settings. Any reader of this document is cautioned that ASHP makes no representation, guarantee, or warranty, express or implied, as to the accuracy and appropriateness of the information contained in this document and will bear no responsibility or liability for the results or consequences of its use.

Director, Special Publishing: Jack Bruggeman
Senior Editorial Project Manager: Dana Battaglia
Editorial Resources Manager: Bill Fogle
Editorial Assistance: Caroline Moyo Myers

Cover and page design: David A. Wade

Library of Congress Cataloging-in-Publication Data

ASHP's pharmprep : interactive case-based board review / [edited by] Diane B. Ginsburg. — 3rd ed.
    p. ; cm.
  Includes bibliographical references.
  ISBN-13: 978-1-58528-148-0
  ISBN-10: 1-58528-148-4
1. Pharmacology—Examinations, questions, etc. 2. Clinical pharmacology—Examinations, questions, etc. I. Ginsburg, Diane B. II. American Society of Health-System Pharmacists. III. Title: Pharmprep. IV. Title: ASHP's pharm prep. V. Title: American Society of Health-System Pharmacists' pharmprep.
[DNLM: 1. Drug Therapy—Case Reports. 2. Drug Therapy—Examination Questions. 3. Pharmaceutical Preparations—Case Reports. 4. Pharmaceutical Preparations—Examination Questions. QV 18.2 A827 2007]

  RM105.A84 2007
  615'.1076—dc22

                2006039333

ISBN: 978-1-58528-148-0

Dedication

This edition is dedicated in loving memory of my Mother, Phyllis B. Ginsburg, and in honor of my dear friends from New Orleans, the Jastram Family.

Table of Contents

Table of Contents: The Book

Disease Management Sections and Cases

Cardiac and Vascular Disorders

Section Editors: James A. Karboski, Steven Marx
See all 21 cases in this section on the CD.

Respiratory and Pulmonary Disorders

Section Editors: Charlotte A. Kenreigh, Linda Timm Wagner
See all 10 cases in this section on the CD.

Gastrointestinal Disorders

Section Editor: Rosemary R. Berardi
See all 10 cases for this section on the CD.

Table of Contents

OB-GYN Disorders and Women's Health

Section Editor: Andrea Coffee
*See the complete section with 9 cases on the CD.

Pediatric Therapy

Section Editor: Lea S. Eiland
*See all 8 cases for this section on the CD,

Diseases of the Eye and Ear

Section Editor: Michael A. Oszko
*See the complete section with 6 cases on the CD.

Skin Disorders

Section Editor: Ellen Rhinard
*See all 6 cases for the section on the CD.

Table of Contents: The CD

Disease Management Sections and Cases

Table of Contents

Table of Contents

Table of Contents

Table of Contents

Federal Law Review
Jesse Vivian

Compounding and Calculations Review
Robert O. Williams, Jason M. Vaughn

Appendixes

Acknowledgments

I was very fortunate to have met some incredibly talented practitioners who were willing to lend their expertise to this endeavor when we produced the first and second editions. What we accomplished was the development and publication of a textbook and software that was different than any other seen, a guide that has helped many students in their quest for licensure and inclusion in our revered profession and a tool to help those refresh their clinical skills and knowledge.

I am grateful and indebted to all of the authors who willingly gave of themselves, their time and expertise, to help create this third edition. As with the first and second editions, all of you continue to exceed what I requested of you. Your commitment to the profession is evidenced by your contributions to this text. To John Blanchett and Kunal Patel, P1 students (during the time of this writing) at the University of Texas at Austin College of Pharmacy, thank you for all of your assisting during the editing process as well as your perspective on the content. It is nice to know this text will be useful to you both when you prepare for boards. Thank you to the College of Pharmacy at the University of Texas at Austin, for their unlimited support and encouragement. My students and colleagues are a continual source of energy that I drew from many times. Thanks for reminding me "why I do what I do" and why it is important to give back to the profession.

A special thank you to two of my section editors, Charles W. Jastram and John L. Woon. You both continue to be incredible supporters and remained enthusiastic throughout this project. I have called on you both for guidance and assistance on so many occasions. Thank you for always being there, and for your amazing support, continuous energy, encouragement, and friendship. This book is a tribute to what you both do on a daily basis.

To my colleagues at ASHP, Jack Bruggeman, Bill Fogle, David Wade, Carol Wolfe, Michael Dodd, Jim Collins, Don Brower, Dean Manke, and especially Dana Battaglia, thank you for all of your unconditional support, understanding, and enthusiasm. All of your contributions make this a reality. It couldn't happen without all of you.

There are special people in my life that continue to inspire me and serve as a source of strength and encouragement. To my dear friends, Darlene Mednick, Janet and Michael Silvester, Debra Devereaux, Teri Bair, Lourdes Cuellar, Jennifer Myhra, Teresa Hudson, Jill Martin, Lynnae Mahaney, Cynthia Brennan, Malcolm Broussard, and Steven Sheaffer, thank you for all of your professional and personal guidance. It means more than you will ever know. To my family, thank you for all of your support and understanding throughout the many months of this endeavor. A special thank you to my husband, Jeffrey Josephs, MD, not only for your professional contributions to this edition but also for your unconditional support and loving understanding of my commitment to this project and giving back to the profession.

Every great dream begins with a dreamer. Always remember, you have within you the strength, the patience, and the passion to reach for the stars to change the world.
Harriet Tubman

Diane B. Ginsburg

Society expects all health professionals, including pharmacists, to achieve and then maintain competency to practice throughout their career. There is no better resource than *ASHP's PharmPrep Interactive Case-Based Board Review* in helping new graduates and practicing pharmacists fulfill this expectation. *PharmPrep* is an excellent resource to assist the pharmacy student and graduate in preparing for practice and the NAPLEX® exam. It is also an invaluable resource for life-long learning. The comprehensive case-based approach to learning is applicable to the student in the classroom or lab, to supplement early and advanced experiential training of Pharm.D. students, for a pharmacist who wishes to brush up clinical skills as he or she takes on new responsibilities or simply as a means of "just keeping up." The new 3rd edition, following just 3 years after the last edition, reflects a huge commitment by editor Diane Ginsburg and very capable chapter authors in making sure the real life cases contributed and what is learned is both current and relevant.

In 2004 the NABP blueprint revision of the content areas of the NAPLEX® exam was completed resulting in their updated competency statements. This update was based on their survey of pharmacy practice and review of various documents developed by the profession. Changes in the NAPLEX® exam based on this new blueprint were implemented in 2005. I was pleased to see that the content covered in the 3rd edition of *ASHP's PharmPrep* reflected the same percentage breakdown as the three major competency areas tested on the revised NAPLEX® exam. The drop in the national passage rate from 97% for first-time candidates in 2004 to 91% for the 2005 exam based on the new blueprint would indicate that the revisions resulted in a more challenging exam. If this trend continues it would suggest even greater importance of being well prepared for anyone taking the NAPLEX® exam. This is especially true of NAPLEX® Area 1; "Assure safe and effective pharmacotherapy and optimize therapeutic outcomes," which now comprises 54% of the exam. Those preparing for this increased focus on pharmacotherapy will particularly benefit from the case-based approach used in *ASHP's PharmPrep*. This book and the accompanying computer based cases cover most of the disease states and conditions likely to be encountered on the NAPLEX® exam. The case-based format also enables readers to utilize real-life situations to hone their knowledge of calculations, dispensing systems and compounding, and in providing drug information and educating patients and other caregivers on medication use issues.

The NAPLEX® exam is not the only area of competency that students must prepare for when entering practice. The Multi-State Jurisprudence Exam (MJPE) usually presents an even greater challenge, given the lower passage rate in most states compared to the NAPLEX® exam results. The Federal Law section provides students with a good foundation to build on for their state specific pharmacy practice laws. Contact information for each state board assists students in accessing and learning state specific laws and in the application process to register for taking the licensure exams.

Today's new and experienced practitioners face an ongoing challenge in keeping up with the growth and complexity of drug therapy. As I noted previously, society expects us to maintain and demonstrate continued competency as a pharmacist. Many in the health professions, including pharmacy, are questioning the effectiveness of mandatory continuing education. Many state and national pharmacy leaders are looking at a new process, Continuing Professional Develop (CPD) as an alternative method to maintain competency. In 2002 the International Pharmaceutical Federation (FIP) defined CPD as "the responsibility of individual pharmacists for systematic maintenance, development and broadening of knowledge, skills, and attitudes, to ensure continuing competence as a professional throughout their careers." Organizations that need to develop and then assess and document the competency of their staff to fulfill JCAHO® standards are already engaged in a similar process. *ASHP's PharmPrep* is an ideal option to consider as state boards of pharmacy and professional organizations look to pilot CPD programs or provider organizations seek to create their own competency development programs to meet individualized needs of their specialists and frontline pharmacists. The scope of topics covered and the extensive selection of cases in the text and on the CD provide for almost unlimited opportunities for professional development.

Diane Ginsburg, the contributing authors, and ASHP should be commended for creating and continuously updating this valuable resource. Regardless of your position or stage of your career, if you deal with the application of drug therapy to patient care, you will benefit from and enjoy the learning process you will experience using this publication. If I was graduating today, I could not think of a better graduation present from a future colleague to support preparation for the "big test" and continued growth of a competent and patient-centered professional.

Steven Sheaffer, Pharm.D., FASHP

Vice Chair for Experiential Learning
Associate Professor of Clinical Pharmacy
Department of Pharmacy Practice and Pharmacy Administration
Philadelphia College of Pharmacy
University of the Sciences in Philadelphia

In both the first and second editions of *ASHP's PharmPrep*, I described the practice of pharmacy like medicine, as an art accompanied by science. Each practitioner approaches a patient differently in the same manner in which an artist approaches the canvas. In the artist's world, there are no true colors of black and white, just many shades of gray. As we know, medicine is the same way. There is not one treatment or manner to manage any disease. The art is to know how to apply the science to hopefully facilitate a positive patient outcome. As we enter clinical practice, we realize that very few patients are "textbook cases" and usually deviate from what we have read in pages. Most patients are a complicated mix of colors requiring analysis of the situation accompanied by the application of our clinical decision-making, or the "art of pharmacy practice."

ASHP's PharmPrep, Interactive Case-Based Board Review, Third Edition, is a multidisciplinary review guide that will provide a comprehensive review of disease states that are covered on the North American Pharmacy Licensure Examination (NAPLEX®). The format is intended to give the student an opportunity to review real cases accompanied by questions that address all of the NAPLEX® competency statements. This text, like the first two editions, differs from other board review books in that it is case-based. The textbook and the accompanying software should help the student identify areas requiring additional study as well as provide a comprehensive review of the types of disease states and therapeutics related issues that pharmacists encounter in practice. In addition, this review guide is an excellent tool for the practitioner who would like to update his or her knowledge of a given disease state.

The authors of *ASHP's PharmPrep, Interactive Case-Based Board Review, Third Edition,* have used "real" patient cases to emphasize that patients seen in practice rarely present in a textbook/black-and-white manner. The goal is for the student to be able to prepare not only for the NAPLEX® but for real practice by exposure to actual patients. The student can practice on the patients provided in this text knowing that no harm will come to them as a result of an incorrect answer.

Many things have been added to the third edition. All cases have been revised, and new cases and diseases states are included. Many sections have been expanded, including Infectious Diseases, Over-the-Counter Medications, Compounding and Calculations, and Federal Law. The software and accompanying textbook contain these new cases and significant revisions from the second edition for additional practice. Cases selected for the textbook represent the most common disease states that the student will encounter in community and hospital practice. All cases and sections are included in the software. The software and textbook is organized based on major therapeutic areas of focus, then tailored into more specific disease states. There are 115 different disease management areas with 2 or 3 cases per topic for a total of 244 patient cases. The Federal Law section has been revised and updated and includes information on the HIPAA regulations. Questions in this section mirror those on the Multistate Pharmacy Jurisprudence Examination (MPJE®).

The layout of each case is presented like a medical chart and includes 10 questions with the NAPLEX® competency statement designated in the answer section. The correct answer is fully explained, including why other answers are incorrect. The software will allow the student to simulate taking the NAPLEX® or enable the student to review a specific disease state.

The authors that have contributed to the third edition represent all facets of pharmacy practice and are experts in their respective disciplines. Two board-certified physicians in psychiatry and neurology have also authored cases. The cases, questions, and answers represent information that the practitioners have taken from their clinical experience. The authors have been careful to recommend therapies that are reflective of current standards and treatment guidelines; however, there may be more than one manner in which to treat the patients seen in this text.

ASHP's PharmPrep, Interactive Case-Based Board Review, Third Edition, is designed not only to assist the student in preparing for licensure but also to facilitate life-long learning. As a professional, a pharmacist must commit to keeping up and must review information to maintain competency. I hope this textbook with its accompanying software will be one mechanism for accomplishing this and wish you the best in your practice.

Diane B. Ginsburg, M.S., R.Ph., FASHP
Editor, *ASHP's PharmPrep, Interactive Case-Based Board Review, Third Edition*
August 2006

Editor-in-Chief

Diane B. Ginsburg, M.S., R.Ph., FASHP
Clinical Professor
Assistant Dean for Student Affairs
Regional Director, Internship Program
The University of Texas at Austin
College of Pharmacy
Austin, Texas

Senior Editor

John L. Woon, Pharm.D., FASHP
Clinical Associate Professor
Idaho State University College of Pharmacy
Clinical Pharmacist, Adult Medicine
Kootenai Medical Center
Coeur d'Alene, ID

Section Editors

Rosemary R. Berardi, Pharm.D., FACCP, FASHP, FAPhA
Professor of Pharmacy
University of Michigan
College of Pharmacy
Ann Arbor, MI

Joseph Bubalo, Pharm.D., BCPS
Oncology Clinical Pharmacy Specialist, Assistant Professor of Medicine
Oregon Health Sciences University Hospital
Portland, OR

Andrea Coffee, Pharm.D., BCPS
Pharmacy Clinical Specialist
Scott & White Memorial Hospital
Temple, TX

Lawrence J. Cohen, Pharm.D., BCPP, FASHP, FCCP
Professor of Pharmacotherapy
Washington State University College of Pharmacy
WIMIRT (Washington Institute for Mental Illness Research and Training)
Spokane, WA

Lourdes Cuellar, M.S., R.Ph., FASHP
Senior Executive Director, Medical Support Services
Director of Pharmacy
Memorial Hermann Hospital - TIRR
Houston, TX

Lea S. Eiland, Pharm. D., BCPS
Assistant Clinical Professor of Pharmacy Practice
Auburn University
Harrison School of Pharmacy
Huntsville, AL

Editors

Katherine C. Herndon, Pharm.D., BCPS
Clinical Education Consultant
Pfizer Pharmaceutical Group U.S. Pharmaceuticals
Birmingham, AL

Teresa Hudson, Pharm.D., FASHP
Health Research Scientist
Center for Mental Health and Outcomes Research
North Little Rock, AR

Beata A. Ineck, Pharm.D., BCPS
Assistant Professor
University of Nebraska Medical Center
Omaha, NE

Charles W. Jastram, Jr., Pharm.D., FASHP
Associate Professor and Department Head,
Clinical and Administrative Sciences
University of Louisiana at Monroe
College of Pharmacy
Monroe, LA

James A. Karboski, Pharm.D.
Clinical Associate Professor
University of Texas at Austin
Division of Pharmacy Practice
College of Pharmacy
Austin, TX

Charlotte A. Kenreigh, Pharm.D.
MLC Solutions, Ltd
Galena, OH

Debra Lopez, Pharm.D., CDE
Clinical Pharmacist
Blackstock Family Practice
Clinical Assistant Professor
University of Texas at Austin
Division of Pharmacy Practice
College of Pharmacy
Austin, TX

Steven Marx, Pharm.D., MS
Associate Director
Global Health Economics & Outcomes Research
Abbott
Abbott Park, IL

Barbara Mason, Pharm.D.
Professor and Vice Chair
Department of Pharmacy Practice
Idaho State University College of Pharmacy
Boise, ID

Jennifer Ridings Myhra, R.Ph.
Assistant Dean for Experiential and Professional Affairs
Clinical Associate Professor
College of Pharmacy
The University of Texas at Austin
Austin, TX

Dannielle C. O'Donnell, Pharm.D., BCPS, CDM
Senior Medical Liaison
Scientific Field Operations, Medical Affairs
Roche Laboratories Inc.
Clinical Assistant Professor
Division of Pharmacy Practice
University of Texas at Austin
College of Pharmacy
Austin, TX

Catherine M. Oliphant, Pharm.D.
Associate Professor of Pharmacy Practice
Idaho State University College of Pharmacy
St. Lukes Internal Medicine
Boise, ID

Ali Olyaei, Pharm.D., BCPS
Associate Professor of Medicine
Director of Clinical Research, Nephrology and Hypertension,
Clinical Pharmacotherapist
Oregon Health Sciences University
Portland, OR

Michael A. Oszko, Pharm.D., BCPS, FASHP
Associate Professor
The University of Kansas Medical Center
School of Pharmacy
Department of Pharmacy Practice
Kansas City, KS

Ellen Rhinard, Pharm.D., BCPS
Assistant Professor of Pharmacy Practice
St. Louis College of Pharmacy
Pharmacy Practice Division
St. Louis, MO

Terry L. Schwinghammer, Pharm.D., FCCP, FASHP, BCPS
Professor and Chair
Department of Clinical Pharmacy
West Virginia University School of Pharmacy
Morgantown, WV

Susan Skledar, Pharm.D., MPH
Associate Professor
School of Pharmacy
Director, Drug Use and Disease State Management Program
Drug Information Center and Investigational Drug Service
University of Pittsburgh and University of Pittsburgh Medical Center
Pittsburgh, PA

Patricia Tabor, Pharm.D., BCPS
Clinical Specialist
Scott & White Hospital, Health Plan, & Clinics
Clinical Assistant Professor
University of Texas at Austin
Division of Pharmacy Practice
College of Pharmacy
Temple, TX

Editors

Holli Temple, Pharm.D., BCPS
Clinical Pharmacist
North Austin Medical Center
Department of Pharmacy
Austin, TX

Jason M. Vaughn, R.Ph., Ph.D.
Associate Director
Analytical R.D. and Product Development
PharmaForm L.L.C.
Austin, TX

Jesse Vivian, J.D., R.Ph.
Professor of Pharmacy Practice
Wayne State University
College of Pharmacy and Health Sciences
Detroit, MI

Linda Timm Wagner, Pharm.D.
MLC Solutions, Ltd
Galena, OH

W. Renee Acosta, R.Ph., M.S.
Clinical Assistant Professor
The University of Texas at Austin
College of Pharmacy
Austin, TX

Robert T. Adamson, Pharm.D.
Corporate Director of Clinical Pharmacy Services
Saint Barnabas Health Care System
West Orange, NJ

Chris Allbritton, Pharm.D.
Assistant Clinical Professor
UAMS College of Pharmacy
Clinical Pharmacy Coordinator
VA Medical Center
Fayetteville, AR

Douglas R. Allington, Pharm.D., BCPS
Associate Professor, Pharmacy Practice
University of Montana
School of Pharmacy and Allied Health Sciences
Missoula, MT

Charles R. Ashton, Pharm.D. (2006)
Idaho State University College of Pharmacy
Boise, ID

Jennifer P. Askew, B.S., Pharm.D.
Coordinator, Outpatient Pharmacy Services
New Hanover Health Network
Wilmington, NC

Nile Barnes, EMT-P, Pharm.D.
Assistant Professor
Feik School of Pharmacy
University of the Incarnate Word
San Antonio, TX

Debra J. Barnette, Pharm.D., BCPS, CDE
Ambulatory Care Clinical Coordinator
Wake Forest University Baptist Medical Center
Winston-Salem, NC

Tawny Bettinger, Pharm.D., BCPP
Assistant Professor
University of Texas at Austin
College of Pharmacy
Austin, TX

Yeshewaneh Beyene, Pharm.D., R.Ph.
Clinical Education Consultant
Pfizer Inc.
Saratoga Springs, NY
Brad Blackwell, M.S., R.Ph.
Sr. Pharmacy Product Manager
Omnicell, Inc.
Mountain View, CA

Contributors

Contributors

Suzanne G. Bollmeier, Pharm.D., BCPS, AE-C
Assistant Professor
St. Louis College of Pharmacy
Pharmacy Practice Division
St. Louis, MO

Scott Bolster, Pharm.D.
Level II Pharmacist, Critical Care
Brackenridge Hospital
Austin, TX

Edward Bornet, M.S., R.Ph.
Director of Pharmacy Services
San Jacinto Methodist Hospital
Baytown, TX

Jennifer Bosworth, Pharm.D.
Coordinator, Pharmacy Continuing Education
University of Texas at Austin
College of Pharmacy
Austin, TX

John D. Bowman, M.S., R.Ph., BCPS
Associate Professor
McWhorter School of Pharmacy
Samford University
Birmingham, AL

Rebekah E. Brunell, Pharm.D., CGP
Clinical Pharmacist
CTXVHS Ambulatory Care Clinic
Clinical Preceptor
University of Texas at Austin
Temple, TX

Helen M. Calmes, Pharm.D., M.B.A.
Clinical Manager
LSU Health Science Center
Earl K. Long Medical Center
Baton Rouge, LA

Bruce Canaday, Pharm.D., FASHP, FAPhA
Director, Department of Pharmacotherapy
Coastal AHEC
Wilmington, NC

Ryan Carnahan, Pharm.D., M.S., BCPP
Assistant Professor
University of Oklahoma
College of Pharmacy
Tulsa, OK

Glenda Carr, Pharm.D.
Assistant Professor of Pharmacy Practice
Idaho State University
College of Pharmacy
Nampa, ID

Jack J. Chen, Pharm.D., BCPS, CGP
Clinical Associate Professor of Neurology
Associate Professor (Neurology)

Loma Linda University
Schools of Medicine and Pharmacy
Loma Linda, CA

Eric Chernin, R.Ph.
Pharmaceutical Care Specialist - OR Pharmacy
Sarasota Memorial Hospital
Sarasota, FL

Vincent W. Chia, Pharm.D.
Clinical Research Scientist I
Altana Pharma US
Florham Park, NJ

Elaine Chiquette, Pharm.D., BCPS
Senior Medical Science Liaison
Amylin Pharmaceuticals
San Antonio, TX

Daniel T. Colley, Pharm.D.
Coordinator
Oncology Pharmacy Clinical Support Services
Kaiser Permanente
Portland, OR

Tenille D. Cowart, Pharm.D.
Idaho State University College of Pharmacy
Boise, ID

Catherine Dennehy, Pharm.D.
Associate Clinical Professor
University of California
San Francisco School of Pharmacy
San Francisco, CA

Victoria S. DeVore-Woodard, Pharm.D.
Consultant Pharmacist
Fort Collins, CO

Andrew J. Donnelly, Pharm.D., M.B.A.
Director of Pharmacy
University of Illinois Medical Center at Chicago
Clinical Professor of Pharmacy Practice
University of Illinois College of Pharmacy
Chicago, IL

Victor G. Dostrow, M.D.
Clinical Associate Professor of Neurology
University of Mississippi School of Medicine
Jackson, MS
Clinical Associate Professor
School of Clinical Pharmacy
University of Mississippi School of Pharmacy
Oxford, MS

Robert Dupuis, Pharm.D., BCPS
Clinical Associate Professor
UNC at Chapel Hill
School of Pharmacy
Chapel Hill, NC

Kim Elliott, Pharm.D.
Manager, Patient Care Services
Children's Hospital
Columbus, OH

Sharon M. Erdman, Pharm.D.
Clinical Associate Professor of Pharmacy Practice
Purdue University School of Pharmacy
Infectious Diseases Clinical Pharmacist
Wishard Health Services
Indianapolis, IN

Nancy Fjortoft, Ph.D.
Associate Dean and Professor
Midwestern University Chicago College of Pharmacy
Downers Grove, IL

M. Patricia Fuhrman, M.S., R.D., CNSD
Area Nutrition Manager
Coram, Inc.
St. Louis, MO

David Fuhs, Pharm.D., M.S., FASHP
Senior Regional Medical Scientist, Cardiovascular/Metabolic
GlaxoSmithKline
Woodbury, MN

Stephanie Garrett, Pharm.D.
Assistant Professor
Nova Southeastern University
Fort Lauderdale, FL

Kathryn Gaudette, Pharm.D.
Clinical Oncology Pharmacist
H. Lee Moffitt Cancer Center & Research Institute
Tampa, FL

Julie Golembiewski, Pharm.D.
Clinical Associate Professor
University of Illinois Medical Center at Chicago
Chicago, IL

Myke R. Green, Pharm.D., BCOP
Clinical Pharmacy Specialist - Adult Oncology
H. Lee Moffitt Cancer Center & Research Institute
Tampa, FL

Karl Gumpper, R.Ph., BCNSP, BCPS, FASHP
Director, Section of Pharmacy Informatics
American Society of Health-System Pharmacists
Bethesda, MD

Thomas C. Hardin, Pharm.D., MBA, FCCP
Associate Director
Anti-Infective Scientific Affairs Liaisons
Ortho-McNeil Janssen Scientific Affairs, LLC
San Antonio, TX

Camtu N. Ho, Pharm.D.
Assistant Clinical Professor

Xavier University of Louisiana
College of Pharmacy at the Medical Center of Louisiana at New Orleans
Harvey, LA

Joseph R. Ineck, Pharm.D.
Clinical Assistant Professor of Pharmacy Practice
Idaho State University
College of Pharmacy
Boise, ID

Jeffrey Josephs, M.D.
Senior Staff Psychiatrist
Austin Travis County MHMR Center
Austin, TX

Audrey Kennedy, R.Ph.
Attending Pharmacist, OR Pharmacy
Massachusetts General Hospital
Department of Pharmacy
Boston, MA

Joseph J. Kishel, Pharm.D., BCPS
Infectious Diseases Specialist
Milton S. Hershey Medical Center
Penn State College of Medicine
Hershey, PA

Catherine Kline, Pharm.D.
Advocate Lutheran General Hospital
Park Ridge, IL

Christine Kurtzeborn, Pharm.D., BCPS
Clinical Pharmacist, Infectious Diseases
Barnes-Jewish Hospital at Washington University Medical Center
Department of Pharmacy
St. Louis, MO

Greg Laine, M.S., R.Ph.
Clinical Coordinator, Critical Care
St. Luke's Episcopal Hospital
Department of Pharmacy
Houston, TX

Julie S. Larsen, Pharm.D.
Director, Clinical Research
MGI Pharma
Bloomington, MN

Pamela Leal, B.S., Pharm.D.
Pharmacy Director
Clinical Pharmacist
Austin Surgical Hospital
Austin, TX

Nancy Letassy, Pharm.D., CDE
Associate Professor
University of Oklahoma Health Sciences Center
College of Pharmacy
Oklahoma City, OK

Contributors

Mary Lewis, Pharm.D.
Assistant Clinical Professor
University of Louisiana at Monroe
College of Pharmacy
Department of Clinical and Administrative Sciences
LSUHSC-Earl K. Long Medical Center
Baton Rouge, LA

Michael Liebl, Pharm.D, BCPS
Clinical Manager
The Methodist Hospital
Pharmacy Department
Houston, TX

Katheleen Louis-Pinto, Pharm.D., R.Ph.
Clinical Coordinator, CV Services and Cardiac Transplantation
Department of Pharmacy
St. Luke's Episcopal Hospital
Adjunct Faculty
Baylor College of Medicine
Houston, TX

Karl Madaras-Kelly, Pharm.D.
Associate Professor of Pharmacy Practice
Idaho State University
College of Pharmacy
Boise, ID

Stephanie Magdanz, Pharm.D.
Affiliate Faculty
ISU College of Pharmacy
Oncology Pharmacist
Saint Alphonsus Cancer Care Center
Boise, ID

Scott Mark, Pharm.D., M.S., M.Ed., FACHE, FASHP, FABC
Director of Pharmacy
University of Pittsburgh Medical Center
Assistant Professor
Director
Pharmacy Practice Management Residency Program
University of Pittsburgh School of Pharmacy
Pittsburgh, PA

Shane Martin, Pharm.D.
Assistant Clnical Professor of Pharmacy
Rudolph H. Raabe College of Pharmacy
Ohio Northern University
Ada, OH

Traci L. Metting, Pharm.D., R.Ph.
Director of Clinical Pharmacy
Broadlane, Inc.
Dallas, TX

Yeruk Lily Mulugeta, Pharm.D.
Pediatric Critical Care Specialist
Children's National Medical Center
Washington, DC

Becky Nagle, Pharm.D.
Senior Director
Clinical Practice & Education
Medco Health Solutions, Inc.
Franklin Lakes, NJ

Sara "Cindy" Noble, Pharm.D.
Clinical Associate Professor of Family Medicine
University of Mississippi School of Medicine
Clinical Education Coordinator
Pfizer, Inc.
Jackson, MS

Karen S. Oles, Pharm.D., M.S., BCPS, CPP
Associate Professor (Clinical Pharmacy)
Wake Forest University
School of Pharmacy
Department of Neurology
Winston-Salem, NC

Venita Papillion, Pharm.D.
Director of Pharmacy
Women's and Children's Hospital
Lafayette, LA

Holly Phillips, Pharm.D.
Multidisciplinary Project Coordinator
University of Colorado Hospital
Clinical Assistant Professor
University of Colorado at Denver and Health Sciences Center
Denver, CO

Jill Polk, Pharm.D.
Assistant Professor of Pharmacy Practice
Texas Tech University School of Pharmacy
Amarillo, TX

Anne Poon, Pharm.D.
Clinical Pharmacist, Allogeneic Bone Marrow & Stem Cell Transplant
Clinical Assistant Professor
University of Washington Medical Center
UW College of Pharmacy
Seattle, WA

Michael Postelnick, R.Ph., BCPS, with Added Qualifications in Infectious
Diseases
Clinical Coordinator
Northwestern Memorial Hospital
Pharmacy Department
Chicago, IL

Nadina J. Powell, Pharm.D.
Mercer Human Resource Consulting
New York, NY

Theresa Prosser, Pharm.D.
Professor
St. Louis College of Pharmacy
Pharmacy Practice Division
St. Louis, MO

Contributors

David J. Ritchie, Pharm.D., FCCP, BCPS
Clinical Pharmacist, Infectious Diseases
Barnes-Jewish Hospital
Professor of Pharmacy Practice
St. Louis College of Pharmacy
Department of Pharmacy
St. Louis, MO

Michael Rivey, M.S. Pharm, BCPS
Professor, Pharmacy Practice
University of Montana
School of Pharmacy and Allied Health Sciences
Missoula, MT

Marc Scheetz, Pharm.D.
Infectious Diseases Pharmacist
Northwestern Memorial Hospital
Chicago, IL

Arvind Shah, R.Ph.
Supervisor, OR Pharmacy
Massachusetts General Hospital Department of Pharmacy
Boston, MA

Stephanie Shamsie, Pharm.D., BCPS
Clinical Specialist
Pflugerville, TX

Sam Shimomura, Pharm.D., FASHP, CGP
Associate Dean, Professional and Student Affairs
Western University of Health Sciences
College of Pharmacy
Pomona, CA

Janet A. Silvester, R.Ph, MBA, FASHP
Director of Pharmacy Services
Martha Jefferson Hospital
Charlottesville, VA

Sherry Smith, Pharm.D., BCPP
Director of RML Strategic Planning and Operations
Amgen, Inc.
Thousand Oaks, CA

Steve Stoner, Pharm.D., BCPS
Regional Assistant Director of Pharmacy
Providence Health System
Portland, OR

Chris Terpening, Ph.D., Pharm.D.
Assistant Professor
Departments of Clinical Pharmacy and Family Medicine
West Virginia University
School of Pharmacy
Charleston, WV

Paula A. Thompson, M.S., Pharm.D., BCPS
Associate Professor
McWhorter School of Pharmacy
Samford University
Birmingham, AL

Nancy Toedter-Williams, Pharm.D.
Associate Professor of Pharmacy Practice
Southwestern Oklahoma State University
College of Pharmacy
Weatherford, OK

Candy Tsourounis, Pharm.D.
Associate Professor of Clinical Pharmacy
UCSF School of Pharmacy
Department of Clinical Pharmacy
San Francisco, CA

Nicholas A. Votolato, R.Ph, BCPP
Clinical Associate Professor
Ohio State University
Department of Psychiatry
Columbus, OH

David Wallace, Pharm.D., R.Ph.
Clinical Assistant Professor
University of Houston
College of Pharmacy
Houston, TX

Gene A. Wetzstein, Pharm.D., BCOP
Clinical Pharmacist-Hematology
H. Lee Moffitt Cancer Center & Research Institute
Tampa, FL

Tara Whetsel, Pharm.D.
Clinical Assistant Professor
Department of Clinical Pharmacy
West Virginia University
School of Pharmacy
Morgantown, WV

Jessica L. White, Pharm.D., BCPS
Clinical Assistant Professor
University of Houston
Houston, TX

Patricia Rozek-Weigel, Pharm.D., BCPS
Assistant Professor
University of Cincinnati
College of Pharmacy
Cincinnati, OH

Robert O. Williams, III, R.Ph., Ph.D.
Professor of Pharmaceutics
The University of Texas at Austin
College of Pharmacy
Austin, TX

Alexandria Garavaglia-Wilson, Pharm.D., BCPS
Assistant Professor of Pharmacy Practice
St. Louis College of Pharmacy
Pharmacy Practice Division
St. Louis, MO

Contributors

Clinton Wright, Pharm.D., BCPP
Senior Area Manager
Medical Science Liaisons
Cyberonics, Inc.
San Antonio, TX

Teri L. Bair, R.Ph., J.D., FASHP

J. Nile Barnes, EMT-P, Pharm.D.

Donna G. Beall, Pharm.D.

Bradley A. Boucher, Pharm.D.

Susan Bruce, Pharm.D., BCPS

Betsy Carlisle, Pharm.D., BCPS

Juliana Chan, Pharm.D.

Keith Christensen, Pharm.D., BCPS

Shelby Corman, Pharm.D.

Sean P. Cosgriff, Pharm.D., BCOP

Denise M. Crow, BS, BCPS

Bonnie A. Falcione, Pharm.D.

Linda A. Felton, Ph.D.

Richard G. Fiscella, R.Ph., MPH

Andrew Grimone, Pharm.D., BCPS

Laura B. Hansen, Pharm.D., FCCP, BCPS

Martin Higbee, Pharm.D.

Ben M. Lomaestro, Pharm.D.

Patricia L. Marshik, Pharm.D.

Margaret McGuinness, Pharm.D., BCOP

Christopher D. Miller, Pharm.D., BCPS

Tera D. Moore, Pharm.D., BCPS

Margie E. Perez, Pharm.D.

Tracy Pettinger, Pharm.D.

Charmaine D. Rochester, Pharm.D., CDE

Carol J. Rollins, M.S., RD, Pharm.D., BCNSP

Gloria Sachdev, Pharm.D., CDE

Laura Carter Smoot, Pharm.D., BCPS

Glen L. Stimmel, Pharm.D., BCPP

Darcie A. Streetman, Pharm.D.

Susie Vasquez, Pharm.D., BCPS

Amy L. Whitaker, Pharm.D.

Dennis M. Williams, Pharm.D.

ASHP's PharmPrep, Interactive Case-Based Board Review, Third Edition is a multidisciplinary review guide that will provide a comprehensive review of disease states that are covered on the NAPLEX® through a review of real patient cases accompanied by questions that address all of the NAPLEX® competency statements (Appendix A). The software will allow the student to review information by specific disease state or simulate the examination with a computer-adapted format similar to that seen on the NAPLEX®.

The layout of each case is presented like a medical chart with subjective patient information and objective data to give a clear depiction of the patient. The physician's assessment of the patient is included, when available, to assist the student in making a decision on the best course of treatment, proper drug therapy, and construction of a plan for the patient. Each case includes a profile similar to those seen in on the NAPLEX® and is followed by 10 questions with the NAPLEX® competency statement designated in the answer section. Explanations for all answers, correct and incorrect, are included.

Format of ASHP's PharmPrep Cases

The patient cases in this review guide are intended to be used as a review of common disease states that are likely to be seen by general pharmacy practitioners as well as several clinical specialties. The format and organization of the cases are meant to mirror what is usually seen in practice in a clinical setting. When using *PharmPrep,* it is recommended that additional resources be accessible to facilitate study, including a comprehensive drug information text (e.g., *AHFS*), medical dictionary, therapeutics text (e.g., *Pharmacotherapy*), and laboratory data reference.

Patient Demographics

The patient's demographical information will include (if known) his or her name (a fictional name to ensure patient confidentiality), address/location, age, height and weight, race, sex, and any known allergies.

Chief Complaint

The Chief Complaint is a brief statement that describes the reason the patient sought medical treatment and presents symptoms in his or her own words.

History of Present Illness

This is a complete chronology and description of the events and symptoms that led up to the patient seeking medical care. Included in this section are:

> Date of onset
> Type of condition, severity, and duration
> Status of any disease state (acute exacerbation or remission)
> Treatments/modalities attempted and their effect
> Impact on system function (e.g., increase/decrease urinary function, etc.)
> Impact on activities of daily living

Past Medical History

Includes all pertinent information related to conditions for which the patient is currently being treated or has been treated for or sought medical care.

Social History

The social history includes the characteristics and habits of the patient that may or may not have contributed to his or her condition. Included in this section are the patient's marital status, drug and alcohol abuse, caffeine intake, and the use of tobacco, among other lifestyle information.

Family History

The family history includes status of the patient's family members, medical conditions, etc., that may provide useful hereditary information (e.g., diabetes, cancer, heart disease).

Review of Systems

This section includes information from the patient describing his or her symptoms with positive and negative findings noted.

Physical Examination

This section denotes the information found on physical examination of the patient. This section usually includes the following information:

GEN: General appearance

VS: Vital signs (including height, weight, blood pressure, heart rate, respiratory rate, and temperature)

HEENT: Head, eyes, ears, nose, and throat status

CHEST: Pulmonary status

CV: Cardiovascular status

ABD: Abdominal status

RECTAL: Rectal area status

GU: Genitourinary systems status

NEURO: Neurologic status

MS: Musculoskeletal status

EXT: Extremities status

Laboratory and Diagnostic Tests

The results of all laboratory and diagnostic tests are included in this section. Normal ranges vary from lab to lab and within different institutions. For information on normal values, consult a laboratory value text.

Diagnosis

All diagnoses for the patient are presented in this section.

Medication Record (Prescription and OTC)

This section includes all prescription and over-the-counter medications the patient is currently taking and/or received in the past. Prescribing physician, prescription number (Rx only), date filled, drug name, strength and quantity, directions for use, and refill information are provided. Medications are presented in a list for hospitalized patients.

Pharmacist Notes and Other Patient Information

Information documented in the patient's record, provided either by the pharmacist of another health care provider, is included in this section.

The software duplicates the environment of the NAPLEX® and will allow the student to simulate taking the NAPLEX® or will allow the student to review a specific disease state. The more practice the student has in the actual test environment, the more the student will relax and feel comfortable during actual testing.

ASHP's PharmPrep, Interactive Case-Based Board Review, Third Edition is a tool to assist with preparation for the NAPLEX® and for pharmacy practice. I hope this text will be a useful addition to your professional library and representative of the patients that you may see in practice.

Nancy F. Fjortoft, Ph.D.

Introduction

After years of preparation, you are ready to begin your career as a pharmacist. Congratulations! To practice pharmacy, individuals must be licensed by the state in which they wish to practice. Licensure ensures a minimum level of competence. Licensure by examination is the method by which new graduates achieve licensure. All state boards of pharmacy require individuals to take and pass the North American Pharmacy Licensure Examination (NAPLEX®) to be licensed.[1] The goal of the NAPLEX® is to ensure that you are competent to safely and effectively provide pharmacy practice services at the entry level. Your state board of pharmacy will use the NAPLEX® score to determine whether you are eligible for a license to practice pharmacy. This chapter will describe the NAPLEX® and assist you in preparing for the NAPLEX® and provide basic test-taking strategies. The objectives of this chapter are to:

1. describe types of questions on the NAPLEX®;
2. describe computer-adaptive testing;
3. review test preparation strategies;
4. describe test-taking strategies; and
5. recognize test-taking anxiety and define how to cope with it.

Description of the NAPLEX® CAT

The NAPLEX® is a 4-hour computer adaptive test (CAT) that consists of 185 multiple-choice test questions. 150,000 of those questions are used to calculate your score, and the remaining 35 are test questions. You will not know which are "real" questions and which are "test" questions. *Computer-adaptive test* simply means that you take the test on a computer, and the computer selects questions based on your level of ability. CAT is a relatively new method of testing. The questions are the same as they would be on a paper and pencil test; however, the computer "selects" questions for you based on whether you answered the previous question correctly. The computer "grades" your answer before presenting the next question. If you answered the question correctly, the computer will then select a more difficult question. If you answered the question incorrectly, the computer will select an easier question for your next question. Because of this format, taking a CAT is different from standard paper-and-pencil tests.

Special Considerations in Taking CAT

CATs are distinct from paper-and-pencil tests in a number of ways. Because of the adaptive nature of the test, you cannot go back and change an answer. In other words, you have one opportunity to answer the question. You may not go back and review your answer.

You may not skip questions. Again, because of the adaptive nature of the test, the computer selects your next question based on your answer to the current question. Therefore, you cannot skip questions. You must answer all questions, even if you need to guess (more on guessing later).

The disadvantage then of CATs is that your practice of answering all the easy questions first to build confidence and ensure that you answer as many questions as you can simply does not work. You need to answer one question at a time, and then leave that question permanently and move on. The questions are all independent and do not build on one another.

Types of Questions on the NAPLEX®

The NAPLEX® is a multiple-choice test. It consists of 185 questions that are either "case-based profile" or "stand-alone" questions. Case-based profile questions present you with a patient profile or brief information regarding a specific situation (typically about a patient). Then you are asked a specific question. You answer the question using the data or case presented immediately above the question. The majority of NAPLEX® questions are case-based profile questions.

The other type of question on the NAPLEX® is the stand-alone question. This is simply a question with a series of potential responses.

These are the types of questions you will see on the NAPLEX®. The responses may either be single-answer or combination. The question that has single-answer responses (probably the most familiar) looks like this:

1. Which of the following antivirals is a pro-drug that is converted to acyclovir?
    a. Famciclovir
    b. Valacyclovir
    c. Ganciclovir
    d. Amprenavir
    e. Lamivudine

The combined-response question (Type K) looks like this:

2. Nonadherence with Zovirax could put JN at risk for which of the following?
    I. Persistence of symptoms
    II. Persistence of viral replication
    III. Possibility of Zovirax resistance

    A. I only
    B. III only
    C. I and II only
    D. II and III only
    E. I, II, and III

Many pharmacy faculty use combined response questions in their examinations partly to give you practice opportunities in answering these kinds of questions.

Preparation for Success

Keep in mind that the NAPLEX® assesses years of education both in the classroom and on rotation. You cannot cram for the NAPLEX®; you must plan a review schedule. This review schedule should cover several months, not just several days. Establish a schedule, with several hours a day set aside for review. Make an outline of topics to be reviewed. Use the NAPLEX® competency statements (Appendix A) to assist you in preparation for the exam. Keep in mind that you need to spend more time on areas in which you are weak. For example, if cardiovascular topics were difficult for you, plan to spend more time studying and reviewing cardiovascular topics. Do not spend large amounts of time on material that you already know.

Establish a study routine and set goals for each study period. Be realistic in setting your study goals. Most people are not effective when they set aside large blocks of time to study. Set aside 3–4 hours a day. Find your best time of day. After years of going to school, you probably have a pretty good idea whether you are a morning person or a night person. Use your best time of day for NAPLEX® study.

Be selective in the books and notes you use. Choose a good review book that is comprehensive and is easy for you to read. A number of review books are available. This book is unique in that it follows a case-based approach and provides plenty of sample questions with in-depth discussion explaining the correct answers.

By now you should also have developed a large library of reference books that will help as you begin your review process. Some suggestions include:

1. McEvoy, GK, ed. *AHFS Drug Information, 2006*. Bethesda, MD: American Society of Health-System Pharmacists; 2006.

2. MedOutcomes Inc. *Ambulatory Care Clinical Skills Program, Core Module*. Bethesda, MD: American Society of Health-System Pharmacists; 1998.

3. Young LY, Koda-Kimble, MA, Guglielmo BJ, Kradjan WA, eds. Applied *Therapeutics: The Clinical Use of Drugs*. 8th ed. Philadelphia: Lippincott Williams & Wilkins, 2004.

4. Traub SL, ed. *Basic Skills in Interpreting Laboratory Values*. 3nd ed. Bethesda, MD: American Society of Health-System Pharmacists; 2004.

5. Hebel SK. *Drug Facts and Comparisons 2006*. Philadelphia: Lippincott Williams & Wilkins; 2006.

6. Trissel, LA. *Handbook on Injectable Drugs*. 14th ed. Bethesda, MD: American Society of Health-System Pharmacists; 2006.

7. Stoklosa MJ, Ansel HC. *Pharmaceutical Calculations*. 11th ed. Philadelphia: Lippincott Williams & Wilkins; 2001.

8. DiPiro JT, ed., et al. *Pharmacotherapy: A Pathophysiologic Approach*. 6th ed. Stamford, CT: Appleton & Lange; 2005.

9. Braunwald E, ed., et al. *Harrison's Principles of Internal Medicine*. 16th ed. New York, NY: McGraw Hill Text; 2004.

10. *Stedman's Medical Dictionary, 27th ed*. Philadelphia, PA: Lippincott Williams & Wilkins; 2000.

11. Strauss S. *Strauss's Federal Drug Laws and Examination Review, 5th ed*. Lancaster, PA: Technomic Pub. Co.; 2000.

12. Goodman LS, ed., et al. *Goodman & Gilman's The Pharmacological Basis of Therapeutics*. 11th ed. New York, NY: McGraw Hill Professional; 2005.

The National Association of Boards of Pharmacy (NABP) prepares extensive information and practice test questions available in the Registration Bulletin. Review all of this information so that you thoroughly understand the NAPLEX®. Make sure you understand and are versatile with the CAT format. Make sure you are absolutely confident in using the mouse, the computer keyboard, and the screen. You do not want to waste any precious time while taking the examination figuring out computer logistics. Above all, practice answering sample questions. Practice test questions are available in the NABP Pre-NAPLEX® exam. This exam uses questions developed by NABP staff and the same CAT format as the NAPLEX®. This is particularly important for the CAT.

Taking the NAPLEX®

You have been preparing and studying for the NAPLEX® for weeks, you are familiar with the NAPLEX® competency statements, and have spent hours answering practice questions and using the CAT format. You are ready for the examination.

Be Prepared

Your first step in achieving success on the NAPLEX® is to arrive for the test well prepared. Arrive at your testing center 30–40 minutes early. This will allow you time to find the rest rooms and get comfortable. If any distracting noises exist, ask for a new seat. You may find that a ticking clock or a neighbor with an annoying cough may distract you from concentrating. Also be aware of blowing air vents and any glare from overhead lights on your computer screen. You do not want any environmental distracters. People have various tolerance levels, so do not hesitate to ask to be moved if you are bothered. This is your test. Please keep in mind that if you arrive at the test center 30 minutes after your scheduled appointment time you may be required to forfeit your appointment time and your fee! It is essential to read the NABP Registration Bulletin very carefully. There are strict rules and procedures that must be followed.

Monitor Your Time

You have 4 hours to complete the examination and the examination consists of 185 questions. Therefore, at the 2-hour mark you should be at the halfway point or have about 90 questions completed. Make yourself a schedule in 15-minute increments. Every 15 minutes you should answer at least 11 questions. You may want to pace yourself during the first 30 minutes of the examination to make sure you are on target for completion.

Read Carefully

Read directions carefully and read each question carefully. Do not rush through the question. You have made yourself a time schedule; now, simply monitor the schedule and do not rush. Do not make assumptions or jump to conclusions. Do not look for answers you have memorized. Read the question and think about the correct answer. Use your mouse to highlight key words in the question. Look for common question words such as how, which, define, and when. Answer the question. Do not assume trick questions. This may sound obvious to you but many careless errors are made because the question was not read carefully.

Guessing

In computer adaptive testing, you must answer the question before you proceed to the next question. Therefore, at times you must guess. Everyone has to guess occasionally. Do not panic. Use the following strategies for intelligent guessing:

1) The most general option is often the correct one because it allows for exception. If four of the five options are specific in nature and one is more general, choose the more general option.

2) The correct choice is often a middle value. If the options range in value from high to low, then eliminate the extreme values and choose from the middle values.

3) The longest option is most often the correct one. If three options are much shorter than the fourth, then choose the longest answer.

4) When two options have opposite meanings, then the correct answer is usually one of these.

5) Look for grammatical agreement between the question and the answer. For example, if the question uses a singular verb tense, then the answer should also be singular. Eliminate the answers that do not produce a grammatically correct sentence.[2]

6) Use your medical terminology. You have learned a whole new language of prefixes and suffixes. You may not recall the exact details of osteoarthritis, but you do know that the prefix "ost" denotes bone. Use that knowledge to help you eliminate responses and increase your chances of guessing the correct response.

7) Use your logic. Think in terms of time sequence, priorities, and severity. Select an appropriate framework, and review the responses in terms of that framework. Then make a logical guess.

The Princeton Review has coined the term process of elimination, or POE.[3] This strategy focuses on eliminating responses to improve your chances of guessing the correct answer. Keep in mind at all times the NAPLEX® competencies (Appendix A). The NAPLEX® is testing only those competencies. In other words, each question and each answer supports and assesses a competency. If a response has nothing to do with a competency area, eliminate it as a choice. By eliminating responses, you increase your chance of guessing the correct response.

Trouble Areas in Objective Tests

There are three trouble areas for people taking objective tests. The first factor to be aware of is specific determiners. These are words that give statements an absolute sense, and, as we know, there are few absolutes in the world. For example, positive specific determiners are words like all, every, everybody, everyone, always, all of the time, invariably, will certainly, will definitely, will absolutely, and the best. Negative specific determiners include the words none, not one, nobody, no one, never, at no time, will certainly not, will definitely not, will absolutely not, the worst, and impossible. When these words are included in an option, that option is usually incorrect.

For example:

Which of the thyroid function tests listed below will always accurately assess euthyroidism?
A. Free thyroxine
B. Total triiodothyronine
C. Free thyroxine index
D. Free triiodothyronine
E. Thyroid-stimulating hormone

An example of specific determiners in the responses or answers follows:

When should KL expect most of her symptoms of hypothyroidism to improve after starting the levothyroxine?
A. Always after 1 week of therapy
B. Never before the third day of therapy
C. After 3 days of therapy
D. After 21 days of therapy
E. After the first dose

Again, you can probably eliminate Response A, always after 1 week of therapy, and B, never before the third day of therapy, because there are no definite guarantees in pharmacotherapeutic treatments. However, some specific determiners are associated with correct statements. Look for more general terms such as often, perhaps, seldom, generally, may, and usually. When you are reading the questions, use your mouse to highlight specific determiners so that you are aware of them. Do not ignore them when answering the question.

The second area to be aware of is negative terms. Statements that contain negatives are more difficult to interpret than those statements without negatives. Here is an example of a double negative statement:

Which of the following are not potential reasons for patients to not adhere to the prescribed anticoagulant regimen?

Strike out the negatives, and read the question again.

Which of the following are ~~not~~ potential reasons for patients to ~~not~~ adhere to the prescribed anticoagulant regimen?"

The question is now easier to read, understand, and interpret.

Coping with Test Anxiety

In spite of the fact that you have been taking examinations for years to obtain your pharmacy degree, you may be anxious about the NAPLEX®. You are not alone. Graduates from pharmacy schools, medical schools, nursing programs, and other professional programs are all preparing to take their licensure examination. It is an exciting and stressful time for graduates all over the country! But do not let the excitement and the stress get the best of you. It has been estimated that half of the nation's students suffer test anxiety and one quarter of them are significantly hampered by it.[4] You may feel faint at heart, apprehensive, nervous, nauseous, or dizzy. Some students even have heart palpitations. Some amount of test anxiety is normal. Performers all feel nervous before they go on stage. It is your body preparing you. Make that anxiety work for you.

To make anxiety work for you, you need to understand it.

There are three components of test anxiety. The first one is fear of failure. Nobody wants to fail the NAPLEX®, but keep in mind that you always have the opportunity to retake it. Nationally, the success rate on the NAPLEX® is more than 90%. That means that less than 1 in 10 students fail the exam on the first attempt. With proper preparation you will not be one of the failures! The second component of test-taking anxiety is fear of running out of time. Again, if you monitor your time during the test as suggested earlier, and use successful guessing strategies, you will not run out of time. Four hours for 185 questions is a minute and a half per question. Again, practice answering questions. You will find that 90 seconds is ample time per question. The third component of test-taking anxiety is test logistics or fear of not understanding how the test is to be conducted. Proper preparation and familiarity with CAT is your solution to this fear.[4]

As discussed earlier, some amount of test anxiety is normal. You may find relaxation techniques helpful in assisting you in focusing on the exam. There are two kinds of relaxation techniques: physical and mental. For physical relaxation, first sit comfortably with both feet on the floor and your hands resting on your thighs. Release all your body tension and close your eyes and count backward from 10 to 1. Count only on each exhalation and breathe very deeply from the abdomen. Alternatively, clench your hands tightly for 5–10 seconds and then slowly relax your hands. Repeat this process using muscles throughout your entire body. Complete the relaxation exercise by taking a deep breath and tensing the entire body, then relaxing it. You may find the first exercise to be particularly helpful during the exam. Mental relaxation techniques include techniques as mental imaging.[5] Picture yourself in a peaceful setting, one that pleases you. For example, picture yourself by the ocean or taking a walk in the woods. Avoid negative thoughts and consequences. Focus your thoughts on the positive outcomes of the NAPLEX®.

Conclusion

The NAPLEX® represents years of education and is the final step before embarking on your career. The success rate of pharmacy students taking the NAPLEX® is very good. Do not think about failure. Think about success. You have had years of excellent education and weeks of review and preparation for the NAPLEX®. You are familiar with the CAT and test-taking strategies. You are ready to be a pharmacist. Congratulations!

References

1. National Association of Boards of Pharmacy. *Survey of Pharmacy Law.* Park Ridge, IL: National Association of Boards of Pharmacy; 1999.
2. Pauk W. *How to Study in College.* 5th ed. Boston: Houghton Mifflin; 1993.
3. Meyers JA. *Cracking the NCLEX-RN.* New York: Random House; 2000.
4. Hill KT. Interfering effects of test anxiety on test performance: A growing educational problem and solutions to it. *Ill Sch Res Dev.* 1983; 20:8–19.
5. Heiman M, Slomianko J. *Success in College and Beyond.* Allston, MA: Learning to Learn Inc.; 1992.

Cardiac and Vascular Disorders

Section Editors: James A. Karboski, Steven Marx

See all 21 cases in this section on the CD.

Case 1

Angina Pectoris

Patient Name: William Pyle
Address: 62 Merbrook Lane
Age: 56   **Height:** 5' 6"
Sex: M   **Race:** White
Weight: 110 kg
Allergies: Cats

Chief Complaint

WP is a 56-yo white male who was transported to the ED by EMS with chest tightness and pressure.

History of Present Illness

WP stated that while raking leaves he started having a feeling of chest pressure, shortness of breath, nausea, and lightheadedness. He rested for about 5 minutes and felt a little better, but the pressure and shortness of breath continued. At that time he took three nitroglycerin (NTG) tablets sublingually at 5-minute intervals but still could not get complete relief and remained short of breath. WP called 911 for help. WP stated that these same symptoms started about 2 months ago when he was cleaning his garage, but they went away with rest. He also states that the symptoms seem to be getting worse every time he works around the yard.

WP also states that he has had "heart problems" in the past; he takes digoxin, verapamil, and a water pill daily. He takes NTG if he has chest pain. His physician has not seen him in the past 6 months.

Before transport, EMS started O$_2$ at 2 L by nasal cannula and administered morphine 2 mg IVP. WP states that he has pain in his jaw and has pressure in his chest as if someone were sitting on him. An admission ECG was obtained that showed a 2-mm ST segment depression and sinus bradycardia.

A presumed diagnosis of unstable angina was made, and serial CPK isoenzymes, CBC and chemistry profile, lipid panel, digoxin level, and troponin-I were ordered. Therapy was initiated with an aspirin, NTG IV infusion at 10 µg/min, and heparin 5000 U bolus followed by 1000 U/h, and WP was transferred to the cardiac care unit.

Past Medical History

CHF, HTN, CAD, PTCA performed about 14 months ago

Social History

Tobacco use: 40 pack-year history

Alcohol use: 6-pack of beer on weekends

Family History

Father died of 'heart problem' at age 60. Mother died of 'clogged arteries' at age 62. Brother died of a heart attack at age 55. Sister had a stroke at age 50.

Review of Systems

Noncontributory

Physical Examination

GEN: Obese (110 kg, 5' 6") white male in distress with SOB

VS: BP 120/63 mmHg, HR 52 bpm, RR 22 rpm, T 98.8°F

CV: Heart rate regular, slow, NL rhythm, no murmurs

LUNGS: CTA, with decreased lung sounds on left at the base

ABD: NT without guarding or rebound, with NL BS

EXT: 2+ Pitting edema in both LE, no clubbing or cyanosis, pulses decreased bilaterally

NEURO: No focal deficits, cranial nerves intact

GU: Noncontributory

RECTAL: NL tone, (-) blood

Labs and Diagnostic Tests

Sodium 141 mEq/L	Potassium 3.2 mEq/L
Chloride 110 mEq/L	CO$_2$ content 29 mEq/L
BUN 24 mg/dL	Serum creatinine 2.8 mg/dL
Glucose 150 mg/dL	WBC 9500/mm^3
HCT 35%	Platelets 195,500/mm^3
PT 12 sec	INR 1.0
Troponin-I 1.4 ng/mL	CPK 60 U/L
CPK-MB 1.0 U/L	MB index 1.6%
TC 258 mg/dL	LDL 150 mg/dL

Digoxin level: 3.0 ng/mL (last dose about 4 hours ago)

CXR: Cardiomegaly, mild blunting with small plural effusion at the left base

Diagnosis

Primary:
    1. Unstable angina

Secondary:
    1. Congestive heart failure
    2. Coronary artery disease
    3. Hypertension
    4. Hypercholesterolemia
    5. Renal insufficiency
    6. Hypokalemia

Case 1

Medication Record

(on admission)

1/28, Simvastatin 20 mg

1/28, K-Dur 20 mEq

1/28, Verapamil-SR 240 mg

1/28, ASA 325 mg

1/28, Furosemide 40 mg

1/28, Heparin 5000 U

1/28, Heparin 25,000 U/D_5W 500 mL

1/28, Nitroglycerin 0.4 mg

1/28, Nitroglycerin 50 mg/D_5W 500 mL

1/28, Famotidine 40 mg

1/28, Morphine 1-2 mg

Pharmacist Notes and Other Patient Information

None available

Questions

1. Why would a toxicology panel be useful in the management of WP?

    I.   The use of cocaine is associated with a number of cardiac complications that can produce myocardial ischemia and can present as unstable angina.

    II. The widespread use of cocaine makes it mandatory to consider this cause, because its recognition mandates special management.

    III. A toxicology panel would either indicate or contraindicate the use of beta-blocker therapy.

    A. I only
    B. III only
    C. I and II only
    D. II and III only
    E. I, II, and III

2. Why is WP's blood glucose (150 mg/dL) a concern?

    I.   Depending on the time of WP's last meal, there is a possibility that he may have diabetes mellitus.

    II. If WP does have diabetes, it is important to consider atypical presentations of unstable angina as well as more traditional signs and symptoms, as diabetic patients may have an atypical presentation due to autonomic dysfunction.

    III. If WP is diabetic, beta-blockers should not be prescribed to treat his angina.

    A. I only
    B. III only
    C. I and II only
    D. II and III only
    E. I, II, and III

3. All of the following are true about nitroglycerin therapy EXCEPT:

    A. Nitroglycerin therapy is clearly associated with improved morbidity and mortality in patients with unstable angina.

    B. Nitroglycerin promotes the dilation of large coronary arteries, resulting in an increase of coronary blood flow to ischemic regions.

    C. Nitroglycerin increases the dilation of peripheral vasculature, thus decreasing myocardial preload.

    D. If WP had used sildenafil (Viagra) within the previous 24 hours, intravenous nitroglycerin therapy would be contraindicated.

    E. Nitrate-free intervals are important because tolerance to the effects of nitrates is dose and duration dependent and typically becomes important after 24 hours of continuous therapy.

4. Which of the following is true with regard to WP's elevated serum digoxin level?

    I.   The level could be elevated as a result of concurrent verapamil therapy.

    II. The serum level of digoxin may be used to assist in evaluating a patient for toxicity, but not to determine the efficacy of the drug.

    III. The principal manifestations of digoxin toxicity include cardiac arrhythmias, gastrointestinal symptoms, and neurologic symptoms such as visual disturbances or confusion.

    A. I only
    B. III only
    C. I and II only
    D. II and III only
    E. I, II, and III

5. Which of the following statements regarding beta-blocker therapy is FALSE?

    A. There is no evidence that any member of this class of agents is more effective than another, except that beta-blockers without intrinsic sympathomimetic activity are preferable.

    B. The choice of beta-blocker for an individual patient is based primarily on pharmacokinetic and side effect criteria with the initial choice of agents including nadolol, timolol, or labetalol.

C. Beta1-selective agents should be initiated cautiously at low doses in patients with significant COPD who may have a component of reactive airway disease.

D. The usual dose of metoprolol for angina is 50-200 mg twice daily.

E. Patients with significant sinus bradycardia or hypotension should not receive beta-blockers until these conditions have resolved.

6. Which of the following is true regarding aspirin therapy?

A. Many trials have directly compared the efficacy of different doses of aspirin in patients who present with unstable angina.

B. Aspirin should be administered as soon as possible after presentation and continued indefinitely.

C. Contraindications to aspirin include intolerance, allergy, active bleeding, hemophilia, severe untreated hypertension, history of stroke, and gastrointestinal or genitourinary bleeding.

D. By reversibly inhibiting cyclooxygenase-1 within platelets, aspirin prevents the formation of thromboxane A2, thereby diminishing platelet aggregation.

E. Daily doses of 75 to 325 mg are the standard of care for patients with angina.

7. WP has been initiated on anticoagulation therapy with intravenous unfractionated heparin (UFH). The recommendation to add anticoagulation with subcutaneous LMWH or intravenous unfractionated heparin (UFH) to antiplatelet therapy with aspirin and/or clopidogrel carries a level of evidence of "A" in the most recent ACC/AHA guidelines for the Management of Patients with Unstable Angina and Non-ST-Segment Elevation Myocardial Infarction. Which of the following is false regarding this level of evidence?

A. "A" is the highest weight of evidence.

B. If recommendations are designated as Level A, the data were derived from multiple randomized clinical trials that involved large numbers of patients

C. Recommendation are given a weight of "A," "B," or "C" based on the amount and quality of published data available for the given recommendation.

D. Level "A" is assigned when "conditions for which there is evidence and/or general agreement that a given procedure or treatment is useful and effective" are present.

E. The use of Level A evidence with carefully reasoned clinical judgment reduces, but does not eliminate, the risk of cardiac damage and death in patients who present with symptoms suggestive of unstable angina.

8. Why was morphine used in the medical management of WP?

A. Morphine sulfate has potent analgesic and anxiolytic

effects, as well as hemodynamic effects that are potentially beneficial in unstable angina.

B. In addition to its efficacy as an analgesic, morphine has been shown to reduce mortality rates in patients with unstable angina.

C. Morphine was chosen for its analgesic properties; however, there are many other fast-acting narcotics that would have been reasonable choices for the treatment of WP's chest pain.

D. Morphine should not have been used as it is contraindicated for this patient.

E. Morphine should not have been used as the major adverse reaction to morphine is nausea and WP presented with nausea accompanying his other symptoms.

9. The cardiologist has recommended that WP quit smoking and asks you to discuss the factors that may influence the success of his cessation and recommend effective smoking cessation products with the patient. Which statement(s) would you include as part of your counseling?

I. Bupropion and nicotine replacement therapies have been shown to be effective when added to brief regular counseling sessions in helping patients to quit smoking

II. Smoking reduces the anti-ischemic effects of beta-blockers and would increase his risks for another cardiac event.

III. Family members who live in the same household should also be encouraged to quit smoking to help reinforce the patient's effort and to decrease the risk of second-hand smoke for everyone.

A. I only

B. III only

C. I and II only

D. II and III only

E. I, II, and III

10. Later in WP's course of care, the decision is made to discontinue unfractionated heparin and initiate enoxaparin therapy. The medical team would like for you to counsel WP on self-injection of enoxaparin. Which of the following statements would you include in your education?

I: It is important to expel the air bubble from the syringe before the injection

II: Avoid injecting too close to the belly button or around existing scars or bruises.

III: To minimize bruising, do not rub the injection site after completion of the injection.

A. I only

B. III only

C. I and II only

D. II and III only

E. I, II, and III

Patient Name: Edward Kline
Address: 4207 Greenbriar Lane
Age: 52   **Height:** 5' 11"
Sex: M   **Race:** White
Weight: 96.4 kg
Allergies: NKDA

Chief Complaint

EK is a 52-yo white male presenting to the ED with shortness of breath. EK claims that he has felt a little short of breath over the past few days but that today it became extremely difficult to breathe and that he generally feels bloated and uncomfortable, had difficulty trying to button his pants and tie his shoes, and notes a 15-lb weight gain over the past week or so. His blood pressure on admission is 138/92 mmHg via arm cuff, with a pulse of 98 bpm.

History of Present Illness

Four days ago, EK's daughter was married, and he claims to have been "on the run" during that time. He claims that his usual dietary restrictions have fallen by the wayside over the past few days, with both food and alcohol indulgences. Additionally, he admits to having missed "about three or four doses" of his heart failure medications, specifically the pill that "sends him to the bathroom" because he did not want to worry about that during his daughter's wedding. He has, since late yesterday, resumed taking his medications regularly but still finds himself extremely short of breath. EK claims that, in retrospect, he has noticed a progression of his shortness of breath, which initially was brought on with physical activity and now occurs even at rest.

Past Medical History

EK was diagnosed with idiopathic heart failure 16 months ago. EK is typically a stable NYHA Class III patient, fairly well-controlled on his current medication regimen. He claims that he sometimes needs to come to the hospital for a "tune-up" once a year, usually during the summer. He used to go to his cardiologist's office occasionally for "some IV medicine," but he stopped going after his cardiologist started him on a new oral medication. There is no other remarkable history.

Social History

Tobacco use: 1 ppd x 15 years, quit 10 years ago

Alcohol use: 1-2 drinks/week

Family History

Father alive and well, 78 yo, MI x 15 years ago

Mother alive and well, 77 yo, no chronic disease

Review of Systems

(+) HJR, hepatomegaly, 3+ pitting edema

Physical Examination

VS: BP 138/92 mmHg, HR 98 bpm, RR 37 rpm, T 37°C, Wt 96.4 kg

HEENT: WNL

CHEST: Inspiratory rales, bilateral rhonchi, decreased breath sounds, decreased percussion

CV: RR, rate 98; S_1, soft S_2, +S_3, 2/6 holosystolic murmur at LLSB

NEURO: A & O x3

Labs and Diagnostic Tests

Sodium 134 mEq/L	Potassium 3.1 mEq/L
Chloride 91 mEq/L	Bicarbonate 29 mEq/L
BUN 18 mg/dL	Serum creatinine 0.9 mg/dL
Glucose 100 mg/dL	Magnesium 1.5 mEq/dL
AST 120 U/L	HGB 12.8 g/dL
HCT 38%	WBC 5500/mm³

ECG: LV hypertrophy

CXR: Cardiomegaly, bilateral pleural effusion

Diagnosis

Primary:

1) Decompensated heart failure

Medication Record

(prior to admission)

Enalapril 20 mg po bid

Furosemide 40 mg po daily

Digoxin 0.25 mg po q am

Carvedilol 6.25 mg po bid

Pharmacist Notes and Other Patient Information

None available

Case 2

Questions

1. Definitive diagnosis of heart failure can be made with which of the following?

   I. B-type natriuretic peptide (BNP) level
   II. Chest x-ray
   III. Echocardiogram

   A. I only
   B. III only
   C. I and II only
   D. II and III only
   E. I, II, and III

2. EK should be counseled on which of the following regarding his drug therapy for heart failure?

   I. Heart failure is curable with proper drug therapy
   II. Most patients with heart failure can be managed on one or two medications
   III. Drug therapy for heart failure must be continued indefinitely

   A. I only
   B. III only
   C. I and II only
   D. II and III only
   E. I, II, and III

3. A dobutamine drip is ordered for EK to start at 5 mcg/kg/min. Your pharmacy stocks premixed dobutamine drips (500 mg/250 mL). At this dose, how long will one bag of dobutamine last?

   A. 2 hours
   B. 4 hours
   C. 8 hours
   D. 15 hours
   E. 17 hours

4. Which of the following drugs is a phosphodiesterase inhibitor?

   A. Dobutamine
   B. Dopamine
   C. Milrinone
   D. Nesiritide
   E. Nitroglycerin

5. Your patient states that his neighbor recommended hawthorn and coenzyme Q10 for his heart failure. Where would you go for the best information on efficacy and safety of these agents?

   A. American Hospital Formulary Service
   B. Trissel's Handbook on Injectible Drugs
   C. Facts and Comparisons
   D. Harrison's Principles of Internal Medicine
   E. Natural Medicines Comprehensive Database

6. Several months later, EK is still experiencing frequent shortness of breath at rest. Which of the following should be added to his regimen?

   A. Bumetanide
   B. Metoprolol XL
   C. Sotalol
   D. Spironolactone
   E. Verapamil

7. Which of the following is a contraindication to using a beta adrenergic blocker in a patient with heart failure?

   I. Second- or third-degree AV block
   II. Severe bradycardia
   III. Diabetes mellitus

   A. I only
   B. III only
   C. I and II only
   D. II and III only
   E. I, II, and III

8. In which of the following circumstances would you recommend Digibind for EK?

   I. Digoxin serum level of 0.4 ng/mL
   II. Digoxin serum level of 4.2 ng/mL and asymptomatic
   III. Digoxin serum level of 3.8 ng/mL with worsening bradycardia

   A. I only
   B. III only
   C. I and II only
   D. II and III only
   E. I, II, and III

9. Over the next few months, EK has numerous episodes of symptomatic paroxysmal atrial fibrillation. Which of the following drugs would be the best choice for EK?

   A. Amiodarone
   B. Flecainide
   C. Quinidine
   D. Propafenone
   E. Procainamide

Case 2

10. If a patient experiences gynecomastia with spironolactone, which of the following drugs could be substituted for spironolactone to achieve the same therapeutic effect with less gynecomastia?

    A. Candesartan
    B. Amiodarone
    C. Hydralazine
    D. Isosorbide mononitrate
    E. Eplerenone

Patient Name: Albert Johnson
Address: 1765 Reed Lane
Age: 72 years   **Height:** 5' 11"
Sex: M   **Race:** African American
Weight: 220 lb
Allergies: Codeine

Chief Complaint

AJ is a 72-year-old African American man who reported to clinic today following his yearly physical examination that showed an elevated blood pressure.

History of Present Illness

One month ago, AJ was seen by his family physician for an annual checkup. At that time he was found to have an elevated blood pressure of 152/85 mmHg. He was informed to return in 2 weeks for a blood pressure follow-up. At that follow-up visit his blood pressure was still elevated at 155/82 mmHg. AJ was provided a home blood pressure monitor and instructions to take his blood pressure at home each day for the next 2 weeks and then return to clinic for evaluation. His at-home blood pressure readings ranged from systolic pressures of 145-155 mmHg and diastolic pressures of 75-85 mmHg.

Past Medical History

Hypercholesterolemia treated for past 10 years

Ankle surgery 5 years ago with secondary osteoarthritis

Seasonal allergic rhinitis: tree pollens

Social History

AJ is a retired postal worker who lives at home with his wife. He has never smoked and currently drinks about 3 beers/week. AJ admits that he consumes a lot of caffeine in the form of coffee (2-3 cups each morning) and soda (2-3 each day). Since retiring 7 years ago, AJ gets very little exercise and has progressively gained weight.

Family History

AJ's mother died in a automobile accident at the age of 53. His father died of a stroke at the age of 65. AJ has two younger brothers and one older sister who are all living. One brother has asthma and angina. The other brother had a CABG 5 years ago. His sister has been on thyroid supplementation therapy for 15 years.

Review of Systems

Unremarkable

Physical Examination

GEN: Overweight, elderly African American male in NAD

VS: BP 153/82 mmHg, HR 82 bpm, RR 15 rpm, T 38.5°C, Ht 5' 11', Wt 220 lb

HEENT: NC/AT, PERRLA, no evidence of retinopathy, neck supple and without masses

CHEST: Lungs CTA bilaterally, heart RRR without murmurs

ABD: Nondistended, nontender, +BS

EXT: Pulses 3+ throughout, normal strength, no evidence of edema

NEURO: CN II-XII intact, no focal deficits

GU/RECTAL: Slightly enlarged prostate, stool heme negative

Labs and Diagnostic Tests

Sodium 140 mEq/L	Potassium 4.1 mEq/L
CO_2 24 mEq/L	Chloride 102 mEq/L
Glucose 85 mg/dL	BUN 15 mg/dL
Serum creatinine 1.2 mg/dL	Uric acid 12 mg/dL
Hemoglobin 15 g/dL	Hematocrit 46%
Total cholesterol 220 mg/dL	LFTs within normal limits
Thyroid panel within normal limits	

Diagnosis

New-onset idiopathic hypertension

H/O osteoarthritis

H/O hyperlipidemia

Pharmacist Notes and Other Patient Information

AJ wanted to purchase ibuprofen last month for a headache and was informed that this drug is similar to the Voltaren that he already takes for osteoarthritis. He did not buy the ibuprofen.

Case 3

 Medication Record

Date	Rx No	Physician	Drug and Strength	Quantity	Sig	Refills
3/1	845693	Walker	Zocor 20 mg	30	1 po q evening	12
3/1			Claritin 10 mg	30	1 po daily	
3/1	845695	Walker	Flonase nasal spray	1	as directed	12
3/1	845696	Walker	Voltaren 75 mg	60	1 po bid	prn

Questions

1. Which of the following is a natural consequence(s) of untreated hypertension?

   I. Ischemic stroke
   II. Congestive heart failure
   III. Renal disease

   A. I only
   B. III only
   C. I and II only
   D. II and III only
   E. I, II, and III

2. What would be the correct classification of AJ's blood pressure?

   A. Normal
   B. High-normal
   C. Stage 1 systolic hypertension
   D. Stage 2 systolic hypertension
   E. Stage 3 systolic hypertension

3. Which of the following lifestyle modifications would be particularly beneficial for lowering AJ's blood pressure?

   I. Lose weight
   II. Reduce dietary sodium
   III. Decrease alcohol intake

   A. I only
   B. III only
   C. I and II only
   D. II and III only
   E. I, II, and III

4. Which of the following factors place AJ at an increased risk of systolic hypertension?

   I. Male
   II. African American
   III. Age

   A. I only
   B. III only
   C. I and II only
   D. II and III only
   E. I, II, and III

5. Which of the following antihypertensive agents is the drug of choice for systolic hypertension?

   A. Thiazide diuretics
   B. Beta-blockers
   C. Calcium channel blockers
   D. ACE inhibitors
   E. Alpha blockers

6. Which of the following antihypertensive drugs should be used with caution in older patients with hypertension?

   I. Terazosin
   II. Clonidine
   III. High-dose loop diuretics

   A. I only
   B. III only
   C. I and II only
   D. II and III only
   E. I, II, and III

7. Which of the following antihypertensive agents should be used with caution in patients with high uric acid levels?

   A. Propranolol
   B. Doxazosin
   C. Verapamil
   D. Hydrochlorothiazide
   E. Lisinopril

8. Which of the following antihypertensive agents can affect serum lipid levels?

   I. Alpha blockers
   II. Beta blockers
   III. Calcium channel blockers

   A. I only
   B. III only
   C. I and II only
   D. II and III only
   E. I, II, and III

9. Which of AJ's current medications can decrease the effectiveness of his antihypertensive medication?

Case 3

    I.   Zocor
    II.   Claritin
    III. Voltaren

    A. I only
    B. III only
    C. I and II only
    D. II and III only
    E. I, II, and III

10. AJ's physician writes a prescription for extended release nifedipine. With which of the following would you fill the prescription?

    A. Procardia XL
    B. Calan SR
    C. DynaCirc CR
    D. Cardizem SR
    E. Toprol XL

Patient Name: Karl Parker
Address: 339 Princeton Drive
Age: 73   **Height:** 5' 6"
Sex: M   **Race:** White
Weight: 258 lb
Allergies: Horse serum

Chief Complaint

KP is a 73-yo white male who presented to the ED this morning with the complaint of chest pain.

History of Present Illness

KP states the chest pain is substernal and started 3 days prior to admission. It has been intermittent but getting more frequent with increasing intensity. Patient states the pain subsided with sublingual nitroglycerin but today the pain is 'the worst pain he has ever felt in his life' and is not relieved by rest or nitroglycerin. The patient also complains of diaphoresis along with nausea associated with the pain.

Past Medical History

The patient's past medical history is significant for CAD, s/p CABG in 1983. KP had a duodenal peptic ulcer 2 years ago that was successfully treated with omeprazole. He has no history of diabetes or HTN.

Social History

Tobacco use: 60 pack-year history

Alcohol use: 2 or 3 servings of beer daily, but a 6-pack on weekends

Family History

Unknown, adopted as an infant

Review of Systems

Negative except as noted previously

Physical Examination

VS: BP 130/78 mmHg, RR 20 rpm, HR 113 bpm, T 97.9°F, Wt 258 lb, Ht 5' 6'

HEENT: Pupils are equal, round, and reactive to light; neck is supple; NT; no jugular venous distention

CHEST: CTA bilaterally

CV: Sinus tachycardia with no murmurs noted

NEURO: Nonfocal

ABD: Soft and NT, (+) BS

EXT: No CCE

ECG: ST elevation in 2, 3, and AVF

X-ray: Chest NL

Labs and Diagnostic Tests

Sodium 141 mEq/L   Potassium 3.8 mEq/L

Chloride 104 mEq/L CO_2 content 25 mEq/L

BUN 22 mg/dL   Glucose 116 mg/dL

H/H 13.3 mg/dL/39.9%   WBC 8.1/mm³

Platelets 289,000/mm³   PT/PTT 18 sec/24 sec

Amylase 54 U/L   Lipase 50 U/L

LFTs WNL

Troponin-I 8.1 ng/mL, 10.5 ng/mL, and 21.4 ng/mL

CPK 230 U/mL   CPK-MB 35.5 U/mL

MB Relative Index 15.4%

Diagnosis

Primary:

1) Acute myocardial infarction

Medication Record

Baby aspirin daily

Nitroglycerin SL prn

Pharmacist Notes and Other Patient Information

None available

Case 4

Questions

1. The cardiology fellow wants to treat KP immediately using alteplase for thrombolytic therapy. Which of the following would be appropriate responses to the physician?

   I. Thrombolytic therapy should not be initiated because the patient is over 70 years of age.
   II. Thrombolytic therapy should not be initiated because the patient has a positive history of a bleeding ulcer.
   III. Thrombolytic therapy should not be initiated because the patient presented more than 24 hours after the start of his chest pain.

   A. I only
   B. III only
   C. I and II only
   D. II and III only
   E. I, II, and III

2. All of the following are absolute or relative contraindications to the use of thrombolytic therapy EXCEPT:

   A. history of CVA.
   B. recent internal bleeding.
   C. current anticoagulation use.
   D. Stage II chronic HTN.
   E. history of intracranial neoplasm.

3. Thrombolytic therapy in the management of acute MI is most efficacious when administered within:

   A. 6 hours since the onset of symptoms.
   B. 12 hours since the onset of symptoms.
   C. 24 hours since the onset of symptoms.
   D. 3 days since the onset of symptoms.
   E. there is no relationship between onset of symptoms and efficacy.

4. Other than receiving a thrombolytic, what medical management could be considered?

   I. Aspirin 325 mg
   II. Morphine
   III. Enoxaparin 1 mg/kg q 12 h

   A. I only
   B. III only
   C. I and II only
   D. II and III only
   E. I, II, and III

5. KP has had a cardiac event even while on aspirin therapy. Which additional antiplatelet agent might be added to his regimen?

   A. Tirofiban
   B. Ticlopidine
   C. Clopidogrel
   D. Abciximab
   E. Amiodarone

6. KP is found to have elevated total cholesterol (250 mg/dL) with LDL (160 mg/dL) during his admission. At discharge you are asked to counsel the patient on appropriate target values, which should include:

   A. LDL = 140 mg/dL.
   B. LDL < 150 mg/dL.
   C. LDL = 130 mg/dL.
   D. LDL < 100 mg/dL.
   E. any value is appropriate if lower than his hospital values.

7. The cardiologist has recommended that KP quit smoking and asks you to counsel the patient on the effects of smoking and his medications. Which of the following statements regarding smoking and smoking cessation are true?

   I. Smoking has a direct effect on the heart and triggers coronary artery spasms.
   II. Smoking reduces the anti-ischemic effects of beta-blockers.
   III. Nicotine gum and patches have been demonstrated to reduce symptoms of nicotine withdrawal.

   A. I only
   B. III only
   C. I and II only
   D. II and III only
   E. I, II, and III

8. Which of the following factors present in KP place him at increased risk of death within 30 days of his AMI?

   I. Age of 73 years
   II. Tachycardia
   III. Male sex

   A. I only
   B. III only
   C. I and II only
   D. II and III only
   E. I, II, and III

9. What patient data in KP's case indicate potential myocardial damage?

Case 4

I.   Troponin-I
II. CPK MB
III. ST segment elevation

A. I only
B. III only
C. I and II only
D. II and III only
E. I, II, and III

10. On discharge, KP has a prescription for Lipitor. What should you do?

A. Fill the prescription with lovastatin.
B. Fill the prescription using atorvastatin.
C. Fill the prescription using simvastatin.
D. Fill the prescription using cerivastatin.
E. Fill the prescription using pravastatin.

Case 5

Patient Name: Lawrence Gold
Address: 6722 Bertner Avenue
Age: 77   Height: 5' 11"
Sex: M   Race: White
Weight: 354 lb
Allergies: Morphine, nifedipine

Chief Complaint

Severe hypotension secondary to cardiogenic shock

History of Present Illness

LG is a 77-year-old white male brought to the emergency department by EMS complaining of shortness of breath, chest pain, and coughing pink frothy sputum. LG had been increasingly short of breath for the past 3 days and unable to sleep at night, requiring five pillows for support. The night before admission, he had been complaining of substernal pain that radiated down his left arm. LG was diagnosed with acute myocardial infarction and underwent emergency three-vessel coronary artery bypass graft surgery. He was weaned from the ventilator but remains hypotensive.

Past Medical History

Coronary artery disease, hypertension, congestive heart failure, osteoarthritis, depression, anxiety, and chronic obstructive pulmonary disease

Social History

Alcohol use: 4 glasses of red wine daily

Tobacco use: 1 pack of cigarettes daily since age 17

Caffeine use: 4 cups of coffee daily

Illicit drug use: denies

Family History

Father died at 49 years old suddenly of unknown cause.

Mother had diabetes, was legally blind, and died at the age of 92.

Review of Systems

General: morbidly obese white male who appears his stated age

Integument: no changes

Neurological: no dizziness, vertigo, or syncope

Vision/hearing: no changes

Respiratory: +pink frothy sputum on night of admission, no recent URI, +dyspnea x3 days prior to admission

Cardiovascular: +chest pain (heaviness) the night before admission, +Raynaud's phenomenon, +orthopnea (5 pillows) x3 days prior to admission, no palpitations

Gastrointestinal: no nausea, vomiting, diarrhea or changes in eating or bowel habits

Gentiourinary: +nocturia (once each night for "years"), no changes

Endocrine: no heat/cold intolerance, no polydipsia, polyphagia or polyuria

Muscoloskeletal: +joint pain (neck, low back and fingers), +crepitation in fingers

Hematologic: no history of anemia, easy bruising or transfusions

Psychiatric: wife reports anxiety and depression since forced retirement at age 72, generally well-managed on Effexor with occasional (1-2 times/month) use of alprazolam

Physical Examination

VS: BP 89/48 mmHg, MAP 59 mmHg, HR 150 bpm, 97.3°F, RR 20 rpm, SpO_2=92 % at FiO_2=0.50

HEENT: Pupils are equal, round, and reactive to light; neck is supple, no jugular venous distention

CHEST: bibasilar coarse crackles

CV: S_1, S_2 clear plus S_3 gallop

EXT: 3 + pitting edema, cool, clammy, and cyanotic

PV: no thrombophlebitis, varicose veins, cold feet, edema or Raynaud's phenomenon

Labs and Diagnostic Tests

Today:

Sodium 134 mEq/L	Potassium 4.5 mEq/L
Chloride 99 mEq/L	CO_2 31 mEq/L
BUN 29 mg/dL	Serum creatinine 1.0 mg/dL
Glucose 166 mg/dL	Hgb 11.0 mg/dL
WBC 12.9/mm²	Platelets 372,000/mm³

ABGs: pH = 7.15, pCO_2 = 31, HCO3 = 17; base excess -6.0

Lactic acid 40 mg/dL	Triglycerides 101 mg/dL

Urinary output 10-20 mL/hour

Cholesterol 164 mg/dL	HDL 47 mg/dL

Case 5

Admitting EKG showed ST segment elevation in leads V1-V6.

On admisson, at 6 and 12 hours the troponin levels were all elevated.

 Diagnosis

Killip Class II cardiogenic shock

 Medication Record

Home medications prior to admission

Aspirin 325 mg po qd

Furosemide 40 mg po bid

Zocor 20 mg po HS

Lisinopril 20 mg po qd

Alprazolam 0.5 mg po tid

Effexor 75 mg po bid

Advair Diskus 250/50 inhaled bid

Albuterol 2 puffs prn

 Pharmacist Notes and Other Patient Information

BMI = 49.5

Questions

1. The mortality rate of untreated cardiogenic shock post-myocardial infarction is approximately:
   A. 10%.
   B. 30%.
   C. 50%.
   D. 70%.
   E. 90%.

2. What is the most likely etiology of cardiogenic shock in this patient?
   I. Hypertension with coronary artery disease
   II. Hyperlipidemia with tobacco and/or caffeine use
   III. Acute myocardial infarction involving over 40% left ventricular damage
   A. I only
   B. III only
   C. I and II only

   D. II and III only
   E. I, II, and III

3. Strategies in the management of cardiogenic shock include all of the following EXCEPT:
   A. aggressive initial fluid resuscitation.
   B. initiation of vasopressors once fluid resuscitation has been optimized.
   C. initiation of inotropic agents to improve cardiac output.
   D. correction of underlying cause.
   E. administration of sodium bicarbonate.

4. What should the initial therapy for LG be, given the above scenario?
   A. 2000-3000 mL NaCl 0.9% infusion
   B. Nesiritide 0.1 µg/kg/min infusion
   C. Dopamine 10 µg/kg/min infusion
   D. Drotecogin alpha 24 µg/kg/hour infusion
   E. Furosemide 10 mg/hour infusion

5. The physician orders insertion of a PA catheter with aggressive fluid resuscitation. Hemodynamic parameters are as follows. PCWP 14 mmHg, CI 2.1 L/min/m², SVR 2591 dyne-sec/cm², BP 103/55 mmHg, MAP 71 mmHg, HR 150 bpm. The physician asks you for your recommendation for the next most appropriate pharmacological intervention. You suggest:
   I. continuing fluid resuscitation.
   II. initiating diuretic therapy.
   III. initiating inotropic therapy.
   A. I only
   B. III only
   C. I and II only
   D. II and III only
   E. I, II, and III

6. The physician wishes to start an inotropic agent. He asks your advice for the most appropriate inotropic agent. You suggest:
   A. dobutamine.
   B. dopamine.
   C. nesiritide.
   D. nitroglycerin.
   E. norepinephrine.

7. A new 12-lead EKG shows ST evidence of extension of his infact. New hemodynamic parameters are as follows. PCWP 18 mmHg, CI 2.1 L/min/m², SVR 2590 dyne-sec/cm², BP 84/50 mmHg, MAP 62 mmHg, HR 112 bpm. What would be the appropriate agent for blood pressure support?

Case 5

    A.   Dobutamine
    B.   Dopamine
    C.   Norepinephrine
    D.   Phenylephrine
    E.   Vasopressin

8. Adverse drug effects for catecholamine vasopressors include all of the following EXCEPT:

    A.   bradycardia.
    B.   extravasation associated tissue necrosis.
    C.   dysrhythmias.
    D.   lactic acidosis.
    E.   myocardial ischemia.

9. LG has been stable on his dopamine infusion 3 µg/kg/min for the last 6 hours and the resident physician wants to turn off the dopamine. All of the following parameters are appropriate for weaning EXCEPT:

    A.   decrease the dopamine by 0.5 µg/kg/min every 30-60 minutes.
    B.   maintain the MAP at least 75 mmHg.
    C.   keep the heart rate less than 110 bpm.
    D.   maintain the urine output at 2 mL/kg/hour.
    E.   maintain a cardiac index above 2.3 L/min/m$^{2.}$

10. Which statement(s) is true regarding dopamine?

    I.   Dopamine 5-10 µg/kg/min is associated with primarily β-adrenergic activity.
    II.   Dopamine doses over 10 µg/kg/min is associated primarily with α-adrenergic activity.
    III.   Tachycardia is a common adverse drug reaction of dopamine.

    A.   I only
    B.   III only
    C.   I and II only
    D.   II and III only
    E.   I, II, and III

Case 6

Patient Name: Mark Jones
Address: 836 Northland Drive
Age: 58   Height: 6' 2"
Sex: M   Race: White
Weight: 85 kg
Allergies: NKDA

Chief Complaint

MJ is a 58-yo male who has been diagnosed with chronic atrial fibrillation.

History of Present Illness

MJ presented to his physician's office complaining of heart palpitations and fatigue earlier in the week, and was diagnosed with chronic atrial fibrillation. MJ refused attempt at elective electrical cardioversion. It was decided that MJ would be initiated on appropriate rate control and anticoagulation.

Past Medical History

MJ has a history of controlled HTN and hyperlipidemia, first diagnosed 5 years ago. He has no other significant medical history.

Social History

Tobacco: quit 3 years ago; 1/2 ppd x20 years before quitting

Alcohol: social, approximately 6 drinks/week

Caffeine use: 1 cup of regular coffee/day

Family History

Father died of melanoma at age 69. Mother AAW at age 77 with hypertension.

Review of Systems

WNL

Physical Examination

GEN: WN/WD male appearing in mild distress

VS: BP 124/83 mmHg, HR 117 bpm, RR 24 rpm, T 37°C, Ht 6' 2", Wt 85 kg

HEENT: WNL

CHEST: Mild crackles bilaterally at the bases

NEURO: A & O x3

Labs and Diagnostic Tests

Sodium 140 mEq/L	Potassium 4.8 mEq/L
Chloride 99 mEq/L	Bicarbonate 26 mEq/L
BUN 20 mg/dL	Serum creatinine 1.0 mg/dL
Glucose 90 mg/dL	Hgb 14 g/dL
Hct 42%	WBC 5000/mm^3
Platelets 200,000/mm^3	TSH 3.0 mIU/mL

Diagnosis

Primary:

    1) Chronic atrial fibrillation

Secondary:

    2) Hypertension

    3) Hyperlipidemia

Pharmacist Notes and Other Patient Information

MJ reports that he enjoys drinking hot green tea and consumes several cups whenever he eats at a Chinese or Japanese restaurant.

Medication Record

Date	Rx No	Physician	Drug and Strength	Quantity	Sig	Refills
8/1	4327	Andrews	Enalapril 20 mg	30	1 po QD	PRN
8/1	4328	Andrews	Warfarin 5 mg	30	1 po QD	PRN
8/1	4329	Andrews	Metoprolol 25 mg	60	1 po BID	PRN
8/1	4330	Andrews	Gemfibrozil 600 mg	60	1 po BID	PRN
8/1	4331	Andrews	Hydrochlorothiazide 25 mg	30	1 po QD	PRN

Case 6

Questions

1. A female patient with atrial fibrillation should receive warfarin if:

   I. the atrial fibrillation has been present for more than 48 hours.
   II. she is 45 years old with a history of hypertension.
   III. she is in her second trimester of pregnancy.

   A. I only
   B. III only
   C. I and II only
   D. II and III only
   E. I, II, and III

2. You are working as a pharmacist in your local community pharmacy when MJ calls to ask about his warfarin and diet. He is inquiring as to which of the following substances will affect his INR level the least.

   A. Green tea
   B. Corn
   C. Spinach
   D. Broccoli
   E. Garlic tablets

3. Which of MJ's medications may cause an increase in his INR?

   I. Hydrochlorothiazide
   II. Metoprolol
   III. Gemfibrozil

   A. I only
   B. III only
   C. I and II only
   D. II and III only
   E. I, II, and III

4. After how many days of therapy is warfarin's full antithrombotic effect achieved?

   A. <1 day
   B. 1 day
   C. 3 days
   D. 8 to 15 days
   E. 30 days

5. MJ calls your pharmacy to report he has had a nosebleed since this morning and he is concerned that it may be related to his warfarin therapy. He inquires if this adverse effect warrants discontinuation of the drug. Which of the adverse effects below are cause for immediate discontinuation and no restart of warfarin?

   I. Epistaxis
   II. Easy bruising
   III. Skin necrosis

   A. I only
   B. III only
   C. I and II only
   D. II and III only
   E. I, II, and III

6. The therapeutic INR range for atrial fibrillation is:

   A. 0.5-1.5.
   B. 1.0-2.0.
   C. 1.5-2.5.
   D. 2.0-3.0.
   E. 3.0-3.5.

7. MJ presents to your clinic for follow-up for his warfarin therapy. He has been therapeutic for the past 4 months. Four weeks ago, his INR was 2.6. Today he reports that his cardiologist added amiodarone to his drug regimen 2 weeks ago and he forgot to call you to inform you of the change. You would expect that today his INR is likely to be which of the following?

   A. Supratherapeutic
   B. No change
   C. Subtherapeutic
   D. Undeterminable
   E. You are not concerned with checking it today because he has been stable for 4 months

8. After being treated with amiodarone, MJ returns to normal sinus rhythm. How long should he continue treatment with warfarin?

   A. For 48 hours
   B. He no longer needs warfarin
   C. For 72 hours
   D. For 4 weeks
   E. For the remainder of his life

9. You are providing counseling to MJ when he arrives to pick up his warfarin prescription. What should you tell him?

   A. Avoid consumption of all foods high in vitamin K.
   B. Increase consumption of foods high in vitamin K.
   C. Maintain current dietary intake of foods high in vitamin K.
   D. Diet does not matter as vitamin K is not absorbed orally.
   E. If consuming foods high in vitamin K, double warfarin dose for that day.

Case 6

10. MJ recently returned from visiting his sister, who is interested in alternative medicines. She is encouraging him to begin taking herbals. MJ would like to know which of the following herbal or nutritional products is least likely to affect his INR.

    A. Cranberry juice
    B. St. John's wort
    C. Vitamin E
    D. Saw palmetto
    E. Coenzyme Q10

Respiratory and Pulmonary Disorders

Section Editors: Charlotte A. Kenreigh, Linda Timm Wagner

See all 10 cases in this section on the CD.

Patient Name: Michael Tarney
Address: 1636 Airflow Lane
Age: 10   **Height:** 4' 8"
Sex: M   **Race:** African American
Weight: 40 kg **Allergies:** NKDA

Chief Complaint

MT is a 10-yo African American male who was seen in the ED yesterday evening, 12/5, during an asthma exacerbation. MT had an uneventful day at school and was working on homework when he began to experience trouble breathing. On arrival at the ED, MT was only able to answer questions with single words and had an O_2 saturation of 89%.

History of Present Illness

MT self-treated his breathing difficulty with an albuterol inhaler that he carries in his pocket wherever he goes. His mother reports that he is using his inhaler at least three to four times every week for the past few months. She states she has had to obtain refills every 2 weeks. This is MT's second reported ED visit this past month due to difficulty breathing. MT's last visit symptoms included watery eyes and a stuffy nose. These symptoms are not present at this visit, however. His mother became concerned when he was disinterested in dinner and experienced trouble speaking.

Past Medical History

MT has had four ED visits since he was age 5 for upper respiratory illness associated with wheezing. All of the visits have occurred in the early fall. With each of these episodes except the latest one he was sent home on an antibiotic and albuterol inhaler. His mother states his episodes of breathing problems are becoming more frequent. His vaccinations are up to date. The rest of his past medical history is negative except for three episodes of otitis media between the ages of 1 and 3 years.

Social History

Tobacco: Denies   Alcohol: Denies

Illicit drug use: Denies   Caffeine use: 1 Coke per day

Family History

Father has multiple allergies and high blood pressure. Mother denies any health problems. Three siblings all healthy by report.

Review of Systems

Occasional wheezes noted on auscultation

Physical Examination

GEN: Tanner stage appropriate for age; appears anxious; moderate respiratory distress

VS: On ED admission: BP 120/75 mmHg, HR 150 bpm, RR 23 rpm, T 38.5°C, Wt 40 kg

HEENT: PERRLA, oral cavity without lesions. Bilateral TM unremarkable.

CHEST: Occasional expiratory wheezes bilaterally

NEURO: Alert and oriented

Labs and Diagnostic Tests

Hemoglobin 15 g/dL

Hematocrit 45%

Platelets 260,000/mm^3 WBC 8000/mm^3 DIFF 60% PMN, 3% bands, 28% lymphocytes, 3% monocytes, 6% eosinophils

pH 7.4 PaO_2 60 $PaCO_2$ 45

Cardiac monitor: Sinus tachycardia

CXR: WNL

Diagnosis

Primary:

1. Asthma exacerbation
2. Seasonal allergic rhinitis

Pharmacist Notes and Other Patient Information

None

Case 7

 Medication Record

Date	Rx No	Physician	Drug and Strength	Quantity	Sig	Refills
9/02	5404	Diller	Albuterol inhaler	1	2 puffs q6h prn	
9/02	405	Diller	Ceftin 250/5	100 mL	1 tsp bid	
10/04	43	Shaw	Albuterol inhaler	1	2 puffs q6h prn	
10/04	544	Shaw	Biaxin 250/5	100 mL	1 tsp bid	
9/02	634	Mark	Albuterol inhaler	1	2 puffs q6h prn	12
9/02	635	Mark	Cedax 180/5	120 mL	2 tsp qd	
9/15	707	Mark	Albuterol inhaler	1	2 puffs q6h prn	
10/01	709	Mark	Albuterol inhaler	1	2 puffs q6h prn	
10/14	710	Mark	Albuterol inhaler	1	2 puffs q6h prn	
10/30	745	Mark	Albuterol inhaler	1	2 puffs q6h prn	
11/15	762	Mark	Albuterol inhaler	1	2 puffs q6h prn	
12/1	808	Fish	Serevent Diskus	1	1 inhalation 30 minutes prior to exercise	
12/1	809	Fish	Prednisone 10 mg	10	1 tab bid x5 days	
12/1	810	Fish	Zyrtec 10 mg tablets	30	1 tab qd daily August through December	
12/1	811	Fish	Albuterol inhaler HFA	1	2 puffs q6h prn	

Questions

1. What type of device might be helpful for MT and his family to self-monitor the status of reactive airway disease?

   A. Sphyngmometer
   B. Peak flow meter
   C. Aero chamber
   D. Blood glucose monitor
   E. InspirEase

2. Based on MT's diagnosis and past medical history, which medication should have been prescribed during his most recent visit?

   A. Nothing
   B. Salmeterol
   C. Fluticasone MDI 44 mcg/puff
   D. Theophylline
   E. Glycopyrrolate

3. Patient education for MT and his parents should include:

   I. Use the albuterol for symptoms of acute asthma
   II. To be cautious of precipitating factors such as viral infections, tobacco smoke, and changes in weather
   III. To discontinue all physical activities, including basketball

   A. I only
   B. III only
   C. I and II only
   D. II and III only
   E. I, II, and III

4. Based on MT's physical exam and past medical history, for what indication was Zyrtec prescribed?

   A. Seasonal allergy relief
   B. Bronchospasm
   C. Inadequate oxygen exchange
   D. Contact dermatitis
   E. Rapid heart rate

5. The use of Serevent would be contraindicated in which of the following situations:

   A. To treat exercise-induced asthma
   B. To treat and reverse an acute asthma exacerbation
   C. When prescribed in children less than 16 years old
   D. If prescribed without a spacer device
   E. If prescribed concurrently with an albuterol inhaler

6. A correct dosing regimen for Serevent would be:

   A. 2 inhalations qid
   B. 1 inhalation qd
   C. 1 inhalations 30 minutes prior to exercise
   D. 2 inhalations at onset of respiratory distress
   E. 1 inhalation q 6 h

7. At his last visit, MT had been switched from a standard chlorofluorcarbon propellant (CFC) albuterol MDI inhaler to a HFA propellant inhaler (hydrofluoroalkane), which is less damaging to the earth's ozone layer. What important items should the pharmacist counsel MT and his mother about concerning the new HFA inhalers?

Case 7

I. The HFA inhaler may feel and taste different than his previous inhalers. This change will not affect efficacy of the product.

II. It is particularly important that inhalers containing HFA be cleaned on a regular basis to assure proper function.

III. HFA inhalers are packaged in foil for moisture resistance and once removed from the foil should be used only up to 3 months.

A. I only
B. III only
C. I and II only
D. II and III only
E. I, II, and III

8. The doctor prescribes a "short burst" of oral corticosteroids for MT secondary to this most recent exacerbation. What is the most important, immediate side effect you should discuss with MT and his parents?

A. Long-term effects on growth
B. Cataracts associated with corticosteroid therapy
C. Buffalo hump
D. Increased appetite and excitability
E. Moon face

9. Patients with a serious asthma exacerbation:

A. always wheeze.
B. may not wheeze.
C. are able to talk in full sentences.
D. should not be given a beta-agonist.
E. always present with cyanosis.

10. The advantages of using a spacer or holding chamber with a MDI aerosol device are:

I. The spacer will decrease systemic absorption by decreasing oral bioavailability of the medication

II. The spacer will decrease the potential systemic side effects of inhaled corticosteroids by reducing potential systemic absorption

III. The spacer allows an MDI device to be used in small children

A. I only
B. III only
C. I and II only
D. II and III only
E. I, II, and III

Case 8   Chronic Obstructive Pulmonary Disease

Patient Name: Brian Greene
Address: 6640 West Tonto Lane
Age: 71   **Height:** 5' 11"
Sex: M   **Race:** White
Weight: 80 kg
Allergies: Reports allergy to nicotine patches

Chief Complaint

BG is a 71-yo white male who comes into the VA clinic 2 months ahead of his scheduled yearly check-up appointment with complaints of worsening SOB, which first started 1 month ago. The SOB appears to be coincidental with daily walks with his granddaughter.

History of Present Illness

About a month ago, BG's wife started to notice that BG was coming home out of breath after a walk around the block with his granddaughter. BG has noticed only a slight nonproductive cough, but no other symptoms. At first he attributed the cough to a cold, but the cold has resolved and the cough remains the same if not worse.

Past Medical History

BG was diagnosed with chronic obstructive pulmonary disease 5 years ago. He was initially started on ipratropium and had recently been maintained on tiotropium with infrequent exacerbations associated with URIs. Two years ago he was diagnosed with BPH. He has been treated for HTN for 8 years. The remainder of his past medical history is unremarkable. He has a 50 pack-year smoking history and continues to smoke a tobacco pipe daily.

Social History

Tobacco use. Daily pipe smoker; 50 pack-year

Alcohol use. 2-3 Beers daily

Caffeine. None

Family History

Father died of lung cancer at age 74.

Mother died of viral cardiomyopathy at age 63.

Sister still living at 72 with HTN and glaucoma.

Review of Systems

No URI symptoms, nonproductive cough

Physical Examination

GEN: Flushed, thin, barrel-chested male, appears anxious, no respiratory distress

VS: On clinic presentation: BP 135/80 mmHg, HR 80 bpm, RR 23 rpm, T 38.5°C, Wt 80 kg

HEENT: PERRLA, lips pursed

CHEST: Diminished breath sounds, scattered rhonchi, minimal wheezes

NEURO: Alert and oriented

Labs and Diagnostic Tests

Baseline PFTs

FEV_1 1.6 L (65% of predicted)   FVC 2.9 L (78% of predicted)

FEV_1/FVC (55%)   Hemoglobin 14 g/dL

Hematocrit 42%   Platelets 250,000/mm^3

WBC 6500/mm^3 pH 7.35

PaO_2 80 $PaCO_2$ 45

CXR:

Extensive air trapping consistent with COPD

Diagnosis

Primary:

1) Chronic obstructive pulmonary disease

2) Benign prostatic hypertrophy

3) Hypertension

Pharmacist Notes and Other Patient Information

4/02 Counseled to take Flomax after the same meal each day, use Spiriva at the same time daily

Case 8

 Medication Record

Date	Rx No	Physician	Drug and Strength	Quantity	Sig	Refills
4/02	678	Hale	Flomax 0.4 mg	30	1 qd	1 year
4/02	679	Hale	Spiriva	1	18 mcg daily via oral inhalation	1 year
4/02	680	Hale	Norvasc 5 mg	30	1 qd	1 year

Questions

1. When BG picked up his prescriptions, he says his buddy has breathing trouble, too, but is on a different inhaler and seems to have better breathing. On further questioning, you discover that the buddy actually has asthma, not COPD. You explain the differences to BG including:

   I.   Asthma is irreversible and COPD is reversible
   II. Family history is an important contributor to COPD
   III. COPD is generally progressive

   A. I only
   B. III only
   C. I and II only
   D. II and III only
   E. I, II, and III

2. Patients receiving a Spiriva inhaler for the first time should receive counseling:

   I.   not to swallow capsules.
   II. that dry mouth may occur.
   III. that symptoms of depression may worsen.

   A. I only
   B. III only
   C. I and II only
   D. II and III only
   E. I, II, and III

3. Tiotropium is in the same class of drugs as:

   A. atropine.
   B. theophylline.
   C. epinephrine.
   D. fluticasone.
   E. isoproterenol.

4. BG is describing increased symptoms and the physician wants to change his therapy. You recommend.

   A. increasing his tiotropium dose to 36 mcg daily
   B. increasing his Flomax to 2 tabs daily.
   C. increasing his Norvasc to 10 mg daily.
   D. adding Combivent 2 puffs qid to the present regimen.
   E. adding an albuterol inhaler.

5. What additional preventative treatment should BG receive?

   I.   Pulmonary function tests
   II. Pneumococcal vaccine
   III. Yearly influenza vaccine

   A. I only
   B. III only
   C. I and II only
   D. II and III only
   E. I, II, and III

6. BG also puchases several over-the-counter products when he picks up his prescriptions. One of these is cause for concern in patients with COPD. It is:

   A. Acetaminophen
   B. Multivitamins with iron and zinc
   C. Robitussin DM
   D. Tums
   E. Saw palmetto

7. The mechanism of action of tiotropium is best described as:

   A. bronchodilation through inhibition of c-GMP.
   B. bronchodilation through stimulation of c-GMP.
   C. bronchodilation through inhibition of c-AMP.
   D. bronchodilation through stimulation of c-AMP.
   E. stimulation of beta receptors.

8. Tiotropium administration exacerbates which of the following conditions?

   I.   Narrow-angle glaucoma
   II. Asthma
   III. Perennial rhinitis (allergic or nonallergic)

   A. I only
   B. III only
   C. I and II only
   D. II and III only
   E. I, II, and III

9. Primary risk factors for COPD include.

   I.   smoking.
   II. a high-fat diet.
   III. female sex.

Case 8

A. I only
B. III only
C. I and II only
D. II and III only
E. I, II, and III

10. BG says he wants to look up information on the Internet about COPD. He says his buddy knows some great sites with information about alternative medicines. You provide the following guidance for him regarding the Internet:

   I. Information about alternative medicines on the Internet is always questionable.
   II. Information on the Internet is generally reliable.
   III. Start with reliable Internet sites, such as the American Lung Association, and use links provided on the site to obtain additional information.

   A. I only
   B. III only
   C. I and II only
   D. II and III only
   E. I, II, and III

Case 9

Patient Name: Theresa Ann Garcia
Address: 102 Breezeway Drive
Age: 10   Height: 4' 4"
Sex: F   Race: Caucasian
Weight: 71 pounds
Allergies: NKDA

Chief Complaint

TG is having ongoing difficulty with stuffy and runny nose, sneezing, and plugged ears.

History of Present Illness

Symptoms of nasal congestion, rhinorrhea, sneezing and plugging of ears have been present since infancy. She occasionally experiences watery eyes. She does well in June and July but symptoms are generally present most of the year. Her sleep is sometimes disturbed by the nasal congestion. TG has tried various medications. Dimetapp and Naldecon syrups have caused insomnia with nightmares. She does not like the "tickly feel" that she experienced when using Flonase nasal spray.

Past Medical History

Past history significant for bilateral ventilation tubes, adenoidectomy, and tonsillectomy. She also has bilateral mild congenital hearing loss and wears hearing aids.

Social History

Patient lives with her family in a 47-year old home with forced air heat. They do have central air conditioning. Her bedroom has carpet and the family dog sleeps on her bed. She does not keep any stuffed toys in her room.

Family History

The father has seasonal allergies in the spring. He does not experience symptoms at other times of the year. TG also has one brother who appears to have spring allergies. The mother does not have any health problems. No one in the family smokes.

Review of Systems

She experiences some dyspnea with exertion but has not had wheezing or coughing. Her mother believes that there may be a history of asthma in the past although she is unclear.

Physical Examination

VS: B/P not done, P 84 bpm, RR 18 bpm

EENT: Was significant for moderately boggy nasal turbinates. Oropharynx and chest were clear.

Labs and Diagnostic Tests

Allergy skin testing revealed positive reactions to dog, house dust mite, tree pollen, and ragweed pollen.

Pulmonary function was within normal limits with an FEV_1 of 2.0 L (92% of predicted).

Diagnosis

Perennial and seasonal allergic rhinitis

Medication Record

Sudafed 1 tablet as needed for congestion or Tavist 1/2 tablet as needed for runny nose

Pharmacist Notes and Other Patient Information

None

Questions

1. Pseudoephedrine is effective in allergic rhinitis by:
   I. blocking histamine receptors.
   II. acting directly on alpha receptors.
   III. indirectly releasing norepinephrine from its storage sites.

   A. I only
   B. III only
   C. I and II only
   D. II and III only
   E. I, II, and III

2. How would you advise this patient to help decrease her exposure to dust mites?
   I. Encase her mattress with plastic protective covers
   II. Wash bedding weekly in hot water (>130°F)
   III. Remove carpeting from bedroom

   A. I only
   B. III only

Case 9

C. I and II only
D. II and III only
E. I, II, and III

3. Her teachers have been reporting that TG has not been doing as well as she used to. She seems to be a little drowsy and sluggish during class. Her doctor has decided to discontinue the Tavist. What are their medication options?

I. An intranasal corticosteroid (e.g., Rhinocort AQ)
II. A second-generation antihistamine (e.g., Claritin)
III. A leukotriene modifier (e.g., Singulair)

A. I only
B. III only
C. I and II only
D. II and III only
E. I, II, and III

4. Which of the following is generally considered one of the safest medications for the treatment of allergic rhinitis in pediatric patients?

A. Fluticasone nasal spray
B. Diphenhydramine
C. Cromolyn nasal spray
D. Pseudoephedrine
E. Oxymetazoline nasal spray

5. TG's family has worked hard at implementing avoidance measures in their home. Although TG does not like the feel of the intranasal fluticasone, they have been compliant with the regimen. If her symptoms are extremely bothersome, her physician has advised them to use loratadine in addition to the fluticasone. Unfortunately, she is requiring the loratadine daily and her symptoms remain uncontrolled. What is the next therapeutic step for this patient?

A. Switch to a different intranasal corticosteroid spray
B. Increase the dose of fluticasone to four sprays each nostril twice a day
C. Consider beginning immunotherapy
D. Add chlorpheniramine in addition to the loratadine and fluticasone
E. Add cromolyn nasal spray in addition to the loratadine and fluticasone

6. What are factors to consider before starting immunotherapy?

I. Specific allergens to which the patient is sensitive have been identified
II. The patient is able to conform to frequent clinic visits to receive the immunotherapy injections
III. All pharmacotherapy and avoidance measures have been exhausted

A. I only

B. III only
C. I and II only
D. II and III only
E. I, II, and III

7. Which of the following are risks of immunotherapy?

I. Small potential for development of an anaphylactic reaction
II. Small potential for development of an infection at the injection site
III. Small potential for development of a hematoma at injection site

A. I only
B. III only
C. I and II only
D. II and III only
E. I, II, and III

8. What is the first line of treatment for a patient who experiences an anaphylactic reaction following the administration of allergy immunotherapy?

A. Administer oxygen
B. Administer injectable diphenhydramine
C. Observe for 10 minutes before beginning any treatment
D. Administer IM or SQ epinephrine
E. Administer nebulized albuterol

9. A few of the suggested mechanisms of action for intranasal corticosteroids include which of the following?

I. Decrease microvascular permeability
II. Decrease mucus secretion
III. Increase nasal edema

A. I only
B. III only
C. I and II only
D. II and III only
E. I, II, and III

10. Which of the following processes have been associated with the development of allergic sensitization?

I. Development of IgE antibodies following exposure to a potential allergen
II. Attachment of IgE antibodies to mast cells and basophils in a genetically susceptible patient
III. Decreased production of eosinophils

A. I only
B. III only
C. I and II only
D. II and III only
E. I, II, and III

Patient Name: Joe Brown
Address: 4588 Parkview Drive
Age: 60 **Height:** 6' 2"
Sex: M **Race:** African American
Weight: 220 lb
Allergies: NKDA

Chief Complaint

JB is in clinic today for a follow-up on his hypertension. He reports feeling short of breath when he cuts the grass or helps his wife carry laundry upstairs. He attributes this "winded" feeling to "being out of shape."

History of Present Illness

JB tried to quit smoking 2 years ago, but relapsed after 4 months. He is worried about weight gain if he does stop again. He currently smokes one-half pack per day of high-nicotine cigarettes. He thinks of quitting from time to time, but doesn't think this is a good time.

The patient states his favorite cigarette is first thing in the morning. He smokes more in the afternoon than morning, especially when watching "Wheel of Fortune" with his wife. Patient states if he is sick in bed all day, he refrains from smoking. His triggers include: stress, coffee, food, driving, watching TV, being "bored" and arguing with his wife. Patient's wife smokes and is not willing to quit at this time.

Past Medical History

JB was diagnosed with coronary artery disease 10 months ago. He has had mild COPD for several years and a long history of hypertension. JB developed erectile dysfunction 2 years ago, which has responded to sildenafil. He has a history of gastroesophageal reflux disease since his early thirties, but he has never taken prescription medications for this.

Social History

Tobacco use: 1/2 pack per day (smoked as much as 1 pack per day in the past) x35 years

Alcohol use: Occasional (1 beer 1-3 times/month)

Recreational drugs: None

Caffeine use: 1-2 cups of coffee daily, (-) soda, tea

Family History

Unknown; was adopted at age 4

Lives with wife and pet bird, Mabel

Review of Systems

JB denies headache, seizures, dizziness, nausea, diarrhea, constipation, or urinary complaints. JB denies chest pain x 6 months. (+) SOB (he can walk up 1 flight of stairs or 1/2 mile without shortness of breath; this is unchanged for the last year), heartburn 1-3 nights per month (after spicy foods)

Physical Examination

GEN: Well-developed, well-nourished male in NAD

VS: BP 140/88 mmHg, HR 64 bpm, RR 18 rpm

HEENT: WNL

CHEST: Mild expiratory wheezes bilaterally

(Assess meter) Peak expiratory flow rate: 350 L/min (best of three with good effort, predicted is 540)

Cardiac: Normal S_1, S_2; no S_3 or S_4. No murmurs or gallop

NEURO: A/O x3

Extremities: No cyanosis, clubbing, or edema

Labs and Diagnostic Tests

(6/05)

Cholesterol panel total 240 mg/dL, LDL 150 mg/dL, HDL 45 mg/dL, TG 235 mg/dL

Na 140 mEq/L   K 4.5 mEq/L

Cl 100 mEq/L   BUN 12 mg/dL

SCr 1.1 mg/dL   Glucose 100 mg/dL

Hemoglobin 16.3 g/dL

Hematocrit 49%

(11/05) Echo: Normal ejection fraction

(11/05) TSH 3.4 mIU/L   PSA 1.2 ng/mL

Diagnosis

1. Tobacco use (35 pack-years)

2. Coronary artery disease

3. Chronic obstructive pulmonary disease over 5 years

4. Erectile dysfunction

5. Mild gastroesophageal reflux disease

6. Hypertension

Case 10

Medication Record

Date	Rx No	Physician	Drug and Strength	Quantity	Sig	Refills
5/20	101		Inderal LA 120 mg	30	1 po q day	3
5/20	102		Viagra 50 mg	9	ud prn	4
5/18	103		Combivent MDI	1	2 p QID	6
5/20			APAP	200	ud prn	
4/20			Pepcid AC	30	ud prn	
4/20			Saw palmetto	100	1 cap q hs	
5/30			Aspirin (enteric coated)		81 mg daily	

Pharmacist Notes and Other Patient Information

5/18 Metered dose inhaler technique assessed. JB has good hand-to-mouth coordination and holds breath for 10 seconds after each puff. Waits 1-2 minutes between puffs.

4/20 JB educated on nonpharmacologic therapy for gastroesophageal reflux disease. Instructed patient to wear lose fitting clothes, elevate the head of the bed with 6-8 inch wood blocks, avoid caffeine and spicy foods, and decrease mints/gum in diet. Also instructed patient to remain upright for at least 3 hours after each meal before laying down. JB voiced understanding.

2/14 Educated patient on importance of smoking cessation. Decreases chance of lung cancer, cardiovascular risks, etc. Patient seemed interested but not willing to quit at this time.

2/14 Pt. denies history of an eating disorder

Questions

1. Which of the following interventions made by the pharmacist would be the most appropriate for JB at this time?

    A. Offer JB nicotine replacement products available over-the-counter
    B. Recommend JB continue to smoke due to his concerns about weight gain
    C. Help JB become motivated towards a quit attempt
    D. Offer relapse prevention techniques
    E. No intervention needed at this time

2. When JB quits smoking, the clearance of which of the following may be altered?

    A. Pepcid AC
    B. Saw palmetto
    C. Combivent
    D. Caffeine
    E. Viagra

3. Which of the following is a common symptom of nicotine withdrawal that JB might experience if he abruptly stops smoking?

    A. Irritability
    B. Insomnia
    C. Heartburn
    D. Palpitations
    E. Dizziness

4. JB calls the pharmacy several months later. He decided to quit smoking by using the "cold turkey" method 48 hours ago. He states he has had a headache for the past 48 hours. If JB's headache is due to nicotine withdrawal, symptoms should resolve within what time frame?

    A. 1-2 days
    B. 3-4 days
    C. 5-6 days
    D. 7-14 days
    E. 15-21 days

5. If JB had severe COPD, which of the following smoking cessation medications should be avoided?

    A. Bupropion
    B. Nicotine gum
    C. Nicotine spray
    D. Nicotine patch
    E. Nicotine lozenge

6. JB now decides he would like to quit smoking. He would like to use a nicotine replacement product. What strength of nicotine patch would you recommend for JB's initial use?

    A. 5 mg
    B. 7 mg
    C. 14 mg
    D. 21 mg
    E. 42 mg

7. JB decided to utilize the 15-mg nicotine patch (Nicotrol) 4 days ago. In a follow-up phone call JB reports a strong urge to smoke on awakening. Which of the following is the best recommendation for JB at this time?

    A. Increase the dose of the Nicotrol patch
    B. Discontinue the patch and switch to bupropion
    C. Begin chewing nicotine gum in the morning in addition to wearing the Nicotrol patch

Case 10

    D.   Change to a similar dose of a 24-hour patch (Nicoderm)

    E.   Discontinue the patch and initiate nicotine spray

8.   Which of the following patient education points would be the most important to explain to JB and his wife regarding the patch?

    A.   No smoking while utilizing the patch

    B.   Proper application of the patch

    C.   Caution regarding new onset seizure activity

    D.   Monitoring for increased frequency of chest pain

    E.   Use of the patch may worsen erectile dysfunction

9.   A week later, JB asks the pharmacist about "the pill he saw on TV that is supposed to help people quit smoking, Zyban." Before recommending Zyban to JB, the pharmacist should rule out:

    A.   Gastroesophageal reflux disease

    B.   Chronic obstructive pulmonary disease

    C.   History of eating disorders

    D.   History of hypertension

    E.   Erectile dysfunction

10. Which of the following is appropriate information to give a patient interested in using nicotine lozenges?

    A.   For maximum benefit, bite and park the nicotine lozenge between the cheek and gum

    B.   Use the 4-mg lozenge if you smoke within 30 minutes of awakening

    C.   The lozenge is a form of nicotine that is safer if patients continue to smoke

    D.   Nicotine lozenges may increase blood glucose levels if you have diabetes

    E.   The maximum recommended number of lozenges a patient can use in a day is 15

Gastrointestinal Disorders

Section Editor: Rosemary R. Berardi

See all 10 cases for this section on the CD.

Case 11

Patient Name: Patrick Duffey
Address: 125 Peninsula Court
Age: 45   **Height:** 5' 10"
Sex: M   **Race:** White
Weight: 185 lb
Allergies: NKDA

Chief Complaint

PD is a 45-yo white male seen in gastroenterology clinic with complaints of recurrent "stomach pain," which occurs daily usually between meals and sometimes awakens him at night.

History of Present Illness

Increasing epigastric pain over the last 3 weeks usually relieved by food or antacids, but relief only lasts for about 1 to 2 hours. Patient states that he experienced similar "stomach pain" about 5 years ago and was treated with Pepcid 20 mg bid x 6 weeks for a "suspected" duodenal ulcer. During the intervening years, he continued to use antacids and over-the counter Tagamet HP when needed for similar symptoms. Endoscopy this morning revealed a duodenal ulcer which was positive for Helicobacter pylori.

Past Medical History

Hypertension x 5 yr

Hyperlipidemia x 3 yr

Social History

Works full time as an air traffic controller

Tobacco use: 1 PPD x 30 yr; quit January 1, 2000

Alcohol use: Occasional glass of red wine with dinner

Caffeine use: 2 cups of coffee every morning with breakfast

Family History

Married with two children, both of whom are healthy

Father: Died at age 65 from MI

Mother: Alive at 71 with HTN and OA

Review of Systems

Occasional headaches relieved with acetaminophen. Otherwise noncontributory except as previously noted.

Physical Examination

GEN: Pleasant, well-nourished, male in moderate distress

VS: BP 148/86 mmHg, HR 80 bpm, RR 22 rpm, T 98.4°F, Wt 185 lb

HEENT: PERRLA

CV: RRR, no murmurs, rubs, or gallops

CHEST: Lungs clear to A/P

ABD: Abdomen soft, mildly tender on palpation between the xiphoid and umbilicus, without masses, organomegaly, or bruits

GU: Deferred

RECTAL: Rectum normal, guaiac-negative

MS/EXT: No clubbing, cyanosis, or edema; normal distal pulses; normal ROM

NEURO: CN II through XII intact; DTR present

Labs and Diagnostic Tests

Sodium 145 mEq/L	Potassium 3.9 mEq/L
Chloride 105 mEq/L	CO2 24 mEq/L
BUN 10 mg/dL	Serum creatinine 1.0 mg/dL
Glucose 110 mg/dL	Hemoglobin 14.5 g/dL
Hematocrit 43.5%	Platelets 260,000/mm³

WBC 7500/mm³, with 66% PMN, 30% lymphocytes, 4% monocytes

EGD: Single 0.5-cm ulcer in duodenal bulb. Ulcer base clear without evidence of active bleeding. Antral gastritis with biopsy positive for Helicobacter pylori.

Diagnosis

Primary:

1. Duodenal ulcer (Helicobacter pylori-positive)

Secondary:

1. Hypertension

2. Hyperlipidemia

Medication Record

Antacids - po various prn stomach pain

Tagamet HP - po prn stomach pain

Hydrochlorothiazide 25 mg po daily in AM

Case 11

Atenolol 50 po mg daily

Simvastatin 20 mg po daily at bedtime

Acetaminophen 650 mg po prn headache

Multivitamin 1 po daily

 Pharmacist Notes and Other Patient Information

None available

Questions

1. What is the most common symptom of peptic ulcer disease (PUD)?

   A. Anorexia often accompanied by weight loss
   B. Substernal pain often accompanied by indigestion
   C. Abdominal pain often accompanied by diarrhea
   D. Epigastric pain often occurring at night
   E. Abdominal pain often radiating to the shoulder

2. Which of the following does NOT reflect the current status of Helicobacter pylori and PUD?

   A. Most individuals infected with Helicobacter pylori are asymptomatic
   B. Most peptic ulcers are Helicobacter pylori-negative
   C. Eradication of Helicobacter pylori heals peptic ulcers
   D. Eradication of Helicobacter pylori reduces ulcer recurrence
   E. Most individuals infected with Helicobacter pylori develop gastric cancer

3. Which of the following is the initial regimen of choice for eradicating Helicobacter pylori, healing the duodenal ulcer, relieving ulcer symptoms, and fostering patient adherence?

   A. Clarithromycin and a proton pump inhibitor
   B. Amoxicillin and a proton pump inhibitor
   C. Clarithromycin, amoxicillin, and a proton pump inhibitor
   D. Clarithromycin, ciprofloxacin, and a proton pump inhibitor
   E. Bismuth subsalicylate, metronidazole, tetracycline, and an H_2-receptor antagonist

4. What is the preferred management of PD's duodenal ulcer if he had a documented allergy to penicillin?

   A. Proton pump inhibitor daily for 4 weeks
   B. Clarithromycin and a proton pump inhibitor
   C. Clarithromycin, tetracycline, and a proton pump inhibitor

   D. Clarithromycin, metronidazole, and a proton pump inhibitor
   E. Clarithromycin, amoxicillin, and a proton pump inhibitor, as there is little chance of cross-sensitivity to amoxicillin when used to eradicate Helicobacter pylori

5. Which alternative drug constitutes an acceptable drug substitution when used as a part of a clarithromycin, amoxicillin, and lansoprazole Helicobacter pylori eradication regimen in a patient with a duodenal ulcer?

   A. You may substitute pantoprazole for lansoprazole
   B. You may substitute famotidine for lansoprazole
   C. You may substitute bismuth subsalicylate for lansoprazole
   D. You may substitute ampicillin for amoxicillin
   E. You may substitute azithromycin for clarithromycin

6. What is the most cost-effective parameter to monitor to assess a positive therapeutic outcome in a patient with a noncomplicated Helicobacter pylori-positive duodenal ulcer?

   A. Serology for antibodies to Helicobacter pylori
   B. Urea breath test
   C. Recurrence of epigastric pain
   D. Abdominal x-ray
   E. Upper endoscopy

7. When metronidazole is part of a Helicobacter pylori eradication regimen, what is the most important information you should convey to a patient regarding the potential for adverse effects?

   A. Do not eat or drink milk products
   B. Do not drink caffeinated beverages
   C. Do not eat or drink citrus foods or beverages
   D. Do not drink carbonated beverages
   E. Do not ingest alcohol (ethanol)

8. Which of the following antacids should be avoided in this patient because of his HTN?

   A. Calcium carbonate
   B. Sodium bicarbonate
   C. Magnesium hydroxide
   D. Magaldrate
   E. Aluminum hydroxide

9. Which of the following agents is most likely to cause diarrhea, especially if this patient used it in high or frequent doses?

   A. Calcium carbonate
   B. Sodium bicarbonate
   C. Magnesium hydroxide
   D. Aluminum hydroxide
   E. Bismuth subsalicylate

Case 11

10. Which of the following medications does NOT interact with cimetidine via the hepatic cytochrome P-450 enzyme system

    A. Atenolol
    B. Theophylline
    C. Warfarin
    D. Phenytoin
    E. Diazepam

Patient Name: Frank Romanoski
Address: 2548 Kings Highway
Age: 55   **Height:** 6' 1"
Sex: M   **Race:** White
Weight: 172 lb
Allergies: Sulfa (rash)

Chief Complaint

FR is a 55-yo white male who presents to his family practice physician with complaints of "worsening heartburn," a hard time swallowing, "dry foods," and "laryngitis." He states that he is concerned that he may have something "serious."

History of Present Illness

FR began experiencing heartburn several times a week 10 years ago. He indicates that the heartburn is located under the sternum and occurs without radiation to the arm or back. During the last 6 months his heartburn has gradually increased in intensity and frequency. In addition, he has developed chronic laryngitis and has had increasing difficulty in swallowing solid foods such as toast and crackers. He states that during the last month he has been awakened from sleep in the middle of the night with coughing or a choking sensation and a feeling of food or liquid in his mouth accompanied by a burning sensation in his throat. He attributes his worsening symptoms to being recently laid off from work, but he is concerned about the possibility of esophageal cancer. Until 6 months ago, FR considered his heartburn to be a minor problem and self-treated with various antacids, Gavison Extra Strength, and more recently with Pepcid Complete. He states that these medications provide satisfactory relief about half of the time. He presents today because of recurrent heartburn 1 week ago after completing a 14-day course of Prilosec OTC. His laryngitis is unrelieved by lozenges.

Past Medical History

Hypertension x 15 years

Coronary artery disease (s/p MI at 52)

Hypercholesterolemia

Gallstones (cholesystectomy 5 yr ago)

Social History

Automobile assembly worker who lost job about 6 months ago; currently unemployed

Tobacco use: Smoked 1-2 PPD for 30 yr; currently smokes ½ PPD x 1 yr

Alcohol use: 1-2 beers a week

Caffeine use: About 6 cups of caffeinated coffee a day

Family History

Married and lives with his wife and two children

Father: Died at 65 from "heart disease"

Mother: Died at age 74 years from lung cancer

Review of Systems

No headache, dizziness, or vertigo; no SOB; frequent episodes of non-radiating substernal CP which patient describes as burning; no N/V/D; otherwise unremarkable except for complaints noted previously

Physical Examination

GEN: Pleasant middle-aged man in moderate distress, somewhat anxious

VS: BP 150/94 mmHg, HR 78 bpm, RR 18 rpm, T 98.4°F, Wt 172 lb

HEENT: PERRLA, EOMI, no AV nicking, hemorrhages or exudates, erythematous throat without exudates

NECK: No lymphadenopathy

CV: RRR with no murmurs

CHEST: CTA and percussion bilaterally

ABD: BS (+), soft and nontender, no masses or organomegaly

GU: Deferred

RECTAL: Guaiac negative; no palpable rectal masses

MS/EXT: No CCE, no rashes

NEURO: A & O x3

SKIN: Warm and dry, no rashes

Labs and Diagnostic Tests

Sodium 139 mEq/L	Potassium 4.0 mEq/L
Chloride 98 mEq/L	CO_2 26 mEq/L
BUN 15 mg/dL	Serum creatinine 1.1 mg/dL
Glucose 110 mg/dL	Hemoglobin 15.1 g/dL
Hematocrit 46%	Platelets 280,000/mm³
WBC 5800/mm³	TC 202 mg/dL

Case 12

LDL 98 mg/dL   HDL 50 mg/dL

Trig 144 mg/dL

EGD: Moderate erosive esophagitis with exudative lesions in distal 4 cm of esophagus (Los Angeles Grade B). No evidence of gastritis or gastroduodenal ulcers. Antral biopsy negative for Helicobacter pylori.

 Diagnosis

Primary:

1. Erosive esophagitis

2. Dysphagia secondary to #1

3. Chronic laryngitis possibly secondary to #1

Secondary:

1. HTN

2. CAD

3. Hypercholesterolemia

 Medication Record

Lopressor HCT 100/25 po bid every AM and PM

Lipitor 20 mg po qd

Aspirin 81 mg po qd

Pepcid Complete 1 tablet po 3 to 4 times a day prn heartburn

Gavison Extra Strength 1 to 2 tablets po every 3 to 4 hours prn heartburn

Halls Mentho-Lyptus Drops po for laryngitis

 Pharmacist Notes and Other Patient Information

A 55-yo man presents with worsening GERD symptoms over the last 6 months. EGD reveals erosive esophagitis. Dysphagia and chronic laryngitis most likely related to worsening GERD.

Questions

1. Which of the following best describes the relationship between heartburn and esophageal mucosal injury (esophagitis)?

   A. Heartburn occurs most often in the absence of esophageal mucosal injury

   B. Most patients with heartburn have some degree of esophageal mucosal injury

   C. Severity of heartburn directly correlates with the severity of esophageal mucosal injury

   D. Frequency of heartburn directly correlates with the severity of esophageal mucosal injury

   E. Most patients with esophagitis do not have heartburn

2. Which of the following is NOT an atypical (extraesophageal) manifestation of GERD?

   A. Dental erosions

   B. Chronic laryngitis

   C. Chronic asthma

   D. Regurgitation (passage of refluxed contents into the oropharynx)

   E. Chronic coughing

3. Which of the following is the preferred drug regimen for healing FR's erosive esophagitis?

   A. Sucralfate 1 g qid

   B. Ranitidine 150 mg bid

   C. Famotidine 40 mg bid

   D. Pantoprazole 40 mg qd

   E. Esomeprazole 40 mg tid

4. FR's physician prescribes a PPI to heal his esophagitis. Which of the following statements most accurately reflects the comparative efficacy of the PPIs when used in recommended dosages to heal erosive esophagitis?

   A. Lansoprazole 30 mg qd is more effective than omeprazole 20 mg qd

   B. Pantoprazole 40 mg qd is more effective than lansoprazole 30 mg qd

   C. Esomeprazole 20 mg qd is less effective than lansoprazole 30 mg qd

   D. Omeprazole 20 mg qd is less effective than esomeprazole 20 mg qd

   E. Pantoprazole 40 mg qd and rabeprazole 20 mg qd provide similar efficacy

5. How should you instruct this patient to take a PPI so that its antisecretory effect is maximized?

   A. Take immediately on rising on an empty stomach

   B. Take in the morning about 30 minutes before breakfast

   C. Take in the morning at least 60 minutes after breakfast

   D. Take in the evening about 30 minutes after dinner

   E. Take at bedtime

6. At his return visit to his physician, FR states that he is "heartburn-free" after 8 weeks of treatment with Protonix 40 mg qd. What is the preferred long-term management of this patient at this time?

Case 12

A. Continue Protonix 40 mg qd and reevaluate in 2 to 3 months
B. Continue Protonix 40 mg qd and add Zantac 300 mg at bedtime for 2 additional months
C. Switch to Prilosec OTC 20 mg and take when needed for recurrent GERD symptoms
D. Discontinue Protonix and begin Zantac 300 mg at bedtime
E. Discontinue Protonix and monitor for recurrent GERD symptoms

D. Alginic acid, aluminum hydroxide, magnesium carbonate
E. Aluminum hydroxide, magnesium carbonate

7. Which of the following responses is most accurate if FR questions you about the long-term safety of PPIs when used as maintenance therapy in GERD?

A. PPIs should not be used beyond 1 year
B. PPIs are likely to cause irreversible acid inhibition once the PPI is discontinued
C. PPI have been linked to esophageal cancer in humans
D. PPIs have not been associated with gastric cancer in humans
E. PPI have been associated with cardiotoxicity in humans

8. Prior to taking Prilosec OTC, FR had been taking Pepcid Complete, which provided less than satisfactory relief of his symptoms. Which of the following best reflects the status of the H_2RAs when used to treat GERD symptoms?

A. Tolerance to the antisecretory effect does not develop
B. Tolerance to the antisecretory effect develops when used prn (occasionally)
C. Tolerance to the antisecretory effect develops when used continuously (daily)
D. Tolerance to the antisecretory effect develops when used in low dosages
E. Tolerance to the antisecretory effect develops when used beyond 8 weeks

9. What is the most important reason why FR should be instructed NOT to chew or crush PPI tablets or granules before swallowing?

A. PPI may cause pharyngitis
B. PPI may injure the esophagus
C. PPI degrades at a low intragastric pH
D. PPI is degraded by salivary bicarbonate
E. PPI tastes bad

10. FR had previously self-treated his heartburn with Gaviscon Extra Strength. What is the primary active ingredient(s) in Gaviscon Extra Strength tablets?

A. Alginic acid
B. Alginic acid, aluminum hydroxide
C. Alginic acid, magnesium carbonate

Patient Name: James Baker
Address: 755 Holland Drive, Apt. #5
Age: 64   **Height:** 5' 9"
Sex: M   **Race:** African American
Weight: 143 lb
Allergies: None

Chief Complaint

JB is 64-yo African American man who presents to urgent care clinic with complaints of "difficult-to-pass stools, abdominal cramping and pain for a long time." He states that he feels "constipated" every day and that "nothing he has tried works very well!"

History of Present Illness

JB states that he has had a problem "moving his bowels" for several years. He indicates that when he was moving his bowels "regularly," he would have about 1 bowel movement every other day. JB states that during the past 6 months he has had as few as 2 bowel movements per week. He describes his stools as usually hard and difficult to pass. Straining and the feeling of incomplete evacuation occur with most bowel movements. Within the last month he reports increased abdominal cramping, pain, and bloating. Patient describes a long history of various nonprescription laxative use with little relief. When he does move his bowels the cramping and pain are usually relieved. On further questioning, JB states that his wife of 40 years died about 1 year ago and he has been living a sedentary life alone with his cat since that time.

Past Medical History

Rheumatoid arthritis x 4 yr

Depression x 1 yr

Benign prostatic hyperplasia

Social History

Recently retired professor

Tobacco use: Smokes a pipe several times a week after dinner

Alcohol use: None

Caffeine use: 1 cup of coffee every morning

Does not go out much since his wife died; meals consist primarily of frozen foods

Does not exercise any more; used to walk every day with his wife

Family History

Widowed 1 year ago; one son in the military

Father: Died of CVA at 72

Mother: Died at 65 of complications secondary to diabetes

Review of Systems

Denies N/V, dizziness, SOB, chest pain, headache, loss of appetite or weight loss; reports minor visual changes corrected with stronger prescription for glasses. Decreased ROM in left hip and both knees, bilateral knee pain; reports morning stiffness every day for about 1 hour. Reports feeling tired and fatigued. Otherwise noncontributory except as previously noted.

Physical Examination

GEN: Slender, elderly black male appearing lethargic and in a moderate degree of discomfort

VS: BP 135/70, HR 75 bpm, RR 22 rpm, T 98.2°F, Wt 143 lb

HEENT: PERRLA

NECK: Supple, no JVD, bruits, palpable lymph nodes

CV: Normal S_1, S_2; no m/r/g

CHEST: CTA bilaterally

ABD: Soft, tender, RUQ pain, no guarding, (+) BS, no organomegaly

GU: Deferred

RECTAL: Guaiac negative

MS/EXT: Hands: mild RA changes; wrists, elbows, shoulders: good ROM; hips: decreased ROM on left; knees: pain bilaterally with decreased ROM; feet: no edema, 3+ pedal pulse

NEURO: Lethargic; oriented to time/place/person, cranial nerves intact, normal DTR

SKIN: Normal, no lesions

Labs and Diagnostic Tests

Sodium 142 mEq/L	Potassium 4.0 mEq/L
Chloride 100 mEq/L	CO_2 15 mEq/L
BUN 5 mg/dL	Serum creatinine 1.1 mg/dL
Glucose 95 mg/dL	AST 28 IU/L
ALT 25 IU/L	Alk phos 71 IU/L
Hemoglobin 15.5 g/dL	Hematocrit 45%

Case 13

Platelets 280,000/mm³   WBC 8500/mm³

Barium enema: Dilated transverse and descending colon

Sigmoidoscopy: Grossly inflamed rectal wall with diffuse pigmentation

 Diagnosis

Primary:

1. Chronic constipation

Secondary:

1. RA

2. Depression

3. BPH

 Medication Record

Celecoxib 200 mg po bid

Esomeprazole 40 mg po qd

Imipramine 100 mg po at bedtime

Colace 100 mg po qd

Senokot 1-2 tablets po 3-5 times/week prn constipation

Magnesium citrate po prn constipation

 Pharmacist Notes and Other Patient Information

A 64-yo man in moderate distress. Constipation not adequately controlled with current mediations. Patient is adherent to medication regimens. RA and depression controlled on current therapy.

Questions

1. Given JB's history of constipation, which of the following best describes whether he has Chronic constipation?

    A. Persistent constipation lasting longer than several days
    B. Persistent constipation lasting longer than 2 weeks
    C. Persistent constipation lasting longer than 1 month
    D. Persistent constipation lasting longer than 6 months
    E. Persistent constipation lasting longer than 1 year

2. It is possible that JB's constipation is related to an underlying condition. Which of the following disorders is NOT usually associated with an increased risk of constipation?

    A. Diabetes mellitus
    B. Ulcerative colitis
    C. Parkinson's disease
    D. Depression
    E. Hypothyroid

3. All of the following tests are important in the evaluation of a patient such as JB with suspected chronic constipation EXCEPT:

    A. Sigmoidoscopy
    B. Barium enema
    C. 24-hour fecal fat
    D. Stool guaiac
    E. Abdominal examination

4. JB takes several nonprescription medications, including magnesium citrate, in an attempt to relieve his constipation. Which of the following statements is INCORRECT regarding the use of saline laxatives such as magnesium citrate?

    A. Avoid use in patients with renal failure
    B. Avoid use in patients with signs and symptoms of dehydration
    C. Avoid use in patients with fluid and electrolyte imbalances
    D. Avoid use in patients requiring prolonged laxative use
    E. Avoid use in patients with drug-induced constipation

5. JB's physician is contemplating the use of Miralax to treat his constipation. What is the primary active ingredient in Miralax?

    A. Docusate sodium
    B. Bisacodyl
    C. Senna
    D. Polyethylene glycol 3350
    E. Mineral oil

6. The long-term use of which of the following agents has been associated with "cathartic colon" (colonic inertia), tolerance, and colonic cancer?

    A. Stimulants
    B. Saline laxatives
    C. Emollients (stool softeners)
    D. Lubricants
    E. Polyethylene glycol 3350

7. The physician instructs the patient to stop taking Colace, Senokot, and magnesium citrate and reviews important dietary and lifestyle modifications. In addition, the physician prescribes a medication to treat JB's constipation. Which of the following medications are preferred when treating chronic constipation?

Case 13

A. Tegaserod, lactulose, or lubiprostone
B. Tegaserod, lactulose, or alosetron
C. Tegaserod, lactulose, or castor oil
D. Alosetron, lactulose, or mineral oil
E. Alosetron, lubiprostone, or polyethylene glycol 3350

8. If JB's physician had prescribed lactulose for his constipation, what would be the most important parameter(s) to monitor to assess the effectiveness of lactulose therapy?

   A. Fluid and electrolytes
   B. Abdominal pain and bloating
   C. Stool frequency and consistency
   D. Stool color
   E. Stool guaiac

9. The physician is considering the use of tegaserod to treat JB's constipation. What is the primary mechanism by which tegaserod acts when used to treat chronic constipation?

   A. $5\text{-}HT_4$ serotonin receptor antagonist in GI tract
   B. $5\text{-}HT_4$ serotonin receptor agonist in the GI tract
   C. $5\text{-}HT_3$ serotonin receptor antagonist in the GI tract
   D. $5\text{-}HT_3$ serotonin receptor agonist in the GI tract
   E. $5\text{-}HT_1$ serotonin antagonist in the GI tract

10. If JB was prescribed tegaserod for his chronic constipation, which of the following statements would BEST characterize the drug when used for this indication?

   A. Severe diarrhea occurs frequently and often requires discontinuation of the drug
   B. Should not be taken for longer than 3 months
   C. Does not relieve abdominal pain and bloating associated with constipation
   D. Advise patients to take tegaserod with meals.
   E. Constipation frequently returns on discontinuation of the drug

Case 14
Diarrhea

Patient Name: Marilyn Dickenson
Address: 555 Golden Parkway
Age: 50   **Height:** 5' 5"
Sex: F   **Race:** White
Weight: 132 lb
Allergies: NKDA; no known allergies to food

Chief Complaint

MD is a 50-yo white woman who visits your pharmacy with complaints of "diarrhea and cramping" and wants to know if there is something she can take for it without having to go to her doctor.

History of Present Illness

MD describes the sudden onset of watery diarrhea (3 bowel movements) and mild abdominal cramping which began approximately 24 hrs ago. During this time she has not had anything to eat or drink except tea and chicken soup. On further questioning, she also complains of a bad headache, increased thirst, dry mouth, some nausea, but no vomiting. When asked, she indicates that there is no blood or mucus in the stool and that she does not have a fever. She denies dizziness, orthostasis, tachycardia (rapid heart rate), and severe abdominal pain. There is no evidence of restlessness or lethargy, but she does note that she has not urinated as much during this time. Patient denies recent travel, antibiotic use, laxative use, use of Mg-containing antacids, and intolerance to specific foods, e.g., dairy or foods containing olestra.

Past Medical History

MD indicates that she has hypertension and high triglycerides.

Social History

Works full time in a day care center for preschool children

Tobacco use: Quit 15 years ago

Alcohol use: Occasional beer with friends (no alcoholic beverages for 24 hr)

Caffeine use: 2-3 cups/day at breakfast and while at work (no coffee for 24 hr)

Diet: Low fat, low carbs, high protein (no solid food for 24 hr)

Family History

Not relevant

Review of Systems

Negative except as previously noted

Physical Examination

GEN: Well-developed, well-nourished, somewhat anxious woman with complaints of diarrhea and abdominal cramping

VS: Patient states that she took her temperature this morning and it was 98.4°F; BP taken in pharmacy is 110/70; no other VS available

Labs and Diagnostic Tests

None available.

Diagnosis

Primary:

1. Acute diarrhea accompanied by mild abdominal cramping

Secondary

1. Hypertension

2. Hypertriglyceridemia

Medication Record

Hydrochlorothiazide 25 mg po q AM

Gemfibrozil 600 mg po bid

Ibuprofen 200 mg po prn headache

Pharmacist Notes and Other Patient Information

Patient complains of diarrhea and abdominal cramping for 24 hr. She wants to know if there is any nonprescription medication she can take so that she does not have to go to her doctor.

Questions

1. What is the most likely cause of this patient's diarrhea?

    A. Infection
    B. Food intolerance
    C. Dietary deficiency
    D. Medication
    E. Medical condition

Case 14

2. Which of the following individuals is NOT at high risk for infectious diarrhea?

   A. Staff at child day care centers
   B. Patients in nursing homes
   C. Individual who recently returned from a camping trip
   D. Individual with lactase deficiency
   E. Homosexual with multiple partners

3. Certain medications may cause diarrhea. All of the following medications may have initiated MD's diarrhea if she had been taking them EXCEPT:

   A. Quinidine
   B. Clindamycin
   C. Sucralfate
   D. Misoprostol
   E. Colchicine

4. What is the best assessment of the severity of this patient's hydration status?

   A. No evidence of dehydration
   B. Mild dehydration
   C. Moderate dehydration
   D. Moderate to severe dehydration
   E. Severe dehydration

5. Evaluate this patient to determine if she has any exclusions to self-treatment. Which of the following is NOT an exclusion to the self-treatment of diarrhea?

   A. Symptoms of 1-2 days duration
   B. Protracted vomiting
   C. Fever and chills
   D. Blood in stool
   E. Pregnancy

6. If MD exhibited signs and symptoms of dehydration, which of the following most accurately describes oral rehydration solutions (ORS) which would most likely be used to rehydrate her?

   A. ORS shorten the duration of the diarrhea
   B. ORS reduce stool frequency
   C. ORS usually contain only electrolytes
   D. ORS usually contain electrolytes and carbohydrates
   E. ORS should only be used under the supervision of a physician

7. What patient education would you provide MD regarding the use of loperamide if she decided to self-treat her diarrhea?

   A. Take 4 mg initially; 4 mg after each bowel movement; up to 16 mg/24 hr
   B. Take 4 mg initially; 2 mg after each bowel movement; up to 16 mg/24 hr
   C. Take 4 mg initially; 4 mg after each bowel movement, up to 12 mg/24 hr
   D. Take 4 mg initially; 2 mg after each bowel movement; up to 12 mg/24 hr
   E. Take 4 mg initially; 2 mg after each bowel movement; up to 8 mg/24 hr

8. What potentially important side effect would you discuss with MD if she decided to self-treat with loperamide?

   A. Flatulence
   B. Skin rash
   C. Increased appetite
   D. Drowsiness
   E. Nausea

9. Antidiarrheal products such as Lomotil contain diphenoxylate and atropine. What is the primary reason for the inclusion of atropine in these preparations?

   A. Contributes to the antidiarrheal effect of diphenoxylate
   B. Deters the use of diphenoxylate for illicit drug purposes
   C. Helps to control symptoms such as abdominal cramping
   D. Reduces the side effects associated with the use of diphenoxylate
   E. Acts to heal the inflammation in the bowel

10. MD wonders whether she should self-treat her diarrhea with Kaopectate. What is the primary active ingredient in Kaopectate antidiarrheal products?

    A. Kaolin and pectin
    B. Attapulgite
    C. Bismuth subsalicylate
    D. Loperamide
    E. Docusate calcium

Case 15

Case 15

Inflammatory Bowel Disease

Patient Name: Carrie Feldman
Address: 490 Portage Road
Age: 35   Height: 5' 7"
Sex: F   Race: White
Weight: 135 lb
Allergies: Sulfa

Chief Complaint

CF is a 35-yo white woman who presents to GI clinic with complaints of increasing "bloody diarrhea and abdominal pain" for approximately 2 weeks.

History of Present Illness

CF has a 7-yr history of diarrhea, abdominal pain, and intermittent weight loss. She was treated initially by her family physician with loperamide while attempting to rule out reasons for her diarrhea and abdominal cramps.

About 3 years ago, she was diagnosed by her family physician with protosigmoiditis and treated with sulfasalazine 3 g/day. Treatment was discontinued after 4 weeks because of a rash which developed on her back and extremities. At that time, the patient complained of headache, nausea, and malaise. Hydrocortisone enemas were prescribed and symptom relief was achieved within 1 month at which time the enemas were discontinued. 6 months later, CF's symptoms returned with accompanying BRBPR and she was referred to the GI clinic for further evaluation and treatment.

The patient underwent a colonoscopy with biopsy which revealed ulcerative colitis. Treatment was begun with oral prednisone (which was tapered over several weeks) and Asacol. Once remission was achieved, the patient was maintained on Asacol until she stopped taking it about 1 month ago.

CF was doing fairly well until 2 weeks ago when she developed bloody diarrhea (now has 5 to 6 bloody stools per day) and abdominal pain. Her clinical course has been complicated by inadequate nutrition and a 10-lb weight loss.

There is no history of out of state/country travel, recent antibiotic or laxative use, or exposure to anyone sick.

Past Medical History

Asymmetrical joint pain of right hip, knee and left wrist x 5 yr

Inadequate nutrition accompanied by intermittent weight loss x 7 yr

Iron deficiency anemia dx 3 yr ago

Social History

Elementary school teacher, works full time

Tobacco use: Denies ever using tobacco

Alcohol use: Occasional glass of wine with dinner

Caffeine use: 1 cup of coffee with breakfast

Family History

Married, lives with husband; no children

Father: Died at 60 of colon cancer

Mother: Alive at 62 with 20 yr history of RA

Review of Systems

Abdominal pain and diarrhea often accompany meals and are usually relieved by defecation. Reports poor appetite, a 10-lb weight loss over 1 month. Negative for N/V, lightheadedness, dizziness, SOB, or chest pain. Denies fever or chills. Joint pain controlled with NSAID. Otherwise noncontributory except as previously noted.

Physical Examination

GEN: Pleasant, cooperative woman, mildly anxious about her condition

VS: BP 140/70 mmHg, HR 90, RR 18, T 99.2°F, Wt 135 lb

HEENT: PERRLA; negative for iritis and conjunctivitis; negative for aphthous ulcers of the mouth; TMs intact

NECK: No lymphadenopathy, bruits, or tenderness.

CV: RRR, normal S_1 and S_2; no S_3, S_4

CHEST: CTA. no rales or rhonchi

ABD: Diffuse tenderness in lower abdomen, no rebound or quadrant pain; hyperactive bowel sounds

GU: Deferred

RECTAL: Deferred

MS/EXT: No cyanosis, clubbing, or edema; pulses 2+

NEURO: A/O x 3

SKIN: Warm and moist

Case 15

Labs and Diagnostic Tests

Sodium 148 mEq/L   Potassium 3.8 mEq/L

Chloride 100 mEq/L CO_2 26 mEq/L

BUN 20 mg/dL   Serum creatinine 1.1 mg/dL

Glucose 70 mg/dL   Hemoglobin 12.5 g/dL

Hematocrit 34%   TP 7.5 g/dL

Alb 4.5 g/dL   AST 32 IU/L

ALT 30 IU/L   Alk phos 75 IU/L

T. bili. 0.9 mg/dL   Platelets 320,000/mm³

WBC 12,500/mm³, with 70% PMN, bands 8%, 18% lymphocytes, 2% mono, 2% eosinophils

FE 48 µg/dL   TIBC 372 µg/dL

Ferritin 22 ng/mL

Colonoscopy: Mucosal surface of transverse, descending, sigmoid colon and rectum irregular and granular in appearance; mucosa friable with spontaneous bleeding. Biopsy consistent with UC. No evidence of fistula, fissures, transmural, or perianal disease.

Diagnosis

Primary:

1. Ulcerative colitis

Secondary:

1. Asymmetrical joint pain of hip, knee, and wrist

2. Nutrition

3. Iron deficiency anemia

Medication Record

Asacol 400 mg po bid (discontinued 1 month ago)

Os-Cal 500 mg + D po bid

Diclofenac 75 mg SR po bid pc

Ferrous sulfate 325 mg po bid

Lo-Ovral po qd

Pharmacist Notes and Other Patient Information

None available

Questions

1. This patient has biopsy confirmed ulcerative colitis. Which of the following INCORRECTLY describes ulcerative colitis?

   A. May affect any part of the GI tract from mouth to anus

   B. Surgery is usually curative

   C. Risk of colon cancer is greater in UC than in the general population

   D. May be associated with extraintestinal manifestations

   E. Predominant signs and symptoms are diarrhea, GI bleeding, and abdominal pain

2. Given CF's clinical presentation and that treatment is based (in part) on disease severity, what is the correct assumption regarding the severity of this patient's UC?

   A. Mild

   B. Moderate

   C. Severe

   D. Life-threatening

   E. Complicated

3. Which of the following was most likely responsible for the exacerbation of CF's disease at this time?

   A. Diet

   B. Stress

   C. Discontinued sulfasalazine

   D. Discontinued Asacol

   E. Discontinued hydrocortisone enema

4. Which of the following is most likely an extraintestinal manifestation of JC's ulcerative colitis?

   A. Poor appetite

   B. Weight loss

   C. Asymmetrical joint pain

   D. Malaise

   E. Headache

5. CF was initially treated with sulfasalazine. Which of the following is NOT a dose-dependent side effect of sulfasalazine?

   A. Dyspepsia

   B. Headache

   C. Nausea

   D. Malaise

   E. Skin rash

6. CF was treated with Asacol until she decided to stop taking it. Which of the following dosage forms best describe Asacol?

Case 15

A. Time-dependent granules release 5-ASA in the small intestine and colon

B. Time-dependent granules releases 5-ASA in the colon and rectum

C. pH-dependent enteric-coated tablet releases 5-ASA in the duodenum

D. pH-dependent enteric-coated tablet releases 5-ASA in the terminal ileum and colon

E. ph-dependent enteric-coated tablet releases 5-ASA in the rectum

7. What is the recommended dosage of Asacol when used to treat CF's active UC?

A. 400 mg bid
B. 800 mg bid
C. 400 mg tid
D. 800 mg tid
E. 1200 mg qid

8. What are the most important endpoints of therapy for CF who is suffering from an acute flare up of UC?

A. Cure the disease so that it does not recur
B. Maintain weight and proper nutrition
C. Induce and maintain remission
D. Avoid anemia and nutritional deficiencies
E. Reduce psychological stress and increase sense of well-being

9. At some point during her life-long illness, CF may become a candidate for treatment with azathioprine or 6-mercaptopurine. Which of the following best describes the use of azathioprine or 6-mercaptopurine when treating patients with IBD?

A. Used to reduce the corticosteroid dose in steroid-dependent patients
B. Used to reduce the 5-ASA dose in patients requiring 5-ASA maintenance therapy
C. Used as first-line therapy in patients with severe acute disease
D. Used as bridge therapy to cyclosporine in steroid refractory patients
E. Used with cyclosporine to decrease severe side effects

10. All of the following medications used to treat inflammatory bowel disease attribute their primary activity to 5-ASA EXCEPT:

A. Olsalazine
B. Infliximab
C. Sulfasalazine
D. Balsalazide
E. Mesalamine

Hepatic and Pancreatic Disorders

Section Editor: Katherine C. Herndon

See all 8 cases for this section on the CD.

Case 16   Adverse Effects of Drugs on the Liver

Patient Name: Lois Welborn
Address: 388 Cypress Lane
Age: 39   Height: 5' 7"
Sex: F   Race: African American
Weight: 162 lb
Allergies: NKDA

Chief Complaint

LW is a 39-yo African American female who presents to the primary care clinic on 5/24 with a chief complaint of "yellow eyes" and itching.

History of Present Illness

LW was last seen in the primary care clinic approximately 2 months ago for her annual physical exam. She was without complaints at that time. Approximately 4 weeks after her last appointment, LW began to experience malaise, anorexia, and nausea. One week later, LW's husband noticed that her sclerae were yellow. Around the same time, she reports the onset of an intense, generalized pruritus.

Past Medical History

Type 2 DM

Hyperlipidemia

Onychomycosis (toenails)

h/o Diabetic foot ulcer

Social History

LW has worked as a registered nurse at a long-term care facility for the past 8 years. She has been married for 10 years and has no children. She denies tobacco, alcohol, and illicit drug use.

Family History

Mother alive at age 65 with type 2 DM. Father alive at age 68 with CAD. She has no siblings. No family history of cancer.

Review of Systems

LW denies fever, rash, and vomiting. Review of systems is positive for mild, diffuse abdominal pain, dark-colored urine, and pale colored stools for the past week.

Physical Examination

GEN: Well-nourished, obese female in no acute distress

VS: BP 150/92 mmHg, HR 80 bpm, RR 16 rpm, T 98.7°F, Wt 162 lb, Ht 67 inches

HEENT: NCAT, PERRLA, EOMI, icteric sclerae, funduscopic exam without hemorrhages or exudates

NECK: Supple, no lymphadenopathy or thyromegaly, no bruits

CV: RRR without m/r/g

CHEST: CTA bilaterally

ABD: Normal bowel sounds, mild abdominal tenderness in upper quadrants, no hepatomegaly or splenomegaly

GU: Deferred

RECTAL: Heme (-)

EXT: No CCE, normal pulses throughout, bilateral onychomycosis of toenails

NEURO: A&O x4, CN II-XII intact

SKIN: No rash, excoriations on arms and chest

Labs and Diagnostic Tests

Sodium 138 mmol/L   Potassium 4.1 mmol/L

Chloride 100 mmol/L CO_2 27 mmol/L

BUN 5.7 mmol/L (16 mg/dL)

Serum creatinine 88.4 µmol/L (1.0 mg/dL)

Glucose 7.8 mmol/L (140 mg/dL)

Albumin 40 g/L

Total cholesterol 5.7 mmol/L (220 mg/dL)

HDL-C 0.98 mmol/L (38 mg/dL)

Triglycerides 2.0 mmol/L (180 mg/dL)

LDL-C (calculated) 3.8 mmol/L (146 mg/dL)

T. bili 120 µmol/L (7.0 mg/dL)

AST 350 U/L   ALT 235 U/L

ALP 1000 U/L   CBC w/ diff wnl

PT/INR wnl

Hepatitis A and B serology - negative

Diagnosis

Primary:

     1. Probable drug-induced hepatotoxicity

Secondary:

     1. Type 2 DM

     2. Hyperlipidemia

     3. Onychomycosis (toenails)

     4. h/o Diabetic foot ulcer

Case 16

Medication Record

Date	Rx No	Physician	Drug and Strength	Quantity	Sig	Refills
10/2	13567	Reilly	Avandia 4 mg	30	1 po qd	12
10/2			Aspirin 81 mg	30	1 po qd	
11/15	13999	Reilly	Glucophage 500 mg	60	1 po bid	12
2/8	17110	Reilly	Niacor 500 mg	90	1 po tid with food	12
3/24	18741	Reilly	Triphasil-28	30	1 po qd	12
3/24	18742	Reilly	Vasotec 10 mg	30	1 po qd	12
4/13	19051	Tucker	Lamisil 250 mg	30	1 po qd x 12 weeks	2
8/18	27839	Poole	Isoniazid 300 mg	30	1 po qd	5
3/24	18743	Reilly	HCTZ 25 mg	30	1 po qd	12
4/25	23768	Reilly	Augmentin 500 mg	28	1 po bid x 14 days	0
2/8	17111	Reilly	Starlix 60 mg	90	1 po tid before meals	12

Pharmacist Notes and Other Patient Information

4/25 Patient presents with diabetic foot ulcer. Fourteen day course of Augmentin prescribed. Education on foot and wound care provided.

8/18 Patient with positive tuberculin skin test during work site screening. She will receive daily isoniazid therapy for 9 months.

Questions

1. LW is presumed to have drug-induced hepatotoxicity. The primary care physician wants to know which of the following medications on LW's profile is known to cause hepatotoxicity.

   I. Niacor
   II. Vasotec
   III. Starlix

   A. I only
   B. III only
   C. I and II only
   D. II and III only
   E. I, II, and III

2. Hepatotoxicity from which of the following medications is consistent with LW's clinical presentation and laboratory values?

   I. Triphasil-28
   II. Lamisil
   III. Augmentin

   A. I only
   B. III only
   C. I and II only
   D. II and III only
   E. I, II, and III

3. Triphasil-28 is temporarily out of stock in the pharmacy. When selecting another agent with the same active ingredients, you choose a product that contains which of the following components?

   A. Mestranol and norethindrone
   B. Ethinyl estradiol and norethindrone
   C. Ethinyl estradiol and ethynodiol diacetate
   D. Ethinyl estradiol and levonorgestrel
   E. Ethinyl estradiol and desogestrel

4. Baseline liver function tests should be obtained prior to initiating therapy with which of the following agents?

   I. Avandia
   II. Glucophage
   III. HCTZ

   A. I only
   B. III only
   C. I and II only
   D. II and III only
   E. I, II, and III

5. The primary care physician wants to read a brief synopsis on the hepatotoxic potential of several drugs in LW's regimen. Which of the following references would you recommend?

   I. AHFS Drug Information
   II. American Drug Index
   III. The Merck Index

   A. I only
   B. III only
   C. I and II only
   D. II and III only
   E. I, II, and III

Case 16

6. According to current guidelines, which of the following should be included in the treatment plan for LW's isoniazid therapy?

   I.   Monitoring for visual disturbances
   II. Baseline liver function tests
   III. Pyridoxine 25 mg po once daily

   A. I only
   B. III only
   C. I and II only
   D. II and III only
   E. I, II, and III

7. Which of the following parameters would be most useful when monitoring for the hepatotoxic effects of isoniazid?

   A. Albumin
   B. Bilirubin
   C. Alkaline phosphatase
   D. GGT
   E. ALT

8. Lamisil would be expected to inhibit the metabolism of other drugs through which of the following cytochrome P450 isoenzymes?

   A. CYP1A2
   B. CYP2C9
   C. CYP2D6
   D. CYP2E1
   E. CYP3A4

9. Which of the following should be included when educating LW about proper foot care?

   I.   Daily monitoring of feet for sores, blisters, calluses, and redness.
   II. Wear protective footwear at all times.
   III. Keep feet clean and dry.

   A. I only
   B. III only
   C. I and II only
   D. II and III only
   E. I, II, and III

10. According to current guidelines, what is the LDL cholesterol goal for LW?

   A. <70 mg/dL
   B. <100 mg/dL
   C. <130 mg/dL
   D. <160 mg/dL
   E. <190 mg/dL

Patient Name: Bart Thomas
Address: 3468 Fulmer Street
Age: 40   **Height:** 5' 8"
Sex: M   **Race:** White
Weight: 167 lb (76 kg)
Allergies: Penicillin

Chief Complaint

BT is a 40-yo white male who presents to your pharmacy with new prescriptions. He has no specific complaints other than general malaise and intermittent bouts of tiredness. He is poised to ask many questions related to his new treatment plan prescribed by his physician.

History of Present Illness

BT was diagnosed with chronic hepatitis C (HCV) infection several years ago. At that time he received interferon-alpha 2b monotherapy but subsequently relapsed. BT states that his primary care physician referred him to a new liver specialist who prescribed a new treatment regimen for his chronic infection.

Past Medical History

BT contracted hepatitis C approximately 10 years ago. The hepatitis was most likely the result of a tattoo application on his back while visiting Thailand. At the time of his hepatitis C diagnosis, HIV and HBV tests were negative. He has had asthma since age 16. Asthma symptoms have been well controlled with pharmacotherapy, with no recent exacerbations requiring ED assistance or hospital admission. BT was also diagnosed with HTN at age 29. Blood pressures have been well controlled with lifestyle modifications and pharmacotherapy. BT does not have any history of depression or other mental illness and denies ever receiving a blood transfusion.

Social History

BT denies injection or use of illicit drugs, body piercing, or promiscuous sexual activity now or in the past. BT says tobacco use is none in the past 8 years. His alcohol use is none since hepatitis C diagnosis. Married for 12 years with no children. BT attends church regularly.

Family History

Mother and father both alive. Mother, age 58, has type 2 DM, HTN, and dyslipidemia. Father, age 62, has medically managed CAD, HTN, and dyslipidemia. Older brother, age 40, has HTN. Younger sister, age 32, has no known medical problems.

Review of Systems

The liver is mildly enlarged and moderately tender on palpation. Otherwise, there are no overt clinical signs or symptoms of chronic hepatitis C other than malaise and tiredness. Since his specialist was very busy today, BT appears anxious to ask questions and learn more about his newly prescribed drug therapy.

Physical Examination

GEN: Well-developed, mildly malnourished, anxious-appearing white male in NAD, alert and oriented to person, place, and time

VS: BP 128/78 mmHg, HR 78 bpm, RR 16 rpm, T 38.3°C, Wt 71 kg, Ht 5' 8'

HEENT: PERRLA, TM clear   CHEST: Clear

ABD: Tender, enlarged spleen   GU: WNL

EXT: No edema or swelling

Labs and Diagnostic Tests

Sodium 138 mEq/L	Potassium 4.0 mEq/L
Chloride 102 mEq/L	CO_2 content 22 mEq/L
BUN 10 mg/dL	Glucose (nonfasting) 88 mg/dL
Serum creatinine 1.1 mg/dL	ALT 150 U/L
PT 15.2	T. bili 1.2 mg/dL
AST 83 U/L INR 1.54	Albumin 3.7 g/dL
ALP 46 U/mL	TSH 3.6 μU/mL

WBC 7000 mm³ without a left shift

Hemoglobin 15.6 g/dL	Hematocrit 47%
Platelets 375,000 mm³	Anti-HCV: Positive

HCV-RNA: Positive (low level; <2 million copies/mL)

HCV genotype 1a liver biopsy: Portal fibrosis with moderate degrees of inflammation and necrosis

Diagnosis

Primary:

1) Chronic hepatitis C   2) Hypertension

3) Mild asthma

Pharmacist Notes and Other Patient Information

None available

Case 17

Medication Record

Date	Rx No	Physician	Drug and Strength	Quantity	Sig	Refills
3/1	824244	Williams	Monopril 10 mg	33	1 po q day	9
3/1	824245	Williams	Advair Diskus 100/50 µg	60	1 puff bid	9
3/1	824246	Williams	Albuterol MDI 17 µg		2 puffs prn	11
3/1	967500	Levinson	PEG-Intron	120 µg/0.5 mL 120 µg SC	weekly	48
3/1	967501	Levinson	Rebetol 200 mg	180	3 po bid	12

Questions

1. Which of the following represents patient specific information that should be discussed with BT when Rebetol is dispensed?

    I.   His wife should not be pregnant or become pregnant during therapy and for 6 months after therapy has been discontinued.
    II. Side effects like nasal itching and stuffiness may represent onset of serious infection since ribavirin commonly hinders immune function.
    III. Fatigue, shortness of breath, and palpitations are common self-limiting side effects of ribavirin that do not represent any underlying serious concern.

    A. I only
    B. III only
    C. I and II only
    D. II and III only
    E. I, II, and III

2. BT has been diagnosed with chronic hepatitis C infection. Which of the following is true regarding infection with the hepatitis C virus?

    I.   Universal vaccination is the primary measure that should be employed to control the spread of this disease and may have prevented BT's infection.
    II. BT is very unfortunate because very few persons who contract acute hepatitis C progress to any form of chronic disease related to the virus.
    III. Historically, non-A, non-B hepatitis was primarily caused by what has now been identified as hepatitis C.

    A. I only
    B. III only
    C. I and II only
    D. II and III only
    E. I, II, and III

3. Which of the following represents some of the patient specific information that should be discussed with BT when PEG-Intron is dispensed?

    I.   Initially, commonly encountered side effects are mild and generally increase in severity after the first several weeks.

    II. Injections should be given by the subcutaneous (SC) route and on the same day of each week.
    III. Pretreatment with ibuprofen or acetaminophen may help minimize some adverse effects.

    A. I only
    B. III only
    C. I and II only
    D. II and III only
    E. I, II, and III

4. Which of the following is true regarding peginterferons?

    I.   They are produced by adding a polyethylene glycol molecule to alpha interferon.
    II. Their side effect profile is similar to standard interferons.
    III. They are equally efficacious with standard interferons against the hepatitis C virus as measured by sustained viral response rates.

    A. I only
    B. III only
    C. I and II only
    D. II and III only
    E. I, II, and III

5. Which of the following information in BT's history and presentation suggest that he is a suitable candidate for combination therapy with PEG-Intron and Rebetol?

    I.   Anti-HCV, HCV RNA with a low level of viral load
    II. Elevated serum ALT and liver biopsy consistent with active disease
    III. Genotype 1a

    A. I only
    B. III only
    C. I and II only
    D. II and III only
    E. I, II, and III

6. BT most likely acquired HCV through a tattoo application overseas. Which of the following represents other known modes of transmission for hepatitis C that should also be considered when evaluating BT as well as other patients with HCV?

Case 17

I. A single intimate sexual encounter
II. Any exposure to a body fluid or secretion other than blood
III. Illicit IV drug use once or just a few times

A. I only
B. III only
C. I and II only
D. II and III only
E. I, II, and III

7. Which of the following would be appropriate monitoring parameters while BT is receiving combination therapy with PEG-Intron and Rebetol?

I. Neuropsychiatric effects such as depression or anxiety
II. Periodic hemoglobin, platelet, and neutrophil counts
III. Paradoxical worsening of the hepatitis

A. I only
B. III only
C. I and II only
D. II and III only
E. I, II, and III

8. In which of the following situations would Monopril NOT be an optimal antihypertensive?

I. Patients who have asthma
II. Patients who have gout
III. Patients who are pregnant or trying to become pregnant

A. I only
B. III only
C. I and II only
D. II and III only
E. I, II, and III

9. Which of the following is true about BT's Advair prescription?

I. It is a combination of a steroid and a long-acting β-agonist.
II. The diskus requires the same breathing coordination as a metered-dose inhaler.
III. It should be used to reverse acute bronchoconstriction.

A. I only
B. III only
C. I and II only
D. II and III only
E. I, II, and III

10. BT's prescription for albuterol MDI could be filled with which of the following?

I. Serevent
II. Atrovent
III. Ventolin

A. I only
B. III only
C. I and II only
D. II and III only
E. I, II, and III

Rheumatic Disorders

Patient Name: Samuel Taylor
Address: 531 S. Washington Street
Age: 56   **Height:** 5' 10"
Sex: M   **Race:** African American
Weight: 225 lb
Allergies: Penicillin (rash)

Chief Complaint

ST is a 56-yo man who presents to the clinic complaining of the gradual worsening of joint pain over the past 4-6 months.

History of Present Illness

The patient states that aspirin is not helping his arthritis pain. The pain is most noticeable in his right knee and hip. The onset of pain has been gradual over the past 4-6 months. He has attempted to treat the pain with aspirin up to 18 tablets per day and has gained some relief from this treatment. He is unsure of the current dosage of aspirin that he is taking. The patient states that he has pain in the morning that improves within about 15 minutes but that the pain worsens with increased use of the affected joints during the day. He also states that he sometimes feels like his knee is going to give out when he is walking, especially when going down stairs.

Past Medical History

Hypertension

S/P appendectomy approximately 30 years ago

Social History

Married and lives with his wife of 30 years; has three grown children who are all healthy. Employed as a carpenter. Quit smoking cigarettes 25 years ago; currently smokes one or two cigars per day. Heavy alcohol intake in the past but claims to have cut back in the past 5 years.

Family History

Father died at age 72 of a CVA; mother alive at age 88 with RA. Patient has no siblings. Family history is otherwise unremarkable.

Review of Systems

Denies shortness of breath, chest pain, fever, chills, or night sweats. No complaints of nausea, diarrhea, constipation, abdominal pain, vomiting, melena, or bloody stools. No dysuria, urgency, or frequency. No skin rashes or changes, intolerance to heat or cold, and no history of any STD. Appetite has been normal.

Physical Examination

GEN: The patient is a W/D African American male in NAD

VS: BP 144/88 mmHg, HR 96 bpm and regular, RR 16 rpm, T 36.9°C, Wt 225 lb, Ht 5' 10"

SKIN: Warm and dry

HEENT: NC/AT, PERRLA; sclerae are anicteric; EOMI; oropharyngeal mucosa is pink, moist, and without lesions. There are multiple dental caries throughout.

NECK: Supple with full ROM. No thyromegaly, lymphadenopathy, or JVD.

CHEST: CTA bilaterally with no wheezes or crackles

CV: Slightly tachycardic with no m/r/g appreciated

ABD: Soft, NT/ND, normo-active bowel sounds

GU/RECT: Deferred

MS/EXT: Full ROM of all extremities. Local tenderness and crepitus noted on right knee. Strength is +4/5 in both UE and +4/5 in both LE. There is no CCE.

NEURO: A & O x3; DTRs 2+ bilaterally

Labs and Diagnostic Tests

Sodium 139 mEq/L

Potassium 3.9 mEq/L

Chloride 101 mEq/L

CO_2 content 26 mEq/L

BUN 19 mg/dL

Serum creatinine 1.1 mg/dL

Glucose 99 mg/dL

ANA titer negative

RA titer negative

Hemoglobin 13.3 g/dL

Hematocrit 39.4%

Platelets 327,000/mm³

WBC 5400/mm³ with 57% PMNs, 3% bands, 1% eosinophils, 36% lymphocytes, 3% monocytes

Hip x-ray: No fractures or dislocations. There is minimal joint space narrowing. Small osteophyte formation at femoral joint margin. No osteopenia or joint erosions are observed.

Knee x-ray: No fractures or dislocations. There is moderate joint space narrowing and osteophyte formation at the joint margins. No osteopenia or joint erosions are observed.

Case 18

Diagnosis

Primary:

1) Osteoarthritis of the hip and knee

2) Hypertension

Secondary:

1) S/P appendectomy

Assessment and Plan:

ST is a 56-yo male with probable OA. We will obtain blood work to rule out other causes of arthritis such as SLE and RA. We will obtain an x-ray of the hip and knee to look for the degenerative changes associated with OA. We will have the patient try acetaminophen 650 mg four times a day (not prn) as initial therapy for OA. We will also recommend glucosamine 1500 mg daily. He should discontinue the high-dose aspirin therapy due to risk of GI toxicity. The patient is scheduled for a follow-up visit in 4 weeks.

Pharmacist Notes and Other Patient Information

10/15 Patient 10 days late for refill of hypertension meds. Discussed importance of compliance with regimen. Recommended a pill box as patient sometimes forgets to take medicine.

11/29 Counseled patient on dosage of acetaminophen. Cautioned patient to avoid alcohol while taking this medication.

1/14 Counseled on adverse effects of ibuprofen. Advised to check blood pressure at home regularly and inform his physician if it increases. Hypertension medications refilled on time. Patient states the pill box helped him remember to take his medication daily.

Questions

1. The drug of choice for initial treatment of OA is:

   A. acetaminophen.
   B. tramadol.
   C. oxycodone.
   D. an NSAID.
   E. intra-articular hyaluronate injections.

2. ST's acetaminophen dose was increased to 1000 mg QID but failed to provide adequate pain relief. The acetaminophen was discontinued and ST was started on an NSAID. What monitoring parameters should be assessed periodically to ensure safety?

   I.   Hepatic enzymes
   II. CBC
   III. Serum creatinine

   A. I only
   B. III only
   C. I and II only
   D. II and III only
   E. I, II, and III

3. How many mg of ibuprofen would it take to compound 50 grams of 5% ibuprofen cream?

   A. 1000 mg
   B. 2500 mg
   C. 5000 mg
   D. 400 mg
   E. 200 mg

4. Which brand/generic pair is correctly matched?

Medication Record

Date	Rx No	Physician	Drug and Strength	Quantity	Sig	Refills
10/15	593847	Williams	Hydrochlorothiazide 25 mg	90	1 po qd	0
10/15	593848	Williams	Lisinopril 40 mg	90	1 po qd	0
11/5			Aspirin 325 mg	100		
11/29		Williams	Acetaminophen 325 mg	200	2 qid	
11/29		Williams	Glucosamine 500 mg	100	1 po tid	
12/28		Williams	Acetaminophen 500 mg	200	2 qid	
1/14	594001	Williams	Ibuprofen 600 mg	90	1 po tid prn	3
1/14	594002	Williams	Hydrochlorothiazide 25 mg	90	1 po qd	3
1/14	594003	Williams	Lisinopril 40 mg	90	1 po qd	3

Case 18

A. Celebrex/piroxicam
B. Daypro/oxaprozin
C. Lodine/ketoprofen
D. Relafen/naproxen
E. Voltaren/nabumetone

5. NSAIDs have the potential to cause clinically significant drug-drug interactions with each of the following medications EXCEPT:

A. warfarin.
B. lithium.
C. phenytoin.
D. lisinopril.
E. ranitidine.

6. Crepitus was noted during this patient's physical exam. What does crepitus mean?

A. Crackling noise
B. Swelling
C. Bruise
D. Thickened cartilage
E. Joint enlargement

7. What adverse effects of ibuprofen should this patient be counseled on?

I. Photosensitivity
II. GI upset
III. Cough

A. I only
B. III only
C. I and II only
D. II and III only
E. I, II, and III

8. Which NSAIDs are specific for inhibition of COX-2?

I. Celecoxib
II. Meloxicam
III. Etodolac

A. I only
B. III only
C. I and II only
D. II and III only
E. I, II, and III

9. Which of the following statements is true regarding glucosamine use for OA?

A. Onset of pain relief can be expected within a few hours.
B. It has not been proven to be effective for OA.
C. The main adverse effect is GI discomfort.
D. It does not require additional blood glucose monitoring in patients with diabetes.
E. It is FDA-approved for treatment of OA.

10. Which of the following non-drug measures could be recommended to this patient for his OA?

I. Rest
II. Weight loss
III. Exercise

A. I only
B. III only
C. I and II only
D. II and III only
E. I, II, and III

Patient Name: Marcella Sarks
Address: 1620 Dewey Street
Age: 52   **Height:** 5' 5"
Sex: F   **Race:** White
Weight: 127 lb
Allergies: Sulfa (rash)

Chief Complaint

MS is a 52-yo woman referred to a rheumatologist on December 26 for evaluation and diagnosis of persistent joint pain, fatigue, malaise, and loss of appetite.

History of Present Illness

The patient has been seen by her PCP twice during the past 6 months because of increasing pain in her hands, wrists, and feet. She states that she initially noticed stiffness in her hands on arising in the morning but that this usually improves within an hour or two. During the past 2 months, the joint pain and stiffness have spread to her wrists and feet. MS states that she has flare-ups of joint pain that last for several days before gradually getting somewhat better. The joint stiffness never totally resolves. When these episodes first began, she self-treated with aspirin 650 mg tid or qid during the flare-ups.

More recently, she has become tired in the late afternoon and is finding it difficult to perform her work productively in the afternoon hours. She does not have pain or stiffness in her neck, elbows, shoulders, hips, knees, or ankles. Six months ago, her PCP prescribed naproxen 500 mg bid for 2 months, from which she obtained only modest pain relief and experienced some GI upset. She was switched to oxaprozin 600 mg 2 tablets daily for the past 4 months, which has helped her joint pain somewhat but has not alleviated the swelling, stiffness, or fatigue.

Past Medical History

Asthma as a child; currently taking no medications

Migraine headaches (occasional)

Social History

Patient is married and lives with her husband. They have two daughters, both of whom are married and live nearby. She works as a secretary in the local city municipal office. She does not smoke and drinks alcohol only on rare occasions.

Family History

Both parents are alive and in their early eighties. Mother has RA and CHF; father has diverticulitis and a history of colonic

polyps. The patient has two siblings who are alive and well, and neither has any rheumatic diseases.

Review of Systems

Negative except for the complaints noted above. No nausea, vomiting, constipation, diarrhea, abdominal pain, or weight loss. No fever, shortness of breath, chest pain, or dry eyes.

Physical Examination

GEN: WD/WN white woman who appears somewhat anxious

VS: BP 138/88 mmHg, HR 72 bpm, RR 18 rpm, T 37.4°C, Wt 127 lb, Ht 5' 5"

SKIN: Warm and dry; normal hair distribution

HEENT: PERRLA; EOMI; disks are flat with no hemorrhages or exudates; TMs intact; nares patent; oropharynx clear

NECK: Supple without JVD, lymphadenopathy, or thyromegaly

CHEST: CTA without wheezes or crackles

CV: RRR, normal S_1 and S_2, no S_3 or S_4

ABD: Soft, NT/ND; normo-active bowel sounds; no organomegaly

GU/RECT: Deferred

MS/EXT: Examination of the hands reveals bilateral soft tissue swelling, erythema, warmth, and tenderness of the second, third, and fourth PIP joints of both hands; there is some mild erythema of the corresponding MCP joints. The DIP joints of both hands appear normal and are without tenderness. Although the patient complains of some stiffness and mild pain during the ROM test of the wrists, there is no obvious swelling. There is mild soft tissue swelling of the second and third MTP joints of both feet. Grip strength is (+) 3/5 bilaterally. There is normal ROM of the shoulders, elbows, hips, and knees. There is no swan-neck or boutonniere deformity and no ulnar deviation. No subcutaneous nodules are observed on the extensor surfaces of the forearms or elsewhere.

NEURO: A & O x3; CN II-XII intact; no focal deficits; DTRs 2+ throughout; Babinski's downgoing

Labs and Diagnostic Tests

Sodium 142 mEq/L	Potassium 4.1 mEq/L
Chloride 106 mEq/L	CO_2 content 23 mEq/L
BUN 12 mg/dL	Serum creatinine 0.8 mg/dL
Glucose 98 mg/dL	Uric acid 5.2 mg/dL

Case 19

ESR (Westergren) 48 mm/h   C-reactive protein 1.47 mg/dL

RF positive 1:1280   ANA negative

Anti-ds DNA negative   Hemoglobin 11.9 g/dL

Hematocrit 36.4%   Platelets 421,500/mm³

WBC 5200/mm³ with 60% neutrophils, 2% bands, 1% eosinophils, 32% lymphocytes, 5% monocytes

Hand x-rays: AP views reveal soft-tissue swelling about the second, third, and fourth PIP joints of both hands. No erosions are observed at the joint margins. There is no obvious osteopenia.

 Diagnosis

Primary:

1) Early but persistent rheumatoid arthritis

Secondary:

1) H/O migraine headaches

2) H/O asthma as a child

 Pharmacist Notes and Other Patient Information

6/15 Advised patient to take naproxen on a regular basis with food, with doses evenly spaced. Patient is not allergic to aspirin or other NSAIDs.

8/20 Possible duplicate therapy. Confirmed with patient that naproxen is to be discontinued and oxaprozin started. Advised patient to take oxaprozin 2 tablets qd with food.

12/26 Instructed patient on proper use of methotrexate dose pack. Advised her of possible adverse effects (e.g., mouth ulcers, diarrhea, nausea, and vomiting). Also advised her to avoid use of alcoholic beverages while taking this medication because of possible adverse effects on the liver.

Questions

1. This patient's signs and symptoms that are consistent with the diagnosis of RA include all of the following EXCEPT:

   A. morning joint stiffness that lasts an hour or more before maximal improvement.
   B. migraine headaches.
   C. swelling of PIP joints.
   D. symmetrical joint involvement.
   E. positive serum rheumatoid factor.

2. This patient with active, persistent RA may require treatment with:

   I.   NSAIDs.
   II. corticosteroids.
   III. DMARDs.

   A. I only
   B. III only
   C. I and II only
   D. II and III only
   E. I, II, and III

3. Which of the following nonpharmacologic treatments should this patient receive at this time?

   I.   Range of motion exercises
   II. Strengthening exercises
   III. Surgery

   A. I only
   B. III only
   C. I and II only
   D. II and III only
   E. I, II, and III

4. What symptoms should this patient self-monitor and report to her physician to assist with the detection of myelosuppression associated with methotrexate use?

 Medication Record

Date	Rx No	Physician	Drug and Strength	Quantity	Sig	Refills
4/3	478923	Dixon	Sumatriptan 5-mg nasal spray	1	1 spray each nostril prn	3
5/5			Aspirin 325 mg	100	2 tablets 3-4 x/day	prn
6/15	489324	Arnold	Naproxen 500 mg	60	1 po bid	3
8/20	673809	Arnold	Oxaprozin 600 mg	60	2 po qd	4
12/26	978212	Levy	Methotrexate 2.5 mg Dose-Pack	1	3 tabs po q week	0
12/26	978213	Levy	Folic acid 1 mg	30	1 po qd	0

Case 19

I. Dark urine
II. Easy bruising
III. Extreme fatigue

A. I only
B. III only
C. I and II only
D. II and III only
E. I, II, and III

5. What parameters will need to be monitored in this patient to determine safety of methotrexate therapy?

I. Liver function tests
II. Chest x-ray
III. Thyroid-stimulating hormone

A. I only
B. III only
C. I and II only
D. II and III only
E. I, II, and III

6. This patient is receiving folic acid along with methotrexate in order to:

A. permit dosage reduction of methotrexate.
B. enhance the efficacy of methotrexate for treatment of rheumatoid arthritis.
C. hasten the onset of action of methotrexate.
D. reduce adverse effects from methotrexate.
E. prevent teratogenicity from methotrexate.

7. When this patient, who has been taking an NSAID, is started on a DMARD such as methotrexate, she may be counseled that the NSAID should be:

A. continued at the current effective dose.
B. discontinued to avoid excessive toxicity.
C. continued but at lower analgesic doses rather than higher anti-inflammatory doses.
D. continued but at a higher dose.
E. given only on days that the DMARD is not taken.

8. Which of the following medications could be considered an appropriate alternative to methotrexate therapy in this patient?

A. Prednisone
B. Hydroxychloroquine
C. Sulfasalazine
D. Adalimumab
E. Infliximab

9. Which of the following statements is true regarding sulfasalazine?

A. The enteric-coated product causes less nausea than the regular tablets.
B. The enteric-coated tablet should be taken with milk or antacids.
C. Sulfasalazine does not cause myelosuppression.
D. The initial dose is 1000 mg three times a day.
E. Diarrhea is the dose-limiting side effect.

10. Which brand/generic pair is correctly matched?

A. Arava/etanercept
B. Humira/anakinra
C. Plaquenil/hydroxychloroquine
D. Enbrel/infliximab
E. Imuran/sulfasalazine

Fluid, Electrolytes, and Nutrition

Section Editor: Charles W. Jastram

*See all 16 cases for this section on the CD.

Case 20

Patient Name: Jenny Schram
Address: 46 Farragut Terrace
Age: 55   Height: 5' 2"
Sex: F   Race: White
Weight: 119.2 kg
Allergies: NKDA

Chief Complaint

Severe lower abdominal pain, nausea, vomiting, and inability to void urine for 12 hours.

History of Present Illness

JS is a 55-yo female who was in her usual state of health until approximately 48 hours prior to admission, when she started complaining of anorexia, mild abdominal pain, inability to urinate, nausea, and one episode of vomiting.

The patient denies fever, diarrhea, or hematemesis. She denies recent alcohol ingestion and/or NSAID use.

Patient has been anorectic for the past 15 hours with an intake of minimal amounts of clear liquids. Her condition has worsened over the past 8 hours, and she presents to the ED appearing very mottled, tachypneic, tachycardic, with marked abdominal distention and in severe respiratory distress.

Shortly after arrival to the ED and during evaluation, the patient developed a full cardiopulmonary arrest requiring endotracheal intubation with mechanical ventilation; external cardiac massage; multiple electrical shocks; numerous medications including lidocaine, epinephrine, dopamine, and sodium bicarbonate; and massive fluid resuscitation. The patient did respond to the above treatment but remains very critically ill.

Past Medical History

The patient has been hypertensive for 20 years and has had type 2 DM for 10 years.

Social History

Patient denies alcohol or tobacco use.

Family History

Married with two living children (25-yo female and 30-yo male). Children are in excellent health. She has two sisters, both in good health. Both parents are living and in their seventies. Mother has gout and has had multiple CVAs. Father has COPD.

Review of Systems

Negative except as noted previously

Physical Examination

GEN: The patient is a morbidly obese female in critical condition at the time of this exam. She is intubated, sedated, and poorly responsive.

VS: BP 60/30 mmHg, HR 140 bpm, RR 24 rpm, T 96.2°F, Ht 62", Wt 119.2 kg

HEENT: Head normocephalic, pupils dilated and reactive prior to arrest

CHEST: Expands poorly, bilateral ronchi

CV: Sinus tachycardia, no m/g/r

ABD: Markedly distended with tenderness in all quadrants, more tender left side; bowel sounds absent

NEURO: Motor and sensory functions are intact. Cranial nerves are intact. Patient responds to verbal commands, but other parameters of mentation cannot be checked.

Labs and Diagnostic Tests

Sodium 120 mEq/L	Potassium 6.4 mEq/L
Chloride 83 mEq/L	CO_2 content 13 mEq/L
BUN 63 mg/dL	Serum creatinine 5.9 mg/dL
Glucose 1358 mg/dL	Anion gap 24
Amylase 1375 U/L	Lipase 24,040 U/L
Calcium 4.6 mg/dL	Magnesium 1.5 mg/dL
Phosphorus 7.8 mg/dL	Uric acid 11.4 mg/dL
Total protein 6.3 g/dL	Albumin 3.5 gm/dL
Lactate 6.3 mmol/L	WBC 21,000/mm³
Hemoglobin 15 g/dL	Hematocrit 43%
pH 7.14	pO_2 164 mmHg
pCO_2 55 mmHg	

Diagnosis

Primary:

1) Acute pancreatitis

2) Intra-abdominal sepsis with multisystem organ dysfunction

Case 20

Medication Record

(Home medications)

Benazepril 10 mg po qd for 5 years

Hydrochlorothiazide 50 mg po qd for 10 years

Glipizide 5 mg po q am for 3 years

Pharmacist Notes and Other Patient Information

None available

Questions

1. The primary parameter for determining whether JS has acidemia or alkalemia includes:

   I.   Arterial pH
   II. Venous bicarbonate concentration
   III. Arterial carbon dioxide concentration

   A. I only
   B. III only
   C. I and II only
   D. II and III only
   E. I, II, and III

2. The primary parameter for determining whether JS has respiratory acidosis versus respiratory alkalosis includes:

   I.   Plasma hemoglobin
   II. Percentage of oxygen saturation
   III. Arterial carbon dioxide concentration

   A. I only
   B. III only
   C. I and II only
   D. II and III only
   E. I, II, and III

3. The primary parameter for determining whether JS has metabolic acidosis versus metabolic alkalosis includes:

   I.   Arterial carbon dioxide concentration
   II. Plasma hemoglobin
   III. Venous bicarbonate concentration

   A. I only
   B. III only
   C. I and II only
   D. II and III only
   E. I, II, and III

4. What is the anion gap for JS?

   I.   24
   II. Serum sodium concentration minus the sum of the chloride and bicarbonate concentration
   III. Must be derived from the Henderson-Hasselbach equation

   A. I only
   B. III only
   C. I and II only
   D. II and III only
   E. I, II, and III

5. The acid-base imbalance in this case is:

   A. metabolic acidosis.
   B. metabolic alkalosis.
   C. respiratory acidosis.
   D. mixed respiratory and metabolic acidosis.
   E. none; no acid-base imbalance is present.

6. Possible etiologies for the acid-base imbalance in this case includes:

   I.   Hypertension
   II. Pancreatitis
   III. Poorly controlled diabetes mellitus

   A. I only
   B. III only
   C. I and II only
   D. II and III only
   E. I, II, and III

7. What is the drug of choice for treating JS's acid-base imbalance?

   A. Shohl's solution
   B. Hydrochloric acid
   C. Oral sodium bicarbonate
   D. IV sodium bicarbonate
   E. Potassium chloride

8. Which of the following should be considered when counseling JS on sodium bicarbonate tablets?

   I.   Possible milk-alkali syndrome may develop
   II. May take if hypocalcemia exists
   III. Treatment alternative for hypokalemia

   A. I only
   B. III only
   C. I and II only
   D. II and III only
   E. I, II, and III

Case 20

9. JS has been taking an ACEI for 5 years. Which of the following precautions are pertinent to her?

   I. Combination of hypovolemia and diuretics predispose a patient to hypotension
   II. Common side effects are cough, rash, and loss of taste
   III. ACEI can contribute to hypokalemia

   A. I only
   B. III only
   C. I and II only
   D. II and III only
   E. I, II, and III

10. The calculated serum osmolarity for JS is:

    A. 137 mOsm/L.
    B. 237 mOsm/L.
    C. 337 mOsm/L.
    D. 437 mOsm/L.
    E. 637 mOsm/L.

Patient Name: Mike Smith
Address: 1234 Main Street
Age: 48   **Height:** 6' 0"
Sex: M   **Race:** White
Weight: 187 lb
Allergies: NKDA

Chief Complaint

MS is a 48-yo male who comes to the clinic requesting a physical exam for employment. MS is under no apparent distress.

History of Present Illness

Noncontributory

Past Medical History

MS was diagnosed with HTN 5 years ago. At that time, he was started on hydrochlorothiazide 25 mg qd and began following a 3-g low-sodium diet. Last year, enalapril was added to better control his HTN. Since then, his blood pressure has been well controlled, and he is not complaining of peripheral edema, orthostasis, dizziness, or vision changes. He complains of left knee osteoarthritis pain. His doctor told him that on x-ray he has mild joint space narrowing.

Social History

Tobacco use: None

Alcohol use: Drinks 4-5 beers every night

Caffeine use: Drinks 1 cup of coffee daily

Drugs of abuse: Denied

Family History

Father died of MI at age 40

Mother alive and well

Review of Systems

Negative except as noted previously

Medication Record

Physical Examination

GEN: Well-developed, overweight male in NAD

VS: BP 148/92 mmHg, HR 80 bpm, RR 28 rpm, T 37.0°C, Ht 6', Wt 85 kg

HEENT: PERRLA, EOMI, wearing corrective lenses

CHEST: CTA

NEURO: A & O x3

Labs and Diagnostic Tests

Sodium 150 mEq/L	Potassium 4.5 mEq/L
Chloride 100 mEq/L	CO_2 content 24 mEq/L
BUN 10 mg/dL	Serum creatinine 1.2 mg/dL
Glucose 100 mg/dL	Hemoglobin 14.5 g/dL
Hematocrit 42%	Platelets 180/mm^3
WBC 6 x 109/L	

Diagnosis

Primary:

1) Hypertension

2) Osteoarthritis

Secondary:

1) Heart disease (primary prevention)

Pharmacist Notes and Other Patient Information

10/1 Advised patient that Advil should only be used for short-term duration as it can contribute to elevated blood pressure.

2/8 Ingredients in each capsule of Glu-droitin: Glucosamine sulfate 500 mg, chondroitin sulfate 400 mg, manganese ascorbate 76 mg, zinc citrate 1.6 mg, sodium chloride 60 mg, potassium chloride 1 mEq

Date	Rx No	Physician	Drug and Strength	Quantity	Sig	Refills
9/01	100231	Jones	Enalapril 5 mg	30	1 po qd	6
9/01	100232	Jones	HCTZ 25 mg	30	1 po qd	6
9/01			Coenzyme Q 10 30 mg	60	1 po tid	
10/01			Advil 200 mg	60	1 po qid prn pain	
1/02			Advil 200 mg	60	1 po qid prn pain	
2/02			Glu-droitin	60	1 po tid prn pain	

Case 21

Questions

1. MS is taking a combination glucosamine product, Glu-droitin. Which of the following is NOT a likely consequence of glucosamine-containing products?

    A. Nausea
    B. Heartburn
    C. Abdominal pain
    D. Hyperglycemia
    E. Flatulence

2. Which of the following statements regarding glucosamine-containing products is true?

    A. Glucosamine-containing products have a rapid onset of analgesia.
    B. Glucosamine-containing products should not be used with NSAIDs.
    C. On discontinuation of glucosamine-containing products, symptoms of pain return within 1-2 days.
    D. Glucosamine-containing products are not absorbed by the GI tract.
    E. Glucosamine-containing products are not effective for rheumatoid arthritis.

3. Glucosamine-containing products contain many different salt forms. Which of the following glucosamine salts has the best evidence to support its use?

    A. Glucosamine chlorhydrate
    B. Glucosamine sulfate
    C. Glucosamine hydrochloride
    D. Glucosamine hydroiodide
    E. N-acetyl glucosamine

4. Combination glucosamine products often contain added ingredients, vitamins, and minerals. Which of the following ingredients is found in amounts far greater than the U.S. recommended dietary intake (RDI)?

    A. Potassium
    B. Zinc
    C. Manganese
    D. Sodium
    E. Copper

5. MS is using Glu-droitin, which is sold in health food stores and many pharmacies. It is considered a dietary supplement and is regulated by the Dietary Supplement Health and Education Act (DSHEA) of 1994. Which of the following statements regarding DSHEA and dietary supplements is FALSE?

    A. Dietary supplements that make 'structure-function' claims must carry the statement, 'This product has not been evaluated by the Food and Drug Administration.

    This product is not intended to diagnose, treat, cure, or prevent any disease.'
    B. Dietary supplement manufacturers may make 'structure-function' claims without FDA authorization but must base these claims on their review and interpretation of the scientific literature.
    C. A dietary supplement manufacturer wishing to use a 'structure-function' claim on their label must notify the FDA within 30 days after a product is marketed.
    D. The Federal Trade Commission (FTC) is responsible for regulating dietary supplement advertising claims.
    E. Under DSHEA, dietary supplement manufacturers must prove that the dietary supplement is safe before it can be marketed to consumers.

6. MS recently started taking Glu-droitin for his mild to moderate knee osteoarthritis. Which of the following statements regarding glucosamine sulfate or chondroitin sulfate are FALSE?

    A. Glucosamine sulfate has been studied in clinical trials for up to 3 years, although long-term safety data are still needed.
    B. Historical and anecdotal evidence supports long-term safety.
    C. Since osteoarthritis can result in cartilage erosion and breakdown, glucosamine sulfate/chondroitin sulfate are thought to strengthen cartilage and prevent further cartilage breakdown.
    D. Chondroitin sulfate has been shown to inhibit cartilage-destroying enzymes in humans with osteoarthritis.
    E. Starting glucosamine sulfate/chondroitin sulfate therapy in severe end-stage knee osteoarthritis may not result in significant improvements in pain and mobility.

7. Glu-droitin contains chondroitin sulfate. Which of the following statements regarding chondroitin sulfate is FALSE?

    A. Chondroitin sulfate is a repeating sequence of glucosamine sulfate and other aminosugars.
    B. Chondroitin sulfate maintains a large molecular weight (MW 50,000) compared to glucosamine sulfate (MW 179).
    C. Chondroitin sulfate has been shown to improve osteoarthritis pain and disability.
    D. Chondroitin sulfate is dosed 200 mg three times daily.
    E. Chondroitin sulfate prevents cartilage breakdown similar to glucosamine sulfate.

8. Research best supports the use of coenzyme Q 10 for which of the following indications?

    A. Hypercholesterolemia

Case 21

B. Hypertension

C. Heart failure

D. Cardiomyopathy

E. Angina

9. Which of the following statements regarding coenzyme Q 10 is FALSE?

A. Patients who begin HMG-CoA reductase inhibitors have higher than normal endogenous coenzyme Q 10 levels.

B. HMG-CoA is a precursor for coenzyme Q 10 formation.

C. Coenzyme Q 10 is reduced to ubiquinol in the blood, which has antioxidant and membrane stabilizing effects.

D. Clinical trials have supplemented coenzyme Q 10 levels to achieve blood levels >2 µg/mL.

E. The antioxidant activity of coenzyme Q 10 is less than that observed with HMG-CoA reductase inhibitors.

10. Which of the following side effects has NOT been associated with coenzyme Q 10?

A. Gastrointestinal distress

B. Maculopapular rash

C. Thrombocytopenia

D. CNS side effects

E. Agranulocytosis

Patient Name: Samuel Morgan
Address: 2206 Dream Lane
Age: 59   **Height:** 5' 10"
Sex: M   **Race:** Caucasian
Weight: 80 kg
Allergies: NKDA

Chief Complaint

Weakness and dizziness

History of Present Illness

SM is a 59-year-old male who presented to the emergency department (ED) complaining of nausea/vomiting, fever, and shortness of breath x1 day. The patient stated that the onset of symptoms started at 11:30 p.m. the night before with episodes of nausea/vomiting and fever of 103°F. The patient's wife stated that she had to give him almost the whole bottle of Advil to reduce his fever. She further commented that he asked for blankets due to chills. Patient also complained of chest pain that was worse with movement. The patient continued to have weakness and dizziness as well as SOB and was brought to the ED by his wife. SM had a temp of 95.4 °F with low blood pressure and consolidation on chest x-ray. While preparing the patient for TEE, the patient was given midazolam and promethazine; the patient became more short of breath, tachypenic with respiratory wheezes, and was intubated in the ED.

Past Medical History

Hypertension

Social History

Ethanol intake of 6 beers daily, smoked 2 packs/day for 10 years, denies illicit drug abuse

Family History

Brother died from a myocardial infarction at unknown age

Review of Systems

White male appearing his stated age. Intubated, sedated, and paralyzed

Physical Examination

GEN: Intubated, sedated, and paralyzed

VS: BP 75/56-163/94 mmHg; P 103-117 bpm; R 24-18 rpm; T 95-98°F

SKIN: No rash

HEENT: No history of headaches, dysphasia, or odynophagia

LUNGS: Crackles, wheezes, no cough, no hemoptysis

CV: Tachycardia, torsades de pointes, chest pain with movement, diaphoresis, SOB

GI: No history of peptic ulcer disease or digestive disorders prior to episodes of vomiting

GU: No history of dysuria

ABD. Positive bowel signs, no masses

EXT: 2 + pulses

Neuro: Hyperactivity

Labs and Diagnostic Tests

Sodium 144 mEq/L	Potassium 4.4 mEq/L
Chloride 101 mEq/L	CO_2 19 mEq/L
BUN 40 mg/dL	Serum creatinine 4.2 mg/dL
Glucose 78 mg/dL	Calcium 7.4 mg/dL
Magnesium 1.2 mg/dL	Phosphorus 4.5 mg/dL
ALT 55 mg/dL	Total protein 7.1 g/dL
Albumin 1.8 g/dL	WBC 14,000 cell

Blood culture gram positive cocci two out of two bottles

Arterial blood gases: pH 7.15, pO_2 49 mmHg, pCO_2 50 mmHg, HCO_3 16 mmol/L

Diagnosis

Sepsis, acute renal failure, pneumonia

Medication Record

Gatifloxacin 200 mg IV qd

Gentamicin 120 IV mg q24h

Pharmacist Notes and Other Patient Information

No pharmacist notes recorded

Case 22

Questions

1. The acid-base imbalance in this case is:

   A. metabolic acidosis.

   B. metabolic alkalosis.

   C. metabolic acidosis and metabolic alkalosis.

   D. respiratory acidosis, metabolic acidosis, and metabolic alkalosis.

   E. none; no acid-base imbalance is present.

2. The calculated anion gap for the patient in this case is:

   A. 17 mmol/L.

   B. 24 mmol/L.

   C. 31 mmol/L.

   D. 37 mmol/L.

   E. 41 mmol/L.

3. Possible etiologies for the acid-base imbalance in this case are which of the following?

   I. Sepsis

   II. Drug inducement

   III. Renal failure

   A. I only

   B. III only

   C. I and II only

   D. II and III only

   E. I, II, and III

4. The lower serum magnesium concentration in SM can be attributed to:

   I. pancreatic insufficiency.

   II. drug inducement.

   III. alcoholism.

   A. I only

   B. III only

   C. I and II only

   D. II and III only

   E. I, II, and III

5. Drugs that can cause SM's drug-induced hypomagnesemia include:

   I. aminoglycosides.

   II. amphotericin B.

   III. pentamidine.

   A. I only

   B. III only

   C. I and II only

   D. II and III only

   E. I, II, and III

6. Treatment options for SM's hypomagnesemia include:

   I. Administration of IV calcium

   II. Magnesium-containing antacid

   III. Administration of IV $MgSO_4$

   A. I only

   B. III only

   C. I and II only

   D. II and III only

   E. I, II, and III

7. Clinical presentation of SM's hypomagnesemia can include the following:

   I. Neuromuscular hyperactivity

   II. Psychiatric effects

   III. Torsades de pointes

   A. I only

   B. III only

   C. I and II only

   D. II and III only

   E. I, II, and III

8. The causes of nonanion gap metabolic acidosis includes:

   I. early renal failure.

   II. posthypocapnia.

   III. ketoacidosis

   A. I only

   B. III only

   C. I and II only

   D. II and III only

   E. I, II, and III

9. Possible causes for SM's increased anion gap include:

   I. renal failure.

   II. ketoacidosis.

   III. methanol poisoning.

   A. I only

   B. III only

   C. I and II only

   D. II and III only

   E. I, II, and III

10. Which of the following are appropriate mixing of magnesium IV for the patient?

    I. 2 g $MgSO_4$ in 100 mL of 0.9% NaCl

    II. 2 g $MgSO_4$ in 100 mL of dextrose 5%

    III. 2 g $MgSO_4$ in 6 mL of 0.9% NaCl

Case 22

A. I only
B. III only
C. I and II only
D. II and III only
E. I, II, and III

Patient Name: Jack Lieberman
Address: 4520 Warren Street
Age: 73   **Height:** 6' 0"
Sex: M   **Race:** Caucasian
Weight: 207 lb
Allergies: NKDA

Chief Complaint

JL is a 73-yo male who comes to the general medicine clinic (3/1) for his biannual physical with his primary care physician. JL and his son are present, and the son relates that JL has been much more anxious over the last few months, especially when he loses things or is unable to recall the topic of recent conversations. JL's son admits that this occurs infrequently and will likely improve now that he has started treating his father with a variety of natural remedies that he obtained at the health food store. JL and his son also relay that JL is scheduled to have bunion surgery in 2 weeks.

History of Present Illness

JL states that he has been feeling well but his urinary problems are getting worse. He uses the restroom frequently and can never seem to empty his bladder completely. JL has trouble sleeping because of his frequent trips to the bathroom. He states that he started using OTC sleeping tablets 2 months ago in combination with a product that his son purchased for him. When he is unable to fall asleep within a half an hour, he also takes one of his wife's prescription sleeping tablets (i.e., alprazolam, Xanax). While these help him to fall asleep, he complains of some drowsiness throughout the day and occasional bed-wetting. JL is aware that in the last month he has been misplacing items around the house more frequently. He relays an incident in which he became confused and could not find his way to the grocery store after getting off of the local bus. He has some difficulty walking due to the bunion on his left foot as well as mild to moderate pain caused by peripheral vascular disease in his legs.

Past Medical History

JL was diagnosed with type 2 diabetes 6 years ago. He also has a long-standing history (i.e., over 10 years) of HTN and hyperlipidemia. He was diagnosed with mild dementia of the Alzheimer's type 1 year ago. He lives with his wife and is currently able to care for himself. His son lives across the street with his family.

Social History

Tobacco use: Smokes 6-8 cigarettes per day

Alcohol use: Drinks 2 glasses of wine while watching television before bedtime

Family History

Mother died of lung cancer at age 70

Father died of myocardial infarction at age 79

Review of Systems

No obvious symptoms

Physical Examination

GEN: Slightly overweight male, appearing slightly sedated

VS: BP 140/64 mmHg, HR 68 bpm, RR 12 rpm, T 37.5°C, Wt 94 kg, Ht 6' 0', BMI 28.1

HEENT: PERRLA, all other systems normal in appearance

CHEST: CTA

NEURO: A & O x3, decreased deep tendon reflexes, decreased sensation in feet by pin prick

Labs and Diagnostic Tests

Sodium 140 mEq/L	Potassium 4.0 mEq/L
Chloride 100 mEq/L	CO_2 content 24 mEq/L
BUN 17 mg/dL	Serum creatinine 1.6 mg/dL
FBG 210 mg/dL	Hg_{A1c} 8.6%
Hemoglobin 16 g/dL	Hematocrit 44%
Platelets 220,000/mm³	

WBC 4500/mm³ with 60% PMN, 4% bands, 30% lymphocytes, 6% monocytes

T. chol. 190 mg/dL	HDL 32 mg/dL
LDL 170 mg/dL	TG 150 mg/dL
UA NML	PSA 3.6 ng/mL

Digital rectal exam reveals uniform moderate enlargement of the prostate.

Lower abdominal bladder distension consistent with urinary retention.

Diagnosis

Primary:

1. Hypertension
2. Hyperlipidemia
3. Type 2 diabetes mellitus
4. Peripheral vascular disease
5. Mild dementia of the Alzheimer's type

Secondary:

1. Anxiety
2. Insomnia
3. Benign prostatic hypertrophy

Case 23

 Medication Record

Date	Rx No	Physician	Drug and Strength	Quantity	Sig	Refills
1/1	65432	Cohen	Simvastatin 10 mg	100	1 po daily	1
1/1	65431	Cohen	Metformin 750 mg	180	1 po bid	1
1/1	65430	Cohen	Benazepril 10 mg	100	1 po daily	1
1/10			Unisom 50 mg	100	1 hs	

Herbal supplements: These were initiated by the patient's son and revealed to the physician on the date of the last clinic visit

3/1 Patient initiated on supplement on date below:

1/1 Garlic (Kwai) 300 mg powdered enteric coated formulation twice daily

1/1 Ginkgo (Ginkoba) 120 mg twice daily

1/1 Valerian officinalis aqueous extract 400 mg capsule at bedtime

1/20 Kava extract 100 mg 3 times daily

2/1 Panax ginseng (Ginsana) 100 mg twice daily

 ## Pharmacist Notes and Other Patient Information

9/20 Refilled prescription for Mrs. Lieberman's alprazolam early; patient states that her husband occasionally uses her medicine when he can't sleep. Instructed wife to inform husband not to use her medication.

Questions

1. How many of the botanicals that JL is using should be stopped prior to surgery?

    A. one
    B. two
    C. three
    D. four
    E. five

2. In reviewing JL's primary and secondary diagnoses, how many of his conditions could be adversely affected by his use of Panax ginseng?

    A. one
    B. two
    C. three
    D. four
    E. five

3. Assuming that JL is adherent to his medications and supplements and is maintaining a low-cholesterol diet, which of the following would be the best therapeutic recommendation, given his current lipid values?

    A. Increase the dose of simvastatin to 20 mg per day
    B. Add niacin
    C. Increase the dose of garlic to 900 mg per day
    D. Increase the dose of ginkgo to 360 mg per day
    E. Add evening primrose oil

4. In addition to JL's history of mild Alzheimer's disease, what other condition might be improved by the use of ginkgo biloba?

    A. Diabetes
    B. Peripheral vascular disease
    C. Hypertension
    D. Hyperlipidemia
    E. Benign prostatic hypertrophy

5. Which of the following botanicals is INCORRECTLY matched with the source of the plant from which it is derived?

    A. Garlic-bulb of the plant
    B. Ginkgo-leaf of the plant
    C. Ginseng-leaf of the plant
    D. Kava-root of the plant
    E. Valerian-root of the plant

6. Which of the following products should not be used by JL because it could exacerbate both his Alzheimer's disease and his benign prostatic hypertrophy?

    A. Alprazolam
    B. Valerian
    C. Kava
    D. Ginseng
    E. Diphenhydramine

7. JL wishes to initiate a saw palmetto product for his benign prostatic hypertrophy, what type of ingredients should this product be standardized to contain?

    A. 85%-95% fatty acids and sterols
    B. 1.3% alliin or 0.6% allicin
    C. 4%-6% ginsenosides
    D. 0.3% hypericin or 5% hyperforin
    E. 70%-80% silymarin

Case 23

8. Which of the following health education tips would be valuable for you to give JL to reduce his risk of a future cardiac event given his positive family history?

   I. Stop drinking
   II. Stop smoking
   III. Diet, weight loss

   A. I only
   B. III only
   C. I and II only
   D. II and III only
   E. I, II, and III

9. What lab test needs to be monitored in JL if he is going to continue to take kava?

   A. WBC
   B. Platelets
   C. BUN, serum creatinine
   D. PSA
   E. AST, ALT

10. Which of the following are appropriate patient education tips for JL regarding his use of ginkgo biloba?

    I. Look for products that are standardized to 24% flavonoids and 6% terpenes.
    II. There is promising evidence that ginkgo is more effective than placebo in improving cognition in mild Alzheimer's disease when used for 4 to 6 weeks.
    III. Ginkgo is also helpful in improving memory and cognition in healthy seniors who do not have dementia.

    A. I only
    B. III only
    C. I and II only
    D. II and III only
    E. I, II, and III

Blood Disorders

Patient Name: Gary Hanes
Address: 7758 W. Queen Road
Age: 66 **Height:** 5' 9"
Sex: M **Race:** White
Weight: 95.7 kg
Allergies: None

Chief Complaint

GH is a 66-yo man seen in the clinic with a 9-kg weight loss in the last year. He describes getting hungry but finding that food tastes bad and that he loses his appetite when he starts to eat. He has had no vomiting, but he does have occasional abdominal cramps and loose stools. He is feeling more irritable than usual.

History of Present Illness

For the last year GH has been irritable and has had occasional tinnitus. For 5 years he has had one to two "dizzy" spells per week, lasting approximately 15 minutes each.

Past Medical History

GH was diagnosed with hypothyroidism approximately 6 months ago and depression approximately 9 months ago. Osteoarthritis complaints have been ongoing for about 3 months. One year ago he was diagnosed with Hashimoto's thyroiditis.

Social History

Tobacco use: none

Alcohol use: none

Caffeine use: 2 cups of coffee per day

Family History

Father died of CVA at age 55. Mother is alive at age 86 with DM.

Review of Systems

(+) dry skin, (-) glossitis, fatigue daily in the afternoon, (-) headache, (-) paresthesias, (+) pallor, (+) anorexia

Physical Examination

GEN: Obese man in NAD

VS: BP 148/84 mmHg, HR 68 bpm, RR 15 rpm, T 38.5°C, Wt 95.7 kg

HEENT: PERRLA, neck supple no adenopathy, thyroid WNL

CHEST: Clear to A & P

CV: RRR, no murmurs

NEURO: A & O x3

ABD: Liver WNL, no masses, bruits, or tenderness

RECTAL: No masses, guaiac negative

Labs and Diagnostic Tests

Sodium 140 mEq/L	Potassium 3.9 mEq/L
Chloride 107 mEq/L	CO_2 content 28 mEq/L
BUN 21 mg/dL	Serum creatinine 0.9 mg/dL
Glucose 116 mg/dL	TSH 1.56 (IU/mL)
Albumin 4.2 g/dL	MCV 123 fL
Hemoglobin 13.8 g/dL	Hematocrit 39.2%
Platelets 180,000/mm³	Serum iron 80 µg/dL

Blood smear: Hypersegmented polys

RBC (folate): 390 ng/mL   Vitamin B_{12} 53 pg/mL

Schilling test - positive, urinary excretion <5%

Diagnosis

Primary:

1) Pernicious anemia

Secondary:

1) Hypothyroidism - s/p Hashimoto's thyroiditis

2) Depression

3) Osteoarthritis

Pharmacist Notes and Other Patient Information

2/24 Counseled patient on self-administration of B_{12} intramuscular injection and appropriate needle disposal, sharps container provided. Counseled on appropriate storage (protection from light) of B_{12}.

Case 24

Medication Record

Date	Rx No	Physician	Drug and Strength	Quantity	Sig	Refills
3/1	29382	Hind	Cyanocobalamin 1000 μg/mL	10 mL	inject 1 mL monthly IM	1
3/1	29383	Hind	Levothyroxine 0.075 mg	30	1 po daily	3
3/1	29384	Lone	Citalopram 20 mg	30	1 po daily	3
3/1	29385	Dane	Naproxen 250 mg	60	1 po BID prn	1

Questions

1. Which symptoms GH is experiencing might be expected to improve with treatment of B_{12} deficiency?

    I.   Irritability
    II. Anorexia
    III. Pallor

    A. I only
    B. III only
    C. I and II only
    D. II and III only
    E. I, II, and III

2. Laboratory findings present in GH that may be associated with pernicious anemia include:

    I.   decreased MCV.
    II. positive Schilling test.
    III. decreased serum B_{12} levels.

    A. I only
    B. III only
    C. I and II only
    D. II and III only
    E. I, II, and III

3. Drug-induced macrocytic anemia may occur due to vitamin B_{12} malabsorption with:

    I.   colchicine.
    II. neomycin.
    III. para-aminosalicylic acid.

    A. I only
    B. III only
    C. I and II only
    D. II and III only
    E. I, II, and III

4. Vitamin B_{12} therapy produces a response:

    I.   in hemoglobin in a week.
    II. in reticulocytes in a week.
    III. in hematocrit levels in a week.

    A. I only
    B. III only

C. I and II only
D. II and III only
E. I, II, and III

5. Vitamin B_{12} deficiency anemia can result from:

    I.   decreased absorption.
    II. inadequate intake.
    III. decreased homocysteine levels.

    A. I only
    B. III only
    C. I and II only
    D. II and III only
    E. I, II, and III

6. Vitamin B_{12} is needed for:

    I.   DNA synthesis.
    II. inflammatory cytokines such as interleukin-1.
    III. oxygen carrying capacity.

    A. I only
    B. III only
    C. I and II only
    D. II and III only
    E. I, II, and III

7. Commercially available cyanocobalamin:

    I.   must be protected from light.
    II. injections are clear, pink to red solutions.
    III. must be reconstituted and primed prior to use.

    A. I only
    B. III only
    C. I and II only
    D. II and III only
    E. I, II, and III

8. In a patient that suspects he (she) may be anemic:

    A. folic acid should be initiated as soon as possible.
    B. erythropoieten should be initiated as soon as possible.
    C. multivitamins should be initiated as soon as possible.
    D. folic acid should be used cautiously.
    E. iron should be initiated as soon as possible.

Case 24

9. Pernicious anemia requires treatment:

   I. with oral vitamin B_{12} 1000 μg if patient refuses parenteral doses.
   II. with oral vitamin B_{12} 50 μg and intrinsic factor.
   III. with intradermal treatment of vitamin B_{12} and intrinsic factor.

   A. I only
   B. III only
   C. I and II only
   D. II and III only
   E. I, II, and III

10. In most cases vitamin B_{12} therapy is administered:

   A. until symptoms of deficiency improve.
   B. for a lifetime.
   C. concurrently with folic acid therapy.
   D. orally and subcutaneously concurrently.
   E. only after results of a Schilling test are obtained.

Patient Name: Earlene Franklin
Address: 1255 South 44th Street
Age: 76   **Height:** 5' 4"
Sex: F   **Race:** African American
Weight: 170 lb
Allergies: Penicillin (rash)

Chief Complaint

EF is a 76-yo African American female that presented to the ED with calf tenderness.

History of Present Illness

EF has complaint of left lower leg swelling with localized pain and tenderness. She complains of difficulty in ambulation. Patient was admitted to the hospital for diagnostic testing to confirm initial diagnosis of a DVT. Patient's venography testing confirmed the development of a DVT of the left lower leg. Patient was started on enoxaparin 80 mg SQ bid and warfarin 10 mg po qd. Patient was discharged home.

Past Medical History

EF was diagnosed with HTN and type 2 DM approximately 20 years ago. Patient diagnosed with Alzheimer's disease 10 years ago. Patient diagnosed with open angle glaucoma 5 years ago.

Social History

Tobacco use: none

Alcohol use: none

Caffeine use: 2 cups of coffee per day

Supportive son, husband hard of hearing, home is cluttered and soiled, family overwhelmed, dependent for meal prep and shopping.

Family History

Father's history unobtainable. Patient lost contact years ago. Mother died of CVA at age 74.

Review of Systems

Negative except as noted previously

Physical Examination

GEN: Well nourished, poor endurance, psychosocial behavior appropriate.

VS: BP 160/70 mmHg, HR 70 bpm, RR 20 rpm, T 98°F oral, Ht 5'4" Wt 170 lb

HEENT: Assessed/no problems noted

CHEST: Symmetrical, lung sounds clear

CV: Regular pulse, no angina

NEURO: Oriented to person, place, and time; situation judgment impaired, forgetful, naps often

ABD: No distention, no ascites, no tenderness, bowel sounds present

GU: Voids incontinent at times, urine clear yellow per patient, no blood

ENDO: Denies numbness or tingling

Labs and Diagnostic Tests

Sodium 142 mEq/L	Potassium 3.6 mEq/L
Chloride 109 mEq/L	CO_2 content 27 mEq/L
BUN 12 mg/dL	Serum creatinine 1.0 mg/dL
Glucose 101 mg/dL	PT 18
INR 1.36	Hemoglobin 11.1 g/dL
Hematocrit 34.2%	Platelets 173,000/mm³
WBC 4.6 k/mm³	RBC 3.98 m/mm³

Diagnosis

Primary:

1) Deep vein thrombosis

Secondary:

1) Hypertension uncontrolled

2) Diabetes mellitus not assessed

3) Alzheimer's disease, significant impairment, poor self-care

4) Open angle glaucoma not assessed

5) Anemia, unknown etiology

Pharmacist Notes and Other Patient Information

None

Case 25

Medication Record

Date	Rx No	Physician	Drug and Strength	Quantity	Sig	Refills
9/4	43682	Granger	Glipizide 2.5 mg	90	1 po qd	3
9/4	43683	Granger	Benazepril 20 mg	90	1 po qd	3
9/4	43684	Upperstrom	Risperidone 0.5 mg	90	1 po qd	3
9/4	43685	Upperstrom	Donepezil 10 mg	90	1 po hs	3
9/4	43686	Auten	Brimonidine tart 0.2%	10 mL	1 gtt OU qd	3
9/4			Aspirin E.C. 325 mg		1 po qd	
9/4	04101	Ewald	Enoxaparin 80 mg	0.8	1 SQ bid	0
9/4	43687	Ewald	Warfarin 5 mg	30	2 po qd	0

Questions

1. Which LMWH(s) are approved for use for the treatment of DVT?

    I.   Dalteparin
    II. Enoxaparin
    III. Tinzaparin

    A. I only
    B. III only
    C. I and II only
    D. II and III only
    E. I, II, and III

2. Which of the following are approved dosage regimens of enoxaparin for the treatment of DVT in the outpatient setting:

    I.   1.0 mg/kg q 24 h
    II. 1.0 mg/kg q 12 h
    III. 1.5 mg/kg q 24 h

    A. I only
    B. III only
    C. I and II only
    D. II and III only
    E. I, II, and III

3. The risk factors for the development of venous thromboembolism in the outpatient setting include all the following EXCEPT:

    A. oral contraceptives and hormone replacement therapy.
    B. extended airline flights.
    C. age >65.
    D. COPD.
    E. any type of surgery or leg trauma.

4. The proper instruction to patient and family on disposal of used enoxaparin syringes and needles is:

    A. to dispose directly into the regular trash.
    B. to administer dose, recap syringe, and dispose directly into the regular trash.
    C. to dispose directly into puncture-resistant container, place bleach into container, seal bag, and place in trash.
    D. to dispose directly into a coffee can, milk jug, or other puncture-resistant container. Then return to prescribing physician's office.
    E. to dispose directly into a coffee can, milk jug, or other puncture-resistant container. Then place in trash.

5. Risk factors for major bleeding include all the following EXCEPT:

    A. renal failure.
    B. heart failure.
    C. Diabetes mellitus.
    D. concomitant use of aspirin.
    E. age less than 70.

6. Which of the following statements is NOT true regarding enoxaparin in the treatment of DVT?

    A. It has ease in dosing and administration and decreased requirement for hospitalization
    B. Its anticoagulant response is predictable
    C. Monitoring for signs and symptoms of bleeding is necessary
    D. Unfractionated heparin is an unacceptable alternative if heparin-induced thrombocytopenia develops
    E. It increases the need for laboratory monitoring

7. The trade name for enoxaparin is:

    A. Plavix
    B. Enoxacin
    C. Fragmin
    D. Lovenox
    E. Arixtra

8. Signs of bleeding include all the following EXCEPT:

    A. rust-colored urine.
    B. black, tarry stools.
    C. unusual pain or swelling.
    D. hypophonia.
    E. fever and chills lasting more than 2 days.

Case 25

9. The goal INR for the treatment of deep venous thrombus without pulmonary embolism is:

    A. a range of 1.0-2.0 with a goal of 1.5.
    B. a range of 1.5-2.5 with a goal of 2.0.
    C. a range of 2.0-3.0 with a goal of 2.5.
    D. a range of 2.5-3.5 with a goal of 3.0.
    E. none; no monitoring of INR required.

10. What test should be performed in the next 1-2 days in this patient?

    A. Venous ultrasound
    B. Anti-Xa levels
    C. PTT
    D. INR
    E. Angioplasty

Endocrine and Metabolic Disorders

Section Editor: Dannielle C. O'Donnell

*See all 10 cases for this section on the CD.

Patient Name: Shirley Wells
Address: 109 Red Berry Drive
Age: 57 **Height:** 5' 5"
Sex: F **Race:** African American
Weight: 218 lb
Allergies: NKDA

Chief Complaint

SW is an obese 57-year-old African American female presenting to her primary care clinic for follow-up of her type 2 diabetes mellitus. She complains of deep burning leg pain.

History of Present Illness

SW was diagnosed with diabetes approximately 8 years ago. For the past year her blood glucose control has steadily worsened. She has been managed on maximum doses of glyburide and metformin (Glucovance) for the past 6 months. Her self-reported home glucose readings are consistently above 200 mg/dL each morning and 2 hours after eating her evening meal. She denies any episodes of hypoglycemia. She describes burning pain below both knees that worsens at night. The pain is somewhat improved, but is not completely relieved despite compliance with her current therapy.

Past Medical History

Hypertension x9 years

Hyperlipidemia x7 years on simvastatin

Obesity (BMI 36.5)

Diabetic polyneuropathy in her legs distally

Depression

Total hysterectomy 15 years ago

Social History

She works on a night shift as an aid. She denies any tobacco use or excessive alcohol intake. For exercise she tries to swim or walk 30 minutes daily; however, she is inconsistent with her exercise program. Her diet has improved over the past month. She has decreased her daily calories and has begun to count her carbohydrate intake. She has limited finances for medications and office visits.

Family History

Her father died of an acute myocardial infarction at age 53. Her mother, who had type 2 diabetes, recently died in a nursing home at age 85. Of her six brothers, two have type 2 diabetes. Her sister, who is 67 years old, has coronary artery disease and is

s/p MI. SW's daughter is 30 years old and has had type 1 diabetes since she was a teenager.

Review of Systems

Remarkable for fatigue, polyuria, nocturia x3, and polydipsia. She denies any visual changes, slurred speech, or unilateral extremity weakness. She denies chest pain with exertion, shortness of breath, or palpitations. She denies any signs or symptoms of infection and she reports that she checks her feet daily. She does report increased leg pain with prolonged walking.

Physical Examination

GEN: Alert and oriented obese female in NAD; flat affect

VS: 142/88 mmHg (R arm sitting, lg cuff), 90 bpm, T 98.0°F, RR 12 rpm. Wt 218 lb, Ht 65 inches (BMI 36.5)

HEENT: PERRLA; optic fundi are clear, the thyroid is not enlarged

CHEST: Clear to auscultation bilaterally

CV: RRR; there are no murmurs or other adventitial sounds

EXT: No edema, normal hair distribution, warm to the touch; peripheral pulses 2+ and symmetric. Feet: without calluses, sores, or ulcers. Hammer toe on the second digit of the left foot. Monofilament shows loss of protective sensation on the plantar portions of both feet.

Labs and Diagnostic Tests

Random office glucose 239 mg/dL 2 hours after eating

Urine dipstick (-) protein, glucose, nitrates, leukocytes

(Fasting labs obtained 2 weeks prior to this visit.)

Sodium 139 mEq/L	Potassium 5.1 mEq/L
Chloride 106 mEq/L	CO_2 content 28 mEq/L
Serum creatinine 1.2 mg/dL (stable)	
Bun 19 mg/dL	Glucose 234 mg/dL
Total cholesterol 167 mg/dL	HDL-C 32 mg/dL
Triglycerides 234 mg/dL	LDL-C 88 mg/dL

LFTs: wnl; TSH: wnl

Hgb_{A1c}: 10.6% (9.4% 6 months prior), urine microalbuminuria 20 µg/mg of creatinine

Case 26

Medication Record

Date	Rx No	Physician	Drug and Strength	Quantity	Sig	Refills
4/1	289	Bell	Glucovance 5/500 mg	120	2 po qAM and qPM	3
4/1	290	Bell	Prinzide 20/12.5	60	2 po qAM	3
4/1	291	Bell	Ibuprofen 600 mg	120	1 po q6h prn	3
4/1	292	Bell	Neurontin 300 mg	360	3 qid	3
4/1	293	Bell	Zocor 20 mg	30	1 po qHS	3
4/1	294	Bell	Desipramine 75 mg	30	1 po qHS	3

Diagnosis

Primary:

Type 2 diabetes mellitus with microvascular complications of diabetic neuropathy

Pharmacist Notes and Other Patient Information

She often receives monthly samples of Prinzide, glucovance, Neurontin and simvastatin because she is unable to afford her insurance copayments.

Questions

1. Which of the following are contraindications for the use of metformin in this patient?

   I.   Elevated serum creatinine and microalbuminuria
   II. Increased risk for developing congestive heart failure
   III. SW does not have any contraindications

   A. I only
   B. III only
   C. I and II only
   D. II and III only
   E. I, II, and III

2. Metformin can cause the rare but very serious side effect of lactic acidosis with inadequate renal function. Which of the following best describes the symptoms of lactic acidosis SW should be warned of?

   A. Rapid onset of nausea, vomiting, and diarrhea
   B. Rapid onset of chills, fever, and malaise
   C. Rapid onset of nausea, vomiting, and shortness of breath
   D. Slow onset of malaise, respiratory distress, and abdominal symptoms
   E. Slow onset of chills, fever, and abdominal distress

3. SW's Hgb$_{A1c}$, fasting blood glucose (BG), and 2-hour postprandial readings are not at goal. Which of the following statements best describes the benefits of a meglitinide (i.e., Repaglinide) or an alpha-glucosidase inhibitor (i.e., acarbose) for this patient?

   A. Adding a meglitinide will help to significantly lower her fasting BG.
   B. Adding a meglitinide should help to further lower her post-prandial BG.
   C. Substituting a meglitinide for the metformin will lower the postprandial BG.
   D. Adding an alpha-glucosidase inhibitor will help to significantly lower the fasting BG.
   E. A meglitinide or an alpha-glucosidase inhibitor will have minimal benefits for this patient.

4. Her primary care provider is concerned about her persistent hyperglycemia and inquires about the addition of a thiazolidinedione. Which of the following best describes the potential side effects of these agents?

   I.   Weight gain
   II. Peripheral edema
   III. Anemia

   A. I only
   B. III only
   C. I and II only
   D. II and III only
   E. I, II, and III

5. If the addition of insulin were considered for SW, which of the following regimens would be the most appropriate initial step to control her fasting blood glucose and provide insulin coverage through the rest of the day?

   A. Add lispro insulin before each meal
   B. Add regular insulin before each meal
   C. Add 70/30 insulin before bedtime
   D. Add NPH insulin at bedtime
   E. Add insulin glargine (Lantus) at bedtime

Case 26

6. It is decided to add insulin to SW's diabetic regimen. Which of the following statements describes appropriate action if the patient experiences symptoms of hypoglycemia?

    I. Drink a half glass of juice, one glass of milk, or a regular soft drink.

    II. Check your BG within 15 minutes of the treatment.

    III. Give yourself an injection of glucagon.

    A. I only

    B. III only

    C. I and II only

    D. II and III only

    E. I, II, and III

7. SW is concerned about her high risk for developing cardiovascular disease. She requests to be placed on hormone replacement therapy (HRT). Which of the following statements are true regarding HRT for SW?

    I. Estrogen replacement therapy increases the HDL-C

    II. Estrogen therapy may increase triglycerides and must be cautiously used in diabetic patients

    III. Estrogen therapy may increase the risk for stroke

    A. I only

    B. III only

    C. I and II only

    D. II and III only

    E. I, II, and III

8. Patient education for proper foot care would include which of the following?

    I. Keep your feet clean and dry.

    II. Wear shoes both indoors and outdoors.

    III. Inspect both feet daily for sores, calluses, redness, or swelling.

    A. I only

    B. III only

    C. I and II only

    D. II and III only

    E. I, II, and III

9. If this patient were taking 30 units of 70/30 insulin, which of the following statements correctly describes the amount of regular and NPH insulin in this regimen?

    A. 21 units of regular and 9 units of NPH insulin

    B. 9 units of regular and 21 units of NPH insulin

    C. 14 units of regular and 16 units of NPH insulin

    D. 14 units of NPH and 16 units of regular insulin

    E. 15 units of regular and 15 units of NPH insulin

10. SW complains of uncontrolled pain related to her diabetic neuropathy. She has been very compliant with her current therapy of ibuprofen 600 mg qid, Neurontin 900 mg tid, and desipramine 75 mg qhs. Which of the following statements describes the most appropriate action to significantly help decrease SW's pain?

    A. Increase her ibuprofen to 800 mg four times a day.

    B. Increase her gabapentin to 1200 mg four times a day.

    C. Change her desipramine to a serotonin reuptake inhibitor.

    D. Soak her feet and legs in hot water several times a day.

    E. Improve her blood glucose control.

Patient Name: John Davis
Address: 203 Smith Avenue
Age: 50   **Height:** 5' 10"
Sex: M   **Race:** Caucasian
Weight: 240 lb
Allergies: NKDA

Chief Complaint

Dyslipidemia

History of Present Illness

The patient first learned of his dyslipidemia 1 year ago when he was diagnosed with type 2 diabetes. He has been trying to manage it with a low-saturated-fat, low-cholesterol diet. Because his lipids remain elevated, he was referred to the Cardiovascular Risk Reduction Clinic.

Past Medical History

The patient has hypertension diagnosed 10 years ago; type 2 diabetes diagnosed 1 year ago; and abdominal aortic aneurysm status post repair 6 months ago.

Social History

The patient is married and has two adult children who no longer live with him. He is a small-business owner. He has smoked one pack of cigarettes per day for the past 30 years. He drinks alcohol socially and drinks two cups of coffee per day. He follows a low-fat, low-cholesterol, diabetic diet but does not exercise.

Family History

His father died at the age of 67 years after an MI. His mother is 74 and has type 2 diabetes. He has one brother who is 47 years of age who has hypertension. He does not know of any family history of high cholesterol or triglycerides.

Review of Systems

Negative for cardiovascular symptoms and symptoms of hyperglycemia and hypoglycemia

Medication Record

Physical Examination

GEN: Obese male in no apparent distress

VS: BP 138/76, Ht 5'10", Wt 240 lb, HR 76 bpm, RR 15 rpm, T 98.6° F

HEENT: EOMI, PERRLA, funduscopic exam negative for signs of diabetic retinopathy

NECK: No JVD, thyromegaly, or bruits

CHEST: Lungs: clear to auscultation

CV: RRR, no murmurs, rubs, or gallops

ABD: Obese with a waist circumference of 42 inches; soft and nontender without masses, organomegaly, or bruits

EXT: No clubbing, cyanosis, or edema; distal peripheral pulses are normal

Labs and Diagnostic Tests

Fasting:

Sodium 145 mEq/L	Potassium 4.0 mEq/L
Chloride 110 mEq/L	CO_2 26 mEq/L
BUN 10 mg/dL	Serum creatinine 0.8 mg/dL
Total cholesterol 208 mg/dL	HDL-C 29 mg/dL
Triglycerides 305 mg/dL	LDL-C 118 mg/dL
ALT 16 mg/dL	Glucose 144 mg/dL
TSH 1.6	HbA_{1c} 7.8%
Uric acid 9 mg/dL	

Diagnosis

Primary diagnoses:
1) Type IIb dyslipidemia
2) Type 2 diabetes
3) Hypertension
4) Abdominal aortic aneurism s/p repair

Pharmacist Notes and Other Patient Information

None available

Date	Rx No	Physician	Drug and Strength	Quantity	Sig	Refills
4/20	515	Smith	Lisinopril 40 mg	30	1 po qd	3
4/20			Aspirin 325 mg	100	1 po qd prn	

Case 27

Questions

1. What factors place this patient in the high risk category of CHD risk equivalent?

   I. His diagnosis of diabetes
   II. His history of abdominal aortic aneurysm
   III. His diagnosis of hypertension

   A. I only
   B. III only
   C. I and II only
   D. II and III only
   E. I, II, and III

2. Based on this patient's high risk status, what are his lipid goals?

   A. LDL-C <160 mg/dL, TG <150 mg/dL, non-HDL-C <130 mg/dL
   B. LDL-C <100 mg/dL, TG <200 mg/dL, non-HDL-C <130 mg/dL
   C. LDL-C <130 mg/dL, TG <200 mg/dL, non-HDL-C <160 mg/dL
   D. LDL-C <100 mg/dL, TG <150 mg/dL, non-HDL-C <160 mg/dL
   E. LDL-C <100 mg/dL, TG <150 mg/dL, non-HDL-C <130 mg/dL

3. JD presents to the Cardiovascular Risk Reduction Clinic for risk factor management. This clinic manages lipids as well as other cardiovascular risk factors. What nondrug therapy would you recommend to JD to help improve his lipids?

   I. Encourage the use of dietary plant stanols/sterols.
   II. Stop smoking.
   III. Initiate an aerobic exercise program.

   A. I only
   B. III only
   C. I and II only
   D. II and III only
   E. I, II, and III

4. Based on this patient's cardiovascular risk factors and secondary causes of dyslipidemia, which of the following options would be the most appropriate initial treatment recommendation to make in a Cardiovascular Risk Reduction clinic?

   A. Optimize therapeutic lifestyle changes (TLC). Do not add lipid drug therapy at this time.
   B. Optimize TLC and initiate metformin concurrently to optimize diabetes control.
   C. Optimize TLC and initiate atorvastatin 10 mg daily concurrently.
   D. Optimize TLC and initiate metformin and atorvastatin 10 mg daily concurrently.
   E. Optimize TLC and initiate metformin and micronized fenofibrate 200 mg daily concurrently.

5. The patient returns for a follow-up visit 3 months after his initial visit and he has implemented all the changes you recommended. His fasting labs are as follows: glucose 91 mg/dL, HbA$_{1c}$ 6.4%, total cholesterol 198 mg/dL, HDL-C 30 mg/dL, TG 273 mg/dL, LDL-C 113 mg/dL. What percent reduction does this patient need to lower LDL-C to approximately 90 mg/dL?

   A. 18%
   B. 20%
   C. 24%
   D. 26%
   E. 31%

6. The patient has a relative contraindication to which of the following medications?

   I. Pravastatin
   II. Niacin
   III. Colestipol

   A. I only
   B. III only
   C. I and II only
   D. II and III only
   E. I, II, and III

7. The patient is initiated on atorvastatin 10 mg daily. Twelve weeks later, he is without any symptoms of side effects and his fasting lab results are as follows: TC 149 mg/dL, TG 227 mg/dL, HDL-C 32 mg/dL, LDL-C 72 mg/dL and AST 20 mg/dL. Based on these results, what are your treatment recommendations?

   A. Stop atorvastatin due to the increase in AST indicating liver toxicity.
   B. Make no changes. All lipids are at goal and AST is within normal limits.
   C. Calculate non-HDL-C level to aid in further treatment decisions.
   D. Increase atorvastatin to 20 mg daily because not all lipids are at goal.
   E. Calculate percent reduction in TG level needed to aid in further treatment decisions.

8. Based on the lab results reported in Question 7, what is this patient's non-HDL-C level?

   A. 40 mg/dL
   B. 117 mg/dL
   C. 130 mg/dL
   D. 160 mg/dL
   E. 190 mg/dL

Case 27

9. This patient is at his goal for LDL-C and non-HDL-C levels but not TG and HDL-C. Further attempts to maximize TLC have been made since initiating atorvastatin yet his lipids remain essentially unchanged. What medication change would likely achieve the greatest reduction in TG while maintaining the same or greater amount of LDL-C reduction?

    A. Increasing atorvastatin to 20 mg daily
    B. Changing to simvastatin 10 mg daily
    C. Adding Niaspan, gradually titrated to 1000 mg at bedtime
    D. Adding fenofibrate 145 mg daily
    E. Adding ezetimibe 10 mg daily

10. This patient has a medical condition known as the metabolic syndrome. Which of the following statements about the metabolic syndrome is/are true?

    I.   This patient exhibits only three of the five risk determinants of the metabolic syndrome.
    II. First-line therapy for the lipid and nonlipid risk factors associated with the metabolic syndrome includes weight reduction and increased physical activity.
    III. Therapies directed against the lipid and nonlipid risk factors of the metabolic syndrome will reduce CHD risk.

    A. I only
    B. III only
    C. I and II only
    D. II and III only
    E. I, II, and III

Case 28

Patient Name: Jennifer Hertz
Address: 271 Painless Lane
Age: 38   Height: 5' 3"
Sex: F   Race: Caucasian
Weight: 200 lb
Allergies: NKDA

Chief Complaint

JH's primary care physician referred her to the weight management clinic after initiating sibutramine 10 mg qd 1 month ago. This is her first visit to the clinic, to evaluate the efficacy and safety of the therapy.

History of Present Illness

JH reports that her weight has risen dramatically since the birth of her second child 5 years ago, and she is now finding it increasingly difficult to get around without becoming breathless. JH reports a 30-lb weight gain since her first pregnancy. She was worried that if she continued to gain weight, she would not be able to be as active. JH states that she already can feel the increased weight in her hips and knees. Because of the knee pain, she had reduced her walking significantly. She takes Tylenol prn for her knee pain. She denies chest pain, SOB at rest, leg edema, swelling or redness of her knees, palpitations, dry mouth, constipation, insomnia, or agitation. She also denies binge eating or purgative behaviors. She reports a 5-lb weight loss since started on sibutramine.

Past Medical History

No previous surgeries. No known allergies. Dyslipidemia x3 years.

Social History

JH is 38 yo, the mother of two children, and has been married for 10 years. She is self-employed as a part-time web site designer. She denies smoking and drinks alcohol occasionally at social functions.

Family History

Patient reports that her parents and siblings are overweight. They are alive and well. No family history of CHD or cancer. Her older brother and her father also have elevated cholesterol. Her older brother was diagnosed with type 2 diabetes within the past year.

Review of Systems

As reported in History of Present Illness.

Physical Examination

GEN: Obese female in NAD

VS: BP 130/80 (increased from primary care clinic visit last month: 127/70), Wt 200 lb, Ht 63 inches, BMI 36 kg/m^2, waist circumference 43 inches, HR 90, T 98°, RR 16

HEENT: PERRLA, mucous membrane moist, teeth normal

NECK: No lymphadenopathy, no palpable thyroid, no JVD

LUNGS: Clear to auscultation bilaterally

CV: Normal S_1, S_2, no murmur, RRR, PMI not displaced

ABD: Bowel sounds normal, no hepatomegaly, bruits, no guarding, no rebound

EXT: Unremarkable

Labs and Diagnostic Tests

Glucose 118 mg/dL	TSH 1.3
Total cholesterol 185 mg/dL	LDL 115 mg/dL
HDL 40 mg/dL	Triglycerides 150 mg/dL
Sodium 145 mEq/L	Potassium 4.0 mEq/L
Chloride 109 mEq/L	BUN/Cr (mg/dL) 11/0.8
ALT/AST (mg/dL): 11/14	

Diagnosis

Primary: Obesity and dyslipidemia

Pharmacist Notes and Other Patient Information

Weight/Diet/Activity History

Patient reports that she has tried the Weight Watchers diet, the Susanne Sommers diet, the Cabbage Soup diet, and the American Heart Diet, but was unable to successfully lose weight (and gained more after discontinuing). She has tried OTC pills, including "Herbal Phen/Fen," but they gave her palpitations. JH is the one responsible for preparing meals at home. She does not rate herself as a good cook. She attempted some of the Weight Watchers recipes but found that her family did not enjoy them, and most of the meal ended up wasted. She reports eating/snacking a lot while working at her computer. She recognizes that she has difficulty controlling her hunger and portion sizes. She denies any regular physical activity plan. She reports following a low-fat, low-calorie diet since she started her new medication and that the medication has helped her control her appetite and portion size.

Case 28

Medication Record

Date	Rx No	Physician	Drug and Strength	Quantity	Sig	Refills
4/02	122	Beet	Pravastatin 20 mg	30	1 po qhs	6
4/02	123	Beet	Tylenol 650 mg	120	1 po qid prn	3
7/02	124	Beet	Sibutramine 10 mg	30	1 po qd	1

Questions

1. Which of the following statements best defines obesity and/or its impact?

   A. A waist circumference greater than 35 inches (88 cm) in women and 40 inches (102 cm) in men is not considered an independent risk factor for type 2 diabetes and cardiovascular disease.

   B. Obesity is defined as a body mass index (BMI) ≥ 30 kg/m², overweight is defined as a body mass index (BMI) 25 to 29.9 kg/m², and desirable weight is a body mass index (BMI) 18.5 to 25 kg/m²

   C. Patients must be 50 lb over ideal body weight (estimated from height and bone structure) to meet the criteria for obesity.

   D. Obesity is not associated with an increased risk for diabetes.

   E. No well-defined height and weight criteria currently exist to define obese patients.

2. Sibutramine should not be taken by individuals with the following conditions EXCEPT those:

   A. already on a monoamide oxidase inhibitor.

   B. suffering from anorexia nervosa.

   C. with uncontrolled high blood pressure.

   D. already using other centrally acting appetite suppressants.

   E. using a beta blocker for blood pressure control

3. Per the NHLBI guidelines, what is considered a reasonable target weight loss at 6 to 9 months?

   A. Reach normal weight

   B. 20% of initial body weight

   C. 15% of initial body weight

   D. 10% of initial body weight

   E. 2% of initial body weight

4. Which of the following obesity treatment approaches is recommended by the American Pharmaceutical Association?

   A. Pharmacotherapy is indicated for all individuals with a BMI >25 kg/m²

   B. Pharmacotherapy should be restricted to overweight individuals (BMI ≥ 25 kg/m²) with comorbidities

   C. Pharmacotherapy combined with low-fat, low calorie diet, increased physical activity, and behavioral therapy is an option in subjects with a BMI ≥ 27 kg/m² and existing comorbidities

   D. Gastric bypass is recommended in all obese individuals (BMI >30 kg/m²)

   E. Herbal weight loss formulas are recommended for overweight subjects who were unable to follow a diet and exercise plan

5. Compared with placebo, sibutramine given to obese adults for six months and combined with a hypocaloric diet is associated with all of the following outcomes EXCEPT:

   A. greater weight loss.

   B. lower blood pressure.

   C. higher incidence of headache.

   D. higher incidence of constipation.

   E. higher incidence of insomnia.

6. Which of the following statements correctly identifies the patient's response to therapy and most appropriate next steps?

   A. JH has not maximized her weight loss potential at 10 mg per day of sibutramine. Sibutramine should be increased to 15 mg qd for better weight loss results.

   B. JH successfully lost more than 4.4 lb in the first 4 weeks and would be considered a responder. No need for further follow-up. Reappoint to clinic in 1 year.

   C. JH had a significant increase in diastolic blood pressure; therefore, sibutramine should be discontinued. JH should be considered for phentermine or orlistat drug therapy.

   D. JH successfully lost more than 4.4 lb in the first 4 weeks and is considered a responder. However, she should be monitored closely for a potential increase in blood pressure secondary to sibutramine.

   E. JH failed to achieve significant weight loss in the first 4 weeks and is unlikely to respond even with an increase in dosage.

7. One week after her visit to your pharmacy, JH presents with a new prescription obtained in the emergency room for an analgesic for her broken toe: Demerol 25mg po q6h as needed for pain.

Case 28

I. You dispense Demerol and make sure to educate JH not to mix with alcohol and how it may make her drowsy.

II. You call the ER physician to change the prescription to a fentanyl patch. You explain to JH how fentanyl is more potent and the patch makes it so much easier.

III. You call the ER physician to change the prescription to acetaminophen with codeine. You explain to JH the potential risk for serotonin syndrome if combining meperidine and sibutramine.

A. I only
B. III only
C. I and II only
D. II and III only
E. I, II, and III

8. Which of the following medications may cause weight gain?

A. Pravastatin
B. Topiramate
C. Metformin
D. Bupropion
E. Rosiglitazone

9. Which of the following statements is true.

A. Chromium picolinate has been shown to induce long term weight loss in randomized controlled trials. Chromium picolinate does not interact with sibutramine and could be used in combination.

B. Ephedra containing weight loss products have been shown to be effective and safe.

C. A cold syrup like Robitussin DM 2 teaspoons bid to diminish dry cough is not a safe combination with sibutramine.

D. Sibutramine should be taken 15 minutes before meals for a better appetite suppressant effect.

E. Once weight loss is achieved, pharmacotherapy should be discontinued.

10. Which of the following statements best describes the mechanism of action of sibutramine?

A. Sibutramine increases release of norepinephrine and serotonin similarly to phentermine and fenfluramine.

B. Sibutramine increases levels of norepinephrine, serotonin and dopamine by interfering with neurotransmitter reuptake.

C. Sibutramine is an appetite suppressant and decreases neuropeptide Y levels.

D. Sibutramine stimulates cholecystokinin gut release which results in increased satiety signals to the brain.

E. Sibutramine decreases CNS serotonin and norepinephrine levels.

Patient Name: Karin Jones
Address: 14 Piersport Way
Age: 57 **Height:** 5' 2"
Sex: F **Race:** Caucasian
Weight: 175 lb
Allergies: NKDA

Chief Complaint

KJ is a 57-yo female seen by her PCP for evaluation of persistent complaints of hair loss, fatigue, depression, constipation, and weight gain. She feels "slow" and is concerned about her heart "not beating normally." She is taking a daily multi-vitamin with iron, but feels like her symptoms are only getting worse.

History of Present Illness

KJ first noted symptoms of fatigue, weight gain, and constipation 3 months ago. At that time, KJ's sister suggested she take a multivitamin with iron. KJ states she has not missed one day of taking this vitamin.

KJ feels very discouraged because she has tried a low-calorie diet and has started exercising, but reports a 20-pound weight gain over the past 2-3 months.

She also is concerned that her temperature is "just not right." She wears heavy sweaters and sits by a floor heater at work, while everyone else is wearing summer-like clothes.

KJ complains of constipation and bloating, and she is now using laxatives every other day.

She is here today because she desperately wants to find out what could be causing all these symptoms.

Past Medical History

KJ's history is remarkable for angina, acid reflux, depression, and hypercholesterolemia. Her angina was discovered 3 years ago and is only brought on by exertion, especially exercise. She takes nitroglycerin before exercise, but lately she has not needed any during her exercise. KJ also takes aspirin and bisoprolol for angina. KJ self-diagnosed herself with acid reflux and takes over-the-counter antacids before meals.

Depression was diagnosed after the birth of her fourth child and she was started on a fluoxetine and has now stabilized.

Hypercholesterolemia (e.g., elevated total cholesterol of 260 mg/dL and low-density cholesterol [LDL] of 190 mg/dL) was discovered at a health fair screening and was verified by her physician about 2 years ago. Her LDL normalized after initiation of atorvastatin. She also underwent a total hysterectomy last year due to benign fibroid tumors and has been maintained on conjugated estrogen therapy.

Social History

Tobacco use: negative

Alcohol use: 1 glass of wine socially

Caffeine use: 3 tall espresso lattes in the morning and 3 cans of Diet Coke per day

Family History

Father is alive and had a heart attack at age 50.

Mother is alive and has type 2 diabetes.

Review of Systems

Fatigue, hair loss, constipation, weight gain, cold intolerance

Physical Examination

GEN: Pale, well-developed, tired-appearing woman

VS: BP 100/85 mmHg, HR 48 bpm, RR 10 rpm, T 36.0°C Wt 79.5 kg (increased 9 kg from 3 months ago)

NEURO: Delayed DTR's, decreased muscle strength in all extremities

HEENT: PERRLA, oral cavity without lesions, TM without signs of inflammation, pale boggy nasal membranes, non-palpable thyroid (thyroid atrophy)

CHEST: Clear to auscultation and percussion, bradycardia, no murmurs

Labs and Diagnostic Tests

Sodium 138 mEq/L	Potassium 4.0 mEq/L
Chloride 100 mEq/L	CO_2 content 29 mEq/L
BUN 10 mg/dL	Serum creatinine 0.7 mg/dL
Glucose 100 mg/dL	Cholesterol 210 mg/dL
HDL 40 mg/dL	Calculated LDL 123 mg/dL
Fasting triglycerides 236 mg/dL	AST 26 IU/L
ALT 20 IU/L	TT_4 3.5 mcg/dL
FT_4 0.7 ng/dL	FT_4I 0.8 U
TT_3 70 ng/dL	FT_3 10 ng/dL
TSH 54 mIU/L	Hemoglobin 12.0 g/dL
Hematocrit 33%	Platelets 25,000/mm³

WBC 4000/mm³ with 60% PMN, 25% lymphocytes, 15% monocytes

PaO_2 70	$PaCO_2$ 39

pH 7.45

Case 29

ECG: Sinus bradycardia

CXR: Normal, no infiltrates, no left ventricular hypertrophy

Diagnosis

Primary:

    1. Primary hypothyroidism

Secondary:

    1. Angina

    2. Acid Reflux

    3. Hypercholesterolemia

    4. Depression

    5. S/p hysterectomy for fibroid tumors

Pharmacist Notes and Other Patient Information

2/12 Explained side effects of fluoxetine.

3/2 Explained how to use NTG and advised about subsequent refills to maintain potency. Told patient if chest pain did not resolve after one pill, call 911 and take another pill. Advised patient to limit or stop caffeine intake to avoid worsening angina symptoms.

3/2 Counseled patient on bisoprolol. Advised her not take with antacids and to not stop it without first talking to Dr. Bates. Advised her to also take her pulse regularly.

3/22 Discussed the correct use of Lipitor and warned patient about muscle weakness and dark urine. Advised patient to not ingest grapefruit or grapefruit juice.

4/10 Recommend at least 1500 mg calcium carbonate to prevent osteoporosis. Advised patient that caffeine intake can interfere with calcium absorption. Recommended that patient do weight bearing exercises when working out.

4/10 Explained risks and benefits of conjugated estrogens. Explained in detail the heart-associated risks of taking hormones and the warning signs.

Questions

1. Which brand name product would you use to fill KJ's prescription for levothyroxine?

    A. Cytomel

    B. Thyrolar

    C. Synthroid

    D. Armour Thyroid

    E. Thyrogen

2. Which medication is KJ's taking that could interact with her levothyroxine and result in her needing to take an increased dose of the levothyroxine?

    A. Conjugated estrogens

    B. Calcium carbonate

    C. Atorvastatin

    D. Magnesium and aluminum hydroxide gel

    E. Multivitamin with iron

3. Which of KJ's medical problems may be aggravated initially by starting low doses of levothyroxine?

    I. Depression

    II. Hypercholesterolemia

    III. Angina

Medication Record

Date	Rx No	Physician	Drug and Strength	Quantity	Sig	Refills
2/12	1543	Bates	Fluoxetine 40 mg	100	1 PO daily	6
3/2	3565	Bates	NTG 0.4 mg	100	1 SL prn chest pain	prn
3/2	3566	Bates	Bisoprolol 5 mg	30	1 PO qam	6
3/2			ASA 81 mg	100	1 PO daily	
3/22	3789	Bates	Lipitor 20 mg	90	1 PO daily	3
4/10	4000	Bates	Bisoprolol 5 mg	90	1 PO qd	1
4/10			Ca Carbonate 500 mg	100	1 PO tid	
4/10	6678	Bates	Premarin 1.25 mg	100	1 PO qd	6
5/12			Magnesium and aluminum hydroxide gel	120 cc	30 cc prn	
5/12			ASA 81 mg	100	1 PO daily	
5/25			Senna laxative tablets	50	1 PO qod	
6/1			Tums	100	1–2 PO prn	
6/15	8540	Bates	Fluoxetine 40 mg	100	1 PO daily	5
6/15			Multivitamins with iron	100	1 PO qd	

Case 29

A. I only
B. III only
C. I and II only
D. II and III only
E. I, II, and III

4. By treating KJ's hypothyroidism, which of her symptoms are likely to improve?

   I.   Hair loss, constipation, and weight gain
   II. Bradycardia, low respiratory rate, and CO_2 retention
   III. High cholesterol

   A. I only
   B. III only
   C. I and II only
   D. II and III only
   E. I, II, and III

5. You want to accurately assess euthyroidism in KJ. Which thyroid function tests would you use?

   A. Free thyroxine
   B. Total triiodothyronine
   C. Free thyroxine index
   D. Thyroid-stimulating hormone
   E. Free triiodothyronine

6. What are the most important counseling points to tell KJ about levothyroxine to ensure she is getting the optimal therapeutic effects?

   I.   Do not take within 4 hours of taking iron.
   II. Do wait 4 hours before taking antacids.
   III. Do not take with dairy products or calcium carbonate.

   A. I only
   B. III only
   C. I and II only
   D. II and III only
   E. I, II, and III

7. After beginning the levothyroxine therapy, when should KJ see some improvements in her symptoms of hypothyroidism?

   A. After the first dose
   B. After 3 days of therapy
   C. After 1 week of therapy
   D. After 10 days of therapy
   E. After 21 days of therapy

8. After 3 months of levothyroxine, her thyroid function tests show a TSH level <0.05 mIU/L and a free thyroxine level of 18 pmol/L. Which of the following adverse effects might be expected, based on these laboratory findings?

   A. No adverse effects are expected because the free thyroxine is normal.
   B. Hypercholesterolemia can be expected.
   C. Decrease in bone density can be expected.
   D. Bradycardia can be expected.
   E. Anemia can be expected.

9. Which of the following factors can alter KJ's thyroxine requirements?

   I.   Renal impairment
   II. Alcohol intake
   III. Excessive weight gain

   A. I only
   B. III only
   C. I and II only
   D. II and III only
   E. I, II, and III

10. Which of the following statements is NOT true when comparing Cytomel and levothyroxine therapy?

    A. T_3 needs to be dosed multiple times a day.
    B. T_3 is more completely absorbed than T_4.
    C. T_3 acts faster than T_4.
    D. The half-life of T_3 is longer than T_4.
    E. T_3 might produce more adverse effects than T_4.

Renal Disorders

Case 30

Patient Name: Tom Truax
Address: 1201 Chase Drive
Age: 64   **Height:** 5' 7"
Sex: M   **Race:** White
Weight: 110 lb
Allergies: Codeine

Chief Complaint

TT, a 64-yo male, is seen in the ED. He complains of weakness and difficulty breathing.

History of Present Illness

TT has not felt well for 3 weeks and has had a poor appetite. He has lost approximately 20 lb in the past month.

Past Medical History

TT has had diabetes for 30 years. Diabetic complications include diabetic nephropathy (which has progressed to ESRD), retinopathy with blindness, and peripheral neuropathy. TT has renal failure secondary to diabetic nephrosclerosis and has been on hemodialysis for 10 years (he is dialyzed 3 times/week). Additionally, TT has a history of CAD s/p CABG, MI, PVD and restless leg syndrome.

TT's past surgical history is significant for CABG x 3 in 2001. AV fistula placed in 1995.

Social History

Remote smoking history. Patient smoked 1 ppd x 30 years. Quit smoking at age 45. Patient denies recent alcohol use. Uses a manual wheelchair.

Family History

Father died of heart disease in his 70s. Mother died of unknown causes. TT is an only child.

Review of Systems

TT is weak, tired, and achy. He has had some shortness of breath (notably increased on exertion). He denies chest pain, cough, or hemoptysis. Denies nausea and vomiting, abdominal pain, and melena. His appetite is very poor. He bruises easily.

Physical Examination

VS: BP 118/72 mmHg, HR 66 bpm, RR 18 rpm, T 97.2°F, Wt 50 kg

GEN: Emaciated, ill-appearing, elderly man who appears older than his stated age.

HEENT: NC/AT, oral mucosa is clean and dry, no JVD

LUNGS: Decreased breath sounds in the right base, he has egophony in the right lower and mid-lung fields with bronchophony, no crackles, left lung field WNL.

CV: Grade 2/6 systolic murmur

ABD: Soft, NT/ND, no hepatosplenomegaly

EXT: Left AV fistula in the upper extremity, good bruits, reduced pulses in lower extremities

Labs and Diagnostic Tests

Sodium 134 mEq/L	Potassium 4.9 mEq/L
Chloride 104 mEq/L	CO_2 content: 19 mEq/L
BUN 58 mg/dL	Serum creatinine 6.0 mg/dL
Glucose 182 mg/dL	Calcium 10.3 mg/dL
Phosphorus 6.6 mg/dL	Albumin 2.4 g/dL
PTH 152 pg/mL	Hgb 10.2 g/dL
Hct 32%	Platelets 218,000/mm³
MCV 89.5 fL	MCH 28.8 pg
MCHC 32.2 g/dL	RDW 19.3%

WBC 8900/mm³ with 91.2% PMNs, 2.5% lymphocytes, 5.1% monocytes, 1.2% eosinophils

PO_2 60.2 mmHg	PCO_2 42.4 mmHg
pH 7.45	O_2 sat 92.2%

CrCl <10 mL/min

Blood cultures (2) & sputum: pending

CXR: Right lower lobe infiltrate consistent with pneumonia

EKG: NSR, no evidence of acute ischemia

Diagnosis

Primary:

    1. Right lower lobe pneumonia

    2. Weight loss

Secondary:

    1. End stage renal disease

    2. Diabetes

Case 30

Medication Record

(scheduled medications only)

09/15, Levofloxacin 500 mg IV x1 given in ED

09/16, Accuchecks bid

09/16, Regular insulin sliding scale SQ bid

09/16, Humulin N 20 units SQ in am and 10 units in pm

09/16, Glyburide 1.25 mg po q AM

09/16, Claforan 2 g IV q 24 h

09/16, Aspirin 325 mg po daily

09/16, Calcium acetate 667 mg, 2 tabs po tid ac

09/16, Centrum multivitamin 1 tab po daily

09/16, Epogen 5,000 units IV with dialysis

09/16, Calcitriol 1 mcg MWF with dialysis

Pharmacist Notes and Other Patient Information

09/15 Codeine causes itching, rash, and hives. Vicodin ordered. Patient has not tried Vicodin. Nursing staff to monitor patient closely for signs of allergy to Vicodin.

Questions

1. PhosLo is the brand name for which of the following products:

    A. Aluminum hydroxide
    B. Calcium acetate
    C. Calcium carbonate
    D. Calcitriol
    E. Sevelamer

2. After reviewing TT's lab values, you see the need for further adjustment in his phosphate binder therapy. Besides considering the actual PO_4 level, you must also consider:

    I.   The calcium X phosphate product
    II. The calcium level
    III. The PTH level

    A. I only
    B. III only
    C. I and II only
    D. II and III only
    E. I, II, and III

3. TT is already receiving PhosLo (calcium acetate) but his PO_4 level is 6.6 mg/dL, his corrected calcium level is 11.6 and Ca x PO_4 product is 76.6 mg^2/dL^2. Your recommendation:

    I.   Change to calcium carbonate
    II. Start aluminum hydroxide
    III. Start sevelamer

    A. I only
    B. III only
    C. I and II only
    D. II and III only
    E. I, II, and III

4. Sevelamer has been shown to have additional beneficial effects on which of the following?

    A. Hypertension
    B. Hyperlipidemia
    C. Hyperkalemia
    D. Metabolic acidosis
    E. Anemia

5. TT's PTH level is currently within the recommended target range for patients with end stage renal disease (ESRD) on dialysis (150-300 pg/mL). However, patients with ESRD can develop PTH levels > 300 pg/ml. Should this occur, which medication would most effectively decrease PTH?

    I.   Cinacalcet
    II. Paricalcitol
    III. Doxercalciferol

    A. I only
    B. III only
    C. I and II only
    D. II and III only
    E. I, II, and III

6. TT's respiratory status has not improved and his CXR shows a more extensive right lower lobe infiltrate. A sputum culture grows out gram positive bacteria, while blood cultures reveal MRSA. The nephrologist has ordered vancomycin 1 g to be given at the end of dialysis. The nurse calls you because she noticed a diffuse rash across TT's face, neck and chest. You suggest:

    A. Switch to another antibiotic
    B. Put note in chart that TT is allergic to Vancomycin
    C. Administer steroids and antihistamine
    D. Change vancomycin dose
    E. Slow down rate of infusion

Case 30

7. TT began to experience hypotension and urticaria with each dialysis session. These reactions were attributed to the use of high-flux dialysis membranes. TT was switched to the conventional low-flux dialysis membranes for each dialysis session. Which of the following vancomycin regimens is appropriate for use with low-flux dialysis membranes?

   A. Continue vancomycin 500 mg IV three times per week after dialysis
   B. Vancomycin 500 mg IV q 24 h
   C. Vancomycin 1 g IV q 12 h
   D. With TT taking other po meds, change vancomycin to 125 mg po qid
   E. Vancomycin 1 g IV q wk

8. After reviewing TT's lab results you notice that his serum CO_2 content is 18 mEq/L. This could be an acute problem but if he requires chronic maintenance therapy, what could you recommend?

   I. Bicitra
   II. $NaHCO_3$
   III. Polycitra

   A. I only
   B. III only
   C. I and II only
   D. II and III only
   E. I, II, and III

9. You notice that TT is receiving a Centrum multivitamin. You would recommend that he start taking Nephrovite in place of this vitamin. What would be the reason(s) for this recommendation?

   I. It contains fat soluble vitamins
   II. It contains water soluble vitamins
   III. It contains folic acid

   A. I only
   B. III only
   C. I and II only
   D. II and III only
   E. I, II, and III

10. What is the leading cause of death in patients such as TT with end stage renal disease and on dialysis?

    A. Anemia
    B. Cardiovascular disease
    C. Hyperkalemia
    D. Metabolic acidosis
    E. Infection

Patient Name: Margaret Parker
Address: Shady Hills Room. 112
Age: 73   **Height:** 5' 3"
Sex: F   **Race:** African American
Weight: 78 kg (IBW 52 kg)
Allergies: NKDA

Chief Complaint

The patient is a 73-yo female, was brought to the ED by EMS from a nursing home. The facility physician had her transported for admission due to "Mental Status Changes." It is difficulty to elicit any complaints due to her compromised mental status. She does appear to have some pain in the area of her right chest.

History of Present Illness

The patient had been convalescing in the extended care facility following a hip replacement. She was scheduled to return home tomorrow but late last night she developed a productive cough and low grade fever. Her local primary care physician called in a prescription for cephalexin 500 mg po tid. In the past 12 hours, she has developed right-sided chest pain and a worsening of the productive cough.

Past Medical History

The patient's significant past medical history includes s/p hip replacement following a fall, diabetes mellitus x 25 years managed with glyburide 10 mg po bid, and mild hypertension with chronic renal insufficiency managed on losartan 25 mg po daily.

Social History

Prior to her hospitalization for the fall and broken hip, the patient lived alone and was doing well. Her son called to speak with her two to three times each week and visited her once a week. Her daughter lived out of town, but called every Sunday.

She does not smoke, drink alcohol or take any illicit drugs. She is widowed and has lived alone in the same house for 12 years. No recent travel. Visitors prior to this hospitalization included her son and two neighbors (all healthy).

Family History

Old medical records suggest that her father died of an apparent stroke at age 70. Mother was diagnosed with diabetes at age 54 and died at age 71 of complications secondary to amputation of a great toe. One brother, 5 years older, died at age 79 of a MI.

Review of Systems

Negative except for some tachypnea, grimacing on inspiration consistent with pleuritic pain, and a productive cough with greenish sputum.

Physical Examination

GEN: Moderately obese female, appearing tired with resting dyspnea, productive cough and in mild distress.

VS: BP 165/109 mmHg, HR 110-120 bpm, RR 25 rpm, T 103.3°F

CHEST: Respirations are shallow and rapid with light crackling rales over right lung base.

CV: Tachycardic with a rate of 120. NSR without murmurs, rubs or gallops.

NEURO: Oriented to person only. Unable to state the correct day of the week or month and thought she was in a nursing home.

Labs and Diagnostic Tests

Sodium 142 mEq/L	Potassium 4.1 mEq/L
Chloride 109 mEq/mL	CO_2 content 23 mEq/L
BUN 40 mg/dL	Serum creatinine 1.7 mg/dL
Glucose 220 mg/dL	Hg_{A1C} 8.5
WBC 18.1 k/mm³	Hgb 10.9 g/dL
Hct 33.5%	Segs 84%
Bands 12%	Lymphs 1%

Respiratory culture: Pending

Gram stain report: Occasional gram-positive cocci in pairs and short chains. Numerous gram-negative rods.

Diagnosis

Primary:

     1. Community-acquired pneumonia (CAP)

     2. R/O Nosocomial pneumonia

Secondary:

     1. Mild renal impairment

     2. Hypertension

     3. Type 2 diabetes-inadequately controlled

     4. S/P hip replacement

Case 31

Medication Record

3/16, Watkins, Ceftriaxone 1 g IV q 24 h

3/16, Watkins, Pantoprazole 40 mg po daily

3/16, Watkins, Glyburide 10 mg po bid

3/16, Watkins, Losartan 25 mg po daily

3/16, Watkins, Acetaminophen 325 mg, 1-2 po q 4 h prn fever

3/16, Watkins, Guaifenesin/hydrocodone syrup 5–10 mL po q 4 h prn cough

3/16, Watkins, Meperidine 50 mg IV q 3 h prn pain

3/16, Watkins, Senna & docusate 2 tabs po daily

3/17, Watkins, Morphine 2-4 mg IV q4h prn pain

3/18, Martin, Metformin 500 mg 1 po bid

3/18, Martin, Increase losartan to 50 mg po qd

3/19, Martin, Gentamicin dosing per pharmacy

3/19. Martin, Piperacillin/tazobactam 4/0.5 IV q6h

Pharmacist Notes and Other Patient Information

3/16 Left note on chart recommending drug dosage adjustments. Called physician and recommended morphine in place of meperidine.

3/19 Final respiratory culture: Pseudomonas aeruginosa.

Questions

1. Using the method of Cockcroft and Gault, estimate this patient's creatinine clearance (use IBW).

   A. 24 mL/min
   B. 28 mL/min
   C. 67 mL/min
   D. 86 mL/min
   E. 100 mL/min

2. Which of the following drugs does not need to be adjusted in renal insufficiency?

   A. Meperidine
   B. Piperacillin/tazobactam
   C. Gentamicin
   D. Guaifenesin/hydrocodone syrup
   E. Metformin

3. Meperidine must be carefully dosed in patients with impaired renal function because:

   I. Meperidine crosses the blood-brain barrier more easily in renal failure.
   II. Meperidine itself is nephrotoxic and can further compromise renal function.
   III. Normeperidine, a metabolite, accumulates during renal failure causing CNS hyperactivity.

   A. I only
   B. III only
   C. I and II only
   D. II and III only
   E. I, II, and III

4. The admitting physician ordered that the patient may have senna & docusate to help prevent constipation. Failing that, which of the following is the next best choice for this patient?

   A. MOM (magnesium hydroxide)
   B. Magnesium citrate
   C. Fleet's Phospho-Soda (sodium phosphates)
   D. Dulcolax (bisacodyl)
   E. Surfak (docusate calcium)

5. After reviewing the respiratory culture results, the physician decided to add an aminoglycoside to therapy. An order is written for gentamicin with pharmacy to dose. Calculate a loading dose for this patient.

   A. 40 mg
   B. 80 mg
   C. 100 mg
   D. 150 mg
   E. 200 mg

6. Which of these would be the best source to find an optimal methodology to calculate estimated creatinine clearance (e.g., Cockcroft-Gault)?

   A. Facts and Comparisons: Drug Interaction Facts
   B. Goodman & Gillman's The Pharmacologic Basis of Therapeutics
   C. Pharmacotherapy: A Pathophysiologic Approach
   D. Stedman's Medical Dictionary
   E. Griffith's 5-Minute Clinical Consult

7. The patient's family members are visiting and one of them comments to you that he did an internet search and discovered that goldenrod can help promote renal function and asks why the patient is not receiving it. You respond:

   A. Goldenrod is not on the formulary so we can not get it.
   B. Information available on the internet is inaccurate.

Case 31

C. Goldenrod is primarily useful in bowel problems, not kidney problems.

D. Goldenrod is a poison that would result in the death of anyone who took it.

E. There are many reports on the internet that lack scientific validity. There is no evidence that goldenrod would be helpful for this patient.

8. Since MP's accucheck blood sugars have been elevated, the physician added metformin 500 mg bid. As the pharmacist you recommend:

A. decreasing metformin to 500 mg po daily.

B. increasing metformin to 850 mg po bid.

C. discontinuing metformin and adding Glynase 3 mg po daily.

D. discontinuing metformin and adding Glucotrol 5 mg po daily.

E. discontinuing metformin and adding Actos 15 mg po daily.

9. The technician you are working with asks you the trade name for losartan. The correct answer is which of the following?

A. Cozaar

B. Hyzaar

C. Diovan

D. Atacand

E. Avapro

10. On completion of the prescribed IV antibiotic therapy, the physician plans to begin an oral antibiotic. Which is an appropriate choice for this patient?

A. Piperacillin 500 mg po qid

B. Ciprofloxacin 500 mg po daily

C. Daptomycin 250 mg po daily.

D. Azithromycin 500 mg po daily.

E. Cefazolin 1 g po daily

Case 32

Patient Name: Ximena Nueve-Orlando
Address: 2836 St Andrews Drive
Age: 38   **Height:** 5' 7"
Sex: F   **Race:** Latin American
Weight: 220 lb
Allergies: NKDA

Chief Complaint

Nausea, vomiting, fever and flank pain.

History of Present Illness

XNO is an obese, 29-yo Latin American female who presented to her OB-GYN last week complaining of dysuria and some mild flank pain. She was prescribed an antibiotic that she believes was amoxicillin. She presents to our ED today with a 2-day history of generalized malaise, myalgias, and fever reaching 103°F with chills. Yesterday she became nauseated and began vomiting. She has vomited 15-20 times since yesterday. She has taken multiple doses of Pepto Bismol without relief. She has been taking naproxen sodium as needed for fever and muscle aches.

Past Medical History

The patient has type 2 DM managed on metformin 850 mg bid and glipizide XL 10 mg daily, GERD for which she takes esomeprazole 20 mg daily and mild hypertension managed on enalapril 10 mg bid.

Social History

The patient is divorced and has no children. She graduated from high school and works as a secretary. She admits to occasional marijuana use but denies other drugs of abuse. She drinks alcohol socially and smokes cigarettes about a half pack per day.

Family History

The patient's father died at age 71 from diabetic complications. Her mother is alive at 74 and has hypertension. Her maternal grandmother also had diabetes. She has two siblings. Her brother is 41 and has diabetes and her sister is 35 yo and in good health.

Review of Systems

In addition to nausea and vomiting as described in the History of Present Illness, the patient complains of weakness, some dysuria and mild flank pain, but otherwise has no complaints. She denies hematemesis, melena, or bright red blood per rectum. She denies rashes, shortness of breath, chest pain, or palpitations.

Physical Examination

GEN: WD/WN Latin American female in mild distress. She is A & O to person only.

VS: BP 78/58 mmHg, HR 110 bpm, RR 16 rpm, T 100°F, Wt 100 kg

HEENT: NC/AT, sclerae anicteric, PERRLA, TMI, mucosa somewhat dry, neck is supple, no adenopathy or thyromegaly

LUNGS: CTA

CV: Sinus rhythm at 124 bpm without m/r/g

ABD: Obese, soft without tenderness, no rebound or guarding, hypoactive BS.

RECTAL: Unremarkable, (-) hemoccult

EXT: Warm, mild tenting, no CCE, strong pedal pulses, no ulcers on feet, monofilament normal.

Labs and Diagnostic Tests

(On admission)

Sodium 124 mEq/L	Potassium 4.9 mEq/L
Chloride 88 mEq/L	CO_2 22 mEq/L
BUN 62 mg/dL	Serum creatinine 6.3 mg/dL
Glucose 300 mg/dL	Calcium 7.7 mg/dL
Phosphorus 1.9 mg/dL	Albumin 3.9 g/dL
HgbA$_{1c}$ 8.9%	Magnesium 1.6 mg/dL
TSH 2.4	Hemoglobin 14.3 g/dL
Hct 43%	Platelets 320,000/mm^3

WBC 8900/mm^3 with 12% bands and 18% segs

Urine analysis:

Color yellow	Specific gravity 1.025
Blood 3+	Protein 2+
pH 5.5	Bili 1+
Urobilinogen 0.3	Hyaline casts 11-14/lpf
Urine output 700 mL/24 hr	

Microbiology:

Blood cultures - no growth

Urine culture - E. coli 50,000-100,000 CFU/mL

Renal ultrasound: Unremarkable, no hydronephrosis or masses seen

Case 32

Medication Record

(Home Medication List)

Date	Rx No	Physician	Drug and Strength	Quantity	Sig	Refills
04/15	62502	Blevins	Glipizide XL 10 mg	60	1 bid	5
04/15	62503	Blevins	Metformin 850 mg	90	1 bid	5
04/15	62504	Blevins	Esomeprazole	20	1 qd	5
05/01	74877	Rhodes	Enalapril 10 mg	60	1 bid	3
06/12	OTC		Aleve 220 mg	12	po prn	OTC

(Inpatient)

07/06, NS x2 liters IV wide open STAT

07/06, Promethazine 25 mg IV STAT

07/06, Regular insulin 10 units IV STAT

07/06, Accuchecks ac hs

07/06, Regular insulin sliding scale SQ ac hs

07/07, Levaquin 500 mg po q 24 h

07/07, TUMS 500 mg po 2 bid

07/07, Magnesium sulfate 1 g IV NOW

07/07, Phenergan 12.5 mg IV q 6 h prn N/V

07/07, Acetaminophen 650 mg po q 4 h prn fever

07/08, Flagyl 500 mg po tid

Diagnosis

Primary:

1. Acute renal failure

2. Mild dehydration

3. Urinary tract infection

Secondary:

1. Type 2 diabetes mellitus

Pharmacist Notes and Other Patient Information

07/06 Serum creatinine = 6.3 (1 year ago, serum creatinine = 0.7)

07/08 Serum creatinine decreased to 3.0

Questions

1. It appears that this patient has acute renal failure. Which of the following best describes the type of renal failure that the patient is experiencing?

   I. Prerenal/functional
   II. Postrenal
   III. Intrinsic renal

   A. I only
   B. III only
   C. I and II only
   D. II and III only
   E. I, II, and III

2. The patient was taking two medications at home for her diabetes, metformin and glipizide. Which of the following are the trade names for metformin and glipizide?

   A. Glucotrol & Glycet
   B. Glucophage & Prandin
   C. Glucophage & Glucotrol
   D. Prandin & Glucotol
   E. Glycet & Prandin

3. Which of the following drugs could have contributed to XNO's acute renal failure?

   I. Metformin
   II. Enalapril
   III. Naproxen sodium

   A. I only
   B. III only
   C. I and II only
   D. II and III only
   E. I, II, and III

4. If the patient becomes hypokalemic (K+ = 3.0) oral potassium would be a viable option. Which of the following is appropriate for potassium replacement?

   A. Potassium chloride 40 mEq PO every 5 minutes for 1 hour
   B. K-Dur 40 mEq PO every hour x 5 doses
   C. K-Dur 40 meq PO bid.
   D. Potassium chloride 100 mEq PO stat
   E. K-Dur 200 meq PO daily

Case 32

5. Based on XNO's most current serum creatinine, calculate her creatinine clearance (base equation on TBW). TBW = 220 lb (Use TBW for easy math); age = 38; serum creatinine on admission = 6.3; serum creatinine two days later = 3.0

   A. 19 mL/min
   B. 22 mL/min
   C. 25 mL/min
   D. 40 mL/min
   E. 47 mL/min

6. You have just received an order for XNO for Synthroid 0.075 mg po daily. You enter the order into the computer and the technician fills the order based on the label printed from your entry. Which is the correct medication?

   A. Levofloxacin
   B. Levorphanol
   C. Levothyroxine
   D. Levonorgestrel
   E. Levodopa

7. Magnesium sulfate injection is commercially available as a 50% solution. The physician wants 2 g added to a 50-mL solution and given IVPB over 30 minutes. How much magnesium in milliliters is added to solution, and at what rate should the nurse run the IVPB (in mL/hr)?

   A. 1 mL of magnesium added; infuse at a rate of 102 mL/hr
   B. 1 mL of magnesium added; infuse at a rate of 1.7 mL/hr
   C. 4 mL of magnesium added; infuse at a rate of 108 mL/hr
   D. 4 mL of magnesium added; infuse at a rate of 1.8 mL/hr
   E. 4 mL of magnesium added; infuse at a rate of 0.03 mL/hr

8. Nurse Cratchett calls the pharmacy requesting information regarding the compatibility of the magnesium solution she must now give with the current IV. Which of the following references will provide the answer to the nurse's question?

   I. Handbook on Injectable Drugs
   II. Basic Skills in Interpreting Laboratory Data
   III. Applied Therapeutics: The Clinical Use of Drugs

   A. I only
   B. III only
   C. I and II only
   D. II and III only
   E. I, II, and III

9. XNO is discharged on the following medications: Glucotrol XL 10 mg bid, Synthroid 0.075 mg daily, Vasotec 5 mg bid, Flagyl 500 mg tid x 5 days, and Levaquin 250 mg daily x 2 days and Tums 2 tablets prn. The pharmacist counsels XNO about her medications and makes the following statements. Please indicate which statements are true.

   I. It is important to finish the full course of Levaquin and Flagyl therapy even if you are feeling completely well.
   II. Levaquin can be taken without regard to food or drink, but avoid taking the Tums within 2 hours before or after a dose.
   III. Avoid alcohol while taking Flagyl and for 3 days after finishing therapy.

   A. I only
   B. III only
   C. I and II only
   D. II and III only
   E. I, II, and III

10. Which of the following lifestyle modifications should be recommended to XNO?

   I. Exercise vigorously for at least an hour each day.
   II. Maintain adequate blood pressure control.
   III. Avoid the use of cigarettes and alcohol; avoid the use of any OTC drugs (especially NSAIDs) unless approved by her physician.

   A. I only
   B. III only
   C. I and II only
   D. II and III only
   E. I, II, and III

Psychiatric Disorders

Section Editor: Lawrence J. Cohen

Patient Name: Kaitlin Townsend
Address: 2131 Keeven Lane
Age: 36   **Height:** 6' 0"
Sex: F   **Race:** White
Weight: 176 lb
Allergies: NKDA

Chief Complaint

KT is a 36-yo white female who goes to the neuropsychiatry clinic for a follow-up appointment to discuss the results of her CT scan. KT has been seen in the neuropsychiatry clinic recently for evaluation of her headaches.

History of Present Illness

KT has been experiencing frequent headaches which she has been attempting to control with OTC medications. In the past 6 weeks her headaches have increased in both severity and number. Besides headaches, KT is also experiencing stomach upset, feelings of restlessness, insomnia, neck pain, and frequently complains of being irritable and stressed out. She states that her husband teases her and calls her "chicken little" because it will not be long until she runs out of things to worry about and moves on to worry about the sky falling. She has always been a worrier but in the last year she feels that her physical health has been on the decline. She adds that her family sees her being just like her grandmother, who has been described as a worry wart.

Past Medical History

KT has been in reasonably good health up until the past few months, when her current symptoms began to escalate.

Social History

Tobacco use: none

Alcohol use: has increased to 2-3 drinks per night over recent months to help her sleep

Caffeine use: 3-5 16-oz Diet Pepsi's per day

Family History

Maternal aunt had 'nervous breakdown' after the birth of her second child. Maternal grandmother described as 'worry wart.'

Review of Systems

Frequent complaints of headache and neck pain

Physical Examination

GEN: WD/WN female who appears anxious and demonstrates psychomotor agitation while waiting for clinician to review the CT scan.

VS: BP 135/90 mmHg, HR 110 bpm, RR 29 rpm, T 38.5°C, Wt 80 kg

HEENT: Normocephalic, PERRLA, neck supple, nasal and throat cavities clear

CHEST: CTA

NEURO: A & O x3

Labs and Diagnostic Tests

Sodium 140 mEq/L	Potassium 3.3 mEq/L
Chloride 110 mEq/L	CO_2 content 27 mEq/L
BUN 19 mg/dL	Serum creatinine 1.0 mg/dL
Glucose 107 mg/dL	Hgb 14.0 g/dL
Hct 42%	Platelets 300,000/mm³
WBC 7500/mm³	AST 100
ALT 210	

CT scan (with and without contrast): WNL

Diagnosis

Primary:

1. Generalized anxiety disorder

2. Rebound headache

Pharmacist Notes and Other Patient Information

2/10 Patient purchased 5 bottles of OTC analgesics

2/29 Refill for Fiorcet okayed by physician and insurance company (neurologist plans to taper her off headache medications)

Case 33

Medication Record

Date	Rx No	Physician	Drug and Strength	Quantity	Sig	Refills
2/10	159086	Evans	Darvocet-N-100	120	1-2 po qid prn	3
2/24	159086	Evans	Darvocet-N-100	120	1-2 po qid prn	2
2/10	159088	Evans	Ambien 5 mg	30	1 po q hs prn	3
2/10			Nuprin 200 mg		1 po q 4-6 h prn	
2/10			Tylenol ES 500 mg		1 po q 4 h prn	
2/10			Citrucel		ud	
2/10			Theragran-M		1 po qd	

Questions

1. Which of the following on KT's medical history does not contribute to the rebound headaches?

   I. Darvocet-N-100
   II. Nuprin
   III. Diet Pepsi

   A. I only
   B. III only
   C. I and II only
   D. II and III only
   E. I, II, and III

2. Which of the following is the primary symptom of generalized anxiety disorder?

   I. Excessive worry
   II. Panic attacks
   III. Depressed mood

   A. I only
   B. III only
   C. I and II only
   D. II and III only
   E. I, II, and III

3. Which of the following educational suggestions would best benefit KT?

   I. Information on medication therapy
   II. Information explaining generalized anxiety disorder
   III. Education of family members on patient's disease state and therapy (with patient's permission)

   A. I only
   B. III only
   C. I and II only
   D. II and III only
   E. I, II, and III

4. Which of the following is a lifestyle change that should be recommended to KT as a non-pharmacological strategy to aid in treating her anxiety?

   I. Change to a job with less stress.
   II. Institute a positive sleep hygiene regimen.
   III. Begin a regular diet and exercise program.

   A. I only
   B. III only
   C. I and II only
   D. II and III only
   E. I, II, and III

5. The agent in KT's medication profile that is most likely to potentiate the side effects of Ambien is:

   I. Alcohol
   II. Darvocet-N-100
   III. Nuprin

   A. I only
   B. III only
   C. I and II only
   D. II and III only
   E. I, II, and III

6. Which of the following would be the best choice of benzodiazepine therapy for KT?

   I. Lorazepam
   II. Temazepam
   III. Prazepam

   A. I only
   B. III only
   C. I and II only
   D. II and III only
   E. I, II, and III

7. The pharmacologic mechanism of benzodiazepines is best described as:

Case 33

A. facilitating influx of chloride ions into the cell.
B. inhibiting influx of chloride ions into the cell.
C. facilitating influx of sodium ions into the cell.
D. inhibiting influx of sodium ions into the cell.
E. inhibiting influx of potassium ions into the cell.

8. Which of the following have GABAnergic mechanisms that may be of benefit in the treatment of anxiety?

    I.   Pre-gabalin
    II. Gabapentin
    III. Valproate

    A. I only
    B. III only
    C. I and II only
    D. II and III only
    E. I, II, and III

9. Abrupt discontinuation of alprazolam therapy in contrast to diazepam therapy results in which of the following symptoms?

    I.   Increased anxiety
    II. Seizures
    III. Rebound insomnia

    A. I only
    B. III only
    C. I and II only
    D. II and III only
    E. I, II, and III

10. KT is started on lorazepam 1 mg tid therapy. Patient arrives at the pharmacy for a refill of lorazepam 7 days earlier than scheduled. She states that she is feeling better but sometimes she needs to take an extra pill or two to keep symptoms at bay. As the pharmacist you carry out which of the following?

    I.   Refuse to refill the scheduled agent before the assigned date
    II. Inquire about patient's symptoms and schedule for taking meds then call physician for override to refill prescription a little early
    III. Counsel patient to address need for modified medication dose and schedule with physician

    A. I only
    B. III only
    C. I and II only
    D. II and III only
    E. I, II, and III

Case 34

ADHD (Child and Adolescent)

Patient Name: Kimberly Shea
Address: 112 Houston Street
Age: 14   **Height:** 5' 1"
Sex: F   **Race:** White
Weight: 98 lb
Allergies: Penicillin

Chief Complaint

KS's maternal grandmother, who is her legal guardian, brought her to the mental health clinic to get help in controlling her behavior.

History of Present Illness

Her symptoms began to cause significant impairment both at home and school around age 6. Symptoms noted include restlessness, impulsivity, distractability, difficulty focusing her attention or staying on task, problems waiting her turn in line and blurting out answers before anyone was called on, forgetfulness, frequent daydreaming, and poor school grades.

She appeared sad most of the time with excessive worrying and nervousness, withdrawing from other children and not wanting to make friends, loss of interest in things she usually enjoyed, irritability, decreased appetite, crying spells and frequent awakenings during the night.

She was started on methylphenidate 10 mg q AM and 10 mg q Noon; and after a few months, the dose was increased to 10 mg TID for re-emergence of symptoms in mid-afternoon. Imipramine 25 mg at HS was added to address depressive symptoms, enuresis, and initial insomnia; and was later increased to 50 mg at HS. Symptoms of depression, insomnia, and enuresis resolved within a month; and Imipramine was discontinued after about a year.

From age 7 to age 13 she was continued on methylphenidate; but last year, to simplify her regimen, short-acting methylphenidate was replaced with Concerta starting at 18 mg and gradually titrated to 54 mg q AM with good results. During those years, symptoms of major depression reemerged 2 or 3 times; and although she was tried on a couple different SSRI's, Bupropion SR, and Venlafaxine XR, they were either ineffective or caused her intolerable side effects. Imipramine was effective in controlling her symptoms each time, and was continued for a year after depressive symptoms resolved.

Past Medical History

Amoxicillin caused a generalized rash and itching. Frequent severe headaches since menarche at age 12. Bilateral PE tubes from age 1 1/2 through age 3 years due to recurrent episodes of otitis media. Primary nocturnal enuresis, organic causes ruled out, which ceased shortly after imipramine was instituted. Immunizations current. Developmental milestones reached at expected ages. Height and weight at 25th percentile.

Social History

Maternal grandparents have been the patient's legal guardians since birth due to the mother having frequent problems with the law, chemical dependence, and several episodes of jail and prison. Patient is in 8th grade in regular classes with B average overall, no suspected learning disability; but precipitous decline in grades and conduct when patient has covertly non-adhered to her medication regimen. No signs of non-adherence since change from short acting methylphenidate to Concerta, until recently.

Family History

Mother suffered from depression since childhood, had chronic conduct problems, started abusing alcohol in junior high and became addicted to cocaine in high school; and was in a psychiatric hospital during her teen years for substance abuse and suicidal ideation. Mother continued alcohol and cocaine abuse into adult years until the present; and has shown no interest in seeking mental health treatment. No information known about the biological father.

Review of Systems

Penicillin allergy, frequent headaches, primary nocturnal enuresis—resolved.

Physical Examination

VS: BP 100/66 mmHg, HR 88 bpm, RR 20 rpm

Mental status examination: She appears her stated age and is attractive and slender, with good grooming and hygiene, neatly and appropriately dressed. Irritable mood, impatient affect, wanted to terminate interview as quickly as possible. Appeared restless and fidgity seated in chair. Poor eye contact. Clear direct speech. Average intellectual and cognitive functioning, No hallucinations, no suicidal or homicidal ideation, no delusional thought content, no abnormality of thought form. Insight and judgment fair to poor.

Patient states she is "sick and tired of having to take medication", reports non-adherence to treatment, and does not recognize the deterioration in her conduct and school work.

Labs and Diagnostic Tests

CBC: WNL	Chem14: WNL
TFTs: WNL	LFTs: WNL
UA: WNL	

EKG: Normal sinus rhythm with mildly increased QT_c interval

Case 34

 Diagnosis

Axis 1: Attention Deficit Hyperactivity Disorder-Combined Type

Major Depression, Recurrent, in Full Remission

Primary Nocturnal Enuresis-Resolved

Intermittent Medication Noncompliance

Axis 2: No Diagnosis

Axis 3: Frequent Headaches

Allergy to Penicillin

Axis 4: Problems with Primary Support Group—Mother

Educational Problems—Deterioration in Schoolwork and Peer Relations off Meds

Axis 5: Current GAF-55

 Medication Record

Concerta 54 mg po q AM

Acetaminophen 325 mg 1 or 2 po q 6 hr prn headache

 Pharmacist Notes and Other Patient Information

EKG changes not clinically significant

Questions

1. In assessing KS's response to treatment for ADHD symptoms, which of the following instruments are useful?

   I.   WISC-R
   II. CBCL
   III. Connors Rating Scales

   A. I only
   B. III only
   C. I and II only
   D. II and III only
   E. I, II, and III

2. Recommending extended release methylphenidate rather than immediate release include all of the following benefits EXCEPT:

A. eliminates the need for multiple daily doses.
B. causes fewer side effects.
C. reduces the potential for diversion or abuse.
D. less expensive than the short-acting forms.
E. eliminates the peaks and troughs of short-acting psychostimulants.

3. What percentage of children diagnosed with ADHD will continue to have difficulty with symptoms of the disorder into adult years?

   A. <2.7%
   B. 5%-10%
   C. 15%-25%
   D. 30%-40%
   E. 60%-70%

4. Usual treatment goals for using stimulant medications in patients with ADHD include:

   I.   decreased impulsivity and distractability.
   II. improved ability to get organized and focus attention.
   III. improved wakefulness.

   A. I only
   B. III only
   C. I and II only
   D. II and III only
   E. I, II, and III

5. What percentage of children with ADHD can be expected to show significant improvement when treated with stimulant medication?

   A. 20%-30%
   B. 40%-50%
   C. 55%-65%
   D. 70%-90%
   E. 96%-100%

6. The postulated mechanism responsible for the therapeutic effect in ADHD of Atomoxetine is:

   A. serotonin reuptake inhibition.
   B. blockade of GABA receptors.
   C. norepinephrine reuptake inhibition.
   D. increasing release of dopamine.
   E. blockade of alpha adrenergic receptors.

7. Criteria that are necessary to make the diagnosis of ADHD that KS meets include which of the following?

Case 34

 I. Clinically significant impairment present in two or more settings before age 7

 II. Symptoms of hyperactivity-impulsivity or inattention persisting at least 6 months

 III. Good response to stimulant medication

 A. I only

 B. III only

 C. I and II only

 D. II and III only

 E. I, II, and III

8. KS weighs 98 pounds, and her current dose of Concerta is 54 mg, what is the rate of methylphenidate administration when she is adherent to her medication as prescribed?

 A. 1 mg/kg/day

 B. 2.5 mg/kg/day

 C. 1.2 mg/kg/day

 D. 0.5 mg/kg/day

 E. 1.8 mg/kg/day

9. Pharmacotherapeutic recommendations to address the insomnia side effect of stimulant medication for ADHD would NOT include:

 A. clonidine.

 B. guanfacine.

 C. trazodone.

 D. mirtazapine.

 E. buspirone.

10. The trade name for modafinil is:

 A. Strattera.

 B. Concerta.

 C. Anafranil.

 D. Provigil.

 E. Dextrostat.

Case 35

Patient Name: Robert Benton
Address: 3215 West Woodruff Avenue
Age: 53   **Height:** 5' 8"
Sex: M   **Race:** Caucasian
Weight: 195 lb
Allergies: Sulfa

Chief Complaint

"I can't keep going on like this." RB is a 53-yo man who is a professor of English at a major university and was admitted for his first psychiatric hospitalization after presenting to his PCP for a routine appointment exhibiting dysarthria and ataxia.

History of Present Illness

RB has been experiencing frequent crying spells, difficulty concentrating, increased drinking, and increased difficulties with his teaching responsibilities over the last 3 years since the loss of his wife do to an acute cardiac event. He also admits to increased irritability with other faculty members. His smoking and time spent alone at home drinking has increased significantly, and he expresses passive suicidal ideation.

Past Medical History

RB has experienced three episodes of depression over the past 15 years, successfully treated with nortriptyline, fluoxetine, and more recently sertraline. He is currently on no psychiatric medication. His nonpsychiatric medical history includes hypertension and hyperlipidemia, which are currently under control with medication.

Social History

Widowed 3 years ago

Tobacco use: 1-2 packs per day for the past 35 years increasing to 2-3 packs recently

Alcohol use: two 6 packs of beer per week with up to 1/2 of a fifth of vodka per week over the last couple of months before bedtime.

Caffeine use: 6-8 cups of coffee every morning

Family History

RB's parents came to the U.S. from England when he was 7 years old. His parents were both professors at a major university but died in an airplane crash while RB was working on his thesis in his late 20s. Both drank alcohol frequently but had no known medical illnesses. RB is an only child.

Review of Systems

Dyspepsia

Physical Examination

PCP chart is reviewed. RB has not been seen for 6 months. Physical examination normal at that time. Blood pressure 130/84 with electrolytes, liver enzymes, lipids, blood sugar, and EKG all normal.

Mental status examination: RB is a moderately obese white male oriented x3. He is cooperative but quiet without volunteering any extra information during the interview. Speech is soft but normal to rate and rhythm. He appears somewhat psychomotor retarded but complains of "anxiety." Thought content is without hallucinations or delusions. His mood is dysphoric, and he admits to suicidal ideation. His judgment is fairly appropriate with insight into his "depression" and "increased drinking" but states that he drinks only because it "helps me sleep." RB complains of fatigue and anhedonia. RB agrees to sign a voluntary admission and be admitted to the psychiatric unit in the hospital.

Labs and Diagnostic Tests

On admission:

Sodium 135 mEq/L	Potassium 3.3 mEq/L
Chloride 98 mEq/L	CO_2 28 mmol/L
BUN 20 mEq/L	Serum creatinine 1.2 mg/dL
Total cholesterol 120	HDL 42
Triglycerides 242	GGT 242
AST 158	ALT 92
Glucose 143	Free T_4 1.6
TSH 5.8	Hb_{A1c} 6.7%
WBC 4.6	RBC 4.14
Hgb 12.4	Hct 38.2
MCV 93.2	Platelet count 159
PT 14.6	INR 1.1
PTT 28	Vitamin B_{12} 341
Folate, serum 16.1 ng/mL	RBC 140

Drug screen, serum alcohol, ethyl 0.22, drug screen, urine, negative for all substances of abuse

Diagnosis

Axis I: Major depressive disorder/recurrent, alcohol abuse, R/O alcohol dependence

Axis II: None

Axis III: Hypertension, hyperlipidemia

Axis IV: Stress at work

Axis V: GAF 35

Case 35

Medication Record

Date	Rx No	Physician	Drug and Strength	Quantity	Sig	Refills
10/18/05	12341	Carter	Hydrochlorothiazide 25 mg	30	qd	5
10/18/05	12342	Carter	Atenolol 100 mg	30	qd	5
10/18/05	12343	Carter	Simvastatin 40 mg	30	qd	5
			Aspirin 81 mg	100	qd	
			Multivitamin	100	qd	

Pharmacist Notes and Other Patient Information

None available

Questions

1. Which of the following is the initial phase of treatment for RB on admission to the hospital?

    I. Detoxification and symptom stabilization

    II. Sobriety and remission of depression symptoms

    III. Establishing support for the recovery and prevention of relapse

    A. I only
    B. III only
    C. I and II only
    D. II and III only
    E. I, II, and III

2. RB continues to complain about anxiety and tremulousness but initially fails to experience other symptoms of alcohol withdrawal associated with other autonomic system symptoms. Which medication in RB's regimen might partially attenuate this syndrome?

    A. Hydrochlorthiazide
    B. Atenolol
    C. Simvastatin
    D. Aspirin
    E. None of RB's medications would be expected to attenuate any of the autonomic symptoms of alcohol withdrawal syndrome

3. After stabilization and the institution of a tapering schedule with chlordiazepoxide, duloxetine is brought up as a possible option for the treatment of RB's depression and anxiety. For which of the following reasons might this NOT be the most appropriate consideration in RB?

    I. It is not recommended first line in patients predisposed to liver disease.

    II. It inhibits cytochrome P-450 enzyme 3A4, significantly raising simvastatin levels and increasing the risk for myopathy.

III. It lacks sedating effects making it a poor candidate for use in a patient with anxiety and insomnia.

    A. I only
    B. III only
    C. I and II only
    D. II and III only
    E. I, II, and III

4. The history of recent response to sertraline contributes to the initiation of sertraline 25 mg qd to RB's regimen. RB's sleep and anxiety continue to be problematic over the next couple of days. What alternatives could be considered for acute symptom relief?

    A. Increase the dose of sertraline to 100 mg which is the target dose in RB

    B. Reevaluate the chlordiazepoxide tapering schedule and consider increasing the dose and/or slowing the taper

    C. Change to fluoxetine since it causes less insomnia

    D. Change to bupropion since it causes less anxiety

    E. Schedule acetaminophen at bedtime to decrease caffeine withdrawal headaches, which could be contributing to the insomnia

5. The treatment plan for RB includes complete abstinence from alcohol. Which of the following are reasons for this recommendation?

    I. Chronic alcohol use without depression more than doubles the likelihood of developing major depression.

    II. Co-morbid alcoholism with depression is associated with more symptoms, longer duration, and more suicide attempts.

    III. Alcohol use is associated with less recovery from depression.

    A. I only
    B. III only
    C. I and II only
    D. II and III only
    E. I, II, and III

6. RB's clinical improvement allows for discharge to an outpatient program. Although he continues to improve, he fails to respond to sertraline as quickly as he had a few years earlier and requests a change. His moderate obesity and

Case 35

hyperlipidemia makes him a candidate to avoid antidepressants that exhibit a greater potential for weight gain. Which agent should be avoided at this time?

A. Fluoxetine
B. Bupropion
C. Venlafaxine
D. Mirtazapine
E. Desipramine

7. RB's multiple drug regimen and previous responses to serotonergic antidepressants influences a change to a serotonergic antidepressant with a less significant effect to inhibit CYP-450 enzymes to minimize the potential for drug-drug interactions. Which of the following agents best meets these characteristics?

A. Venlafaxine
B. Bupropion
C. Duloxetine
D. Paroxetine
E. Fluoxetine

8. RB's antidepressant is changed to venlafaxine XR 75 mg, which is slowly increased over the month to 300 mg with continued improvement of mood and work and social functioning. RB starts to date another faculty member and, for the first time in many years, starts to have an intimate relationship with this individual. At his regular appointment with his PCP he describes this improvement but also relates problems at times with libido and delayed orgasm and wants an explanation for the problem. The most likely explanation for this problem would be which of the following?

A. RB has started drinking alcohol again.
B. Increase the dose of venlafaxine because these sexual symptoms are residual symptoms of depression.
C. Venlafaxine is probably the problem since serotonergic antidepressants do this in a dose-dependent manner.
D. Simvastatin has significant effects on libido and orgasmic functioning.
E. Atenolol has a significant effect on libido and orgasmic functioning.

9. RB is given a prescription for venlafaxine-XR 75 mg three capsules each morning. RB decides that he does not need antidepressants anymore and that his problem is just related to his previous excessive alcohol use. Instead of starting on the lower dose of venlafaxine, RB decides that maybe he should take some other type of antidepressant and starts taking 900 mg of St. John's wort since he heard that it works the same and does not have any sexual problems. Two days after starting St. John's wort, RB calls his pharmacist and asks if there are any drug interactions with St. John's wort since he is experiencing dysphoria, paresthesias,

and vivid dreams. What is the probable explanation for these problems?

A. St. John's wort induces several CYP-450 isoenzymes and is causing a drug interaction and this problem.
B. This is a discontinuation syndrome associated with the abrupt cessation of venlafaxine.
C. This is part of the discontinuation syndrome associated with long-term alcohol use.
D. This is a hypertensive reaction associated with the initiation of St. John's wort.
E. These are just somatic symptoms that RB is expressing as a part of his depression.

10. After RB recovers from his event, he decides that maybe he does need to take antidepressants for awhile longer but asks his pharmacist for his opinion on how long he will need to take antidepressants. The best response by the pharmacist would be which of the following?

A. Given RB's recent reaction, he should stop his medication as soon as possible but first talk to his PCP.
B. The AHCPR guidelines for the treatment of depression in primary care states that maintenance therapy should continue for 6 months after symptoms remit, so RB should continue antidepressants for another few months anyway.
C. Given RB's alcohol history, he must take this medication for about a year.
D. Given the three episodes of depression, RB will probably need to continue to take antidepressants indefinitely and must work out the details with his PCP.
E. RB should continue to take antidepressants unless his BMI is greater than 30 or his lipids become elevated again.

Case 36

Patient Name: Mark Dunn
Address: 3E-Room 25
Age: 48 **Height:** 6' 1"
Sex: M **Race:** White
Weight: 193 lb
Allergies: Sulfa

Chief Complaint

MD is a 48-yo SWM who was seen in the ED yesterday with complaints of nausea, vomiting, diarrhea, sweating, increased heart rate, dehydration, fever, and auditory hallucinations. He reports long-term daily use of heroin, alcohol, and marijuana. He was admitted to the inpatient substance abuse unit for treatment of withdrawal.

History of Present Illness

MD reports a $100-$200/day habit of heroin use for approximately 16 years, 10 quarts of beer/day since the age of 15, and daily use of marijuana since Vietnam. His longest period of sobriety was from 1986 to 1987, and he has had multiple detoxifications over the past 14 years. He has a positive history of delirium tremens, withdrawal seizures, and blackouts. He has decided that he is finished with all drugs and has come into the hospital requesting detoxification. His last use of all substances was approximately 8 hours before admission. His symptoms upon admission were three to five recent episodes of both vomiting and diarrhea, "the shakes," sweating, fever, dehydration, and hearing voices screaming that he was going to die.

Past Medical History

The patient has been diagnosed with heroin dependence, alcohol dependence, and marijuana dependence with multiple detoxifications over the past 14 years. He was diagnosed with hypertension in 1992 and suffers from back pain secondary to a MVA in 1996. He had a positive PPD in 1994 and denies any other psychiatric illness.

Social History

MD has never been married and has no children. He currently lives with his mother, is unemployed, and has a girlfriend of 7 years. He has a long-term history of heroin use, alcohol use, and marijuana use, and he smokes 1 ppd (35 pack-year history).

Family History

Father committed suicide (mixed substance overdose). Mother has HTN and denies alcohol or illicit drug use.

Review of Systems

Negative except as noted previously

Physical Examination

GEN: Patient arousable but gives only one word answers, oriented to place, date was 1 year off, disheveled, poor hygiene

VS: (on admission) BP 145/92 mmHg, HR 94 bpm, T 100°F, RR 24 rpm, Wt 193 lb

HEENT: PERRLA, poor dentition, dry mucous membrane

CHEST: CTA bilaterally

ABD: Prominent scar down midline of abdomen (+) BS

EXT: 2+ radial pulse, 2+ dorsalis pedis pulse bilaterally, <2 sec capillary refill

Labs and Diagnostic Tests

Sodium 134 mEq/L	Potassium 4.0 mEq/L
Chloride 93 mEq/L	BUN 5 mg/dL
CO_2 content 23 mmol/L	Serum creatinine 0.5 mg/dL
Glucose 91 mg/dL	WBC 6800/mm³
Hct 41.4%	Hgb 13.7 g/dL
Platelets 241,000/mm³	Alk phos 85 U/L
SGPT 98 U/L	T. bili 0.8 mg/dL
GGT 170 U/L	SGOT 82 U/L
Amylase 43 U/L	EKG: Sinus tachycardia

Chest x-ray: Clear

Urine drug screen: (+)opiates, (+)THC, (-)alcohol

Diagnosis

Primary:

1. Heroin dependence

2. Heroin withdrawal

3. Alcohol dependence

4. Alcohol withdrawal

5. Marijuana dependence

Secondary:

1. Hypertension

2. Back pain

Case 36

Medication Record

Normal saline at 250 cc/h x1 L then, D$_5$ NS at 120 cc/h x3 L

Diazepam 5 mg 1 tab po prn q 6 h W/D sxs

Folic acid 1 mg po qd

Thiamine 100 mg po qd

Ranitidine 150 mg po q hs

Clonidine 0.1 mg q 6 h prn W/D sxs

Haloperidol 0.5-2.0 mg po/IM q 4 h prn agitation

Methadone 30 mg po stat

Ocean Nasal Spray 1-2 prn dry mucosa

Hydrochlorothiazide 25 mg qd

Pharmacist Notes and Other Patient Information

None available

Questions

1. Which of the following presenting symptoms is attributable to opioid withdrawal?
    I.   Auditory hallucinations
    II. Nausea and vomiting
    III. Diaphoresis
    A. I only
    B. III only
    C. I and II only
    D. II and III only
    E. I, II, and III

2. Withdrawal from which of the following substances is most likely to be deadly if untreated?
    A. Alcohol
    B. Haloperidol
    C. Heroin
    D. Marijuana
    E. Nicotine

3. Which of the following is FDA-approved for the treatment of opiate dependence?
    I.   Talwin
    II. Dolophine
    III. Subutex
    A. I only
    B. III only
    C. I and II only
    D. II and III only
    E. I, II, and III

4. Which of the following is NOT a sign of alcohol withdrawal?
    A. Diaphoresis
    B. Increased blood pressure and pulse
    C. Sedation
    D. Tremor
    E. Hyperthermia

5. MD is discharged to an outpatient methadone clinic, and you are the pharmacist. He is eventually tapered off of methadone, and the remainder of his prescription is returned to your pharmacy. How would you dispose of the remainder of his prescription?
    I.   The drug may be destroyed by two responsible parties employed or acting on behalf of the registrant when there are factors that preclude an onsite destruction witnessed by DEA personnel.
    II. The drug may be held until the DEA can witness the destruction of the substances.
    III. The drug may be forwarded to the appropriate state agency for destruction.
    A. I only
    B. III only
    C. I and II only
    D. II and III only
    E. I, II, and III

6. Which of the following adverse reactions is more common with haloperidol than olanzapine?
    I.   EPS
    II. Sedation
    III. Anticholinergic side effects
    A. I only
    B. III only
    C. I and II only
    D. II and III only
    E. I, II, and III

Case 36

7. Which benzodiazepine is most appropriate in a patient with hepatic failure because it has no active metabolites and is not oxidatively metabolized?

   A. Chlordiazepoxide
   B. Clonazepam
   C. Diazepam
   D. Lorazepam
   E. Quazepam

8. MD is receiving which of the following to prevent Wernicke-Korsakoff syndrome (a type of potentially irreversible brain/nerve damage)?

   A. D_5 NS
   B. Diazepam
   C. Folate
   D. Methadone
   E. Thiamine

9. Three months after discharge MD is undergoing methadone maintenance treatment and develops depression. Which of the following antidepressants is will result in increased methadone concentrations due to inhibition of CYP450 2D6?

   I. Mirtazapine
   II. Paroxetine
   III. Bupropion

   A. I only
   B. III only
   C. I and II only
   D. II and III only
   E. I, II, and III

10. Examples of nonmedication treatment strategies for substance dependence are:

   I. Alcoholics Anonymous.
   II. cognitive behavioral therapy.
   III. motivational enhancement therapy.

   A. I only
   B. III only
   C. I and II only
   D. II and III only
   E. I, II, and III

Patient Name: Blake Bennett
Address: 27 Hidden Valley Road
Age: 16   **Height:** 5' 3"
Sex: F   **Race:** White
Weight: 32 kg
Allergies: NKDA

Chief Complaint

BB is a 16-yo white female who came to the hospital with the following complaint: "My mother is making me do this." Her appearance is that of an extremely malnourished young woman.

History of Present Illness

BB began dieting at age 13. When she tried out for the cheerleading squad, one of the other girls had made a comment that she was "too fat to possibly make the team." From that point on her family noticed that BB picked at her food during mealtimes. Her diet consisted of primarily vegetables when she did eat, but many times she would go for a few days without joining the family for dinner. She started running on a daily basis and had taken to running long distances even when the family advised her to skip a day because of weather, cold, or their worries about exhaustion. BB has isolated herself for the past 6 months from both friends and family. She was elated when someone recently yelled at her when she was running, "look at the anorectic." In her assessment, it finally meant that she was skinny.

Past Medical History

Tonsillectomy at age 8

Fractured ulna at age 7

Social History

Denies alcohol and/or drugs

Mother is concerned about drugs because of recent declines in schoolwork and socialization

Family History

History of depression in mother, diabetes in maternal grandmother, and alcohol/drug use in the older brother. Father deceased from suicide approximately 3 years ago. One brother and one sister alive and well with no reported problems. BB is the second of four children.

Review of Systems

No complaints

Physical Examination

GEN: Pale, underdeveloped white female with significant weight loss, emaciated appearance with rough, scaly discolored skin

VS: BP 70/40 mmHg, HR 43 bpm, T 96°F, Ht 5' 3", Wt 70 lb, IBW 49 kg

HEENT: Fine, downy hair

GU: Amenorrhea for the past 6 months, minimal breast tissue

Mental status examination:

Appearance: 16-yo very thin, cachectic white female, disheveled with pale skin and thinning hair

Mood: Angry with irritability, suicidal ideation

Affect: Appropriate to mood

Sensorium: Oriented to person, place and time

Intellect: WNL

Insight: Denies a problem with weight or the need for treatment; refuses to attend outpatient eating disorder group

Thought content: Preoccupied with weight and fears of gaining weight in the hospital, no psychosis, hallucinations, or paranoia

Thought process: Slightly tangential WNL of age

Labs and Diagnostic Tests

Hgb 9 g/dL

Hct 30%

MCV 105 fL

Diagnosis

Primary:

1) Anorexia nervosa

Medication Record

Denies herbal use but mother reports Metabolife 356 in patient's possessions at home

Pharmacist Notes and Other Patient Information

None available

Case 37

Questions

1. Which of the following tests would be most appropriate to give you more information regarding the patient's condition at the time of admission?

   I.   Electrolytes
   II. Urine drug screen
   III. Estradiol concentration

   A. I only
   B. III only
   C. I and II only
   D. II and III only
   E. I, II, and III

2. At the patient's admitting weight, at what percentage of IBW is the patient currently (round to the closest whole number)?

   A. 60%
   B. 65%
   C. 70%
   D. 75%
   E. 80%

3. Which of the following over-the-counter products has been used for weight loss?

   I.   Emetine
   II. Ephedra
   III. Phenolphthalein

   A. I only
   B. III only
   C. I and II only
   D. II and III only
   E. I, II, and III

4. All of the following drugs have been used in the treatment of anorexia. Which of the following drugs is NOT approved by the FDA for the treatment of this disorder?

   I.   Desipramine
   II. Lithium
   III. Cyproheptadine

   A. I only
   B. III only
   C. I and II only
   D. II and III only
   E. I, II, and III

5. Which of the following patient characteristics qualifies the patient for inpatient treatment?

   I.   Weight loss of 30% or greater of IBW
   II. Denial of the need for help with the existence of electrolyte abnormalities
   III. Bradycardia

   A. I only
   B. III only
   C. I and II only
   D. II and III only
   E. I, II, and III

6. Given the patient's suicidal ideation and family history, the decision was made to start the patient on an antidepressant. Imipramine was chosen. Which of the following side effects of imipramine could be potentially fatal in this patient?

   I.   Sedation
   II. Constipation
   III. Cardiac arrhythmia

   A. I only
   B. III only
   C. I and II only
   D. II and III only
   E. I, II, and III

7. Which of the following may explain why patients with anorexia nervosa may not respond acutely to an SSRI, but patients with bulimia nervosa do?

   I.   Anorexia nervosa patients have too much serotonin and therefore the SSRI is unable to block the reuptake adequately, versus bulimia nervosa patients who have normal amounts of serotonin which can easily be blocked.
   II. Serotonin has not been shown to be involved in the pathogenesis of anorexia nervosa, but plays a role in bulimia nervosa.
   III. Anorexia nervosa patients have very low levels of serotonin versus bulimia nervosa patients. The SSRI will not work in this hypo-serotonergic state.

   A. I only
   B. III only
   C. I and II only
   D. II and III only
   E. I, II, and III

8. Many patients with anorexia nervosa have associated obsessive-compulsive features. When the obsessions and compulsions are not related to food, body shape, or weight, an additional diagnosis of OCD may be made. What would be the best antidepressant choice for the treatment of OCD in patients with a comorbid diagnosis of anorexia nervosa?

Case 37

A. Clomipramine
B. Fluvoxamine
C. Bupropion
D. Nefazodone
E. Amitriptyline

9. Medication use in anorexia will assist in which of the following parameters?

I. Comorbid obsessive-compulsive disorder
II. Improvement in mood
III. Maintenance of target weight

A. I only
B. III only
C. I and II only
D. II and III only
E. I, II, and III

10. The overall treatment goals of treating patients with anorexia nervosa include:

I. preventing relapse.
II. restoring healthy eating habits.
III. resolving physical complications.

A. I only
B. III only
C. I and II only
D. II and III only
E. I, II, and III

Patient Name: Leonard Ferrell
Address: 3802 W. 45th Street
Age: 29   **Height:** 5' 10"
Sex: M   **Race:** Caucasian
Weight: 86.5 kg
Allergies: NKDA

Chief Complaint

LF is a 29-yo married man who is being evaluated by psychiatric emergency services after trying to assault his wife. He states, "She would not let me arrange the plants and furniture. So I got mad and tried to hit her." Although LF has had obsessive-compulsive behaviors for several years, he states that recently, he has been hearing voices telling him to arrange the plants and furniture.

History of Present Illness

LF says that he gets stressed when the house does not look organized. "My wife just does not understand. There needs to be order to this world, and it begins in my house." In the past few months, his obsessions have focused around being organized, particularly organizing items in his house. He believes there is a certain order in which the furniture and plants in the house should be set. If it is not set up accordingly, LF feels that chaos will result and his household will fall apart. Subsequently, he spends several hours each night moving the furniture and plants in the living room area. Although he is rarely satisfied with the finished arrangement, he becomes exhausted and eventually falls asleep.

Over the last month, LF reports that he has been hearing the voice of an older man, whom he believes to be his late father. The voice repeatedly tells him that the arrangement of the furniture and plants is not satisfactory and needs to be redone. LF states that because of the voice telling him to do so, he is more determined to reorganize. He feels that if he does not do as the voice says to, there will be serious consequences.

His wife has become increasingly worried about LF's behaviors and says that "his obsessions and compulsions have become so bad that their marriage is about to break up." He states that he was taking fluoxetine (maximum of 60 mg/day), which was prescribed by his primary care physician (Dr. Humphries), for almost 3 years. The beneficial effects "wore off," and he stopped taking the medication one year ago. LF says that he took sertraline 100 mg/day for approximately 6 months, which was prescribed by his psychiatrist (Dr. Becker). He stopped taking sertraline 2 months ago as he did not like the side effects, namely, a decrease in his sexual libido and delayed ejaculation.

Dr. Becker was also providing psychotherapy for his OCD, but he did not feel that he gained much from the visits and thus stopped seeing her 2 months ago.

Past Medical History

LF was diagnosed with OCD approximately 4 years ago. He states that initially, his obsessive-compulsive behaviors were restricted primarily to ritualistic hand washing. As the years passed, he found himself engaging in other odd behaviors, such as checking his door locks a number of times before going to bed. Several months ago, he found the need to rearrange things on a daily basis, primarily plants and furniture around the house. More recently, LF states that voices in his head tell him to organize the plants and furniture each day. His wife states that his OCD is disrupting their marriage, and she tries to stop him on occasion. When she attempts to do so, he becomes increasingly agitated and sometimes becomes violent. Medical records from his primary care physician showed that he has a history of anxiety, which resolved with fluoxetine in the past. There are no prior psychiatric hospitalizations. Most recently, he has received treatment at an outpatient psychiatric clinic. LF's medical history is positive for HTN that was diagnosed 1 year ago. His HTN is controlled by hydrochlorothiazide. The remainder of his history is unremarkable.

Social History

LF was born and raised in a small town in Texas. He is the younger of two children, which include his 31-yo sister. As a child, LF was very organized with his schoolwork and performed very well. He was a straight "A" student throughout his high school and undergraduate college years. LF recently was awarded a doctorate in business administration. He married his wife 5 years ago. They do not have any children and do not plan to have any for several more years. LF denies any physical, sexual, or emotional abuse when he was a child or adolescent. He has worked for a marketing firm for the past 2 years in a management position. LF had emotional difficulties when his father passed away last year but has since been able to cope and move on with his life. He denies any alcohol, tobacco, or illicit drug use.

Family History

Father died of acute myocardial infarction at age 64. Mother, who is 65 and has mild Alzheimer's disease, lives in an assisted living facility. Sister, who is 31 years old, has HTN and DM, both controlled pharmacologically.

Review of Systems

He reports a recent onset of auditory hallucinations commanding him to rearrange his plants and furniture; complains of occasional tension headaches (one every 2-3 months), with no visual changes (aura); no changes in appetite, changes in sleep patterns; no cough, dyspnea, chest pain, or edema; no constipation, diarrhea, or abnormal stools; no dysuria or nocturia.

Case 38

Physical Examination

GEN: Alert, cooperative male in NAD, oriented x3

VS: BP 134/83 mmHg, P 78 bpm, RR 20 rpm, T 98.6°F, Wt 86.5 kg

HEENT: PERRLA, EOMI, normal fundi, TMs clear, nares clear, pharynx WNL

CHEST: Breath sounds clear throughout

NEURO: No localizing signs, negative Babinski and Romberg, DTRs active and equal bilaterally

Labs and Diagnostic Tests

Sodium 140 mEq/L	Potassium 4.2 mEq/L
Chloride 108 mEq/L	CO_2 content 25 mEq/L
BUN 16 mg/dL	Serum creatinine 0.8 mg/dL
Glucose 80 mg/dL	Hgb 17.3 g/dL
Hct 49.5%	Platelets 258 x 103/mm³
WBC 8.0 x 103/mm³	TSH 1.64 µIU/mL

Urinalysis: Color yellow, appearance clear, (-) glucose, (-) bili, (-) ketones, specific gravity 1.02, (-) blood, (-) urobilinogen, (-) nitrite, (-) leukocyte esterase

EKG: NL sinus rhythm, unremarkable

CXR: NL CXR, unremarkable

Diagnosis

Primary diagnoses:

1. Obsessive-compulsive disorder (OCD)

2. Psychotic disorder, not otherwise specified (NOS)

3. Hypertension (HTN)

Medication Record

(Medication record compiled by patient's wife.)

Date	Rx No	Physician	Drug and Strength	Quantity	Sig	Refills
6/01-2/02		Humphries	Fluoxetine 20	30	1qd	3
2/02-7/02		Humphries	Fluoxetine 20	60	2 q am	3
7/02-2/04		Humphries	Fluoxetine 20	90	3 q am	2
8/04-1/05		Becker	Sertraline 50	30	1 q am	3
1/05-2/05		Becker	Sertraline 100	30	1 q am	0
2/05-7/05		Becker	Sertraline 100	30	1 q am	0
2/05-7/05		Becker	Sertraline 100	45	1 1/2 q am	1
7/05		Becker	Sertraline 100	30	1 q am	1

Pharmacist Notes and Other Patient Information

Based upon prescription history, it is likely that this patient is non-compliant with his medications. Patient may be noncompliant with medications as his insight into his illness is poor. He feels his obsessive-compulsive behaviors are justified and it is his obligation to fulfill his needs.

Questions

1. Which of the following is used in making a diagnosis of obsessive-compulsive disorder (OCD)?

    A. Covi Anxiety Scale

    B. Brief Psychiatric Rating Scale (BPRS)

    C. Hamilton Anxiety Rating Scale (HAM-A)

    D. Diagnostic and Statistical Manual of Mental Disorders, Fourth Edition, Text Revision (DSM-IV-TR)

    E. Simpson-Angus Scale

2. In LF's case, what symptoms are present that indicate a diagnosis of OCD?

    I. Aggression

    II. Auditory hallucinations

    III. Obsessions and compulsions

    A. I only

    B. III only

    C. I and II only

    D. II and III only

    E. I, II, and III

3. Which of the following medications would be considered an appropriate first-line agent for the treatment of OCD?

    I. Fluvoxamine

    II. Buspirone

    III. Nefazodone

A. I only
B. III only
C. I and II only
D. II and III only
E. I, II, and III

4. Identify the INCORRECT recommended starting dose in OCD for the following medications.

   A. Clomipramine: 25 mg
   B. Fluoxetine: 20 mg
   C. Paroxetine: 40 mg
   D. Fluvoxamine: 50 mg
   E. Sertraline: 50 mg

5. After LF is seen by the psychiatry emergency services physician, it is determined that the patient be initiated on paroxetine. You are the pharmacist at the pharmacy where LF's wife fills his prescriptions. She is concerned that paroxetine will not work as well as fluoxetine did in the past. She would like some information about paroxetine and its use in OCD. All the following are part of your discussion with her EXCEPT:

   A. it may take 10-12 weeks for the paroxetine to work.
   B. individuals with OCD usually respond to lower doses of paroxetine than individuals with major depression.
   C. paroxetine and fluoxetine are thought to work in a similar fashion.
   D. paroxetine has been shown to be an effective medication for patients with OCD and is FDA-approved medication for the treatment of OCD.
   E. paroxetine has a similar side effect profile to that of fluoxetine.

6. LF has been taking paroxetine for 4 months and just last month it was increased to 60 mg/day. Dr. Becker calls in a new prescription to the pharmacy today for paroxetine 40 mg/day. After reviewing LF's profile, you call Dr. Becker back to verify the dose and she confirms the need for a dose decrease. When asked why, she states "because of side effects." Which of the following is not a common side effect related to paroxetine?

   I. Increase in diastolic blood pressure
   II. Nausea
   III. Sexual dysfunction

   A. I only
   B. III only
   C. I and II only
   D. II and III only
   E. I, II, and III

7. LF continues to have side effects from the paroxetine, and Dr. Becker considers using fluoxetine again. She asks you about the generic substitutes available for fluoxetine.

Specifically, she wants to know whether or not the generic fluoxetine is the same as the brand name (Prozac). All of the following regarding generic drugs are true EXCEPT:

   A. generic drugs are bioequivalent to the brand name drugs.
   B. generic drugs do not have to contain the same inactive ingredients as the brand name drugs.
   C. generic drugs must be identical to the brand name drugs in dosage form and route of administration, but can come in varied strengths.
   D. generic drugs must have the same use indications as the brand name drugs.
   E. generic drugs must have similar pharmacokinetic profiles as the brand name drugs.

8. Dr. Becker calls you and says that LF's serum sodium concentrations have dropped. She wants to know whether any cases of hyponatremia with fluoxetine have been reported. Which of the following resources would help you identify whether or not fluoxetine caused hyponatremia?

   I. MEDLINE
   II. Facts and Comparisons
   III. Micromedex

   A. I only
   B. III only
   C. I and II only
   D. II and III only
   E. I, II, and III

9. After several months on the fluoxetine, LF continues to complain of auditory hallucinations. Dr. Becker determines that LF needs antipsychotic therapy. Which of the following agents would be the best choice for LF's case?

   A. Haloperidol
   B. Thioridazine
   C. Clozapine
   D. Risperidone
   E. Buspirone

10. Which of the following CYP P450 enzyme systems are responsible for the drug-drug interaction between risperidone and fluoxetine?

   I. CYP2D6
   II. CYP1A2
   III. CYP2C19

   A. I only
   B. III only
   C. I and II only
   D. II and III only
   E. I, II, and III

Patient Name: Richard McWilliams
Address: 1631 E. Second Street
Age: 43   Height: 5' 9"
Sex: M   Race: African American
Weight: 237 lb
Allergies: NKDA

Chief Complaint

RMcW reports recent recurrence of command auditory hallucinations and feelings of paranoia.

History of Present Illness

RMcW was admitted to the acute psychiatry inpatient unit after presenting to the outpatient mental health clinic complaining of bothersome auditory hallucinations and paranoid delusions.

His symptoms take the form of several male voices criticizing him and a feeling that unknown people are plotting to harm him, progressive disorganization of his thought processing, deterioration in self care, social isolation and withdrawal, and restlessness advancing to agitation.

He has been prescribed olanzapine 20 mg q HS; but has episodes of non-adherence to treatment due to side effects of daytime sedation and weight gain. Most of the time he can be convinced to start back on his med; but some episodes progress to serious loss of insight and judgment with thoughts of wanting to end his life and threatening behavior toward others requiring rehospitalization.

Past Medical History

RMcW had the onset of his symptoms around age 20; and was hospitalized for several weeks on an acute care psychiatric unit until his symptoms were brought under control with haloperidol 20 mg q HS and benztropine 1 mg BID to prevent extrapyramidal side effects.

He had occasional episodes of medication non-adherence with rapid recurrence of psychotic symptoms requiring rehospitalization until his treatment was changed to haloperidol decanoate 100 mg IM q 4 weeks.

About 8 years ago, after taking haloperidol for 15 years, he started showing signs of tardive dyskinesia; and his treatment was changed to olanzapine 20 mg q HS. The signs of dyskinesia resolved; but the patient again had occasional problems with non-adherence, rapid return of symptoms and resulting rehospitalization.

In the years since being on olanzapine his fasting blood glucose, serum cholesterol, triglycerides, and LDL have become increasingly elevated. As his weight increased he also developed hypertension; and has attempted unsuccessfully many times to modify his diet and be consistent with regular physical exercise.

Social History

Patient graduated high school and attended college for 2 years prior to the onset of his symptoms; and he has never been able to complete his higher education or train for a vocation due to the deterioration in his cognitive functioning.

He has never been married, but is heterosexual in orientation; and has been involved in several significant relationships over the years with women he has met while hospitalized.

He receives Social Security Disability income, Medicare, and Medicaid due to his psychiatric disability, and lives in his own apartment supported by Section 8 housing.

He has no history for abuse of drugs or alcohol, and no arrests or warrants for any problem with the law, except for peace officer's emergency commitments to psychiatric facilities when decompensated.

Both parents are alive and well, and he has two older brothers and a younger sister, all of whom are emotionally supportive of the patient.

Family History

Three siblings without medical or psychiatric problem. Both parents have HTN, father developed type II diabetes at age 47. No known relatives with psychiatric or substance abuse disorder, learning disability or mental retardation.

Review of Systems

Hypertension, hypercholesterolemia, obesity, hyperglycemia.

Physical Examination

(Patient has appointment in primary care clinic where he is followed for hypercholesterolemia and HTN)

VS: BP 180/95 mmHg, P 76 bpm, RR 22 rpm, BMI 35.

Mental Status Examination: 43-yo African American male who appears a little older than stated age, noticeably overweight, dressed in hospital pajamas, hair is uncombed, and he is unshaven. Poor eye contact, but cooperative with interview.

Mood: Uncomfortable, dysphoric.

Affect: Tense, anxious.

Psychomotor activity: Restless, paces the floor.

Cognitive function: Oriented to person and location only; states he does not know why he was brought to the hospital.

Thought process: Mildly tangential, appears distracted. Clear, coherent speech, not pressured.

Thought content: Reports hearing a single male voice saying

Case 39

that pt. is going to die and pressuring him to harm himself. Describes feeling extremely fearful due to "being watched" and followed by "bad people." Poor insight. Judgment impaired secondary to nonadherence to medication. Concrete interpretation of proverbs.

Labs and Diagnostic Tests

CBC-WNL, EKG-normal sinus rhythm, normal QT$_c$ interval, Lipid profile: cholesterol-275, triglycerides-360, HDL-35, LDL-140, Chem 14: FBS-120, all the rest-WNL, TFT's-WNL, toxicology screen-negative.

Diagnosis

Axis 1: Schizophrenia, paranoid type

    Noncompliance with treatment

    History of neuroleptic induced tardive dyskinesia - resolved

Axis 2: No diagnosis

Axis 3: Hypercholesterolemia

    Hypertension

    Obesity

    Hyperglycemia

Axis 4: Occupational problems - unemployed

Axis 5: GAF 40

Medication Record

Olanzapine 20 mg q HS

Pharmacist Notes and Other Patient Information

Hospital course: Olanzapine discontinued due to daytime sedation, weight gain, and metabolic abnormalities.

Risperidone started to see if it would control patient's symptoms and cause minimal side effects with intention of having patient start injections q 2 weeks of Risperdal Consta to address medication adherence problem.

Pt. saw his primary care physician in clinic, and enalapril 10 mg q AM started for hypertension, and atorvastatin 10 mg q HS started for hypercholesterolemia.

Nutrition consult to teach patient how to establish a reduced calorie diet, and physical rehabilitation started for weight loss exercise program to be continued as an outpatient.

Questions

1. A potentially life-threatening condition termed neuroleptic malignant syndrome can occur when treating a patient with an antipsychotic medication; and includes the following signs and symptoms EXCEPT:

    A. muscle rigidity and elevated CPK.
    B. fever and dehydration.
    C. leukopenia.
    D. tachycardia and labile or elevated blood pressure.
    E. diaphoresis, tremor.

2. Risperdal Consta for injection q 2 weeks is commercially available in which of the following doses?

    I.   25 mg
    II. 37.5 mg
    III. 50 mg

    A. I only
    B. III only
    C. I and II only
    D. II and III only
    E. I, II, and III

3. Which of the following instruments is used to assess degree of symptoms in individuals with schizophrenia?

    A. YBOCS
    B. Positive and Negative Symptom Scales (PANSS)
    C. Abnormal Involuntary Movement Scale (AIMS)
    D. Barnes Akathisia Scale
    E. Global Assessment of Functioning (GAF)

4. Risperidone was prescribed for RMcW. Which of the following counseling information should he receive?

    I.   Risperidone can cause dizziness and even syncope on changing position suddenly.
    II. Risperidone may be taken either with or without food.
    III. White blood cell counts must be measured on a weekly basis.

    A. I only
    B. III only
    C. I and II only
    D. II and III only
    E. I, II, and III

5. Common herbal preparations that have been implicated or associated with psychotic symptoms that can appear like schizophrenia include the following EXCEPT:

    A. periwinkle.
    B. kava-kava.
    C. Ma Huang.

Case 39

D.   mandrake.

E.   Rauwolfia serpentine.

6.   Which of the following strategies might be useful to improve medication adherence in RMcW?

   I.   Change to a long-acting depot antipsychotic medication.
   II. Change to an antipsychotic medication that causes fewer side effects.
   III. Change to an every other day regimen.

   A.   I only
   B.   III only
   C.   I and II only
   D.   II and III only
   E.   I, II, and III

7.   The brand name for ziprasidone is:

   A.   Risperdal.
   B.   Zyprexa.
   C.   Seroquel.
   D.   Geodon.
   E.   Clozaril.

8.   Negative symptoms of schizophrenia noted in RMcW's record are:

   A.   social withdrawal.
   B.   paranoid delusions.
   C.   disorganized thought process.
   D.   visual hallucinations.
   E.   auditory hallucinations.

9.   Patients with schizophrenia should be educated from the onset of antipsychotic medication treatment about nutrition, regular physical exercise, and proper medical care, since both schizophrenia and antipsychotic medications are associated with significantly increased risks for which of the following?

   I.   Gastrointestinal disorders
   II. Diabetes, obesity, and hyperlipidemia
   III. Cardiovascular disease and metabolic syndrome

   A.   I only
   B.   III only
   C.   I and II only
   D.   II and III only
   E.   I, II, and III

10. Four months after discharge on risperidone with change to IM Risperdal Consta, RMcW is diagnosed with depression and treated with paroxetine controlled release 25 mg qd. Three weeks later RMcW is brought back to the clinic because he is sleepy all day, dizzy when he stands, restless, and has muscle stiffness. The most likely explanation for these symptoms is:

   A.   inhibition of CYP 2D6 by paroxetine.
   B.   induction of CYP 2C9 by paroxetine.
   C.   inhibition of CYP 2D6 by risperidone.
   D.   induction of CYP 1A2 by risperidone.
   E.   inhibition of CYP 3A4 by paroxetine.

Neurological Disorders

Section Editor: Teresa Hudson

See all 12 cases for this section on the CD.

Patient Name: Ruby Matlock
Address: 123 Sunrise Drive
Age: 70   **Height:** 5' 4"
Sex: F   **Race:** White
Weight: 135 lb
Allergies: None

Chief Complaint

RM is a 70-yo white female brought to the clinic by her daughter for evaluation for Alzheimer's disease. Yesterday, when her daughter went to check on RM, she found her trying to heat food in a plastic container on the gas stove.

History of Present Illness

RM's daughter reports that during the past 5 years, RM has become increasingly forgetful. About 2 years ago she started having so much difficulty with her checkbook that her daughter had to start managing RM's finances. In the past 12-18 months RM has had a great deal of difficulty taking her medication correctly. Three months ago she had an episode of confusion associated with a urinary tract infection.

Past Medical History

Limited information is available regarding past psychiatric history. According to the daughter, RM was treated with some kind of antidepressant 1 year ago after her husband died. Other health problems include hypertension, type 2 diabetes mellitus, atrial fibrillation, hypothyroidism, osteoarthritis, osteoporosis and vitamin B_{12} deficiency.

Social History

Tobacco use: none

Alcohol use: none

Illicit drug use: none

Patient has had a high school education and 2 years of community college. She worked as an administrative assistant. Patient lives alone. She has 2 children.

Family History

Both of RM's parents are deceased. RM's daughter reports that she does not know much about RM's family, but one of RM's sisters was in a nursing home because she was too senile to care for herself.

Review of Systems

Negative except as noted previously

Physical Examination

VS: BP 154/87 mmHg, HR 72 bpm, RR 19 rpm, Ht 5'4", Wt 135 lb

EXT: Enlarged joints of her hands

Mini Mental State Examination: 22/30 correct (probably mild dementia), Geriatric Depression Scale is 8/30 (normal but some depressive symptoms).

The patient is a WD, thin white female in NAD. She knows the approximate time and the day of the week. When asked where she is, she cannot name the clinic but knows she is at the doctor's office. She maintains good eye contact. There is no psychomotor agitation or retardation. Speech is normal tone and pressure. Thought content contains no suicidal or homicidal ideation, with no auditory or visual hallucinations. Patient has the delusion that when she watches TV, the people on the TV can see and talk with her. She describes her mood as fine; and her affect is appropriate. Patient displays fair judgment in that she did attend today's appointment. However, her insight is impaired because she does not feel she has any problems and says she does not know why her daughter insisted she come to the clinic today. When asked about her hobbies and free time activities, she says she used to knit sweaters and hats but cannot do it anymore.

Labs and Diagnostic Tests

(performed 8/12)

Na 130 mEq/L	K 4.3 mEq/L
Ca 9.2 mg/dL	SCr 1.2 mg/dL
BUN 7 mg/dL	Glucose 144 mg/dL
LFTs WNL	CBC/differential WNL
INR 2.5	Hb_{A1c} 7
Ferritin 50 ng/mL	ESR 11 cc/h
Folic acid 340 ng/mL	Vitamin B_{12} 377 pg/mL
RPR nonreactive	

Diagnosis

Axis I: Alzheimer's disease

Axis II: None

Axis III: Osteoporosis, isolated systolic hypertension, atrial fibrillation, type 2 diabetes mellitus, hypothyroidism, osteoarthritis, vitamin B_{12} deficiency

Axis IV: Difficulty living alone

Case 40

Medication Record

Date	Rx No	Physician	Drug and Strength	Quantity	Sig	Refills
7/10	98765	Cody	Levothyroxine 0.1 mg	30	1 qd	3
7/10	98766	Cody	Alendronate 70 mg	4	1 weekly	3
7/10	98768	Cody	Vitamin B$_{12}$ 1 mg	30	1 qd	3
7/30	98926	Cody	Acetaminophen 500 mg	90	1-2 po tid prn pain	2
7/30	98777	Cody	Hydrochlorothiazide 25 mg	30	1 in AM	3
7/30	98761	Cody	Glyburide 5 mg daily	30	1 in AM	2
7/30	98778	Cody	Warfarin 7 mg	31	1 in PM	1

Pharmacist Notes and Other Patient Information

None available

Questions

1. RM was evaluated for dementia, which included drawing a vitamin B$_{12}$ concentration, RBC folate, ferritin, syphilis screen, erythrocyte sedimentation rate, complete blood count, and complete chemistries. This was done because:

    A. symptoms of dementia can be seen in individuals with certain diseases such as hyperthyroidism, hypothyroidism, vitamin deficiencies, and neurosyphilis.
    B. these tests can be used as a screening test for patients with treatable versus nontreatable dementia.
    C. these are baseline measurements done before placing the patient on an acetylcholinesterase inhibitor.
    D. these tests are markers for patients at risk for vascular dementia which has different treatments from Alzheimer's disease.
    E. these tests can be used as prognostic indicators for patients with Alzheimer's disease.

2. The health professional who is most likely to provide current information about services, placement, and respite care for patients with dementia is:

    A. an occupational therapist.
    B. a social worker.
    C. a physical therapist.
    D. a neuropsychologist.
    E. a physician.

3. During the work-up of RM, a magnetic resonance imaging (MRI) scan of her head is done to look for infarcts which can cause vascular dementia. An important risk factor for vascular dementia in this patient is:

    A. osteoarthritis.
    B. uncontrolled hypertension.
    C. hypothyroidism.
    D. family history.
    E. female gender.

4. Current hypotheses for the etiology of Alzheimer's disease include which of the following?

    I. Alzheimer's disease is a natural part of the aging process, not a pathologic process.
    II. Depletion of brain cholesterol results in neuronal damage and disease progression.
    III. Alzheimer's disease results from the accumulation of beta-amyloid causing neuronal damage.

    A. I only
    B. III only
    C. I and II only
    D. II and III only
    E. I, II, and III

5. When considering the use of acetylcholinesterase inhibitors for Alzheimer's disease it is important to consider warnings. These include:

    I. asthma and COPD.
    II. peptic ulcer disease.
    III. heart block.

    A. I only
    B. III only
    C. I and II only
    D. II and III only
    E. I, II, and III

6. RM's physician would like to prescribe a medication to treat Alzheimer's disease. You would recommend:

    A. tacrine (Cognex) 10 mg 1 po qid.
    B. donepezil (Aricept) 5 mg 1 po daily.
    C. rivastigmine (Exelon) 3 mg 1 po bid.
    D. galantamine (Razadyne) 8 mg 1 po bid.
    E. memantine (Namenda) 5 mg daily.

Case 40

7. RM's daughter tells the nurses that she heard use of several other medications or vitamins may be helpful in decreasing the progression of Alzheimer's disease and is interested in trying these therapies. Which of the following is appropriate information for the pharmacist to provide to the daughter and the nurses?

 I. Nonsteroidal anti-inflammatory agents have been associated with a reduced likelihood of developing Alzheimer's disease, but these agents may cause gastrointestinal bleeding, renal impairment, hypertension, and fluid retention.

 II. Estrogens were once thought to have been associated with improvement in cognitive function; clinical trial data have so far shown an increased risk of dementia in patients who already have Alzheimer's disease.

 III. Vitamin E, at a dose of 1000 IU bid, has been shown to improve cognition in controlled clinical trials.

 A. I only
 B. III only
 C. I and II only
 D. II and III only
 E. I, II, and III

8. RM's daughter would like to know if starting donepezil earlier would have been helpful. A recent randomized trial evaluated the benefit of starting donepezil 10 mg daily in mild cognitive dysfunction. Mild cognitive dysfunction is a state of impaired cognition that is believed to precede development of Alzheimer's disease in some patients. In this study, after 24 months of therapy, the hazard ratio for donepezil compared to placebo was 0.64, 95% confidence interval 0.44-0.95 and p = 0.03. There was no benefit found at 3 years. The Mini-Mental State Examination (MMSE, a 30-point scale with higher scores indicating better function) showed a change in score from baseline of -0.98 compared to the change seen with placebo of -1.49. Which of the following is the most appropriate interpretation of these results?

 A. 6-24 month results are not important since there is no benefit at 36 months

 B. The results are controversial; donepezil delays progression to Alzheimer's disease over at least 2 years though the benefit when measured by specific cognitive testing is small

 C. At 24 months, patients on donepezil had a MMSE score one point higher than patients on placebo

 D. A p-value of 0.03 means that 3/100 patients benefit from donepezil

 E. A hazard ratio of 0.64 means that patients are 64% less likely to develop Alzheimer's disease when taking donepezil

9. RM had a urinary tract infection and became markedly more confused. You would call her confusion:

 I. delirium.
 II. depression.
 III. worsening of dementia.

 A. I only
 B. III only
 C. I and II only
 D. II and III only
 E. I, II, and III

10. Three days later RM's daughter calls. RM is taking donepezil (Aricept) 5 mg qd. RM has developed nausea and vomiting. The daughter is very concerned. You recommend:

 A. no change in the medication regimen because nausea and vomiting are a transient problem; you still plan to increase her dose to 10 mg after 6 weeks to maximize benefit.

 B. she stops donepezil and avoids use of acetylcholinesterase inhibitors.

 C. she stops donepezil and, after she feels better, initiates therapy with either rivastigmine or galantamine.

 D. she changes to a liquid formulation of rivastigmine or galantamine; donepezil has no liquid formulation.

 E. no change in the medication regimen; nausea and vomiting are not known side effects of acetylcholinesterase inhibitors.

Case 41

Patient Name: Greg Smith
Address: 4343 Woodrow Court
Age: 48   **Height:** 6' 1"
Sex: M   **Race:** White
Weight: 176 lb
Allergies: Penicillin, rash; codeine, itching

Chief Complaint

GS is a 48-yo male who is currently in the postoperative recovery room following a splenectomy and fixation of his fractures. He is complaining of abdominal pain and pain in his fractured areas with a verbal pain intensity score of 9 out of 10.

History of Present Illness

GS was involved in an MVA in which he sustained multiple fractures (a fracture of his right collar bone, two right ribs, right tibia, and an open [compound] fracture of his left ankle) as well as a ruptured spleen.

Past Medical History

GS' PMH is significant for depression, of which he was diagnosed approximately 1 year ago and has been in ongoing counseling since that time. He also has a history of mild renal insufficiency from polycystic kidney disease and a history of seasonal allergies that are controlled with antihistamines and steroid inhalers. He is currently not on any medication for his allergies.

Social History

Tobacco use: none

Alcohol use: social, approximately 3 servings of beer/week

Caffeine use: 1-2 cups of coffee daily, occasional soft drinks

Family History

Father, age 75, recent MI

Mother, age 70, polycystic kidney disease, kidney transplant 14 years ago

Review of Systems

Complaining of severe pain in chest, right upper extremity, and left lower extremity

Physical Examination

GEN: WD male, slightly sedated but agitated

VS: BP 90/60 mmHg, HR 120 bpm, RR 30 rpm, T 99.0°F, Wt 80 kg

HEENT: PERRLA, multiple small lacerations on right forehead

CHEST: Clear to auscultation and percussion, collar-bone tender to touch

ABD: Soft, ND, incision tender to touch

EXT: Grade I fracture of R ulna, grade II fracture L tibia

NEURO: Alert and oriented x3

Labs and Diagnostic Tests

Sodium 135 mEq/L	Potassium 4.1 mEq/L
Chloride 101 mEq/L	CO_2 content 25 mEq/L
BUN 41 mg/dL	Serum creatinine 2.4 mg/dL
Glucose 120 mg/dL	WBC 11 000/mm³
Platelets 353,000/mm³	Hgb 14.1 g/dL
Hct 31.1%	PT 18.2 sec
INR 1.8	PaO_2 95
$PaCO_2$ 30	pH 7.45

CXR: Fractured collar bone, no puncture to the lung

UE XR: Grade I fracture R ulna

LE XR: Grade II fracture L tibia

Diagnosis

Primary:

     1. Multitrauma with multiple fractures

     2. S/P splenectomy

Medication Record

(prior to admission)

Prozac 20 mg qd po

(hospital orders)

3/1, ED, Morphine 15 mg IVP x1 at 11:00 PM

3/1, ED, Cefazolin 1g IVPB x1 at 11:00 PM

3/1, ED, Metronidazole 500 mg IVPB x1 at 11:00 PM

3/1, OR, Propofol IV infusion at 11:00 PM

3/1, OR, Fentanyl IV infusion at 11:00 PM

3/2, PACU, Morphine 5 mg IVP x1 at 4:00 AM

Case 41

Pharmacist Notes and Other Patient Information

None available

Questions

1. Which of the following modalities is most appropriate for the initial analgesic approach for this patient?

   I.   Intermittent IM morphine q 6 h prn
   II. Epidural analgesia with morphine
   III. Intravenous patient-controlled analgesia with morphine

   A. I only
   B. III only
   C. I and II only
   D. II and III only
   E. I, II, and III

2. When evaluating the best dose of morphine for GS, you would consider which of the following?

   I.   An initial dose should be calculated on a mg/kg basis because weight is the most important parameter in determining dose.
   II. The manufacturer's maximum recommended dose/day is 200 mg of IV morphine.
   III. After a loading dose to comfort, an appropriate initial PCA regimen would be morphine IV 1 mg bolus, 10-minute lockout interval.

   A. I only
   B. III only
   C. I and II only
   D. II and III only
   E. I, II, and III

3. Which of the following medications is the best selection for this patient's multiple bone fractures and abdominal pain?

   A. Meperidine
   B. Ketorolac
   C. Codeine
   D. Hydromorphone
   E. Ibuprofen

4. Two weeks after his accident, GS is tolerating food and the physicians would like to convert his pain medications to an oral regimen. On review of his medication profile, his consumption of analgesic is equivalent to 60 mg IV morphine over a 24-hour period. Based on this information, which of the following is an equivalent conversion to an oral regimen?

   I.   15 mg morphine po q 6 h prn
   II. 5 mg oxycodone po q 6 h prn
   III. 30 mg morphine po q 4 h prn

   A. I only
   B. III only
   C. I and II only
   D. II and III only
   E. I, II, and III

5. Of all the listed regimens, which of the products is available in an immediate release tablet formulation in the exact size of the dose being prescribed?

   I.   15 mg morphine po q 6 h prn
   II. 5 mg oxycodone po q 6 h prn
   III. 30 mg morphine po q 4 h prn

   A. I only
   B. III only
   C. I and II only
   D. II and III only
   E. I, II, and III

6. When GS is discharged, you will be asked to counsel him on the use of his analgesics, which will include an opioid analgesic. Which of the listed information is true to explain to GS?

   I.   This type of medication will likely cause constipation and often a laxative will be required to maintain regularity.
   II. Acetaminophen may be taken with opioid analgesics and may provide further analgesic efficacy, although you should generally not exceed 4 g/day.
   III. Promethazine is an anti-nausea medication that may be used to potentiate the analgesic effects of the opioid analgesics.

   A. I only
   B. III only
   C. I and II only
   D. II and III only
   E. I, II, and III

7. The mechanism by which opioid analgesics are believed to provide analgesic activity is:

   I.   via opioid receptors in the brain.
   II. via opioid receptors in the spinal column.
   III. direct action on serotonin receptors in the spinal cord and periphery.

   A. I only
   B. III only
   C. I and II only
   D. II and III only
   E. I, II, and III

Case 41

8. A morphine PCA was ordered. When the pharmacy made the syringe to be administered through the PCA device, 0.6 mL of a 50-mg/mL morphine solution is diluted with sterile normal saline to a total volume of 30 mL. What was the final morphine concentration in the syringe?

    A. 1 mg/mL
    B. 2 mg/mL
    C. 3 mg/mL
    D. 5 mg/mL
    E. 10 mg/mL

9. On GS' discharge, a family member comments that narcotics are dangerous and wants to know the risk of GS becoming addicted. As you counsel this family member about GS' medication, you explain that opioid analgesics are used to treat pain and that psychologic dependence (addiction) develops in what percentage of patients?

    A. 50 percent
    B. 40 percent
    C. 25 percent
    D. 10 percent
    E. <1 percent

10. Which of the following is true regarding the use of NSAIDs in GS?

    I.   NSAIDs may be very beneficial in pain associated with fractures.
    II.   All NSAIDs may negatively affect GS's renal function and should be used with caution, if at all.
    III. NSAIDs may provide additive analgesic activity when used in combination with opioid analgesics.

    A. I only
    B. III only
    C. I and II only
    D. II and III only
    E. I, II, and III

Case 42

Patient Name: Starbuck Jones
Address: 2005 Linda Avenue
Age: 63   **Height:** 5' 8"
Sex: M   **Race:** White
Weight: 170 lb
Allergies: NKDA

Chief Complaint

SJ is a 63-yo male with Parkinson's disease who reports feeling moderately nauseated after each dose of carbidopa/levodopa. Other than the nausea, he feels fine. SJ is also requesting information on the drug amantadine, which he heard is useful for Parkinson's disease.

History of Present Illness

SJ was diagnosed with Parkinson's disease about 3 years ago and has been maintained on trihexyphenidyl and ropinirole with good effect. On examination, SJ's signs and symptoms include moderate rest tremor; lack of arm swing; a slow, shuffling gait; micrographia; difficulty arising from a chair from sitting to standing; and moderate rigidity of the lower and upper extremities. The signs and symptoms affect both sides of his body but his right side more than his left. SJ is an avid golfer and also reports that his golf game has progressively deteriorated over the past several months (more so than when he was first diagnosed). His wife also reports that SJ had become increasingly "clumsy" and that because SJ takes "forever to get dressed in the mornings," they have been late for church services on several occasions. Despite treatment with the trihexyphenidyl and ropinirole at maximally tolerated doses, SJ's signs and symptoms are worsening and are having a negative impact on the couple's quality of life. Therefore, SJ was initiated on carbidopa/levodopa 10/100 mg po qd, which was titrated to 10/100 mg po tid over 3 weeks. SJ has been on the 10/100 mg tid regimen for 1 week now.

Past Medical History

1) Parkinson's disease

Social History

Occupation: retired, formerly an auctioneer

Martial status: married with two grown children

Tobacco use: none

Alcohol use: none

Caffeine use: none

Family History

No family history of parkinsonism or tremor

Review of Systems

Well-developed, well-nourished white male

Neurologic exam: Findings as noted

Physical Examination

Slow and rhythmic "pill rolling" tremor at rest; no postural or action tremor noted. Rigidity in both upper and lower extremities noticeable upon passive flexion and extension. Signs and symptoms affect right-side greater than left-side of body. No postural instability. Remainder of neurologic exam unremarkable.

Labs and Diagnostic Tests

None available

Diagnosis

Primary:

1) Parkinson's disease

Pharmacist Notes and Other Patient Information

Higher doses of ropinirole not tolerated due to nausea

Higher dose of trihexyphenidyl not tolerated due to confusion

Medication Record

Date	Rx No	Physician	Drug and Strength	Quantity	Sig	Refills
5/31	50001		Trihexyphenidyl 1 mg		1 po tid	2
5/31	50002		Ropinirole 4 mg		1 po tid	2
5/31	50003		Sinemet 10/100 mg		1 po tid	2

Case 42

Questions

1. Which of the following are common signs/symptoms of Parkinson's disease?

   I.   Tremor
   II. Rigidity
   III. Bradykinesia

   A. I only
   B. III only
   C. I and II only
   D. II and III only
   E. I, II, and III

2. Which of the following statements regarding carbidopa/levodopa is true?

   I.   The 25/100-mg tablet contains 25 mg carbidopa and 100 mg levodopa.
   II. Dyskinesias can be relieved by decreasing the carbidopa/levodopa dosage.
   III. Carbidopa/levodopa is contraindicated with nonselective monoamine oxidase inhibitors (e.g., phenelzine and tranylcypromine).

   A. I only
   B. III only
   C. I and II only
   D. II and III only
   E. I, II, and III

3. The prescribing clinician attributes SJ's nausea to the carbidopa/levodopa product. You agree. Which of the following is an appropriate recommendation(s)?

   I.   Change the dose of carbidopa/levodopa to 25/100 mg tid.
   II. Suggest metoclopramide.
   III. Suggest prochlorperazine.

   A. I only
   B. III only
   C. I and II only
   D. II and III only
   E. I, II, and III

4. Which of the following statements regarding trihexyphenidyl is true?

   I.   Cogentin is the brand name of trihexyphenidyl.
   II. Trihexyphenidyl is a centrally acting anticholinergic agent.
   III. Trihexyphenidyl is also useful for relieving neuroleptic-induced acute dystonia.

   A. I only
   B. III only
   C. I and II only
   D. II and III only
   E. I, II, and III

5. When counseling SJ on his ropinirole prescription, you should explain that common side effects that may be expected are:

   I.   nausea.
   II. drowsiness.
   III. pulmonary fibrosis.

   A. I only
   B. III only
   C. I and II only
   D. II and III only
   E. I, II, and III

6. In response to SJ's drug information request, which of the following statements regarding amantadine is true?

   I.   Amantadine can cause livedo reticularis.
   II. Flumadine is a brand name for amantadine.
   III. Amantadine is an antiviral agent used to treat symptoms of influenza type A and is not effective for Parkinson's disease.

   A. I only
   B. III only
   C. I and II only
   D. II and III only
   E. I, II, and III

7. Carbidopa/levodopa is available as a standard release tablet (Sinemet) and a sustained release tablet (Sinemet CR). Which of the following statements is true?

   I.   Sinemet CR is less bioavailable than Sinemet.
   II. Administering Sinemet CR with food improves bioavailability.
   III. Sinemet CR may be crushed, chewed, or dissolved.

   A. I only
   B. III only
   C. I and II only
   D. II and III only
   E. I, II, and III

8. The prescribing clinician asks you to provide a list of drugs that can antagonize the effects of levodopa. In addition to metoclopramide and prochlorperazine, which of the following drugs should be included on that list?

   I.   Apomorphine
   II. Chlorpromazine
   III. Haloperidol

Case 42

A. I only
B. III only
C. I and II only
D. II and III only
E. I, II, and III

9. Two months later, SJ is doing well on his carbidopa/levodopa regimen of 25/100 mg tid. However, on several occasions, SJ has forgotten to take his afternoon dose of carbidopa/levodopa. The prescribing clinician calls and asks for your advice on converting SJ over to sustained-release carbidopa/levodopa (Sinemet CR). According to the product insert, you recommend that when converting to Sinemet CR, the daily levodopa dosage should be increased by approximately 10%-30% and the dosing frequency decreased by approximately 30%. Choose the appropriate dosing regimen:

A. Sinemet CR 50/200 mg: 1 tablet po bid
B. Sinemet CR 25/100 mg: 1 tablet po qid
C. Sinemet CR 25/100 mg: 1 tablet po bid
D. Sinemet CR 50/200 mg: 1/2 tablet po qid
E. Sinemet CR 25/100 mg: 1 tablet po tid

10. SJ and his wife are interested in learning more about Parkinson's disease to help them cope and adapt. Which of the following is NOT appropriate?

A. Recommend that they read a medical textbook on the subject.
B. Remind them that their prescriber or pharmacist can help with questions.
C. Suggest that they attend a local Parkinson's disease support group.
D. Suggest that they contact a nonprofit educational organization, such as the National Parkinson's Foundation or the American Parkinson's Disease Association, for supplemental information.
E. Suggest that they visit the public library.

Patient Name: Steven Booker
Address: 1485 Hampton Place
Age: 12 years   **Height:** 4' 0"
Sex: M   **Race:** White
Weight: 42 kg
Allergies: Sulfa; hives

Chief Complaint

SB is a 12-yo WM who was brought to the emergency room for a seizure that lasted 3-5 minutes while playing in a soccer game.

History of Present Illness

During the second half of the soccer game, SB fell to the ground, was stiff at first and then began having rhythmic contractions of his arms and legs. EMS was called to the scene. The mother reports the seizure only lasted about 3-5 minutes. She was not able to get his attention during the seizure and he would not look at her when she called his name. After the seizure stopped, SB was very confused and wanted to go to sleep.

In the ER, SB has another witnessed seizure involving both arms and legs which lasted 2 minutes. SB again lost consciousness. No medication was needed to stop the seizure.

His mother reports SB has never had a seizure before. He is a very active boy and loves soccer. On asking about recent trauma, his mother states that SB did fall off his bike about 1 month ago and bumped his head. He had bruises and scratches on his arm, but he was fine overall. She did not think anything of it as he did not complain.

Mom reports no sick contacts recently and that SB has been feeling fine and eating like normal.

The pediatric emergency department physician believes SB is having generalized tonic-clonic seizures and admits the child for observation and neurology consult.

Past Medical History

Chicken pox at 7 years old, Mild persistent asthma diagnosed at age 8, ADHD diagnosed at age 10

Immunizations: UTD

Social History

SB lives with both parents in a single story home along with 3 brothers and sisters. He rides his bike to school daily and enjoys playing soccer on the weekends.

Family History

Father has diabetes mellitus type 2. Brother had febrile seizures growing up but none since age 5.

Review of Systems

Negative except as noted previously

Physical Examination

GEN: Well appearing male, sleepy but arousable, no acute distress

VS: T 97.3°F, HR 72 bpm, RR 22 rpm, BP 99/65 mmHg, O_2 sat. 99 room air, Wt. 42 kg,

HEENT: PERRLA, EOMA, Moist membranes, oral mucosa clear, no hemorrhages, exudates, or papilledema

CHEST: Lungs clear to auscultation & percussion bilaterally

CV: RRR, NL heart sounds, no murmur

ABD: Positive bowel sounds, no masses, soft

GU: WNL

NEURO: Symmetric, positive reflexes

Labs and Diagnostic Tests

(In ER)

Sodium 136 mEq/L	Potassium 4.1 mEq/L
Chloride 101 mEq/L	CO_2 content 25 mEq/L
BUN 14 mg/dL	Creatinine 0.5 mg/dL
Calcium 10.1 mEq/L	Glucose 94 mg/dL
WBC 9.4 mm³	RBC 4.8 mm³
HCT 38.5%	Hgb 13.7g/dL
Platelet 305 mm³	Neutrophils 54%
Eosinophils 3%	Lymphocytes 38%
Monocytes 4%	Basophils 1%

CT scan - no affirmative focal lesions identified

EEG - slow, generalized pattern

Tox screen - negative

U/A - clear

Case 43

Diagnosis

Generalized tonic-clonic seizure disorder

Medication Record

(Home Medication)

Albuterol MDI 2 puffs q4h PRN wheeze/cough

Flovent 110 mcg MDI 1 puff BID

Adderall XR 20 mg PO daily

(On admission)

Lorazepam 4mg IV PRN seizure > 5 minutes

Carbamazepine 100 mg chew tabs PO BID

Albuterol MDI 2 puffs q4h PRN wheeze/cough

Flovent 110 mcg MDI 1 puff BID

Pharmacist Notes and Other Patient Information

None available

Questions

1. SB complains that the chewtab does not taste good. His mother asks if there is another form of carbamazepine that SB could try. Which of the following is true regarding carbamazepine formulations?

   I.   There is an extended-release tablet or capsule that SB could take, but swallow whole.
   II. There is a citrus-vanilla flavored suspension but SB will have to take this three or four times a day.
   III. There is an extended-release capsule which can be opened and placed on applesauce.

   A. I only
   B. III only
   C. I and II only
   D. II and III only
   E. I, II, and III

2. In the hospital, SB has a seizure and requires a dose of lorazepam. There is a new nurse on the floor and she asks you which of the following vials should she administer. Which vial is lorazepam?

   A. Valium
   B. Klonapin
   C. Xanax
   D. Ativan
   E. Versed

3. The nurse then asks you how much she should give the patient. Lorazepam is available in a 2 mg/mL and 4 mg/mL vial. The nurse has the 2 mg/mL vial in her hand. How many mL do you tell her to administer to the patient?

   A. 0.5 mL
   B. 1 mL
   C. 1.5 mL
   D. 2 mL
   E. 2.5 mL

4. SB tolerates his carbamazepine therapy in the hospital and the neurologist decides to place him on chronic therapy. When would you have SB return to clinic to have a carbamazepine level obtained?

   A. 3 days
   B. 7 days
   C. 14 days
   D. 28 days
   E. 2 months

5. SB and his family need to be counseled on carbamazepine use. Which of the following adverse effects do you tell the family?

   I.   Carbamazepine may cause a rash. If he develops one, stop the medication and call the neurologist.
   II. SB may experience some dizziness and drowsiness on initiation and at times of dose increases.
   III. Carbamazepine may cause an increase in kidney stone formation. SB should stay well hydrated especially when playing soccer.

   A. I only
   B. III only
   C. I and II only
   D. II and III only
   E. I, II, and III

6. SB returns to clinic and has his carbamazepine level drawn. What is the therapeutic concentration range for carbamazepine?

   A. 1-5 mcg/mL
   B. 4-12 mcg/mL
   C. 10-20 mcg/mL
   D. 10-40 mcg/mL
   E. No therapeutic range is defined. Clinical outcome does not correlate to levels.

Case 43

7. When counseling the parents on what to do if SB has a seizure at home, you tell them all of the following EXCEPT:

   A. take any sharp objects out of his hands.
   B. loosen any restrictive clothing.
   C. turn him on his side or turn his head to the side.
   D. place an object in his mouth for stabilization.
   E. cushion his head to protect from hard surfaces.

8. A few months later, SB returns to the neurologist. SB's seizures have decreased in frequency but he is still having a few every month on carbamazepine monotherapy. The neurologist is debating to change monotherapy drugs or add an adjunct agent. Which of the following anticonvulsants should NOT be considered when adjusting SB's current therapy?

   A. Lamotrigine
   B. Topiramate
   C. Phenytoin
   D. Valproic acid
   E. Zonisamide

9. Which of the following supplement should SB take while on anticonvulsant therapy?

   A. Vitamin C
   B. Vitamin D
   C. Vitamin B_{12}
   D. Vitamin B_3
   E. Vitamin E

10. SB's mom asks if he will ever come off anticonvulsant therapy completely and if so, when? You reply that SB may be given a trial off his medication when all of the following are met EXCEPT:

    A. SB must be seizure free for a least 2 years.
    B. SB must have a EEG that normalized with treatment.
    C. SB has only one seizure type.
    D. SB has remained on the same dose of medication for the last 6 months.
    E. SB has a normal IQ.

Neoplastic Disorders

Patient Name: Jillian Jackson
Address: 123 Whitehall Drive
Age: 44   **Height:** 5' 2"
Sex: F   **Race:** Caucasian
Weight: 189 lb
Allergies: NKA

Chief Complaint

Chronic myelogenous leukemia with hematologic, but not a cytogenetic, remission after 6 months of imatinib mesylate therapy.

History of Present Illness

JJ presented to her family physician 7 months ago with a several month history of increasing abdominal girth and a history of an unintentional 40-lb weight loss over 6 months. Her complete blood count was remarkable for a white blood count of 414,000, hematocrit 27.3%, and platelets of 205,000 with 10% blastic neutrophilic forms. A bone marrow biopsy was performed and was positive for a major bcr/abl fusion product with no other cytogenetic abnormalities found.

She was initally treated with hydroxyurea and then started on imatinib mesylate 400 mg po daily. Within 1 week her white blood count had fallen to 107,000 and her platelets to 94,000. Over the following weeks, her white blood count continued to fall, but she was unable to maintain adequate platelet counts, and her imatinib dose was reduced to 300 mg po daily. JJ had resumed her usual activites of daily living including running her household and has regained some of her lost weight. At 3 months into her therapy her bone marrow studies revealed > 50% persistant metaphases positive for bcr/abl, so her siblings were HLA typed to evaluate her for allogeneic bone marrow transplant. One of her younger brothers is a full HLA match, and JJ has decided to proceed with an allogeneic bone marrow transplant.

Past Medical History

Her medical history is otherwise notable for a cholecystectomy and hysterectomy. She was pregnant once and delivered a healthy child.

Social History

She currently resides within the city. Her one child is alive and well. She does not smoke or drink alcohol and has never used illicit drugs.

Family History

Noncontributory. She has four brothers and four sisters all alive, and one brother is a 6/6 HLA match.

Review of Systems

Except as listed in the other areas of the history, all systems are negative.

Physical Examination

GEN: Well developed, middle aged female in no apparent distress. Wt is 86 kg and ht 158.5 cm. T 36.4°C, pulse 80 bpm, BP 108/72 mmHg, RR 18 rpm, HR 80 bpm. Oxygen saturation of 99% on room air, pain is 0/10.

HEENT: No sinus tenderness, normal fundoscopic exam, tympanic membranes are clear bilaterally, oropharynx is clear of lesions, and dentition is good.

CHEST: Clear to ascultation and percussion bilaterally

CV: Normal S_1, S_2 with no murmurs, rubs, gallops, or heaves

ABD: Soft, nontender, with no palpable hepatospleenomegaly

EXT: Free of edema

SKIN: Free of rash

NEURO: She is alert and oriented with cranial nerves II through XII intact. Motor and sensory are 5/5 bilaterally.

Labs and Diagnostic Tests

Sodium 138 mEq/L	Potassium 3.9
BUN 19 mg/dL	Serum creatinine 0.8 mg/dL
Glucose 107 mg/dL	Calcium 9.6 mg/dL
CO_2 25 mEq/L	AST 29 U/L
ALT 39 U/L	Total bilirubin 1.3 mg/dL
Direct bilirubin 0.2 mg/dL	Total protein 7.4 g/dL
Albumin 4.1 g/dL	White blood cells 3900/mm³
Hemoglobin 12.8 g/dL	Hematocrit 36.9%
Platelets 156,000/mm³	
Absolute neutrophil count 2,500,000/mm³	
INR 1.04	aPTT 28.3 seconds

Case 44

Diagnosis

Primary:

1. Philadelphia chromosome-positive chronic myeloid leukemia

Plan:

To undergo a conditioning regimen and receive an allogeneic bone marrow transplant from her HLA matched brother

Medication Record

Lansoprazole 30 mg po daily

Ursodiol 300 mg po bid

Itraconazole solution 200 mg po bid

Ciprofloxacin 500 mg po bid

Valacyclovir 500 mg po bid

Cyclosporine (Neoral) 300 mg po bid

Prednisone 25 mg po bid

Transplant conditioning chemotherapy:

Busulfan 1 mg/kg (actual body weight with target AUC 1315-1500 micromol*minutes) po Q6H x 16 doses

Cyclophosphamide 60 mg/kg (ideal body weight) IV daily x 2 days

Mesna 60 mg/kg (ideal body weight) continuous IV infusion daily x 2 days

Pharmacist Notes and Other Patient Information

None available

Questions

1. You are reviewing the transplant conditioning regimen prior to JJ beginning conditioning. Orders for which of the following agents would be required to be scheduled with the listed regimen at this time?

   I.   Antiemetics
   II. Anticonvulsants
   III. Antidiarrheals

   A. I only
   B. III only
   C. I and II only
   D. II and III only
   E. I, II, and III

2. When reviewing JJ's medications, you notice that there will be significant drug interactions between:

   I.   cyclosporine and itraconazole.
   II. ciprofloxacin and valacyclovir.
   III. lansoprazole and prednisone.

   A. I only
   B. III only
   C. I and II only
   D. II and III only
   E. I, II, and III

3. Eight days after her BMT, JJ's blood pressure is up to 178/96 mmHg, and the attending physician is requesting a medication review to see if there is a drug-induced cause. You reply:

   A. no, none of her agents are likely to cause this.
   B. no, but this is a frequent side effect of BMT.
   C. yes, it is a relatively frequent side effect of cyclosporine.
   D. yes, this occurs late due to cyclophosphamide toxicity.
   E. yes, it is due to prednisone, which was started the day before.

4. To treat JJ's newly documented hypertension (BP is 178/96 mmHg), you recommend:

   A. clonidine 0.1 mg patch, apply once weekly.
   B. nifedipine XL 30 mg po qd.
   C. methyldopa 250 mg po tid.
   D. apply 1-inch nitroglycerin paste to chest wall every 4 hours.
   E. verapamil SR 240 mg po qd.

5. On the basis of her actual body weight of 86 kg you calculate JJ's busulfan dose at 86 mg po every 6 hours. The floor nurse calls and complains that the central pharmacy has delivered each dose as 43 of the 2-mg tablets. You respond:

   A. they should have used eight 10-mg and three 2-mg tablets.
   B. it would be fine to substitute 86 mg of the injectable busulfan dosed at the same frequency.
   C. 2-mg tablets are the only available oral size, so the dose is correct.
   D. the oral liquid should be used for tranplant regimens.
   E. intravenous once daily dosing should be used instead of tablets.

6. Methotrexate 15 mg/m^2 will be given the day after bone marrow infusion to help prevent graft versus host disease. What dose should JJ receive?

   A. 23.9 mg
   B. 27.9 mg

Case 44

C. 29.2 mg

D. 30.8 mg

E. 32.3 mg

7. Does this dose of methotrexate require you to add sodium bicarbonate to JJ's intravenous (IV) fluids?

    A. Yes, you need to alkalinize her to prevent tumor lysis.

    B. No, the methotrexate is more soluble at normal blood pH.

    C. Yes, she is at high risk for precipitation of methotrexate in the urine.

    D. No, the dose is low, and it will not be needed for renal protection.

    E. Yes, all intravenous doses of methotrexate require IV bicarbonate.

8. JJ is having trouble sleeping and requests to use valerian root to help with her insomnia as she had done prior to transplant. You explain that:

    A. the use of valerian is fine and she should watch for persistent drowsiness the next day.

    B. valerian is not a good idea since it may inhibit the metabolism of her cyclosporine causing unpredictably high drug levels.

    C. valerian doesn't work for insomnia but SAMe would be a great choice.

    D. herbal agents are FDA reviewed for efficacy and that one is currently not indicated for insomnia.

    E. a benzodiazepine like trazodone would be a better choice as a sleep aid.

9. JJ is having trouble taking her cyclosporine capsules and has decided to switch to the oral solution form. The proper way for her to take it is:

    A. mixed in a glass container and stirred into milk with a metal spoon.

    B. mixed with milk in a plastic cup stirred with a plastic spoon.

    C. only mixed with hot liquids.

    D. undiluted in a plastic dosing syringe.

    E. once daily in the AM due to its superior absorption over the capsules.

10. You receive a call from JJ's community pharmacy regarding substitutable products for the cyclosporine micro-emulsion capsules she had been receiving. You respond that:

    A. all of the current cyclosporine preparations are equivalent.

    B. the generic substitute should be a Neoral equivalent.

    C. the generic substitute should be a Sandimmune equivalent.

    D. only generics in the liquid form are equivalent.

    E. only generic forms in the capsule form are equivalent.

Patient Name: Cassie Fernandez
Address: 1034 Gandy Drive
Age: 55   Height: 5' 7"
Sex: F   Race: Hispanic
Weight: 101 kg
Allergies: Penicillin (rash)

Chief Complaint

CF is a 55-yo female who presents to the oncology clinic with a newly diagnosed right breast cancer.

History of Present Illness

While performing her monthly breast self-exam, CF found a hard, round lump in her right breast in November 2005. She subsequently saw her gynecologist who felt a hard, mobile mass in the 10 o'clock position without associated skin change, pain, or nipple discharge. The gynecologist ordered a mammogram of the breasts. CF had no other complaints at that time. A mammogram demonstrated a mass, suspicious for carcinoma, in the 10 o'clock position of the right breast. A core biopsy of the mass was positive for infiltrating ductal carcinoma. CF underwent a right modified radical mastectomy in January 2006, which revealed a 3.5-cm x 2.1-cm lesion with 4 positive lymph nodes out of 20 removed. All other staging was negative.

Past Medical History

CF was diagnosed with hypertension 6 years ago during a routine physical exam. She has been able to control her hypertension with Dyazide daily. CF began menses at age 11. She is G-1, P-1, and A-0, with one living child. Her age at first birth was 27 years old. She took oral contraceptives consecutively for 5 years from age 21-26 years. She is post-menopausal and took Prempro as hormone replacement therapy for 2 years until November 2005 when breast lump was discovered. The remainder of her history is unremarkable.

Social History

Tobacco use: none

Alcohol use: occasional glass of wine with dinner

Illicit drug use: none

Family History

Mother deceased with breast cancer diagnosed at age 72 .

Paternal grandmother deceased with ovarian cancer at age 61.

Review of Systems

In February, 2006, the patient has slight tenderness at the surgical site on the right chest wall. She denies any other symptoms.

Physical Examination

March 2006

GEN: Ambulatory in NAD

VS: T 37.1°C, HR 88 bpm, RR 16 rpm, BP 118/83 mmHg, Wt 101 kg, Ht 5',7" HEENT: PERRLA, oral cavity without lesions. No cervical lymphadenopathy or thyromegaly.

CHEST: Lungs CTA bilaterally. Heart RRR, w/o murmurs. She has a well-healed mastectomy scar on the right. She has slight erythema, but no edema or drainage noted from this site. There are no palpable lesions in the left breast. No palpable axillary lymphadenopathy bilaterally.

ABD: Normo-active BS, soft, nontender, non-distended. No organomegaly.

EXT: No cyanosis, clubbing, edema

NEURO: A & O x3, no focal neurologic findings

Labs and Diagnostic Tests

Sodium 141 mEq/L	Potassium 3.7 mEq/L
Chloride 104 mEq/L	CO_2 content 29 mEq/L
Magnesium 2.1 mg/dL	Calcium 9.1 mg/dL
BUN 8 mg/dL	Serum creatinine 0.8 mg/dL
Glucose 124 mg/dL	Phosphorous 2.6 mg/dL
CA-2729 24.4 units/mL	T. bili 0.7 mg/dL
ALP 64 IU/mL	LDH 666 IU/mL
SGPT 28 IU/mL	

WBC 6300/mm^3 with 55% PMN, 37% lymphocytes, 6% monocytes, 1% eosinophils

Hemoglobin 12.4 g/dL	Hematocrit 37.2%

Platelets 262,000/mm^3

CT abdomen: No evidence of metastatic disease

CXR: Negative for active disease

Bone scan: No active bony metastases, mild degenerative changes in joints consistent with patient's age

Mastectomy specimen-right breast: A 3.5-cm x 2.1-cm lesion was identified with 4 positive lymph nodes out of 20; infiltrating ductal carcinoma of the breast, modified Black's nuclear grade 3 (poorly differentiated). Estrogen receptor, positive (80%); progesterone receptor, positive (40%); Her2/neu overexpression, IHC-2+, FISH (fluorescence in situ hybridization) pending.

Echocardiogram: Left ventricular ejection fraction is 56% with normal wall motion

Case 45

Diagnosis

Primary:

    1. Stage IIB right breast cancer ($T_2N_1M_0$)

Secondary:

    1. Controlled hypertension

    2. Asymptomatic degenerative joint disease

Assessment and Plan:

Due to the positive lymph nodes found at surgery, CF will receive chemotherapy, then radiation to the chest wall and lymphatics followed by Arimidex for 5 years. The chemotherapy HB will receive consists of Adriamycin (doxorubicin) and Cytoxan (cyclophosphamide) for four courses followed by Taxol (paclitaxel) weekly for 12 weeks concurrently with Herceptin if patient is Her2/neu (+) by FISH.

AC Chemotherapy regimen as follows:

    1. Dexamethasone 20 mg IV before chemotherapy (anti-emetic)

    2. Ondansetron 16 mg po 30 minutes before chemotherapy (anti-emetic)

    3. Doxorubicin 60 mg/m^2 IVP

    4. Cyclophosphamide 600 mg/m^2 IV

This regimen will be given in a dose-dense fashion every 14 days with growth factor support.

Paclitaxel and Herceptin treatment regimen:

    1. Dexamethasone 20 mg po 12 and 6 hours before chemotherapy

    2. Diphenhydramine 50 mg IV before chemotherapy

    3. Ranitidine 50 mg IV before chemotherapy

    4. Paclitaxel 80 mg/m^2 IV over 1 hour weekly x 12 weeks

    5. Herceptin 4 mg/kg loading dose IV week 1, followed by Herceptin 2 mg/kg loading dose IV weekly x 51 weeks if Her2/neu positive by FISH.

Pharmacist Notes and Other Patient Information

12/05 Patient noted breast lump. Advised to immediately see gynecologist. Advised patient to discuss the use of conjugated estrogens and medroxyprogesterone with her gynecologist.

Medication Record

3/06 Patient instructed regarding the dosing, administration, side effects, drug-drug, and drug-food interactions with AC and paclitaxel chemotherapy regimens. AC course #1 initiated.

6/06 Taxol and Herceptin week #1 initiated. During paclitaxel infusion, the patient was instructed to notify the nurse if she experiences any rashes; itching; flushing; swelling around the face, lips, or neck; wheezing; coughing; trouble breathing; or chest pain. Patient also educated about a reaction that may occur with the first dose of Herceptin including chills and fever that may persist up to 24 hours after the infusion.

Questions

1. CF is about to start her first cycle of AC chemotherapy. Which of the following is NOT a side effect of Adriamycin (doxorubicin)?

    A. Mucositis

    B. Heart failure

    C. Peripheral neuropathy

    D. Leukopenia

    E. Alopecia

2. One of Cytoxan's (cyclophosphamide) metabolites is a compound called Acrolein, which can cause hemorrhagic cystitis. At doses >1.5-2 g/m^2 cyclophosphamide regimens may contain what medication to prevent hemorrhagic cystitis?

    A. Dexrazoxane

    B. Naloxone

    C. Leucovorin

    D. Flumazenil

    E. MESNA

3. Which of the following statements is most accurate regarding chemotherapy-induced nausea and vomiting (CINV)?

    A. All chemotherapy agents cause nausea and vomiting to the same degree.

    B. Palonosetron is the 5-HT$_3$ antagonist with the longest half-life.

    C. Nausea and vomiting is not life-threatening but uncomfortable for patients.

    D. Chemotherapy-induced nausea and vomiting is not preventable.

    E. Chemotherapy-induced nausea and vomiting lasts for approximately 6 hours.

Date	Rx No	Physician	Drug and Strength	Quantity	Sig	Refills
2/1	674582	Hillman	Dyazide	30	1 po qd	6
2/1	674583	Hillman	Prempro 0.3/1.5 mg	30	1 po qd	6
3/1	675870	Parker	Prochlorperazine caps 10 mg	30	1 po q 6 h	4
7/1	678960	Parker	Dexamethasone 4 mg	10	5 tablets (20 mg) po 12 and 6 h prior to chemo	3

Case 45

4. CF is having some delayed nausea/vomiting despite use of scheduled dexamethasone 4 mg PO BID x 2 days following chemotherapy and breakthrough compazine 10 mg PO Q 6 hours. What additional anti-emetics may be prescribed to prevent delayed nausea/vomiting with subsequent courses?

   I.   Emend 125 mg PO day 1 of chemotherapy, Emend 80 mg PO days 2,3
   II. Ativan 1 mg PO Q 6 hours prn nausea/vomiting
   III. Zofran 8 mg (ondansetron) PO Q 8 hours prn nausea/vomiting

   A. I only
   B. III only
   C. I and II only
   D. II and III only
   E. I, II, and III

5. After 4 cycles of AC chemotherapy and verification of Her/neu positivity by FISH, CF will start taxol Q week x 12 weeks and Herceptin Q week x 52 weeks. Why would she not start the Herceptin during the AC treatment?

   I.   Increased risk of cardiac toxicity
   II. Increased risk of myelosuppression
   III. Increased risk of hepatotoxicity

   A. I only
   B. III only
   C. I and II only
   D. II and III only
   E. I, II, and III

6. CF's BSA calculates to 2.19. The Taxol dose is 80 mg/m². The concentration of Taxol is 6 mg/mL.

   The total taxol dose she will be receiving is 175 mg in 0.9% normal saline 250 mL over 1 hour.
   Calculate the rate at which the Taxol is to infuse.
   A. 279 mL/h
   B. 304 mL/h
   C. 558 mL/h
   D. 608 mL/h
   E. 250 mL/h

7. Why does the oncologist want to give CF anastrazole (Arimidex) after her chemotherapy?

   I.   CF tumor was poorly differentiated
   II. CF tumor was positive for estrogen receptors
   III. CF is post-menopausal

   A. I only
   B. III only
   C. I and II only
   D. II and III only
   E. I, II, and III

8. Tamoxifen is associated with which of the following adverse events?

   I.   Endometrial cancer
   II. Hot flashes
   III. Deep venous thrombosis

   A. I only
   B. III only
   C. I and II only
   D. II and III only
   E. I, II, and III

9. During CF's chemotherapy she starts having symptoms of extreme fatigue. Routine labs were drawn and her hemoglobin value was 10.1 g/dL, Fe-23 mcg/dL, Ferritin-89 ng/mL, and transferrin saturation of 15%. Since the patient has chemotherapy-induced anemia, which of the following would be the most appropriate treatment option for her anemia.

   A. Procrit 40,000 units SC Q week
   B. Procrit 40,000 units SC Q 2 weeks
   C. Aranesp 200 mcg SC Q 2 weeks
   D. Aranesp 200 mcg SC Q 2 weeks + ferrous sulfate 325 mg PO TID
   E. Ferrous sulfate 325 mg PO TID

10. According to the American Cancer Society women at average risk of developing breast cancer should follow which screening guidelines?

    I.   Mammograms annually starting at age 40.
    II. Clinical breast examinations (CBE) about every 3 years for women in their twenties and thirties and annually for women 40 and older. They should be part of a woman's periodic health examination.
    III. Women in their twenties should be told about the benefits and limitations of breast self-examinations (BSE). It is acceptable for women to choose not to do BSE or to do it occasionally. Women should report any breast change promptly to their healthcare provider.

    A. I only
    B. III only
    C. I and II only
    D. II and III only
    E. I, II, and III

Case 46

Patient Name: Michael Williams
Address: 8745 Lands End Way
Age: 48   **Height:** 5' 10"
Sex: M   **Race:** White
Weight: 184 lb
Allergies: PCN

Chief Complaint

MW is a 48-yo male with Stage II adenocarcinoma of the rectum diagnosed 4 weeks ago. He comes in today for consideration of adjuvant chemotherapy. He was discharged from the hospital 3 weeks ago, status post an abdominoperineal resection with colostomy. Today he complains of mild epigastric pain and mild incisional pain. Patient states he has done nothing but lie around since the surgery. However, he does note that he hasn't had a bowel movement in 4 days. The plan is to start him on concomitant radiation and adjuvant chemotherapy with 5-fluorouracil and leucovorin calcium.

History of Present Illness

MW presented to the ED 4 weeks ago with rectal bleeding, fatigue, and crampy abdominal pain. After admission to the hospital, a colonoscopy showed a large mass 6 cm from the anal verge. Biopsy revealed moderately differentiated adenocarcinoma. Based on the pathologic and radiographic staging, MW has a stage IIa ($T_3N_0M_0$) rectal cancer. His hospital course was uneventful and he was discharged 5 days post-op.

Past Medical History

MW has a history of PUD.

Social History

Tobacco use: none

Alcohol use: occasional

Family History

Mother died of colon cancer at age 58. Father is alive with a diagnosis of prostate cancer. Sister died of breast cancer at age 42.

Review of Systems

Well-appearing male with appropriately healing midline incision.

Medication Record

Date	Rx No	Physician	Drug and Strength	Quantity	Sig	Refills
9/1	24878	Smith	Hydrocodone/APAP 7.5/500	30	1-2 q 4-6 h prn	0
6/10	19935	Jones	Pantoprazole 40 mg	30	1 po qd	2

Physical Examination

On current admission:

VS: BP 140/85 mmHg, pulse 78 bpm, T 37.6°C, Ht 70", Wt 184 lb

ABD: Firm, nontender

Labs and Diagnostic Tests

Sodium 143 mEq/L	Potassium 3.9 mEq/L
Chloride 106 mEq/L	Bicarbonate 24 mEq/L
BUN 16 mg/dL	Serum creatinine 0.9 mg/dL
Glucose 125 mg/dL	Magnesium 1.8 mg/dL
T. bili 0.9 mg/dL	SGPT 35 u/L
CEA 2.4 ng/mL	WBC 5600/mm^3
Hgb 12.6 g/dL	Hct 37.3%
Plt 223,000/mm^3	Neutrophils 73%
Lymphs 12%	Monos 7%
Baso 5%	Eosi 3%

Diagnosis

Primary:

   1. Colon cancer

Secondary:

   1. Peptic ulcer disease

Pharmacist Notes and Other Patient Information

None available

Questions

1. 5-Fluorouracil is which type of chemotherapeutic agent?

   A. Alkylating agent
   B. Pyrimidine antimetabolite
   C. Purine antimetabolite
   D. Intercalating agent
   E. Antitumor antibiotic

Case 46

2. 5-Fluorouracil is also known as

   A. FUDR.
   B. 5-FC.
   C. 5-FU.
   D. UFT.
   E. CPT-11.

3. 5-Fluorouracil is to be administered to MW at a dosage of 425 mg/m²/day x5 days, repeated every 28 days along with leucovorin at a dosage of 20 mg/m²/day x5 days. What is MW's daily 5-fluorouracil dose (rounded to the nearest tenth)?

   A. 740 mg
   B. 860 mg
   C. 1000 mg
   D. 1130 mg
   E. 1260 mg

4. When administered in combination with 5-fluorouracil in the treatment of colon cancer, leucovorin should be administered:

   A. 24 hours after 5-fluorouracil.
   B. based on 5-fluorouracil levels.
   C. prior to 5-fluorouracil.
   D. immediately following 5-fluorouracil.
   E. mixed together with 5-fluorouracil to allow co-infusion.

5. The main dose-limiting toxicity of 5-fluorouracil plus leucovorin is:

   I. nausea and vomiting.
   II. alopecia.
   III. myelosuppression.

   A. I only
   B. III only
   C. I and II only
   D. II and III only
   E. I, II, and III

6. If MW was to develop metastatic disease during his adjuvant therapy, which of the following chemotherapy agents would be considered appropriate next-line therapy?

   A. Cytarabine
   B. Alpha interferon
   C. Oxaliplatin
   D. Paclitaxel
   E. Doxorubicin

7. MW needs his pantoprazole prescription refilled. You can refill it utilizing which of the following products?

   A. Prilosec
   B. Zantac
   C. Pepcid
   D. Protonix
   E. Prevacid

8. 5-Fluorouracil and leucovorin is considered to be of level 2 mild-moderate emetogenicity. Which of the following regimens would be the most efficacious, cost-effective antiemetic treatment?

   A. Ondansetron 8 mg IV prior to each 5-fluorouracil + leucovorin dose
   B. Granisetron 2 mg po prior to each 5-fluorouracil + leucovorin dose
   C. Ondansetron 8 mg po q 6 h prn nausea
   D. Prochlorperazine 10 mg po or IV prior to each 5-fluorouracil + leucovorin dose and every 6 h prn
   E. Diphenhydramine 25 mg po or IV prior to each 5-fluorouracil + leucovorin dose and every 6 h prn

9. According to the American Cancer Society Guidelines for Screening and Surveillance For Early Detection of Colorectal Polyps and Cancer, MW should have had a sigmoidoscopy/colonoscopy at what age (given his family history)?

   A. 30
   B. 40
   C. 50 (and, therefore, did not need one yet)
   D. 60 (and, therefore, did not need one yet)
   E. Screening is of no benefit in colorectal cancer

10. Which of the following statements would be inappropriate when counseling MW on his prescription for hydrocodone/APAP (Vicodin)?

   A. If the medication is not working, you should try taking a higher dose.
   B. APAP is an abbreviation for acetaminophen.
   C. You can try taking Vicodin with food or milk if it causes upset stomach.
   D. You should not drive until you know how Vicodin will affect you.
   E. You should not drink alcohol while taking this medication.

Case 47

Patient Name: Benjamin Martin
Address: 33 Nutt Road
Age: 28   **Height:** 6' 0"
Sex: M   **Race:** White
Weight: 185 lb
Allergies: NKDA

Chief Complaint

BM is a 28-yo male seeking treatment for his newly diagnosed acute lymphocytic leukemia (ALL).

History of Present Illness

BM presented to his PCP last week complaining of fatigue, shortness of breath, and joint pains lasting approximately 2 months. He felt it was just the flu, but when it seemed to get worse he sought medical advice. In addition, he noticed bruises on his lower extremities that did not go away and has recently had several nose bleeds. A routine blood test revealed that BM was anemic and thrombocytopenic. He was transfused with platelets and packed red blood cells. A bone marrow aspiration was obtained and revealed ALL.

Past Medical History

BM was well until the diagnosis of ALL.

Social History

Tobacco use: none

Alcohol use: social drinker

Occupation: full-time student, working on his MBA

Hobbies: swam varsity in high school and continues to swim daily at the co-rec pool

Family History

Family history is negative. He has a brother and sister who will be given kits to be HLA typed.

Review of Systems

Complains of frequent nose bleeds, easy bruising, shortness of breath, and aching joints. He has lost approximately 10 lb over the past 2 months. Denies fever, night sweats, or change in eating habits.

Physical Examination

GEN: Young male in NAD

VS: BP 108/68 mmHg, HR 87 bpm, RR 20 rpm, T 36.9°C, Ht 72 inches, Wt 185 lb

HEENT: PERRLA, neck supple and no lymphadenopathy.

CHEST: Lungs clear and resonant; heart RRR, S_1 and S_2 with no m/g/r.

ABD: Soft and nontender to palpation. No guarding or rebound. No hepatosplenomegaly.

LYMPHS: Negative

NEURO: A and O x3

EXT: No clubbing, edema, or cyanosis. Ecchymoses present on both lower extremities.

Labs and Diagnostic Tests

Sodium 138 mEq/L	Potassium 4.1 mEq/L
Chloride 139 mEq/L	CO_2 content 25 mEq/L
BUN 9 mg/dL	Serum creatinine 0.9 mg/dL
Magnesium 1.8 mEq/L	Uric acid 7.4 mg/dL
LDH 1280 U/L	Calcium 9.3 mg/dL
Phosphate 3.5 mg/dL	Glucose 87 mg/dL
Albumin 3.8 g/dL	T. bili 1.0 mg/dL
Hgb 9.5 g/dL	Platelets 46,000/mm³
WBC 6500 mm³	

Differential: neutrophils 63%, bands 3%, lymphocytes 20%, eosinophils 1%, basophils 1%, myelocytes 2%, nucleated red blood cells 6%, blasts 6%

Chest x-ray: Lungs clear, no evidence of an acute pulmonary process. Mediastinal lymph nodes are clearly distinguishable. Double lumen central venous catheter is in place.

CT abdomen: Negative

Bone marrow aspiration:

BM total cells 500	Blasts 38%
Progranulocytes 5%	Myelocytes 1%
Metamyelocytes 4%	Segs, neutrophils 26%
Eosinophils 1%	Basophils 1%
Lymphocytes 11%	Plasma cell 0%
Monocytes 1%	Reticulum cell 0%
Pronormoblast 1%	Normoblast 21%
ME/Ratio, BM-BX 1.2	Cellularity: 80%

Peroxidase stain: Negative (0.3%)

TDT stain: Strongly positive (98%)

Periodic acid Schiff: Positive

CD2: Positive	CD5: Positive
CD7: Positive	CD13: Negative
CD33: Negative	CD38: Positive

Case 47

Bone marrow interpretation: Hypercellular marrow consistent with acute lymphocytic T-cell leukemia.

Chromosome bone marrow interpretation: Ph+ metaphases 45,XY,t(9;22)(q34;q11)2

Two abnormal and 19 normal male metaphases are analyzed. The Philadelphia + clone is observed in bone marrow.

FISH interpretation: 400 interphase/metaphase analyzed. A nuclear fusion signal was seen in 13.7% of the interphase/metaphase indicating Ph+ cells. 86.3% of the cells were Ph-.

 Diagnosis

Primary:

    1. Acute lymphocytic leukemia

Plan:

    BM has acute lymphoblastic T-cell leukemia and will be admitted to receive the following chemotherapy regimen listed in the medication record.

 Medication Record

Hyper CVAD chemotherapy

Cyclophosphamide 300 mg/m² IV q 12 h x6 doses, days 1-3

Vincristine 2 mg IV on day 4 and 11

Doxorubicin 50 mg/m² IV on day 4

Dexamethasone 40 mg po qd on days 1-4 and 11-14

Mesna 600 mg/m² CIV days 1-3

 Pharmacist Notes and Other Patient Information

None available

Questions

1. BM will need to receive an intrathecal treatment prior to starting chemotherapy. Which of the following medications is suitable for intrathecal administration?

    I.   Methotrexate
    II. Cytarabine
    III. Vincristine

    A. I only
    B. III only
    C. I and II only
    D. II and III only
    E. I, II, and III

2. Cyclophosphamide-induced hemorrhagic cystitis is caused by which metabolite?

    A. Chloracetaldehyde
    B. Acrolein
    C. 4-Hydroxycyclophosphamide
    D. Difluorodeoxyuridine
    E. Uracil arabinoside

3. Which of the following agents may be administered to prevent hemorrhagic cystitis?

    A. Dexamethasone
    B. Allopurinol
    C. Mesna
    D. Dolasetron
    E. Methylene blue

4. A pharmacist is preparing the dose of doxorubicin. Which of the following chemotherapeutic agents can he or she use?

    A. Adriamycin
    B. Idarubicin
    C. Daunorubicin
    D. Doxil
    E. Mitoxantrone

5. BM wonders how important it is to call the doctor's office for a fever greater than 100.5 °F when his white blood cell counts are low?

    I.   It is fine to wait until the next convenient time to call.
    II. He must call right away due to increased risk of infection.
    III. He should always call for a suspected fever since antibiotics are needed to prevent an acute septic event from occurring.

    A. I only
    B. III only
    C. I and II only
    D. II and III only
    E. I, II, and III

6. In the middle of the night, BM trips and pulls out his double lumen central venous catheter. A new catheter cannot be placed until tomorrow and his doxorubicin dose is due. It is decided that it will be given peripherally. BM complains of burning during the infusion. The nurse stops the infusion and examines his arm. The chemotherapy has extravasated. The appropriate treatment is to:

    A. wait a few minutes and restart the infusion at a slower rate.
    B. aspirate any drug via the intravenous cannula before it is removed; call a plastic surgery consult; and apply a warm compress; and apply 1/6 or 1/3 M sodium thiosulfate.
    C. aspirate any drug via the intravenous cannula before it

Case 47

is removed; call a plastic surgery consult; apply a warm compress; and apply a baking soda paste to the affected area.

D. aspirate any drug via the intravenous cannula before it is removed; call a plastic surgery consult; apply a cold compress; and apply DMSO (dimethylsulfoxide) 50%-99% (w/v) topical solution.

E. administer a dose of hydromorphone intravenously and restart the infusion immediately at the previous rate.

7. Which of the following are standard ways to ensure the preparation of a safe, sterile product when preparing an intrathecal chemotherapy medication?

I. Filtration of the final product with a 0.22-μm filter
II. Using a bacteriostatic diluent
III. Preparing each dose in a class II horizontal flow hood

A. I only
B. III only
C. I and II only
D. II and III only
E. I, II, and III

8. BM has completed his induction treatment and has no evidence of disease. It is decided that he will receive consolidation treatment consisting of high-dose methotrexate and high-dose cytarabine. A methotrexate level is drawn 24, 48, and 72 hours after methotrexate was administered. His 24-hour level was higher than desired. Which of the following agents would you administer to BM in an attempt to reduce toxicity from occurring?

A. Levamisole
B. Leucovorin
C. Dexrazoxane
D. Filgrastim
E. Dolasetron

9. BM is to receive sodium bicarbonate 150 mEq/L mixed in Normal saline. The physician is concerned about the sodium load and asks you to calculate the percent saline in the resultant solution. 1 mEq = 5.7 mg sodium. You reply that it is:

A. 1.05% saline.
B. 1.76% saline.
C. 2% saline.
D. 1.9% saline.
E. 3% saline.

10. BM has run out of his leucovorin and wants to replace it with the folic acid that is available over the counter. He has a prescription for 1-mg folate tablets but his insurance doesn't cover it anyhow. You respond:

A. Leucovorin is not the same as folic acid but he can get the folate 1 mg without a prescription.
B. Leucovorin isn't the same as folic acid but he can get 0.4-mg tablets of folic acid over the counter.
C. Leucovorin isn't the same as folic acid but he can get 0.8-mg folic acid tablets over the counter.
D. Leucovorin isn't the same as folic acid but he can get 0.4- and 0.8-mg folic acid tablets over the counter.
E. It is fine to just take the folic acid and but he can get only 0.4- and 0.8-mg tablets over the counter.

Patient Name: Janice Brown
Address: 1940 Hidden Valley Road
Age: 61   **Height:** 5' 2"
Sex: F   **Race:** African American
Weight: 135 lb
Allergies: NKDA

Chief Complaint

JB is a 61-yo female who returns to the clinic for her third dose of vinorelbine and cisplatin for stage IIIB non-small-cell lung carcinoma. She has tolerated the past two cycles, except for mild nausea and vomiting. Today she appears more anxious and wants to take a break from her chemotherapy regimen.

History of Present Illness

Two months ago JB went to her local doctor with upper respiratory symptoms, a productive cough with yellow secretions, and pleuritic chest pain. She was started on Augmentin 500 mg po tid for 7 days. Her symptoms did not improve and she telephoned her doctor 1 week after completing her course of antibiotics. A prescription for Zithromax was telephoned into her local pharmacy. She returned to her physician 2 weeks later with no improvement in URI symptoms and stated that she is slightly winded after climbing a flight of stairs. A chest x-ray revealed a left lower lobe mass with obstructive changes. A CT of her chest and bronchoscopy with cervical mediastinoscopy were performed. Her diagnosis was confirmed with tissue obtained from this procedure as adenocarcinoma.

Past Medical History

JB has had several episodes of pulmonary congestion and cough since she was a child. Several chest x-rays were obtained over the years, all negative for a mass. She was diagnosed with HTN 10 years ago that is now controlled with medication. Other than a hysterectomy at age 35, the remainder of her history is unremarkable.

Social History

Tobacco use: 1 ppd for 40 years, has not quit as of this visit

Alcohol use: none

Illicit drug use: marijuana use 35 years ago

Occupation: worked for a company which removes asbestos; retired 5 years ago

Family History

Unknown, patient was adopted

Review of Systems

No complaints except persistent cough, chest pain, and DOE; denies hemoptysis, anorexia, and weight loss.

Physical Examination

VS: BP 132/79 mmHg, HR 89 bpm, RR 21 rpm, T 36.5°C, Wt 135 lb, Ht 157.48 cm

HEENT: PERRLA, oral cavity without lesions and mucositis, head atraumatic and normocephalic, neck supple without JVD and without lymphadenopathy

CHEST: Bilateral wheezes and decreased breath sounds, heart NSR

ABD: Soft, nontender, positive bowel sounds

EXT: Negative for cyanosis, clubbing and edema

NEURO: A & O x3

LYMPHS: Negative

Labs and Diagnostic Tests

Sodium 136 mEq/L	Potassium 4.8 mEq/L
Chloride 104 mEq/L	CO_2 content 26 mEq/L
Serum creatinine 0.9 mg/dL	T. bili 2.3 mg/dL
Alk Phos 78 U/L	LDH 698 U/L
SGPT 58 U/L	

WBC 42,000/mm³ with 88% neutrophils

Hemoglobin 9.6 g/dL, hematocrit 29.2%

Platelets 251,000/mm³

Chest x-ray: Left lower mass with obstructive changes

CT chest: 8-cm mass in medial aspect of LLL and a 2.5-cm cavity within mass consistent with tumor necrosis. Left hilar and subcarinal lymphadenopathy.

Bone scan: Negative

Bronchoscopy and cervical mediastinoscopy: Invasive poorly differentiated squamous cell carcinoma

Case 48

 Medication Record

Date	Rx No	Physician	Drug and Strength	Quantity	Sig	Refills
7/2	42099	Brown	Premarin 0.625 mg	30	1 po qd	3
7/2	42100	Brown	Vasotec 5 mg	30	1 po qd	2
7/2	42101	Jones	Prochlorperazine 10 mg	30	1 po q 4 h prn N/V	3

Physician orders:

Vinorelbine 30 mg/m^2 IV weekly

Cisplatin 100 mg/m^2 IV q 28 days

Zofran 8 mg IV premedication for cisplatin

Decadron 20 mg IV premedication for cisplatin

Compazine 10 mg IV premedication for vinorelbine

 Diagnosis

Primary:

   1. Stage IIIB non-small-cell lung carcinoma, adenocarcinoma

Secondary:

  1. Hypertension

  2. Anxiety

  3. S/P hysterectomy

Plan:

JB has been instructed about the importance of keeping her chemotherapy on schedule. She agrees to proceed and is given a prescription for lorazepam to take as needed for anxiety associated with her disease and for anticipatory nausea and vomiting. On reviewing her labs, it is noticed that her bilirubin is elevated. This necessitates a 50% dose reduction of her vinorelbine.

 Pharmacist Notes and Other Patient Information

None available

Questions

1. The dose of vinorelbine JB should receive today is:
   - A. 25 mg.
   - B. 49 mg.
   - C. 50 mg.
   - D. 60 mg.
   - E. 73 mg.

2. JB has expressed a desire to stop smoking. Which of the following medications could be a potentially helpful therapeutic modality for smoking cessation?
   - I.   Zyban
   - II. Nicoderm
   - III. Niacin
   - A. I only
   - B. III only
   - C. I and II only
   - D. II and III only
   - E. I, II, and III

3. The mechanism of action of vinorelbine is:
   - I.   incorporation of FUTP into RNA and inhibition of thymidylate synthase.
   - II. production of intrastrand crosslinks and formation of DNA adducts.
   - III. the inhibition of the polymerization of tubulin.
   - A. I only
   - B. III only
   - C. I and II only
   - D. II and III only
   - E. I, II, and III

4. The emetogenicity of vinorelbine is:
   - A. high.
   - B. moderate to high.
   - C. moderate.
   - D. moderate to low.
   - E. low.

5. When preparing chemotherapy, a pharmacist should:
   - I.   use proper aseptic technique.
   - II. prepare the chemotherapy in a class I biologic safety cabinet.
   - III. clean up a small solid spill with dry absorbent gauze.

Case 48

A. I only
B. III only
C. I and II only
D. II and III only
E. I, II, and III

6. The dose-limiting toxicity of vinorelbine is:

A. mucositis.
B. neutropenia.
C. cardiotoxicity.
D. neuropathy
E. pulmonary fibrosis.

7. JB returns for her next course of vinorelbine and cisplatin. Three days later she is admitted to the hospital with severe nausea and vomiting and stomatitis. Which of the following antiemetics could have been prescribed for JB to prevent delayed emesis?

I. Lorazepam around the clock for up to 1 week after chemotherapy
II. Metoclopramide in tapering doses for 4 days
III. Aprepitant and dexamethasone with chemotherapy and for 3 and 4 days respectively along with a serotonin antagonist on the chemotherapy day

A. I only
B. III only
C. I and II only
D. II and III only
E. I, II, and III

8. JB is unable to take anything orally because of her nausea and stomatitis. It is decided that a Dilaudid PCA would be in the best interest for JB. A physician orders a basal rate of 0.5 mg/h and a demand rate of 0.3 mg every 20 minutes. The pharmacist should dispense:

A. hydrocodone.
B. propoxyphene.
C. fentanyl.
D. hydromorphone.
E. acetaminophen.

9. JB is unable to take anything orally because of her nausea and stomatitis. It is decided to start a Dilaudid PCA. A physician orders a basal rate of 0.5 mg/h and a demand rate of 0.3 mg every 20 minutes. Over the course of 24 hours, JB hits the PCA 34 times but only receives 11 extra doses of Dilaudid. What is the total dose of Dilaudid JB received over 24 hours?

A. 3.3 mg
B. 12 mg
C. 15.3 mg
D. 19.2 mg
E. 22.2 mg

10. JB returns to the clinic 2 weeks after being discharged from the hospital for nausea and vomiting and stomatitis. She complains of mild pain in the RUQ, but is otherwise feeling well (though not looking forward to more cisplatin). Restaging reveals liver metastases and new contralateral mediastinal lymph nodes. She would like to know which of the following agents would provide the best chance of response.

A. Vinblastine
B. Carmustine
C. Tamoxifen
D. Cytarabine
E. Docetaxel

Case 49

Lymphoma

Patient Name: Karen Levy
Address: 2950 Alamo Drive
Age: 37   **Height:** 5' 5"
Sex: F   **Race:** Caucasian
Weight: 60.1 kg
Allergies: Sulfa

Chief Complaint

KL presents to the hematology clinic for evaluation and treatment of newly diagnosed nodular sclerosing Hodgkin's disease.

History of Present Illness

KL began experiencing an assymmetric neck and a "choking" sensation that had been getting progressively worse over the last six weeks. In addition, KL had been experiencing drenching night sweats, persistent fevers, and had lost ~15 pounds over the last two months. She visited her primary care physician who appreciated significant lymphadenopathy and referred her to an ENT specialist. A fine needle aspirate of one of the neck lymph nodes was obtained and CAT scans were performed. CT of the neck showed multiple large soft tissue attenuation masses in the lower neck and upper chest with extension to the left hemithorax. There was narrowing and displacement of the trachea, and encasement of the left common carotid and left subclavian artery all consistent with lymphadenopathy. CT of the chest showed extensive supraclavicular adenopathy. There was a large anterior mediastinal mass measuring approximately 9.5 x 7.1 cm. CT of the abdomen and pelvis were without lymphadenopathy.

Past Medical History

Cesarean section (11/04)

History of frequent urinary tract infections

History of infectious mononucleosis and Epstein-Barr virus

Social History

The patient is married. She is a registered nurse and her husband is a psychiatrist. The patient denies any tobacco, alcohol, or illicit drug use. She has 1 child born a couple months prior to diagnosis. Patient has a twin brother.

Family History

Mother and father alive and well. Mother with history of hypertension controlled on drug therapy. Father with history of diabetes controlled on diet alone. No history of malignancy in the family.

Review of Systems

Patient denies any headache. No blurry vision or lightheadedness. No sore throat. Positive neck discomfort, especially on the left side (post-surgical). Patient denies any chest pain. No shortness of breath, cough, or abdominal pain. Mild discomfort/burning on urination. No nausea/vomiting or diarrhea/constipation. No swelling of the lower extremities. No easy bruising or bleeding. The patient denies any hemoptysis or hematemesis. No bright red blood per rectum or black stools. Patient denies any skin rash.

The patient does report having drenching night sweats and persistent fevers. In addition, patient report losing ~15 pound over the last month. She does report having a burning feeling on urination, but beyond that has no other significant symptomatology.

Physical Examination

GENERAL: Patient is awake, alert and orientated x 3, in no acute distress.

HEENT: Pupils are round, reactive to light and accommodation. Extraocular movement intact. Conjunctivae pink, moist. Schlerae nonicteric. Mouth: No oral lesions. Throat: No exudates. Neck: Supple. No jugular venous distention. The patient has bilateral neck lymphadenopathy. Patient has surgical scar on left side which is slightly tender to palpation. Patient does have supraclavicular lymphadenopathy.

LUNGS: Clear to auscultation bilaterally.

CARDIAC: Regular rhythm, no murmurs or gallops

AXILLARY AREA: No evidence of lymphadenopathy.

ABDOMEN: Bowel sounds positive. Soft, nontender. No guarding. No rebound. No splenomegaly.

BACK: No costovertebral angle tenderness. No spinal tenderness.

GROIN: No lymphadenopathy.

EXTREMITIES: No cyanosis. No clubbing. No edema.

NEUROLOGICAL: Grossly nonfocal. Strength 5/5 in all extremities. Sensation to touch is intact bilaterally.

Labs and Diagnostic Tests

Sodium 144 mEq/L	Potassium 4.1 mEq/L
Chloride 105 mEq/L	BUN 10 mg/dL
Creatinine 0.8 mg/dL	Total bilirubin < 0.3 mg/dL
Direct bili <0.1 mg/dL	Alkaline phos 80 u/L
Glucose 93 mg/dL	TSH: 1.81 uIU/mL

Case 49

Urine HCG- negative

The immunoperoxidase stains negative for CD-20; CD 45 positive. Cytospin shows lymphocytosis composed predominantly of small mature cells with scattered large atypical cells. The large atypical cells have prominent nucleoli and abundant amophilic cytoplasm. Many are binucleated resembling Reed-Sternberg cells. Findings most consistent with Hodgkin's lymphoma.

Bilateral bone marrows were normocellular with no involvement of malignant cells.

MUGA: Ejection fraction was 65%.

PULMONARY FUNCTION TESTS: FVC was 3.51 L or 97% predicted. The FEV1 was 2.93 or 96% of predicted. The flow volume loop had normal contours. The total lung capacity was 4.95 L or 98% predicted. The diffusing capacity was 17 or 70% of predicted. Overall, spirometry and lung volumes are normal. The diffusing capacity was mildly reduced. Urinalysis - 10-20 WBC's, 3+ bacteria; culture- 80 K E. Coli

Diagnosis

Nodular schlerosing Hodgkin's lymphoma,

Medication Record

Multivitamin One by mouth daily

Dexamethasone 4 mg by mouth daily for 1 week until next clinic visit which was initiated because of the tracheal displacement secondary to the significant lymphadenopathy.

Protonix 40 mg by mouth daily for 1 week while on dexamethasone

Pharmacist Notes and Other Patient Information

Patient characteristics for chemotherapy dosing:

Height: 165.1   Weight: 60.1 kg

BSA: 1.67 m²

Dosage schedule:

Ondansetron 16 mg PO 30 minutes pre-chemo, days 1 and 15

Dexamethasone 20 mg IVPB 30 minutes pre-chemo, days 1 and 15

ABVD:

Doxorubicin 25 mg/m² x 1.67 m² = 42 mg IV, days 1 & 15

Prior to bleomycin, give acetaminophen 650 mg PO and diphenhydramine 50 mg PO, then bleomycin 10 units/m² x

1.67 m² = 17 units in 50 mL NS IVPB over 30 minutes, days 1 & 15 slow IV push

Vinblastine 6 mg/m² x 1.67 m² = 10 mg in 100 mL NS IVPB over 10 minutes

Dacarbazine 375 mg/m² x 1.67 m² = 630 mg in 500 mL NS IVPB over 2 hours, days 1 & 15

Bleomycin test dose 2 units (total dose) in 50 mL NS IVPB over 15 minutes on course 1, day 1 only. If no reaction proceed with remainder of total dose (i.e., Bleomycin 15 units, total remainder dose) in 50 mL NS IVPB over 30 minutes.

Repeat every 28 days for 6 cycles

Questions

1. How is KL's Hodgkin's lymphoma classified according to the Ann Arbor staging system?

    A. Stage IA
    B. Stage IIA
    C. Stage IIB
    D. Stage IIIA
    E. Stage IVA

2. The best drug therapy option for this patient is:

    A. CHOP + rituximab.
    B. CHOP x 3 cycles, then radiation therapy.
    C. ABVD x 6 - 8 cycles, then with or without radiation therapy.
    D. MOPP x 6 - 8 cycles.
    E. ABVD/ MOPP alternating plus rituximab for 6 - 8 cycles, then with or without radiation therapy.

3. A MUGA demonstrated an ejection fraction of 71%. What organ and which drug is the MUGA monitoring?

    A. Kidney, rituximab
    B. Liver, vincristine
    C. Lung, cyclophosphamide
    D. Heart, doxorubicin
    E. Bone, prednisone

4. Pulmonary function tests (PFTs) were obtained prior to initiating chemotherapy. What chemotherapy drug is the potential concern with?

    A. Doxorubicin
    B. Bleomycin
    C. Vinblastine
    D. Dacarbazine
    E. All of the above

Case 49

5. B symptoms, when present, typically have a negative impact in patients with Hodgkin's lymphoma. B symptoms include:

    I.   backache, bronchospasm, and bells palsy.
    II. fever, night sweats, and bulky disease.
    III. fever, night sweats, and weight loss.

    A. I only
    B. III only
    C. I and II only
    D. II and III only
    E. I, II, and III

6. ABVD combination chemotherapy may be preferred over a MOPP or MOPP/hybrid regimen for which of the following reasons?

    I.   ABVD has shown superior response rates in all clinical trials to date
    II. ABVD has less likelihood of causing sterility
    III. ABVD is associated with a decreased risk of secondary malignancies

    A. I only
    B. III only
    C. I and II only
    D. II and III only
    E. I, II, and III

7. Which of the following treatments would you recommend for doxorubicin extravasation?

    A. Heat plus hyaluronidase
    B. Alternating cold and hot packs
    C. Topical lidocaine
    D. Topical DMSO with cold packs
    E. Topical dexrazoxane

8. KL has a history of frequent urinary tract infections and is currently symptomatic. Her urinalysis is suggestive of an active infection with increased WBC's and bacteria. In addition, she has bacteria in her urine culture. What would be the best antibiotic treatment option in this patient?

    A. Sulfamethoxizole/trimethoprim alone
    B. Fluconazole alone
    C. Ciprofloxacin alone
    D. Amoxicillin/clavulinic acid and ciprofloxacin
    E. Metronidazole

9. Factors considered in the etiology of Hodgkin's lymphoma in this patient may include:

    I.   history of mononucleosis and Epstein-Barr virus.
    II. familial history.
    III. being of the female gender.

    A. I only
    B. III only
    C. I and II only
    D. II and III only
    E. I, II, and III

10. What is the most appropriate information to tell KL about taking dexamethasone?

    I.   Agent is indicated for weight gain
    II. Hypoglycemia is a frequent side effect
    III. Establish her tolerance to and understanding of dexamethasone

    A. I only
    B. III only
    C. I and II only
    D. II and III only
    E. I, II, and III

Patient Name: Phillip Nielson
Address: 5 London Avenue
Age: 60   **Height:** 5' 9"
Sex: M   **Race:** African American
Weight: 94 kg
Allergies: PCN (rash), morphine (nausea/vomiting)

Chief Complaint

PN, a 60-year-old male, presents to clinic for follow-up.

History of Present Illness

PN was in his usual state of health until 6 months ago when he presented to his primary provider with complaints of mild irritation upon urination. He was otherwise asymptomatic. Routine labs and urine culture at that time were unremarkable except for an elevated PSA level of 20 ng/mL. The digital rectal exam showed a small mass. Following further diagnostic work-up, PN was diagnosed with early localized Stage 2B prostate cancer. He received a nerve-sparing radical prostatectomy 2 months ago. Follow-up PSA levels were undetectable 1 month following surgery.

Past Medical History

Significant medical history includes HTN (well controlled with diuretic and calcium channel blocker therapy), diabetes mellitus type II (moderately controlled with insulin), h/o basal cell carcinoma on his back (surgically removed 5 years ago), and vasectomy.

Social History

Tobacco use: 20 pack-year history, quit smoking 10 years ago

Alcohol use: occasional

Family History

Father deceased at age 50 (metastatic prostate cancer)

Mother alive, with HTN and type 2 DM

Two brothers alive, healthy

One sister alive, healthy

Review of Systems

No constitutional, gastrointestinal, cardiac, or neurological symptoms. He reports occasional episodes of urinary incontinence.

Physical Examination

Date of exam: 2/1/06

GEN: Slightly obese, alert man

VS: BP 172/87 mmHg, HR 76 bpm, RR 20 rpm, T 36.8°C, Wt 94 kg, Ht 175.3 cm

HEENT: Normocephalic, atraumatic, PERRLA, moist oral mucosa without lesions

CHEST: Lungs clear to auscultation and percussion bilaterally. Heart with regular rate and rhythm, no m/g/r.

ABD: Soft, nontender, no organomegaly, masses, or ascites

EXT: No clubbing, cyanosis, or edema; lymphatic survey is negative

NEURO: Normal mental acuity, cranial nerves and motor function

GU: Palpable nodule, about 1 cm in diameter on posterior side of prostate

Labs and Diagnostic Tests

CBC WNL   Chem-7 panel WNL

PSA 15 ng/mL   BP: 172/87 mmHg

Transrectal ultrasound: Positive for 0.9-cm mass. Biopsy recommended.

Transurethral resection of prostate tissue: Positive for 0.9-cm adenocarcinoma, confined to 60% of single lobe.

Diagnosis

Primary:
     1. Stage B prostate cancer

Secondary:
     1. Hypertension
     2. Diabetes mellitus, type II
     3. h/o basal cell carcinoma status post resection

Medication Record

Furosemide 40 mg po qd   Amlodipine 5 mg po qd

ECASA 325 mg po qd   NPH insulin 20 units sq bid

Lispro insulin 5 units sq qac

Pharmacist Notes and Other Patient Information

None available

Case 50

Questions

1. PN has several risk factors which increase his risk for developing prostate cancer. Besides, age and a positive family history, which additional risk factor does PN have?

   A. Smoking history
   B. Race
   C. Alcohol use
   D. History of basal cell carcinoma
   E. Vasectomy

2. PN started prostate screening at age 50. What age should his brothers start prostate screening?

   A. 35 years
   B. 40 years
   C. 45 years
   D. 50 years
   E. 55 years

3. Besides PSA measurement, what other screening tool is used for early detection of prostate cancer?

   A. Ultrasound guided fine needle biopsy
   B. Labs
   C. Pain on urination
   D. Digital rectal exam
   E. Age

4. The following are abnormal PSA levels EXCEPT:

   A. <4 ng/mL.
   B. >4-10 ng/mL.
   C. >10-25 ng/mL.
   D. >20-30 ng/mL.
   E. >30 ng/mL.

5. Which of the following is (are) true statements?

   I. Prostatectomy and radiation are viable approaches for prostate cancer management.
   II. Radical-prostatectomy is preferred to nerve-sparing prostatectomy.
   III. Prostatectomy and radiation are devoid of complications.

   A. I only
   B. III only
   C. I and II only
   D. II and III only
   E. I, II, and III

6. Terazosin is used in the treatment of hesitancy, impaired urinary stream, nocturia, and urgency. It belongs to which pharmacological class?

   A. Alpha blocker
   B. Beta blocker
   C. Calcium channel blocker
   D. 5HT-$_3$ blocker
   E. ACE inhibitor

7. Impotence is a common complication of prostatectomy. PN is receiving alprostadil urethral suppositories for this complication. He is interested in a medication that is available orally. Which of the following agent(s) would be appropriate?

   I. Sildenafil
   II. Tadalafil
   III. Vardenafil

   A. I only
   B. III only
   C. I and II only
   D. II and III only
   E. I, II, and III

8. 5-alpha reductase inhibitors prevent the conversion of testosterone to dihydrotestosterone, the primary androgen in the prostate. In the Prostate Cancer Prevention Trial, what 5-alpha reductase inhibitor was studied to reduce the risk of prostate cancer?

   A. Sildenafil
   B. Dutasteride
   C. Gemcitabine
   D. Finasteride
   E. Tolterodine

9. The Prostate Cancer Prevention Trial randomized men to daily finasteride vs. placebo. The following statement(s) is(are) true EXCEPT:

   A. Can be taken regardless of food
   B. Should be taken with food
   C. Incidence of high-grade prostate cancer is higher in the finasteride arm
   D. Decreased libido is a common side effect
   E. Daily dose of finasteride studied in this trial was 5 mg

10. In the event of disease progression, LHRH agonists are utilized for androgen ablation. Which of the following is an example of an LHRH agonist?

    A. Aminoglutethimide
    B. Bicalutamide
    C. Goserelin
    D. Estramustine
    E. Pamidronate

Patient Name: William Wallace
Address: 3405 Falkirk Lane
Age: 18   **Height:** 6' 1"
Sex: M   **Race:** White
Weight: 80 kg
Allergies: Ceclor (hives)

Chief Complaint

WW is an 18-yo male who presents to the oncology clinic with a new diagnosis of melanoma of the left neck lymph nodes from a primary scalp lesion.

History of Present Illness

WW noticed a lump in his left neck after an ear piercing. Since the mass in the neck did not resolve after a course of antibiotics, a physician performed a fine-needle aspiration of the mass revealing unusual cells. A computed tomography (CT) scan performed revealed diffuse lymphadenopathy. He underwent an excisional biopsy of the large node in his neck and this revealed melanoma. Several skin lesions were also removed and were negative for melanoma. Finally, a scalp lesion was biopsied a second time and revealed a melanocytic nevus compound type with atypia and was found to be Clark Level III. A left modified neck dissection revealed melanoma in 2 of 32 lymph nodes with a large metastasis measuring at least 1.3 cm with evidence of extranodal extension within the parotid gland. The patient comes to the clinic today for discussion of systemic adjuvant treatment options.

Past Medical History

Unremarkable

Social History

Currently attends junior college and has 5 siblings.

Tobacco use: none

Alcohol use: none

He is a left-handed pitcher on a baseball team.

Family History

Grandmother: melanoma at age 36 on leg; surgically removed; she is currently alive and well with no evidence of disease.

Review of Systems

The patient denies headaches, stiff neck, fevers, chills, nausea, diarrhea, or weight loss. He has some limitation in his left upper extremity mobility related to his recent neck dissection.

Physical Examination

GEN: WD/WN white male in NAD.

VS: T 35.7°C, HR 54 bpm, RR 18 rpm, BP 132/70 mmHg, Wt 80 kg, Ht 180 cm.

HEENT: Skin examination reveals fineness in the middle of the left neck dissection scar that may be postoperative changes. No other palpable lymphadenopathy. Total body skin examination reveals no suspicious lesions.

CHEST: Lungs CTA bilaterally. Mild expiratory wheezing noted.

CV: RRR

ABD: Soft, nontender, and nondistended; bowel sounds were present.

EXT: No edema. Within normal limits.

Labs and Diagnostic Tests

Sodium 143 mEq/L	Potassium 3.6 mEq/L
Chloride 104 mEq/L	CO_2 content 26 mEq/L
Magnesium 2.1 mg/dL	Calcium 8.9 mg/dL
BUN 10 mg/dL	Serum creatinine 0.9 mg/dL
Glucose 104 mg/dL	Phosphorous 2.7 mg/dL
T. bili 0.4 mg/dL	Alk phos 89 u/L
LDH 474 IU/mL	SGPT 30 IU/mL

WBC 11,900/mm³ with 78% PMN, 14% lymphocytes, 7% monocytes, 2% eosinophils

Hemoglobin 14.6 g/dL   Hematocrit 41.9%

Platelets 163,000/mm³

CT chest: No evidence of pulmonary metastatic disease.

CT abdomen: No metastatic disease identified in the abdomen or pelvis.

MRI head: The sagittal images demonstrate almost 1 cm of tonsillar ectopia of the cerebellum, indicating Chiari 1 malformation. No evidence for metastatic tumor.

Left modified neck dissection, left neck contents: Metastatic malignant neoplasm consistent with metastatic melanoma in 2 of 32 lymph nodes; largest measures at least 1.3 cm with extranodal extension.

Excisional biopsy scalp lesion: Melanocytic nevus, compound type, completely excised. The architectural pattern suggests congenital onset. Architectural disorder moderate cytologic atypia of melanocytes.

Case 51

Medication Record

Date	Rx No	Physician	Drug and Strength	Quantity	Sig	Refills
12/04	641987	Bruce	Cetirizine 10 mg	1 tablet	po daily prn	
6/05	726988	Bruce	Albuterol MDI	1 MDI (17 g)	1 puff every 4 hours as needed for wheezing	PRN
10/05	752120	Bruce	Methylprednisolone Dosepak	1 Dosepak	UAD for asthma exacerbation	0

Diagnosis

Primary

    1. Stage III melanoma with lymph node involvement

Secondary

    1. Chronic sinusitis

    2. Reactive airway disease

Assessment and plan: WW has stage III melanoma of the left neck. He is recovering from primary surgery. After which time, he will receive systemic adjuvant high-dose interferon per FDA-dosing recommendations.

Pharmacist Notes and Other Patient Information

None available

Questions

1. Which route(s) may interferon-alpha 2b be administered?

    I. IV

    II. SQ

    III. Oral

    A. I only

    B. III only

    C. I and II only

    D. II and III only

    E. I, II, and III

2. The ABCD rule for differentiating melanomas from benign moles stands for which series of words?

    A. Asymmetry, border irregularity, color variation, and diameter >6 mm

    B. Actinic keratoses, border irregularity, congenital nevi, and diameter <6 mm

    C. Asymmetry, biopsy positive, completely excised, and dysplastic appearance

    D. Actinic keratoses, biopsy positive, color variation, and dysplastic appearance

    E. Actinic keratoses, biopsy positive, congenital nevi, and dysplastic appearance

3. The approved dose of interferon for the adjuvant treatment of melanoma is.

    A. 30 mg/m^2 SQ three times weekly x2 years

    B. 20 million units/m^2/day IV x5 days/week x4 weeks, then 10 million units/m^2 SQ three times weekly x48 weeks

    C. 20 million units/m^2 po three times weekly x12 weeks

    D. 10 mg IV x5 days/week x12 weeks, then 3 mg SQ three times weekly x2 years

    E. 30 mg/m^2/day SQ x5 days/week x1 year

4. Which of the following should be included when counseling a patient who will receive interferon alpha-2b?

    A. The majority of toxicities will resolve on discontinuation of interferon alpha-2b

    B. May cause alterations in thyroid function. Thyroid function tests may be necessary while receiving treatment.

    C. Flu-like symptoms are the most likely adverse effects seen from interferon alpha-2b. This often includes fever, headaches and fatigue. These symptoms may occur within 2 hours of administration and last up to 24 hours.

    D. CNS toxicity, such as depression, somnolence or confusion may occur.

    E. All of the above should be included in patient counseling

5. Which agent has NOT shown activity in melanoma?

    A. Aldesleukin

    B. Interferon-alpha 2b

    C. Cisplatin

    D. DTIC

    E. Capecitabine

6. If WW were found to have metastatic (Stage IV) melanoma and receive high-dose aldesleukin (600,000 units/kg IV every 8 hours x 14 doses) for therapy, which of the following would be appropriate to tell him on providing counseling?

    A. May cause temporary flare of melanoma lesions

    B. May increase chance of secondary malignancy 3-5 years

    C. May cause neutropenia. Wear mask in public and avoid contact with those with signs/symptoms of infection

Case 51

D.   Discontinue methylprednisolone to allow aldesleukin
         to have full effect
    E.   This regimen is given every 21 days for 6 cycles

7. Which of the following is recommended to be given before
    each dose of interferon-alpha 2b to reduce incidence of
    adverse reactions?

    A. Fluoxetine
    B. Diphenhydramine
    C. Acetaminophen
    D. Epinephrine
    E. Oxycodone

8. Which of the following are risk factors for developing skin
    cancer?

    I.   Fair skin
    II.   Sunburn easily
    III. Light-colored hair

    A. I only
    B. III only
    C. I and II only
    D. II and III only
    E. I, II, and III

9. Which of the following screening tools are useful for early
    detection of skin cancers?

    A. Total body PET scan
    B. Total body CT scan
    C. Total body MRI
    D. Total body skin examination
    E. Total body ultrasound

10. While receiving his adjuvant interferon, WW's LFTs begin
    to rise. What is the most appropriate recommendation to
    make regarding the interferon?

    A. Discontinue the interferon and never give WW
        interferon again.
    B. Discontinue the interferon until the LFTs return to
        normal, and resume at half the dose.
    C. Continue the interferon at the current dose and
        continue to monitor the LFTs.
    D. Continue the interferon at half the dose and continue
        to monitor the LFTs.
    E. Continue the interferon at one quarter the dose and
        continue to monitor the LFTs.

Infectious Diseases

Section Editors: John L. Woon, Catherine Oliphant

*See all 38 cases for this section on the CD.

Case 52

Patient Name: Lee Reeves
Address: 101 Broken Arrow Drive
Age: 18   **Height:** 5' 10"
Sex: M   **Race:** Caucasian
Weight: 165 lb
Allergies: NKDA

Chief Complaint

LR presents to the emergency room complaining that his left arm is hurting and swollen.

History of Present Illness

LR broke his left radius playing football 14 days ago. He required surgery and placement of a metal plate to hold the bones in place. He states that all has been well until 2 days ago, when he bumped his arm on a door frame. A few hours later, he noticed the swelling, and it has gotten worse with increasing pain.

Past Medical History

Past medical history is unremarkable except for normal childhood illnesses.

Social History

LR is a high school senior who lives at home with his sister, little brother, mother, and father. He is very active physically. He denies drinking alcohol and using tobacco products.

Family History

Mother and father are living. Sister and brother are also living at home. There are no significant medical illnesses known at this time.

Review of Systems

Left arm is notably swollen, red, and hot to the touch. No other systems reviewed.

Physical Examination

GEN: Alert and oriented. Cooperative, pleasant, and animated in conversation.

VS: Ht 5' 10", Wt 165 lb, HR 77 bpm, RR 19 rpm, T 101.8° F, BP 122/75 mmHg

HEENT: Unremarkable

CHEST: Lungs CTA, heart RRR

ABD: Soft, nondistended

NEURO: Not checked

Labs and Diagnostic Tests

CBC: WBC 11,000 no diff., RBC 4500

ESR 52 mm/hr

CRP 10 mg/dL

X-ray: Possible but not definitive blurring of margins of left radius at point of fx

Bone scan: Positive for inflammation in the left radius

Blood cultures are pending

Diagnosis

Primary: Possible osteomyelitis of left radius

Medication Record

None, except for minor pain medications provided at time postsurgery

Pharmacist Notes and Other Patient Information

None available

Questions

1. What information presented supports the diagnosis of osteomyelitis?

    I.   Elevated temperature
    II. Elevated WBC
    III. Elevated ESR

    A. I only
    B. III only
    C. I and II only
    D. II and III only
    E. I, II, and III

Case 52

2. The most likely microbiologic etiology for the suspected osteomyelitis is:

   A. Candida albicans.
   B. Pseudomonas aeruginosa.
   C. Staphylococcus aureus.
   D. Enterococcus faecalis.
   E. E. coli.

3. Complications of osteomyelitis include:

   I. bone necrosis.
   II. sepsis.
   III. amputation.

   A. I only
   B. III only
   C. I and II only
   D. II and III only
   E. I, II, and III

4. The patient appears very agitated and preoccupied. He explains that he has tickets to a sold-out concert for that evening and was hoping to get a "shot of some kind" and then be sent home with oral antibiotics. His classmate was recently prescribed oral ciprofloxacin for a wound infection, and he was hoping to get a similar prescription. How would you counsel the patient regarding treatment of his osteomyelitis?

   I. Only parenteral antibiotics are used in the management of osteomyelitis.
   II. Early antibiotic therapy may reduce the need for surgery.
   III. Ciprofloxacin has poor activity against staphylococci.

   A. I only
   B. III only
   C. I and II only
   D. II and III only
   E. I, II, and III

5. While awaiting culture results, the physician empirically prescribes ceftriaxone. What is the most appropriate initial dose and route of adminstration for this agent and infection?

   A. Ceftriaxone 1 g orally once daily
   B. Ceftriaxone 2 g orally twice daily
   C. Ceftriaxone 500 mg IV every 24 hours
   D. Ceftriaxone 2 g IV every 24 hours
   E. Ceftriaxone 1 g IM every 24 hours

6. Which of the following is NOT a commonly recognized adverse effect of ceftriaxone?

   A. Thrombocytopenia
   B. Rash
   C. Phototoxicity
   D. Diarrhea
   E. Nausea

7. Culture results come back positive for MRSA, and the patient is switched to vancomycin 1000 mg IV every 12 hours. The patient currently has only peripheral IV access. To minimize thrombophlebitis, the pharmacist wants to dilute the vancomycin solution to a concentration of 4 mg/mL. Therefore, the vancomycin should be added to what volume of dextrose 5% in water?

   A. 50 mL of dextrose 5% in water
   B. 100 mL of dextrose 5% in water
   C. 250 mL of dextrose 5% in water
   D. 500 mL of dextrose 5% in water
   E. 1000 mL of dextrose 5% in water

8. LR does not tolerate the vancomycin, so the physician decides to change his antibiotic regimen to IV linezolid. Which of the following statements is correct regarding linezolid therapy?

   I. There is no oral formulation of linezolid available.
   II. SSRIs, such as fluoxetine, may cause a serotonin syndrome when administered with linezolid.
   III. Thrombocytopenia is a recognized adverse effect of linezolid.

   A. I only
   B. III only
   C. I and II only
   D. II and III only
   E. I, II, and III

9. After receiving 7 days of parenteral antibiotics, the physician decides to switch LR to oral therapy. Which criteria should be present before using oral antibiotics to complete therapy for acute osteomyelitis?

   I. Afebrile
   II. At least 1 day of parenteral antibiotics
   III. Elevated CRP

   A. I only
   B. III only
   C. I and II only
   D. II and III only
   E. I, II, and III

Case 52

10. Approximately 2 weeks later, the patient visits with you and states a desire to discontinue his antibiotic therapy. He explains that at his last doctor's appointment 2 days ago, the physician told him that he had no fever, his WBC count was back to normal, and the physical exam was unremarkable with no swelling, redness, or tenderness at the surgical wound site. How would you counsel this patient?

A. "Don't ask me; you should ask your doctor."

B. "Two weeks should be sufficient; I think you can quit the antibiotics."

C. "Despite your lack of symptoms, 2 weeks is not long enough for treating osteomyelitis. I would strongly advise you to continue your antibiotic therapy for at least 4 to 6 weeks."

D. "Two weeks should be sufficient. I think you can quit the antibiotics, but I recommend speaking with your physician first."

E. "Despite your lack of symptoms, 2 weeks is not long enough treatment for osteomyelitis. An additional 6 to 8 weeks of low-dose antibiotics is recommended for treatment of osteomyelitis."

Patient Name: Tommy Chicago
Address: 251 E. Huron St.
Age: 18 **Height:** 6' 2"
Sex: M **Race:** White
Weight: 220 lb
Allergies: Sulfa-rash

Chief Complaint

"I have the worst headache of my life."

History of Present Illness

TC is an 18-yo college freshman who was brought to the ED by his roommate on 10/20 due to decreased energy, general malaise, and an excruciating headache since last night. His symptoms were of sudden onset and have persisted about 6 hours. The patient attended a party the night of the onset of symptoms but denies illicit drug use. The subject consumed three cans of beer prior to symptoms.

On admission to the ED the patient continues to complain about headache, sensitivity to light, and neck stiffness. The patient has vomited once since presenting to the ER and is continually nauseous.

Past Medical History

TC has a past medical history of seasonal allergies as well as intermittent insomnia.

Social History

Travel history: Prior to attending university this fall, the patient spent the summer backpacking across Western Europe (France, Germany, Spain, and Italy)

Tobacco use: Social smoker (approximately 1 pack every 2 weeks), began smoking at the age of 17

Alcohol use: Approximately 12 drinks per week with use mainly on the weekends

Recreational drug use: Denied by patient and roommate

Caffeine use: 2 cups of coffee per day; use is tripled during exams

Family History

Father: 50-yo male alive and well with mild hypertension

Mother: 51-yo female alive and well with no known medical problems

Review of Systems

Exam reveals an ill-appearing young male who is only able to respond to questions intermittently with yes/no answers but denies any focal pain. The patient appears somnolent but is arousable.

Physical Examination

GEN: Pale, well-nourished, lethargic male in NAD

VS: On ED admission: BP 110/68 mmHg, HR 120 bpm, RR 22 rpm, T 102°F, Ht 6'2", Wt 220 lb

HEENT: No papilledema on exam. Pupils equally round and reactive to light. Patient with photophobia.

CHEST: Clear to auscultation

CV: RRR with normal S_1/S_2 and no audible murmur

SKIN: Petechiae present as noted below

NEURO: Intermittently alert; oriented to self (patient is unable to state where he is or what day it is). Nuchal rigidity present, positive Brudzinski's sign, positive Kernig's sign

EXTREM: Notable for several petechial skin lesions on arms

Labs and Diagnostic Tests

Sodium 140 mEq/L	Potassium 4 mEq/L
Chloride 106 mEq/L	CO_2 content 28 mEq/L
BUN 30 mg/dL	Serum creatinine 1.3 mg/dL
Glucose 106 mg/dL	Hemoglobin 16.2 g/dL
Hematocrit 49%	Platelets 281,000/mm³

WBC 20,600/mm³ with 75% PMN, 18% bands, 3% lymphocytes, 4% monocytes

Blood toxicology/alcohol screen: Negative

Head CT: Normal   CXR: Normal

Lumbar puncture/cerebral spinal fluid: WBC 2700/mm³, 88% segs, 6% lymphocytes, 6% monocytes, 10 RBCs, glucose 7 mg/dL, protein 610 mg/dL

CSF Gram stain: Gram-negative diplococcus

Diagnosis

Primary:

1. Acute bacterial meningitis

2. Dehydration

Case 53

Medication Record

Date	Rx No	Physician	Drug and Strength	Quantity	Sig	Refills
08/12	150652	Moffett	Fluticasone 50 mcg	1	1 spray per nostril daily	5
08/12	150653	Moffett	Zolpidem 10 mg	30	1 tablet prn insomnia	2

(Admission profile)

Vaccination history:

1. Influenza vaccine: Receives annually

2. Hepatitis B: Series complete 8/12

2. Tetanus diptheria: 8/12

3. Polio: series complete 1993

4. Measles mumps rubella: series complete 1993

Pharmacist Notes and Other Patient Information

None available

Questions

1. Identify the terms that are properly matched with their definitions.
   - I. Nuchal rigidity/stiff neck
   - II. Petechial rash/large flat red rash area with small confluent bumps
   - III. Photophobia/fear of photography
   - A. I only
   - B. III only
   - C. I and II only
   - D. II and III only
   - E. I, II, and III

2. Which of the following are consistent with bacterial meningitis?
   - I. Elevated protein count in the CSF
   - II. Polymorphonuclear cell predominance in the CSF
   - III. Elevated glucose in the CSF
   - A. I only
   - B. III only
   - C. I and II only
   - D. II and III only
   - E. I, II, and III

3. Which pair of organisms represent the most likely pathgens in our 18-yo immunocompetent patient with suspected community-acquired meningitis?
   - A. Listeria monocytogenes/Haemophilus influenzae
   - B. Group B Streptococci/Esherichia coli
   - C. Neisseria meningitidis/Streptococcus pneumoniae
   - D. Staphylococcus aureus-Bacteriodes fragilis
   - E. Pseudomonas aeruginosa-Acinetobacter baumannii

4. Which anti-infectives would provide optimal (yet the most narrow spectrum) empiric coverage for meningitis prior to microbiology laboratory findings in this patient?
   - A. Cefazolin, gentamicin, and metronidazole
   - B. Ceftriaxone and vancomycin
   - C. Vancomycin, ceftazidime, and metronidazole
   - D. Oxacillin, azithromycin, and acyclovir
   - E. Daptomycin, ampicillin, and fluconazole

5. After 3 days of therapy, the pathogen is determined to be N. meningitidis. Which statement most accurately summarizes the utility of corticosteroids in this patient?
   - A. Dexamethasone should be initiated in this patient since the culture confirmed N. meningitidis.
   - B. Dexamethasone should be initiated in this patient in order to decrease inflammation associated with concomitant enterovirus infection.
   - C. Dexamethasone should have been initiated early in this patient but delay in therapy and uncertain efficacy of dexamethasone in N. meningitidis preclude its current utility at this point in the clinical course.
   - D. Since the culture confirmed N. meningitidis, dexamethasone should not be initiated in this patient as it will decrease the penetration of vancomycin, and vancomycin will be unable to treat the N. meningitidis.
   - E. Dexamethasone should not be initiated in this patient due to the patient's leucocytosis. This is a black box warning and an absolute contraindication.

Case 53

6. Which of the following is the most appropriate prophylaxis for household contacts of a patient diagnosed with community-acquired meningitis caused by N. meningitidis?

    A. Daptomycin 300 mg po x 1 dose
    B. Trimethoprim/sulfamethoxazole IV 15 mg/kg/day x 4 weeks
    C. Rifampin 600 mg po q 12 h x 4 doses
    D. Vancomycin 500 mg po x 1 dose
    E. No prophylaxis is ever recommended for N. meningitidis meningitis

7. TC has been in close contact with his sister, who is currently 8 months pregnant. What prophylaxis should she receive?

    A. Rifampin 600 mg po x 4 doses
    B. Ciprofloxacin 500 mg po x 1 dose
    C. Ceftriaxone 250 mg IM x 1 dose
    D. Chloramphenicol 75 mg/kg/day po divided in 4 doses x 7 days
    E. Sulfamethoxazole/trimethoprim 800/160 mg po QD x 7 days

8. The N. meningitidis vaccine is currently recommended for

    I.   pre-adolescents and young adults.
    II. pediatrics before the age of 10.
    III. the elderly (age>65).

    A. I only
    B. III only
    C. I and II only
    D. II and III only
    E. I, II, and III

9. The most appropriate route of therapy for vancomycin in community acquired meningitis is

    A. IM
    B. Oral
    C. Intrathecal
    D. IV-push
    E. Slow IV infusion

10. Which answer matches the correct gram stain and colony morphology with the correct genus and species?

    A. Staphylococcus aureus/gram negative bacillus
    B. Neisseria meningitidis/gram positive bacillus
    C. Haemophilus influenzae/gram positive cocci
    D. Streptococcus pneumoniae/gram negative bacillus
    E. Listeria monocytogenes/gram positive bacillus

Case 54   Drugs Used to Counter Biological Warfare

Patient Name: Thomas Carter
Address: 105 Harris Street
Age: 56   **Height:** 5' 10"
Sex: M   **Race:** African American
Weight: 180 lb
Allergies: NKDA

Chief Complaint

TC is a 56-yo African American man who was brought to the emergency department by his wife for evaluation. He was confused and in obvious respiratory distress. TC has been unable to work for the last couple of days at the local UPS distribution center.

History of Present Illness

TC's wife reported that TC had no complaints prior to this illness, which started about 4-5 days ago. At that time, he began feeling generally fatigued with fever and chills progressing to soaking sweats, nausea and vomiting, mild nonproductive cough, and shortness of breath. This morning, his wife found him to be confused and experiencing significant shortness of breath, and she proceeded to bring him to the emergency department.

Past Medical History

TC suffers from hypertension, which is controlled with medication

Social History

Alcohol: Social

Tobacco: Denied

Caffeine: 1-2 cups of coffee daily

Family History

Parents and sibling alive. Father w/ hypertension. No pertinent history.

Review of Systems

Negative except as noted previously

Physical Examination

GEN: Well-nourished adult male in apparent respiratory distress

VS: On ED admission: BP 108/61 mmHg, HR 135 bpm, RR 20 rpm, T 38.5°C, Wt 82 kg, Ht 5' 10'

HEENT: Normal

CHEST: Rales at the right base with diffuse wheezing and tachycardia

NEURO: Not oriented to place and time

Labs and Diagnostic Tests

WBC 9900/mm³ w/ 83% neutrophils, 4% bands, 6% lymphocytes, and 7% monocytes

Hematocrit 43%	Sodium 130 mEq/L
Potassium 5.3 mEq/L	Chloride 99 mEq/L
Serum creatinine 1.6 mg/dL	Arterial pH 7.42
$PaCO_2$ 25	PaO_2 66

O_2 sat 93% on 2 L O_2/min nasal

Chest x-ray: Mediastinal widening, right hilar and peritracheal soft tissue fullness w/ right, middle, and lower lobe infiltrates and right pleural effusion

CSF: Microscopic exam showed many gram-positive bacilli; Bacillus anthracis was isolated after 7 hours of incubation

Blood cultures: Bacillus anthracis was isolated after 15 hours of incubation

Diagnosis

Patient was admitted to the hospital with an initial diagnosis of meningitis, which was changed to inhalation anthrax once cultures were available.

Medication Record

Initial admission orders:

Cefotaxime 2 g IV q 4 h

Enalapril 5 mg qd

Acetaminophen 650 mg po q 4 h prn fever

Pharmacist Notes and Other Patient Information

None available

Case 54

Questions

1. Which of the following might be appropriate antimicrobials to include in a treatment regimen for this patient?

   I. Cefotaxime
   II. Ciprofloxacin
   III. Rifampin

   A. I only
   B. III only
   C. I and II only
   D. II and III only
   E. I, II, and III

2. Which of the following antimicrobials is FDA approved for treatment of inhalation anthrax?

   I. Ciprofloxacin
   II. Doxycycline
   III. Chloramphenicol

   A. I only
   B. III only
   C. I and II only
   D. II and III only
   E. I, II, and III

3. On the basis of the Consensus Statement on Anthrax as a Biological Weapon, 2002, it is advocated that two or three antibiotics be used in combination for the treatment of inhalation anthrax based on susceptibility testing with epidemic strains. Which of the regimens below would be best for this patient empirically?

   A. Ciprofloxacin, vancomycin, rifampin
   B. Doxycycline, penicillin, ceftriaxone
   C. Clindamycin, levofloxacin, ceftazidime
   D. Ciprofloxacin, gentamicin, ampicillin
   E. Trimethoprim-sulfamethoxazole, levofloxacin, metronidazole

4. What is the appropriate duration of antimicrobial treatment for inhalation anthrax?

   A. 10 days
   B. 14 days
   C. 28 days
   D. 30 days
   E. 60 days

5. Which of the following statements about anthrax is true?

   I. Inhalation anthrax results from the deposition of B anthracis spores into alveolar spaces.
   II. Inhalation anthrax is thought to present as a two-phase illness with the initial phase of fever, fatigue, malaise and nonproductive cough lasting 1-4 days followed by a fulminant phase of respiratory distress, diaphoresis, and shock.
   III. Anthrax infection occurs in humans by three major routes. inhalation, cutaneous, and gastrointestinal with the inhalation route being associated with the greatest morbidity and mortality.

   A. I only
   B. III only
   C. I and II only
   D. II and III only
   E. I, II, and III

6. All of the following are possible diagnostic indicators for anthrax EXCEPT:

   A. malaise and fever as presenting symptoms.
   B. abnormal chest x-ray, including mediastinal widening, infiltrates, and pleural effusions.
   C. hemorrhagic pleural fluid.
   D. blood cultures positive for B anthracis in patients who have not received antibiotics prior to cultures.
   E. runny nose.

7. Which of the following is the appropriate infusion time for ciprofloxacin 400 mg IV?

   A. 15 minutes
   B. 30 minutes
   C. 60 minutes
   D. 90 minutes
   E. IV push

8. What would be the rationale for adding rifampin to the ciprofloxacin regimen for this patient?

   I. TC had B anthracis in the cerebrospinal fluid, and rifampin has better CNS penetration than ciprofloxacin.
   II. There is the possibility that an engineered strain of B anthracis resistant to one or more antibiotics might be used in a future attack.
   III. The use of two or more antibiotics confers a survival advantage.

Case 54

    A. I only
    B. III only
    C. I and II only
    D. II and III only
    E. I, II, and III

9.   During a grand rounds presentation at your hospital you are asked what the median time period was from presumed time of anthrax exposure to the onset of symptoms based on the 2001 cases. Your answer is:

    A. 7 days.
    B. 10 days.
    C. 4 days.
    D. 14 days.
    E. 2 days.

10. Which of the following are appropriate resources for information on bioterrorism?

    I.   Centers for Disease Control and Prevention
    II. Americal Society of Health-System Pharmacists
    III. American Pharmaceutical Association

    A. I only
    B. III only
    C. I and II only
    D. II and III only
    E. I, II, and III

Case 55

Patient Name: Jose Baccaro
Address: 232 Lynden Road
Age: 71   **Height:** 5' 7"
Sex: M   **Race:** Hispanic American
Weight: 78 kg
Allergies: NKA

Chief Complaint

JB is a 71-yo Hispanic male who was admitted to the hospital with general weakness, fever with night sweats, and dyspnea. JB states he feels weak and has no appetite. His daughter states he usually is a big eater and her father has complained of being too warm for the past 2 days.

History of Present Illness

Over the past 3-4 days, JB has been short of breath when completing activities of daily living. His activity has decreased substantially, and he has been sitting in his chair most of the day. He stated he was chilled and sweating last night. This morning, his daughter felt his forehead and he felt warm, so she gave him two acetaminophen tablets.

Past Medical History

JB has a history of mitral valve prolapse with regurgitation approximately 3 years ago. He was admitted about 11 months ago for an infective endocarditis. He spent 2 weeks in the hospital, followed by 2 weeks of home health care. The remainder of his history is unremarkable.

Social History

Tobacco use: None

Alcohol use: None

Caffeine use: 1-2 Cups of coffee in the morning

Drug abuse: None

Family History

Mother died of an MI at age 66. Father died of complications of surgery at age 58.

Review of Systems

Unremarkable

Physical Examination

GEN: Pale, WD, NAD except for general weakness

VS: BP 138/95 mmHg, HR 90 bpm, RR 28 rpm, T 100.1°F, Wt 78 kg

HEENT: Unremarkable

CHEST: Heart murmur

NEURO: Alert and oriented x3

Labs and Diagnostic Tests

Sodium 145 mEq/L	Potassium 3.8 mEq/L
Fasting blood glucose 79 mg/dL	WBC 14,000 cells/mm³
RBC 4.6 cells/mm³	Hgb 12.1 g/dL
Hct 42%	Reticulocyte count 0.5%
TIBC 223 mg/dL	Fe 49 µg/dL

Blood cultures: Microbiology reports 5 of 6 BacTec cultures are positive for Streptococcus viridans, penicillin-susceptible

Diagnosis

Primary:

    1. Infective endocarditis

    2. Anemia

Secondary:

    1. Hypertension

Medication Record

(Prior to admission)

Hydrochlorothiazide 25 mg po q am

Tylenol prn

Pharmacist Notes and Other Patient Information

None available

Case 55

Questions

1. Select the clinical manifestations in this patient that are commonly associated with endocarditis.

    I.   Shortness of breath
    II. Sweating, felt warm
    III. Heart murmur

    A. I only
    B. III only
    C. I and II only
    D. II and III only
    E. I, II, and III

2. Prior to receiving microbiology blood culture reports, which of the following pathogens would you consider when selecting treatment options for this patient with suspected infective endocarditis?

    I.   Meningococci
    II. Streptococci
    III. Staphylococci

    A. I only
    B. III only
    C. I and II only
    D. II and III only
    E. I, II, and III

3. Empiric drug(s) of choice for the two most likely pathogens for infective endocarditis in this patient would include?

    I.   Ceftriaxone
    II. Erythromycin
    III. Nafcillin

    A. I only
    B. III only
    C. I and II only
    D. II and III only
    E. I, II, and III

4. Which of the following is a risk factor(s) for endocarditis?

    I.   Mitral valve prolapse with regurgitation
    II. IV drug abuse
    III. Family history of an MI

    A. I only
    B. III only
    C. I and II only
    D. II and III only
    E. I, II, and III

5. If aqueous penicillin G 20 MU vial is reconstitution with 33 mL of sterile water and the powder displaces 7 mL of fluid. How many mL of the above aqueous penicillin G concentration and which solution should used to provide 24 mu IVPB in four equally divided doses?

    A. 6 mL into 100 mL 0.9% sodium chloride
    B. 6 mL into 100 mL 0.9% sodium chloride
    C. 12 mL into 100 mL 0.9% sodium chloride
    D. 18 mL into 100 mL 0.9% sodium chloride
    E. 18 mL into 100 mL 0.9% sodium chloride

6. Which type of sterile environment should intravenous solutions per prepared?

    I.   Horizontal laminar flow hood
    II. Vertical laminar flow hood
    III. Diagonal laminar flow hood

    A. I only
    B. III only
    C. I and II only
    D. II and III only
    E. I, II, and III

7. Aqueous penicillin G IVPB may be administered through?

    I.   Compatible continuous intravenous solution tubing y-site
    II. Heparin lock
    III. Non-compatible primary IV solution y-site with primary solution stopped and tube is flushed before and after with saline solution

    A. I only
    B. III only
    C. I and II only
    D. II and III only
    E. I, II, and III

8. What potential electrolyte imbalance may be seen with administration of aqueous penicillin G sodium?

    I.   Sodium
    II. Potassium
    III. Phosphorous

    A. I only
    B. III only
    C. I and II only
    D. II and III only
    E. I, II, and III

Case 55

9. What would you recommend if a patient experiences an allergic reaction to the aqueous penicillin G?

   I. Oxygen
   II. Intravenous steroids
   III. Airway management

   A. I only
   B. III only
   C. I and II only
   D. II and III only
   E. I, II, and III

10. If the physician believes this patient experienced a penicillin-induced nonanaphylactoid type allergic reaction during the patient's last admission, which antibiotic would you recommend?

   A. Aqueous penicillin G
   B. Cefazolin
   C. Vancomycin
   D. Nafcillin
   E. Oxacillin

Case 56

Patient Name: Martha Babcock
Address: 921 S. Washington
Age: 52   **Height:** 5' 2"
Sex: F   **Race:** White
Weight: 158 lb
Allergies: Erythromycin

Chief Complaint

MB is a 52-year-old female who was admitted 15 days ago for a small bowel obstruction. She has remained in the surgical intensive care for 15 days. MB is currently on vancomycin, meropenem, tobramycin, and fluconazole for a nosocomial pneumonia and MRSA wound infection. Her WBC count has been increasing over the past 3 days, and this morning, she spiked a temperature to 103.4°F, and her blood pressure dropped to 85/46 mmHg.

History of Present Illness

MB was admitted 15 days ago for a small bowel obstruction. She underwent a small bowel resection on the day of admission. MB was emergently taken back to the operating room 4 days later with a perforation. She has subsequently had multiple other trips to the OR secondary to this perforation. MB developed a MRSA wound infection 7 days ago and was placed on vancomycin. She then developed a nosocomial pneumonia 5 days ago and was placed on ceftazidime. Three days ago, her WBC increased and her ceftazidime was discontinued, and she was placed on meropenem and tobramycin. Today, her WBC is 32,000 with 62% segs and 18% bands. She is hypotensive and requiring 100% oxygen via mechanical ventilation. She has central venous access. MB has been in the surgical intensive care unit since admission.

Past Medical History

MB suffers from arthritis, hypertension x 8 years, and impaired glucose tolerance (recently diagnosed) and has a history of urinary tract infections. Gravida 3, para 3.

Social History

Alcohol: None   Tobacco: None

Married x 22 years

Three children: Ages 16, 18, 21

Family History

Mother: Hypertension, hypothyroidism

Father: Deceased 1997, MVA

Brother: Hypertension, diabetes

Sister: No known medical problems

Review of Systems

Negative except as noted previously

Physical Examination

GEN: Critically ill female, intubated, in moderate distress

VS: BP 86/50 mmHg, HR 132 bpm, RR 28 rpm, T 103.2°F, Wt 71.8 kg

HEENT: PERRLA, intubated, fundoscopic exam-negative

CHEST: Diminished breath sounds bilaterally, rales at both bases

ABD: Mild erythema around surgical incisions, colostomy pink, mild hepatomegaly

EXT: 2+ Pitting edema, no rash

LYMPH: No nodes

Labs and Diagnostic Tests

Sodium 132 mEq/L   Potassium 3.8 mEq/L

Chloride 114 mEq/L CO_2 22 mEq/L

BUN 24 mg/dL   Serum creatinine 1.1 mg/dL

Glucose 210 mg/dL   Hemoglobin 11.1 g/dL

Hematocrit 34%   Platelets 372,000/mm³

WBC 32,000/mm³ with 62% segs, 18% bands

CXR: Consolidation in both lower lobes-unchanged from prior exam

Micro: Blood cultures-negative x 2 days; sputum-2+ yeast; urine-yeast

Diagnosis

1. S/p small bowel obstruction/resection

2. S/p small bowel perforation/repair

3. MRSA abdominal wound infection

4. Nosocomial pneumonia

5. R/o disseminated (systemic) candidiasis

Case 56

Medication Record

4/1 ampicillin/sulbactam 3 g IVPB q 6 h

4/1 Morphine sulfate prn

4/1 Midazolam drip IV

4/4 TPN

4/8 Vancomycin 1 g IVPB q 12 h

4/8 Levofloxacin 500 mg IVPB q 24 h

4/8 Metronidazole 500 mg IVPB q 8 h

4/8 D/C Ampicillin/sulbactam

4/10 Ceftazidime 2 g q 8 h

4/10 D/C Levofloxacin

4/10 Fluconazole 400 mg IV Q24 h

4/13 Meropenem 1 g q 8 h

4/13 Tobramycin 170 mg q 8 h

4/13 D/C ceftazidime

4/13 D/C metronidazole

4/15 Dopamine drip IV

Pharmacist Notes and Other Patient Information

Tobramycin levels:

4/14 1200 1.1 µg/mL-trough

4/14 1400 8.2 µg/mL-peak

Questions

1. Risk factors for disseminated (systemic) candidiasis include all of the following EXCEPT:

    A. total parenteral nutrition.
    B. hypertension
    C. central venous catheter.
    D. broad-spectrum antibiotic use.
    E. immunosuppression.

2. Which one of the following antifungal agents is most appropriate for MB?

    A. Ketoconazole
    B. Voriconazole
    C. Fluconazole
    D. Amphotericin B
    E. Nystatin

3. Amphotericin B is compatible with which of the following solutions?

    I.   0.9% NaCl
    II. Lactated ringers
    III. Dextrose

    A. I only
    B. III only
    C. I and II only
    D. II and III only
    E. I, II, and III

4. Adverse effects of amphotericin B include all of the following EXCEPT:

    A. nephrotoxicity.
    B. rigors.
    C. aplastic anemia.
    D. thrombophlebitis.
    E. nausea.

5. MB's physician stops you in the hall and wants to know how to minimize the nephrotoxicity secondary to the amphotericin B. MB's serum creatinine has increased by 0.8 mg/dL since beginning therapy 1 week ago. You reply:

    I.   sodium loading.
    II. avoidance of diuretics.
    III. ACEI (angiotensin-converting enzyme inhibitor).

    A. I only
    B. III only
    C. I and II only
    D. II and III only
    E. I, II, and III

6. MB experienced fever, chills, and rigors during her infusion yesterday. What can you recommend to prevent or minimize these infusion-related toxicities?

    I.   Slow the amphotericin B infusion rate
    II. Acetaminophen
    III. Meperidine

    A. I only
    B. III only
    C. I and II only
    D. II and III only
    E. I, II, and III

Case 56

7. Advantages of lipid-formulated amphotericin B over amphotericin B deoxycholate include:

   I. reduced nephrotoxicity.
   II. larger doses can be administered.
   III. improved efficacy.

   A. I only
   B. III only
   C. I and II only
   D. II and III only
   E. I, II, and III

8. Which of the following laboratory parameters should you follow while MB is receiving amphotericin B?

   I. Potassium
   II. Serum creatinine
   III. Magnesium

   A. I only
   B. III only
   C. I and II only
   D. II and III only
   E. I, II, and III

9. MB's blood culture and susceptibility testing reveal Candida albicans that is susceptible to voriconazole. Adverse effects of voriconazole include all of the following EXCEPT:

   A. lepatotoxicity.
   B. gynecomastia.
   C. skin rash.
   D. visual disturbances.
   E. N/V.

10. All of the following antifungals are active against Aspergillus species EXCEPT:

    A. fluconazole.
    B. amphotericin B.
    C. itraconazole.
    D. caspofungin.
    E. voriconazole.

Patient Name: Jon Jamison
Address: 332 W. Claybourn
Age: 37 **Height:** 5' 5"
Sex: M **Race:** White
Weight: 135 lb
Allergies: NKDA

Chief Complaint

JJ is a 37-year-old white male who comes to the HIV clinic with a new diagnosis of HIV infection. He was discovered to be HIV positive when donating blood at his company's last blood drive. He has had some weight loss and fatigue but nothing serious as far as he was able to tell.

History of Present Illness

JJ has been well, without any major complaints other than having the 'flu' about 6 months ago and a 15-lb weight loss and some increased fatigue over the past 2 months. He does not have a regular physician and has not had any reason to see a physician in the past 10 years.

Past Medical History

JJ's past medical history is quite unremarkable. He has received all childhood vaccinations, reports that he had chickenpox at the age of 7, has no chronic diseases, and has no surgical history.

Social History

JJ works as a commodities trader at the Chicago Board of Trade. He denies tobacco and injection drug use. He is a social drinker (no more than 5 drinks/week). He is quite conscious of his appearance and works out 5 days/week at the local health club. JJ is homosexual and has had a number of brief sexual encounters over the past 5 years but is not in a committed relationship. He states that he usually practices safe sex; however, he does admit to numerous lapses in this practice.

Family History

Mother is alive and well at age 62.

Father died 5 years ago at age 69 of a massive MI. He had a history of hyperlipidemia which was being managed by diet.

JJ has a sister, age 30, with no medical problems.

Review of Systems

Unremarkable, except for increasing fatigue, decreased appetite, and weight loss, which concerns the patient. With these issues he has found it difficult to keep his workout schedule.

Physical Examination

GEN: Slightly cachetic male in NAD

VS: BP 120/70 mmHg, HR 60 bpm, RR 12 rpm, T 99.0°F, Wt 135 lb, Ht 69'

HEENT: WNL

CHEST: Lungs clear

CV: Normal, no murmurs, rubs, or gallops

ABD: WNL

EXT: WNL

Labs and Diagnostic Tests

Sodium 140 mEq/L	Potassium 3.9 mEq/L
Chloride 100 mEq/L	Bicarb 22 mEq/L
BUN 10 mg/dL	Serum creatinine 1.0 mg/dL
Total cholesterol 180 mg/dL	Triglycerides 160 mg/dL
WBC 2500	90% Neutrophils
10% Lymphocytes	CD4 count 150 cells/mL

HIV viral load > 1,000,000 copies/mL

Diagnosis

1. HIV infection

2. AIDS

Medication Record

No prescription medications. Patient takes the following herbal remedies:

> St. John's wort: 1 capsule daily
>
> Garlic capsules: 3 with each meal

Pharmacist Notes and Other Patient Information

None available

Case 57

Questions

1. JJ has been diagnosed with HIV infection and AIDS. Which of the following factors along with his positive HIV test entered into his AIDS diagnosis?

   I.   Recent flu-like illness
   II. WBC count of 2500/mm³ with 90% neutrophils, 10% lymphocytes
   III. CD4 count of 150/mm³

   A. I only
   B. III only
   C. I and II only
   D. II and III only
   E. I, II, and III

2. JJ should be initiated on antiretroviral therapy. Which of the following clinical factors indicate that JJ is a candidate for antiretroviral therapy?

   I.   Fatigue
   II. Weight loss
   III. Diagnosis of AIDS

   A. I only
   B. III only
   C. I and II only
   D. II and III only
   E. I, II, and III

3. One of the primary areas of concern for a pharmacist when antiretroviral therapy is initiated is the potential for serious drug interactions. Which of the following antiretrovirals is NOT likely to be involved in significant drug interactions?

   A. Lamivudine
   B. Delavirdine
   C. Amprenavir
   D. Ritonavir
   E. Nevirapine

4. Adherence is critical to successful antiretroviral therapy. When counseling JJ on this antiretroviral regimen, which of the following statements regarding adherence would be most accurate?

   A. To achieve the best outcome, you must never miss a dose. If you miss a dose, resistance will develop, and we will not be able to treat your HIV infection.
   B. Everyone misses doses occasionally. If you miss a dose or two every couple of days, it is no big deal.
   C. Everyone misses doses occasionally; however, research has shown that to achieve the best control of your HIV infection, you need to take 95 out of every 100 doses as prescribed by your doctor.

   D. Everyone misses doses occasionally; however, research has shown that if you take 80% of your prescribed doses, your HIV therapy should work just fine.
   E. Make sure that you take your zidovudine and lamivudine exactly 12 hours apart.

5. You receive the following prescriptions for antiretroviral therapy for JJ from Dr. Jones.

   > Zidovudine 300 mg po bid
   > Stavudine 40 mg po bid
   > Efavirenz 600 mg po at bedtime

   What would be the most appropriate action to take?

   A. Fill the prescriptions and counsel JJ on the importance of adherence to his antiretroviral regimen.
   B. Contact Dr. Jones to discuss the use of efavirenz, as only a protease inhibitor containing regimen has been shown to be efficacious in patients with advanced HIV disease.
   C. Fill the prescriptions and counsel JJ regarding adherence and potential adverse effects such as anemia, peripheral neuropathy, and vivid dreams.
   D. Fill the prescriptions and counsel JJ to continue taking St. John's wort, as efavirenz has been associated with some mental depression.
   E. Contact Dr. Jones to discuss the use of zidovudine and stavudine concurrently, as this combination is not recommended due to potential antagonism.

6. Dr. Jones has decided to place JJ on Combivir (zidovudine 300 mg/lamivudine 150 mg) 1 po bid, indinavir 400 mg 2 po q 12 hours, and ritonavir 100 mg 2 po q 12 hours. Which of the following counseling points are critical to the success of JJ's antiretroviral therapy?

   I.   JJ should consume plenty of fluids (at least five 8-ounce glasses of water per day).
   II. JJ should stop taking his St. John's wort and garlic capsules, as both of these herbal remedies have been shown to decrease blood levels of protease inhibitors.
   III. Indinavir should be taken 1 hour before or 2 hours after meals.

   A. I only
   B. III only
   C. I and II only
   D. II and III only
   E. I, II, and III

7. JJ initiates therapy and returns to Dr. Jones' office in 4 weeks. He is tolerating the regimen of zidovudine/lamivudine and indinavir plus ritonavir well. Laboratory tests drawn in Dr. Jones' office indicate that his viral load is now 1000 copies/mL and his CD4 count is 180 cells/mL. A fasting lipid profile reveals a total cholesterol of 295 mg/dL

Case 57

and triglycerides of 245 mg/dL. All other laboratory values are within normal limits. JJ indicates that there has been no change in the low-fat diet that he has always followed. Because of JJ's family history and his good dietary habits, Dr. Jones wishes to initiate therapy with an HMG-coA reductase inhibitor. Given JJ's antiretroviral therapy, which of the following would be the safest medication to prescribe?

A. Lovastatin
B. Simvistatin
C. Atorvostatin
D. Pravastatin
E. Fluvastatin

8. On JJ's initial office visit, other than antiretroviral therapy, what other medication issues related to JJ's current infection status should be addressed?

I. Prophylaxis for cytomegalovirus infection with ganciclovir
II. Prophylaxis for Mycobacterium avium complex infection with azithromycin
III. Prophylaxis for Pneumocystis carinii infection with trimethoprim/sulfamethoxazole

A. I only
B. III only
C. I and II only
D. II and III only
E. I, II, and III

9. Which of the following outcomes would be expected to result from JJ's antiretroviral regimen?

A. Eradication of the HIV virus from his body
B. Maintaining his CD4 count at the current level
C. A decline in viral load but little to no change in his CD4 count
D. A decline in viral load to undectable levels and a significant increase in his CD4 count
E. At best, to prolong his life by about 6-12 months

10. JJ returns to Dr. Jones' office for a visit 6 months after initiating therapy. He has stopped his St. John's wort and garlic capsules and is taking trimethoprim/sulfamethoxazole on Monday, Wednesday, and Friday for Pneumocystis carinii pneumonia prophylaxis. He reports feeling well. He has gained 8 lb in the last 6 months and reports having more energy than before. His only complaint is an increase in thirst and an increase in frequency of urination. Pertinent laboratory values indicate a viral load of less than 50 copies/mL and a CD4 count of 250 cells/mL. Other chemistries are within normal limits except for a blood glucose level of 250 mg/dL. Dr. Jones calls you to ask if there are any

medication-related reasons that may be responsible for JJ's increase in blood glucose. Your response is.

A. On the basis of the medication history available to you, no potential medication-related reasons that you can determine.
B. Zidovudine has been associated with hyperglycemia.
C. Lamivudine has been associated with hyperglycemia.
D. Trimethoprim/sulfamethoxazole has been associated with hyperglycemia.
E. Protease inhibitors have been associated with hyperglycemia.

Case 58

Patient Name: George McReady
Address: 1350 Duncan Loop South
Age: 5   **Height:** 4' 0"
Sex: M   **Race:** African American
Weight: 20 kg
Allergies: NKDA

Chief Complaint

GM is a 5 year-old African American male who has developed burning on urination and fever to 38.5°C.

History of Present Illness

GM has had these symptoms for the past 24 hours.

Past Medical History

GM has a history of bilateral kidney stones with resulting hydronephrosis 1 year and 6 months ago. The acute event resolved with no symptoms until 24 hours ago. GM also has a history of generalized tonic-clonic seizures.

Social History

Attends kindergarten 3 days per week

Family History

Mother and father are alive and in good health

Review of Systems

Abdomen is non-tender and non-distended. Bowel sounds are present. Genital exam reveals no abnormalities or deformities.

Physical Examination

GEN: well-nourished, healthy-appearing child

VS: BP 100/60 mmHg, HR 100 bpm, RR 100, Temp 38.5°C, Wt 20 kg

NEURO: A & O x 3, anxious

Medication Record

Date	Rx No	Physician	Drug and Strength	Quantity	Sig	Refills
1 year ago	45698	Dr. Reed	Ampicillin 250 mg	30	TID	0
6 mos. ago	Unknown	Unknown	Bactrim (dose unknown)	?	?	?
Current	42356	Dr. Reed	Pediatric mulitvitamin	30	daily	11
Current	41020	Dr. Reed	Phenytoin 50 mg	90	TID	11

Labs and Diagnostic Tests

Na 145 mEq/L	K 4 mEq/L
Cl 101 mEq/L	CO_2 22 mEq/L
BUN 7 mg/dL	Scr 0.5 mg/dL
Gluc 100 mg/dL	

UA:

color: straw	appearance: cloudy
nitrite: positive	leukocyte esterase: positive
WBC: 10-50	RBC: 1-4
bacteria: many	

Culture

>100 CFU gram negative rods

E. coli

Sensitive to gentamicin, piperacillin, cefepime, sulfamethoxazole/trimethoprim

Resistant to ciprofloxacin, ampicillin, cefazazolin, tetracycline

Diagnosis

1. Complicated urinary tract infection

2. Further work-up required

Pharmacist Notes and Other Patient Information

Refills of MVI on time every month

Questions

1. Which of the following medications is most likely to cause a cytochrome P450 drug interaction with ciprofloxacin?

    A. Furosemide
    B. Phenytoin
    C. Ampicillin
    D. Hydrochlorothiazide
    E. Linezolid

Case 58

2. Which of the following antibiotics requires a dosing adjustment in the presence of renal dysfunction?

   A. Doxycycline
   B. Clindamycin
   C. sulfamethoxazole/trimethoprim
   D. Itraconazole oral
   E. Nafcillin

3. The organism growing in GM's urine culture has developed resistance to ciprofloxacin. What is the most likely means of ciprofloxacin resistance?

   A. Modification of DNA gyrase
   B. Beta lactamase production
   C. Altered antibiotic binding site
   D. Drug hydrolysis
   E. Supernatant production

4. What factors are likely to contribute to antibiotic resistance?

   I. Long-term broad spectrum antibiotic use
   II. Spontaneous bacterial mutation
   III. Medication dosing optimized for age, weight, and renal function

   A. I only
   B. III only
   C. I and II only
   D. II and III only
   E. I, II, and III

5. If this patient were to receive sulfamethoxazole/trimethoprim 6 mg/kg/day what would be the proper dose?

   A. Sulfamethoxazole 240 mg/trimethoprim 18 mg oral suspension BID
   B. Sulfamethoxazole 120 mg/trimethoprim 9 mg oral suspension BID
   C. Sulfamethoxazole 300mg /trimethoprim 60 mg oral suspension BID
   D. Sulfamethoxazole 600mg/trimethoprim 180 mg oral suspension BID
   E. Sulfamethoxazole/trimethoprim is contraindicated in children less than 6 years old

6. What organisms are most likely to produce an extended spectrum beta lactamase (ESBL)?

   I. Streptococcus pneumoniae
   II. Eschericia coli
   III. Klebsiella pneumoniae

   A. I only
   B. III only
   C. I and II only
   D. II and III only
   E. I, II, and III

7. Generally speaking, what are common mechanisms of bacterial resistance?

   I. Chromosomal mutation
   II. Plasmid transfer from viral DNA
   III. Superoxide formation in the bacterial cell membrane

   A. I only
   B. III only
   C. I and II only
   D. II and III only
   E. I, II, and III

8. If this patient was intially seen in the emergency department with symtoms of a UTI, with an indwelling Foley catheter but no labs or culture data, what is an alternative to antibiotic therapy?

   I. Remove or replace the Foley catheter and reculture
   II. Delay antibiotic therapy until a urine analysis is performed confirming infection
   III. Lavage the bladder with an ethanol solution

   A. I only
   B. III only
   C. I and II only
   D. II and III only
   E. I, II, and III

9. Why are restrictions and criteria for use placed on new or broad-spectrum antibiotics in the inpatient setting?

   I. To prevent the spread of bacterial resistance
   II. To prevent injudicious use of new antibiotics
   III. To prevent renal disease

   A. I only
   B. III only
   C. I and II only
   D. II and III only
   E. I, II, and III

10. If the E. coli in this case was reported as being resistant to cefpodoxime and ceftazidime, what is the implication for therapy?

    A. The E. coli must be a non-lactose fermenting gram-negative rod
    B. The E. coli is likely to be resistant to all carbapenems and quinolones.
    C. The E. coli is likely to susceptible to all glycopeptide antibiotics except teicoplanin.
    D. The E. coli is likely to susceptible to all other antibiotics
    E. The E. coli is an extended spectrum beta-lactamase producing organism

Patient Name: Donna Hundley
Address: 19 Lincoln Parkway
Age: 33   **Height:** 5' 5"
Sex: F   **Race:** Caucasian
Weight: 145 lb
Allergies: Sulfa and latex

 ## Chief Complaint

DH is a 33 year-old woman who presented to the ambulatory clinic at Shady Lane Hospital complaining of fatigue and joint pain. She states that she feels like she has the "flu" and is asking for an antibiotic prescription.

 ## History of Present Illness

DH recently returned from camping in New Hampshire approximately 10 days ago when she first felt very tired. The next morning she began to feel muscle aches and a headache. She felt that she was developing the flu and began to self-medicate with over the counter strength naproxen with no success. Her husband noticed she had a large red circular area on her back near the right shoulder. She then presented to the internal medicine clinic for evaluation.

 ## Past Medical History

Noncontributory

 ## Social History

Tobacco use: yes

Alcohol use: socially

Patient has been sexually active with multiple partners over the past 13 years.

Is married with a 4-year-old son.

 ## Family History

Mother is in good health. Father died 3 years ago from a heart attack. Patient has no siblings.

 ## Review of Systems

Fatigue, muscle ache, and annular lesion

 ## Medication Record

Currently not taking any medications

Date	Rx No	Physician	Drug and Strength	Quantity	Sig	Refills
05/16	125489	McGhee	Doxycycline 100 mg	28	Take 1 capsule twice a day	0

 ## Physical Examination

GEN: Well-developed, well-nourished young caucasian female with fatigue, myalgia, and annular lesion on right shoulder

VS: BP 118/68 mm Hg, HR 86 bpm, RR 20/min, T 98.6°F, Wt 145 lb.

HEENT: Within normal limits

CARDIAC: Normal sinus rhythm

CHEST: Right shoulder reveals an annular lesion with bright red borders warm to the touch, which was consistent with erythema migrans.

 ## Labs and Diagnostic Tests

Serum Chemistry

Sodium 138 mEq/L	Potassium 4.1 mEq/L
Chloride 103 mEq/L	CO_2 content 26 mEq/L
BUN 11 mg/dL	Serum creatinine 0.8 mg/dL
Glucose 84 mg/dL	CBC with Differential
Hemoglobin 11.7 g/dL	Hematocrit 37%

Platelets 278,000/mm³

WBC 9000/mm³ with 50% PMNs, 2% bands

Miscellaneous Results

CXR: Unremarkable

Erythrocyte sedimentation rate 45 mm/hr

Enzyme-linked immunoabsorbent assay (ELISA) negative

Pregnancy test: negative

 ## Diagnosis

Early disseminated Lyme borreliosis disease

 ## Pharmacist Notes and Other Patient Information

None

Case 59

Questions

1. What risk factors does DH have for developing Lyme disease?

    I.   Female
    II. Outdoor activity
    III. Living in a Lyme disease-endemic area

    A. I only
    B. III only
    C. I and II only
    D. II and III only
    E. I, II, and III

2. Which of DH's physical findings are consistent with Lyme disease?

    I.   Muscle ache
    II. Fatigue
    III. Erythema migrans

    A. I only
    B. III only
    C. I and II only
    D. II and III only
    E. I, II, and III

3. Which of the following lab results are consistent with a Lyme disease presentation?

    I.   Elevated sedimentation rate
    II. Platelets within normal limits
    III. Substantial elevation in white blood cell count

    A. I only
    B. III only
    C. I and II only
    D. II and III only
    E. I, II, and III

4. What are the possible treatment options for DH?

    I.   Doxycycline 100 mg BID
    II. Cefuroxime 500 mg PO BID
    III. Amoxicillin 500 mg PO TID

    A. I only
    B. III only
    C. I and II only
    D. II and III only
    E. I, II, and III

5. DH's physician decides to treat her with amoxicillin. What is the appropriate length of therapy for this patient?

    I.   5-10 days
    II. 21-28 days
    III. 14-21 days

    A. I only
    B. III only
    C. I and II only
    D. II and III only
    E. I, II, and III

6. DH asks, "How can I prevent this from happening in the future?" Your reply would be:

    I.   Ceftriaxone 1 g IM x 1 dose
    II. Administration of Lyme disease vaccine
    III. Administation of tick repellent containing DEET or picaridin

    A. I only
    B. III only
    C. I and II only
    D. II and III only
    E. I, II, and III

7. The organism responsible for Lyme disease, Borrelia burgdorferi, is which of the following?

    A. Virus
    B. Trophozoite
    C. Cryptosporidium
    D. Spirochete
    E. Protozoa

8. You are asked to council DH about taking her doxycycline prescription. What information are you going to provide to her?

    I.   Birth control pills may not work while you are on doxycycline to keep from getting pregnant use another form of birth control
    II. Avoid the use of antacids while taking doxycycline
    III. Avoid direct sunlight or use a sunscreen

    A. I only
    B. III only
    C. I and II only
    D. II and III only
    E. I, II, and III

9. Which of the following is important to educate DH about doxycycline administration and storage?

    I.   Take each dose with a full glass of water or food
    II. Avoid alcohol and maintain adequate hydration (2-3 L/day)
    III. Store in a warm area in direct sunlight

    A. I only
    B. III only
    C. I and II only
    D. II and III only
    E. I, II, and III

Case 59

10. You receive a prescription for doxycycline 100 mg PO bid. You could fill this prescription with any one of the following dosage forms EXCEPT:

    A. capsule.
    B. tablet.
    C. oral suspension.
    D. syrup.
    E. chewable tablet.

Case 60

Sepsis and Septic Shock

Patient Name: Jill Shay
Address: 361 S. 8th Street
Age: 64 **Height:** 5' 5"
Sex: F **Race:** Caucasian
Weight: 185 lb
Allergies: Sulfa

 Chief Complaint

JS is a 64-year-old white female who presented to the emergency room complaining of increasing abdominal pain over the last 3 days. Besides the pain she also complains of nausea and vomiting for the last 48 hours.

 History of Present Illness

JS was in her usual state of health up until 3 days ago. She awoke in the middle of the night due to acute abdominal pain and cramping. She took an H₂ blocker without relief. The pain continued over the next day and a half. In the last 12 hours, the pain has intensified, and she has not been able to keep anything down. At the time of presentation to the emergency department, JS was febrile and diaphoretic. She had severe lower right quadrant pain with rebound and guarding. She was evaluated by surgery for possible appendicitis.

JS underwent an emergency appendectomy. At surgery she was found to have a perforated appendix with diffuse peritonitis. During surgery she became acutely hypotensive and required massive fluid replacement. Postoperatively, she was transferred to the intensive care unit. She is intubated and continues to be hypotensive despite receiving 2 L of fluid over the last 4 hours.

 Past Medical History

JS has a 10-year history of hypertension, treated with various antihypertensives. Three years ago, she was diagnosed with breast cancer and underwent a left mastectomy with radiation therapy.

 Social History

JS has a 40 pack/year history of smoking.

 Family History

Noncontributory

Review of Systems

Review of systems noncontributory except for physical exam findings

 Physical Examination

GEN: 64-year-old intubated, diaphoretic female, in significant distress. Pulmonary artery and arterial lines in place.

VS: BP (S/D/M) 70/50/57 mmHg, HR 120 bpm, RR 20 rpm, T 103°F, Wt 200 lb

HEMODYNAMIC PARAMETERS: CO 8 L/min (normal 4-7), CI 3.5 L/min/m² (normal 2.5-4.2), PCWP 10 mmHg (normal 5-12), CVP 4 mmHg (normal 2-6), SVR 530 dyne/sec/cm⁻⁵ (normal 800-1440)

LUNGS: Reduced breath sounds bilaterally

URINE OUTPUT: 30 mL/h over the last 2 hours

 Labs and Diagnostic Tests

Sodium 132 mEq/L   Potassium 5.1 mEq/L

Chloride 105 mEq/L   CO₂ content 22 mEq/L

BUN 30 mg/dL   Serum creatinine 2.1 mg/dL

Glucose 120 mg/dL   Hemoglobin 12.2 g/dL

Hematocrit 32%   Platelets 110,000/mm³

WBC 20,000/mm³   PMNs 42%, bands 9%

Arterial blood gases (fraction of inspired oxygen 60%): pH 7.29, PaO₂ 100 mmHg, PaCO₂ 42 mmHg, bicarbonate (HCO₃) 19 mEq/L

 Diagnosis

1. Perforated appendicitis

2. Septic shock

 Medication Record

Medications prior to admission:

Hydrochlorothiazide 50 mg qd   Atenolol 50 mg qd

Aspirin 80 mg qd   Atorvastatin 20 mg qd

Lisinopril 20 mg qd

Medication record:

Heparin 5000 units, SQ, q 12 h

Furosemide 40 mg, IV, q 12 h

Piperacillin/tazobactam 4.5 g, IV, q 6 h

Gentamicin 60 mg, IV, q 12 h

Pantoprazole 40 mg, IV, q 24 h

ASHP's PharmPrep

Case 60

Morphine 1-4 mg, IV, q 1-2 h

D₅LR/50 mEq sodium bicarbonate at 200 mL/h

Pharmacist Notes and Other Patient Information

5/11 Pharmacy aminoglycoside note:

s: Patient hypotensive and in acute pain

o: See flowsheet for labs and estimate CrCl

a: On the basis of renal function and current dose of gentamicin, estimated peak: 5-6 mg/dL, trough < 2.0; however, renal function may be deteriorating. Dose of Zosyn high for renal function.

p: Recommend peak/trough gentamicin after third dose. Monitor serum creatinine daily. Will adjust gentamicin dose based on levels. Recommend decrease Zosyn to 2.25 g q 6 h. JP

Questions

1. The goal for the initial therapy (first 6 hours) of septic shock in JS should be directed at correcting all of the following parameters EXCEPT:

   A. central venous pressure. 8-12 mmHg.
   B. mean arterial pressure of equal to or greater than 65 mm Hg.
   C. temperature < 39° C.
   D. urine output equal to or greater than 0.5 mL/kg/h.
   E. Central venous (superior vena caval) or mixed venous oxygen saturation of equal to or greater than 70%.

2. Based on the 2003 consensus guidelines for goal-directed therapy, which of the following should be initiated in JS as soon as possible?

   A. Methylprednisolone 2 g IV
   B. Change from gentamicin to aztreonam 2 g IV every 8 hours
   C. Dopamine 5 µg/kg/min
   D. Norepinephrine 0.1 µg/kg/min
   E. 500 cc normal saline bolus

3. Appropriate antimicrobial therapy continues to play a prominent role in the treatment of severe sepsis. Pharmacists can significantly impact outcomes from sepsis through their appropriate use. According to the 2003 guidelines, appropriate antimicrobial therapy should be initiated in which of the following time frames?

   A. Within 1 hour
   B. Within 2 hours
   C. Within 4 hours
   D. Within 8 hours
   E. Initiation of antimicrobial therapy is not an initial goal for the treatment of severe sepsis; therefore, efforts should be placed on other therapies rather than initiation of antimicrobial therapy. Antimicrobial therapy can be ordered once the patient is stabilized and admitted to the intensive care unit.

4. In evaluating whether to use normal saline (crystalloids) or albumin (colloids) for the fluid resuscitation in JS, the medical team turns to you and asks you for your recommendation. Based on your analysis of the literature your response should be.

   A. Fluid resuscitation in patients with severe sepsis should be initiated with crystalloids as opposed to colloids due to the leakage that can occur into lung parenchymal tissue with the use of colloids.
   B. Fluid resuscitation in patients with severe sepsis should be initiated with colloids as they require less volume for the same increase in central venous pressures.
   C. Fluid resuscitation in patients with severe sepsis should be initiated with colloids, but they may result in more edema than with the use of crystalloids.
   D. Fluid resuscitation in patients with severe sepsis may be initiated with either crystalloids or colloids as outcomes are similar with each.
   E. Fluid resuscitation in patients with severe sepsis should be initiated with colloids as use of crystalloids will result in severe edema.

5. After fluid resuscitation, JS has the following hemodynamic parameters. mean arterial pressure 55 mmHg (goal equal to or greater than 65 mmHg), CVP 10 mmHg (goal 8-12 mmHg), cardiac index 3.0 L/min/m² (normal 2.5 - 4.2).

   The decision is made to administer a vasopressor. According to the 2003 consensus guidelines, which of the following are appropriate to administer in JS?

   I.   Dopamine
   II. Norepinephrine
   III. Dobutamine

   A. I only
   B. III only
   C. I and II only
   D. II and III only
   E. I, II, and III

Case 60

6. The decision is made to initiate JS on dopamine at 5 μg/kg/min. On the basis of a standard dopamine IV admixture of 400 mg in 500 cc of normal saline, calculate the appropriate infusion rate in mL/h.

   A. 10 mL/h
   B. 26 mL/h
   C. 32 mL/h
   D. 34 mL/h
   E. 40 mL/h

7. Appropriate monitoring parameters for the use of IV dopamine include:

   I. hemodynamic parameters, i.e., PCWP, SVR, CVP, and CI.
   II. mean arterial pressure (MAP).
   III. urine output.

   A. I only
   B. III only
   C. I and II only
   D. II and III only
   E. I, II, and III

8. A discussion occurs regarding the appropriateness of using drotrecogin alfa in this patient. The attending physician asks you the significance of the PROWESS and ADDRESS trials, which evaluated the use of drotrecogin in severe sepsis. In order to answer his question, which type of drug information source would you need to review in order to respond to his question?

   I. Primary reference sources
   II. Secondary reference sources
   III. Tertiary reference sources

   A. I only
   B. III only
   C. I and II only
   D. II and III only
   E. I, II, and III

9. The results of the gentamicin levels come back with a peak level of 5.5 μg/mL and a trough level of 2.4 μg/mL. On the basis of these levels an appropriate response would be to:

   I. decrease the dose.
   II. increase the dosing interval.
   III. increase the dose and the dosing interval.

   A. I only
   B. III only
   C. I and II only
   D. II and III only
   E. I, II, and III

10. The critical care nurse asks you whether she can run the dopamine with the IV containing sodium bicarbonate. Which of the following references would help you answer the question?

    I. DiPiro's Pharmacotherapy: A Pathophysiologic Approach
    II. Micromedex
    III. Trissel's Handbook on Injectable Drugs

    A. I only
    B. III only
    C. I and II only
    D. II and III only
    E. I, II, and III

Case 61

Patient Name: Rachel Clark
Address: 4775 Cheshire Court #107
Age: 23   Height: 5' 4"
Sex: F   Race: White
Weight: 136 lb
Allergies: NKDA

Chief Complaint

RC is a 23-yo white female who presents to the urgency care clinic with a chief complaint of increased frequency and dysuria for 3 days. She reports that she has been having to get up in the middle of the night to urinate more frequently during this time and has been experiencing painful voiding as well. She reports that painful urination is the most bothersome the first thing in the morning and is accompanied by a mucopurulent discharge, with dysuria improving during the day but never quite resolving. She notes that she believes that she has a UTI.

History of Present Illness

RC noted that she had no problems with urination until 3 days ago when she noted an intense internal burning sensation when going to the bathroom the first thing in the morning. The problem persisted throughout the day with some resolution in pain. That night she had to get out of bed to urinate twice, each time accompanied by dysuria. The following morning she noted that the dysuria was accompanied by a mucopurulent discharge. She notes that the problem has gradually gotten worse over the ensuing 2 days, culminating in presentation today. She denies the presence of flank pain, fever, or other accompanying symptoms.

Past Medical History

RC reports a history of two previous UTIs while she was in college, occurring 2 and 4 years ago. She also reports being diagnosed with genital HSV about a year ago. The remainder of her history is unremarkable with the exception of occasional allergies and is noncontributory.

Medication Record

Date	Rx No	Physician	Drug and Strength	Quantity	Sig	Refills
11/12	12345	Jones	OrthoNovum 7/7/7	3	ud	3
8/27	7572	Jones	Cetrizine 10 mg	30	1 po daily	2
			Multivitamin OTC			
			Ferrous Sulfate OTC			

Social History

Single, never married, and lives alone. Sexually active and currently involved in a monogamous, heterosexual relationship. Involved with new partner for around 4 weeks. Currently taking oral contraceptives; partner does not use condoms.

Tobacco use: None

Alcohol use: Infrequent, 2-3 drinks/month

Caffeine use: 1-2 cups of coffee per day

Family History

Father alive, age 48. Mother alive, age 50. One brother, age 27, one sister, age 19.

Review of Systems

Normal

Physical Examination

GEN: Well-nourished, white female in NAD

VS: BP 117/68 mmHg, HR 65 bpm, RR 18 rpm, T 37.2°C, Ht 5' 4", Wt 62 kg

HEENT: Normal

LUNGS: Clear breath sounds

CV: RRR with normal S_1/S_2 and no audible murmur

SKIN: No erythema or petechiae

GU: Mild erythema of external genitalia, moderate cervical erythema with mucopurulent discharge, no lesions

Labs and Diagnostic Tests

Hemoglobin 13.5 g/dL

Hematocrit 41%

Case 61

Platelets 321,000/mm³

WBC 7600/mm³ with 75% PMN, 20% lymphocytes, 4% monocytes, 1% eosinophils

Urinalysis: Appearance cloudy, color yellow, ketones neg, specific gravity 1.020, urobilinogen 0.2, blood trace, bilirubin negative, glucose negative, protein negative, pH 6.00, WBC 65/hpf, RBC 5/hpf, bacteria few, nitrite negative, leukoesterase negative

Cervical smear: Gram stain 4 + WBC, 4+ gram-negative diplococci

 Diagnosis

Primary:

1. Infectious urethritis

2. Seasonal allergic rhinitis

 Pharmacist Notes and Other Patient Information

None available

Questions

1. The cervical gram stain for this patient most likely reflects which organisms?

   A. Chlamydia trachomatis
   B. Bacteriodes fragilis
   C. Neisseria gonorrhea
   D. Candida albicans
   E. Treponema pallidum

2. Empiric antimicrobial coverage should include agent(s) which are active against which of the following?

   A. Chlamydia trachomatis and Candida albicans
   B. Neisseria gonorrhea and Candida albicans
   C. Chlamydia trachomatis and Neisseria gonorrhea
   D. Candida albicans and Neisseria gonorrhea
   E. Treponema pallidum and Candida albicans

3. Select the most appropriate medication(s) to be dispensed to RC to adequately treat her and her sexual partner.

   I. Cefixime 400 mg #2 tablets
   II. Cefixime 400 mg #2 tablets; doxycycline 100 mg #14 capsules
   III. Ciprofloxacin 500 mg #2 tablets; azithromycin 250 mg #8 tablets

   A. I only
   B. III only
   C. I and II only
   D. II and III only
   E. I, II, and III

4. A patient should be counseled to avoid sun exposure and/or use sunscreen with which of the following agents?

   A. Azithromycin
   B. Cefuroxime
   C. Ofloxacin
   D. Amoxicillin
   E. Doxycycline

5. This patient should be counseled to abstain from sex:

   I. for 24 hours.
   II. for 3 days.
   III. for 7 days.

   A. I only
   B. III only
   C. I and II only
   D. II and III only
   E. I, II, and III

6. Select the most appropriate diluent(s) and volume for administration of a single 125-mg IM dose of ceftriaxone.

   I. 2 mL of a 1% lidocaine in sterile water solution
   II. 10 mL of sterile water for injection
   III. 5 mL of 5% dextrose solution

   A. I only
   B. III only
   C. I and II only
   D. II and III only
   E. I, II, and III

7. Which of the following patients may receive ciprofloxacin for the treatment of N. gonorrhea?

   A. Recent travel to Asia
   B. Resident of Hawaii
   C. Resident of California
   D. Resident of New York
   E. Recent travel to the Pacific Islands

8. If this patient is prescribed ciprofloxacin, she should be counseled to take ciprofloxacin:

   A. with a meal.
   B. with an antacid to reduce GI upset.
   C. spaced from the administration of Ortho Novum 7/7/7.
   D. with a glass of milk.
   E. spaced from the administration of the multivitamin.

Case 61

9. If this patient were to experience another outbreak of
   genital HSV, which of the following may be recommended?

   A. Valacyclovir 1 g po bid x 10 days
   B. Acyclovir 400 mg IV q8h x 10 days
   C. Valacyclovir 1 g po qday x 5 days
   D. Famciclovir 250 mg po tid x 5 days
   E. Valganciclovir 900 mg po bid x 5 days

10. A prescription for Valtrex should be filled with:

    A. famciclovir.
    B. ganciclovir.
    C. valganciclovir.
    D. acyclovir.
    E. valacyclovir.

Skin and Soft Tissue Infection

Patient Name: Derrick Hazard
Address: 1234 Ski-Doo Drive
Age: 58   **Height:** 6' 2"
Sex: M   **Race:** Caucasian
Weight: 96.1 kg
Allergies: NKDA

Chief Complaint

DH, a 58-year-old male, presents to the emergency department with complaints of a reddened and swollen right knee after striking it on a tree while snowmobiling.

History of Present Illness

DH was in his usual state of health until about a week ago. One day he went snowmobiling and accidentally bumped his knee on a tree. Later that day he went swimming in a natural hot springs. The next day he noticed an ingrown hair with associated edema on his right knee. He describes "picking off a scab" and then noticing increased erythema. He was seen in a clinic and given a prescription for cephalexin 500 mg po qid. for 7 days. Three days after starting the cephalexin, a silver dollar sized area of skin on his knee is missing, and the area is now more erythematous and edematous. He was seen in clinic a second time and given a prescription for dicloxacillin 250 mg po qid. for 10 days. Wound cultures were obtained, which subsequently grew 4+ coagulase-positive Staphylococcus. Two days after starting the dicloxacillin DH noticed the edema and erythema moving up his leg to mid-thigh over the weekend and drove to the ER for further evaluation.

Past Medical History

Impotence

Peptic ulcer disease with history of H. Pylori (treated with triple therapy)

Osteoarthritis

Bilateral arthroscopic knee surgery (1998)

Hyperlipidemia

Left partial kidney resection due to complicated cyst

Social History

DH lives out of town with second wife. He has three grown children. Retired from the Air Force where he worked in a missile silo. No tobacco, occasional alcohol. No illicit drug use.

Family History

Father died at age 72 of myocardial infarction. Mother and all siblings still alive. History of congenital heart defects in siblings.

Review of Systems

Positive only for joint aches.

Physical Examination

GEN: NAD, well-nourished male

VS: T 39.3°C, BP 121/73 mmHg, P 90 bpm, RR 20

HEENT: NC/AT, EOMI, PERRLA, OP clear, mucus membranes moist, no LAD or masses; Normocephalic, atraumatic

LUNGS: CTAB, no wheezes or crackles

CV: RRR, normal S_1 and S_2, no murmur, rubs, or gallops

ABD: soft, no organomegaly, no masses or tenderness. Normal BS

NEURO: CN II-XII grossly intact. 5/5 upper and lower extremity strength. Negative Romberg.

EXT: 90-degree flexion only on right knee. Full ROM all other joints. No tenderness to palpation in calf.

SKIN: Silver dollar sized skin tear on right knee cap. Entire knee erythematous and edematous. Erythema to mid-calf and mid-thigh.

Labs and Diagnostic Tests

Obtained 12/1

Total cholesterol: 190 mg/dL

LDL-C: 123 mg/dL	HDL-C: 61 mg/dL

Triglycerides: 77 mg/dL

AST: 45 IU/L	ALT: 33 IU/L
Alkaline phosphatase: 68 IU/L	Bilirubin: 1.2 mg/dL

Albumin: 4.7 g/dL

Obtained in ED on day of admission

Chemistry Panel

NA: 142 mEq/L	K: 3.9 mEq/L
CL: 108 mEq/L	CO_2: 26 Mmol/ L
BUN: 18 mg/dL	Creatinine 1.1 mg/dL
Glucose 94 mg/dL	WBC: 9.4 K/uL
RBC: 5.07 m/uL	Hgb: 15.1 g/dL
Hct: 45.0%	Plt: 345 K/uL
Neut%: 76.2	Lymph%: 12.6
Mono%: 9.8	Eos%: 1.2

Baso%: 0.2

Case 62

Medication Record

Acetaminophen 650 mg q 4-6 h prn pain or fever

Date	Rx No	Physician	Drug and Strength	Quantity	Sig	Refills
12/1		Dr. Smith	Simvastatin 40 mg	90	1 po qd	
1/14		Dr. Smith	Cephalexin 500 mg	28	1 po q.i.d.	
1/18		Dr. Polaris	Dicloxacillin 250 mg	40	1 po q.i.d.	
1/20		Dr. Zupp	Vancomycin 1 g		1 IV q12h	
1/20		Dr. Zupp	Piperacillin/tazobactam 3.375 g	8	1 IV q6h	
1/24		Dr. Zupp	Linezolid 600 mg	28	1 po b.i.d.	

Vancomycin and zosyn started for empirical coverage of severe cellulitis of unknown origin not responsive to Gram-positive coverage with beta-lactam antibiotics. Renal function normal. Vancomycin trough ordered post 3rd dose.

Microbiology

Specimen source: knee swab

Coagulase-positive Staphylococcus aureus

Susceptibility:

amp/sulbactam R	cefazolin R
cefpodoxime R	cefuroxime R
erythromycin R	gatifloxacin S
gentamicin S	linezolid S
oxacillin R	TMP/SMZ S
vancomycin S	

Diagnosis

Cellulitis of the right leg associated with community acquired methicillin resistant Staphylococcus aureus (CA-MRSA). No evidence of joint infection.

Pharmacist Notes and Other Patient Information

None available

Questions

1. Community acquired methicillin resistant Staph aureus skin infections CANNOT be treated with which of the following antibiotics as an outpatient?

    A. Vancomycin 1000 mg po bid
    B. SMZ/TMP DS po tid
    C. Linezolid 600 mg po bid
    D. Minocycline 100 mg po bid
    E. Clindamycin 300 mg po qid

2. What potential drug-drug, drug-food, drug-herb interactions should the pharmacist warn DH about? He is to receive a 2-week prescription for linezolid 600 mg po bid.

    I.   He should avoid eating excessive tyramine-containing foods (chocolate, wine, cheeses, dried meats) while on linezolid and for 2 weeks after.
    II. He should not take any antidepressants, over-the-counter cough and cold preparations, or appetite suppressants while on linezolid.
    III. He should stop taking his simvastatin while on linezolid.

    A. I only
    B. III only
    C. I and II only
    D. II and III only
    E. I, II, and III

3. Bacteria that should be considered in a patient with an uncomplicated cellulitis include:

    I.   Staphylococcus aureus.
    II. Streptococcus pyogenes.
    III. Escherichia coli.

    A. I only
    B. III only
    C. I and II only
    D. II and III only
    E. I, II, and III

4. Skin infections involving furuncles, carbuncles, or abscesses are usually caused by:

    I.   Streptococcus pyogenes.
    II. Escherichia coli.
    III. Staphylococcus aureus.

    A. I only
    B. III only
    C. I and II only
    D. II and III only
    E. I, II, and III

Case 62

5. A patient presents to the emergency room with a cut on the bottom of his foot that look infected. He has fever and chills and an elevated white blood count. The patient states that he stepped on a piece of broken glass at the bottom of a pond and that the glass went through his tennis shoe and cut his foot. The physician wants to prescribe cephalexin as empiric treatment for this skin and soft tissue infection. The pharmacist disagrees, stating that:

I. infections that occur where the foot is punctured through a tennis shoe are possibly caused by Pseudomonas auerginosa (a common pathogen that lives in tennis shoes). Cephalexin does not posess activity against Pseudomonas aeruginosa.

II. Pseudomonas aeruginosa has high intrinsic resistance and can produce inducible AmpC beta-lactamases capable of hydrolyzing cephalosporins. Moxifloxacin should be used to treat the infection.

III. his foot infection is likely caused by a food and water contaminant like Shigella or Salmonella and should be treated with IV vancomycin.

A. I only
B. III only
C. I and II only
D. II and III only
E. I, II, and III

6. DH was placed on vancoymcin intravenously for his community-acquired MRSA infection. The pharmacist is responsible for adjusting the dose based on levels. After three doses at 1000 mg IV q 12 h, his serum trough vancomycin level is 3.0 mg/dL. What should the pharmacist do?

A. Decrease the patient's dose to 750 mg IV q 12 h
B. Decrease the patient's dose to 500 mg IV q 12 h
C. Increase the patient's dose to 1500 mg IV q 12 h
D. Decrease the patient's dosing interval to 1000 mg IV q 8 h
E. Do nothing. The trough level is satisfactory.

7. Which of the following skin infections can be treated with topical antibiotics?

I. Cellulitis
II. Impetigo
III. Recurrent furunculosis

A. I only
B. III only
C. I and II only
D. II and III only
E. I, II, and III

8. What is a possible side effect of vancomycin?

I. Grey-baby syndrome
II. Red-man syndrome
III. Renal toxicity

A. I only
B. III only
C. I and II only
D. II and III only
E. I, II, and III

9. A doctor calls the pharmacy to ask what beta-lactam type PO antibiotic has the best anti-staphylococcal activity. The pharmacist answers:

A. Cephalexin
B. Ampicillin
C. Levofloxacin
D. Dicloxacillin
E. Penicillin

10. In the hospital DH is placed in contact isolation due to his MRSA infection in an attempt to prevent other patients from becoming infected. Which of the following infection control procedures should be followed while DH is in the hospital?

I. Private room or shared room with other MRSA positive patient
II. Gloves and gown when touching patient or close environment
III. Washing hands prior to and after entering room

A. I only
B. III only
C. I and II only
D. II and III only
E. I, II, and III

Patient Name: Melinda Blake
Address: 153 Carmel Avenue
Age: 53   Height: 5' 6"
Sex: F   Race: Caucasian
Weight: 155 lb
Allergies: NKDA

Chief Complaint

MB is a 53-yo white female seen in her doctor's office yesterday afternoon complaining of weight loss and shortness of breath with exertion.

History of Present Illness

MB notes that for the past few months she has had a low-grade temperature, has been awakened often during the night because of excessive sweating, and has had a weight loss of about 20 lb over the past 2 months. MB's husband complains that during this period of time she has also been coughing constantly. MB admits to occasionally coughing up blood during these coughing attacks.

Past Medical History

MB is postmenopausal and has a diagnosis of mild hypertension and hypothyroidism.

Social History

MB is married and has a grown daughter and 5 grandchildren who live with her. She is not a smoker but regularly drinks at least one glass of wine or beer with dinner.

Family History

Noncontributory

Review of Systems

Negative except as noted previously

Physical Examination

VS: T 99.8°F, HR 84 bpm, RR 24 rpm, BP 135/72 mmHg

SKIN/EXTREMITIES: No rash, cyanosis, clubbing, or edema

NECK: Supple, no lymphadenopathy

LUNGS: Bibasilar rales and apical "crackles" on deep inspiration

NEURO: Alert and oriented x3

Labs and Diagnostic Tests

WBC 9800/mm^3

Hemoglobin 12 g/dL

Hematocrit 38%

Serum creatinine 1.3 mg/dL

Serum bicarbonate 26 mEq/L

Glucose 142 mg/dL (non-fasting)

T-4 (free) 1.5 ng/dL

TSH 1.6 MIU/L

AST 45 IU/L

ALT 30 IU/L

CXR: Right lower lobe infiltrate with bilateral hilar and right paratracheal adenopathy; evidence of old cavitary lesions in both apices

Diagnosis

Primary:

    1. Pulmonary tuberculosis

Secondary:

    1. Postmenopausal female - stable

    2. Hypertension - treated

    3. Hypothyroid - treated

Medication Record

Premarin (conjugated estrogen) 1.25 mg qd

Enalapril 5 mg qd

Levothyroxine 0.15 mg qd

Pharmacist Notes and Other Patient Information

None available

Case 63

1. On the basis of the information provided, tuberculin screening skin tests (PPD) should be given to:
   I.   MB's husband.
   II. MB's grown daughter.
   III. MB's grandchildren.

   A. I only
   B. III only
   C. I and II only
   D. II and III only
   E. I, II, and III

2. The patient's husband has a positive reaction within 48 hours of administration of a PPD skin test. Which of the following is considered a positive reaction?

   A. >1 mm area of induration
   B. <5 mm area of induration
   C. >5 mm area of induration
   D. Any area of induration regardless of size
   E. Any area of erythema and induration regardless of size

3. A medical student asks you why MB's husband was also given mumps and Candida antigen skin tests when he received his PPD skin test. What is your response to the medical student?

   A. To confirm he is not anergic
   B. To increase the potency of the TB test antigen
   C. To prevent an allergic reaction to the TB test antigen
   D. To test for potential concomitant infection with either Candida or mumps
   E. To boost the immune response to the TB test antigen

4. The Mycobacterium tuberculosis strain isolated from MB's sputum culture was susceptible to isoniazid, rifampin, and pyrazinamide. Which of the following represents an appropriate treatment recommendation for MB's pulmonary TB disease?

   A. Isoniazid + rifampin + pyrazinamide for 2 months followed by 4 months with isoniazid and rifampin
   B. Isoniazid + rifampin for 2 months followed by 4 months with pyrazinamide
   C. Isoniazid + pyrazinamide for 2 months followed by 4 months with rifampin
   D. Isoniazid + rifampin + pyrazinamide for 3 months
   E. Isoniazid and rifampin for 2 months

5. In addition to the specific anti-TB regimen selected, what other therapy should be considered for MB at this time?

   A. Ferrous sulfate, 325 mg po tid
   B. Vitamin E, 400 units po qd
   C. Alendronate, 70 mg po q week
   D. Pyridoxine, 25 mg po qd
   E. Vitamin C, 500 mg po qd

6. When MB's medications are dispensed to her, which of the following issues should be addressed with her as part of her medication counseling?

   I.   Pyrazinamide may cause optic neuritis, so she should notify her physician if she starts having blurred vision or trouble distinguishing red and green colors.
   II. Ethanol consumption can increase the risk of INH-induced hepatotoxicity, so she should refrain from drinking during therapy.
   III. Rifampin may cause orange discoloration of body fluids, including tears, urine, and sweat.

   A. I only
   B. III only
   C. I and II only
   D. II and III only
   E. I, II, and III

7. MB's liver function tests (LFTs) increase to two times the original concentrations after 1 month of therapy with isoniazid, rifampin, and pyrazinamide. MB does not have any complaints regarding her drug therapy, other than having to take so many drugs in a single day. Which of the following should NOT be a recommended change to her drug therapy?

   A. Decrease the dose of isoniazid to half the starting dose; discontinue the rifampin
   B. Interview the patient monthly for symptoms of hepatotoxicity
   C. Inform the patient of symptoms of hepatotoxicity and tell her to report these to her doctor if they occur
   D. Maintain the original doses of isoniazid, rifampin, and pyrazinamide
   E. Routine monitoring of liver function tests for the entire course of therapy

8. One of MB's grandchildren has a positive reaction to the PPD skin test. What therapy, if any, should be initiated in this 6-year-old male who is otherwise healthy and without clinical evidence of TB?

   A. INH, 10-20 mg/kg/d for 9 months
   B. Rifampin, 50 mg/kg/d for 6 months
   C. Ethambutol, 50 mg/kg/d for 12 months
   D. Moxifloxacin, 200 mg po qd for 12 months
   E. No therapy is indicated at this time

Case 63

9. MB comes into your pharmacy and complains of pain in her right large toe. This is her only complaint, and she states that she is pleased that the night sweats have disappeared. What is a likely cause of this toe pain?

    A. Tuberculous osteomyelitis
    B. Cartilage destruction secondary to rifampin therapy
    C. Increase in uric acid concentration secondary to pyrazinamide therapy
    D. Osteomyelitis with Staphylococcus aureus secondary to immunosuppression caused by tuberculosis
    E. Arthritis secondary to isoniazid therapy

10. MB and her family members want to learn about TB and ask you for recommendations as to where they can seek out additional patient/family information. You refer them to which of the following agencies?

    A. Local chapter of the American Cancer Society
    B. Infectious Diseases Society of America
    C. Local chapter of the American Heart Association
    D. Local branch library
    E. Local chapter of the American Lung Association

Case 64 — Upper and Lower Respiratory Tract Infection

Patient Name: Adam Smith
Address: 221 Wood Street
Age: 76   **Height:** 5' 11"
Sex: M   **Race:** White
Weight: 177 lb
Allergies: NKDA

Chief Complaint

AS is a 76-yo male who was admitted 13 days ago for coronary artery bypass surgery. Post CABG the patient had a slow recovery and remained in the ICU because he was unable to be extubated. Two days ago, he developed a fever and severe abdominal pain. He was subsequently taken to the operating room where a perforated duodenal ulcer was repaired. He has been stable postoperatively in the ICU. Last night, he became agitated, spiked a temperature, and had increasing oxygenation demands.

History of Present Illness

Last evening, AS became agitated, spiked a temperature to 102.8° F, and had increasing oxygen requirements (FIO_2 increased from 40% to 80%). Two sets of blood cultures were drawn, and a sputum sample was sent for gram stain and culture. A stat chest x-ray revealed an infiltrate at the left lower lobe.

Past Medical History

Myocardial infarction 1 month ago

CABG 5-13 days ago

Hypertension

Hyperlipidemia

Diabetes mellitis type 2 x 27 years

Benign prostatic hypertrophy

COPD

Social History

Tobacco use: quit 35 years ago

Alcohol use: occasional

Marital status: married

Family History

Mother died of complications of diabetes in 1979

Father died of heart disease in 1975

Review of Systems

Negative except as previously noted

Physical Examination

GEN: Elderly male, sedated, intubated

VS: BP 151/87 mmHg, P 93 bpm, RR 28 rpm, T 102.6°F, Wt 81.6 kg

HEENT: PERRLA, intubated

CHEST: Diminished breath sounds, rales LLL, incision pink, no drainage, healing

ABD: Incision pink, no drainage, some tenderness around incision

Labs and Diagnostic Tests

Sodium 136 mEq/L	Potassium 4.2 mEq/L
Chloride 116 mEq/L	CO_2 18 mEq/L
BUN 24 mg/dL	Serum creatinine 1.2 mg/dL
Glucose 228 mg/dL	Hemoglobin 10.2 g/dL
Hematocrit 32.6%	Platelets 376,000/mm³

WBC 23,500/mm³ with 68% segs, 20% bands

CXR: Left lower lobe infiltrate

Micro: Blood cultures negative (at 12 hours)

Sputum gram stain: 4+ WBC, 3+ gram-negative bacilli

Diagnosis

1. S/p CABG x 5

2. S/p perforated duodenal ulcer with repair

3. Probable nosocomial pneumonia

Medication Record

3/16, Regular insulin sliding scale

3/16, Famotidine 20 mg IVPB q 12 h (added to TPN 3/25)

3/23, Ampicillin/sulbactam (Unasyn) 3 g x 1, 1.5 g q 6 h

3/24, Midazolam prn

3/25, Morphine sulfate prn

3/25, TPN

3/25, Enoxaparin 30 mg SQ bid

3/25, Enalaprilat 1.25 mg IV q 6 h prn

Case 64

Pharmacist Notes and Other Patient Information

None available

Questions

1. Which of the following organisms is least likely to be a pathogen in AS?

    A. Pseudomonas aeruginosa
    B. Streptococcus pneumoniae
    C. Staphylococcus aureus
    D. Enterobacter spp.
    E. Klebsiella spp.

2. Which of the following parameters should be monitored to assess response to therapy?

    I.   WBC
    II. Temperature
    III. Oxygenation

    A. I only
    B. III only
    C. I and II only
    D. II and III only
    E. I, II, and III

3. Which one of the following empiric treatment regimens is most appropriate for AS?

    A. Ceftazidime plus gentamicin
    B. Vancomycin
    C. Ceftriaxone
    D. Piperacillin/tazobactam plus gentamicin
    E. Levofloxacin plus metronidazole

4. What are risk factors for the development of antibiotic resistance?

    I.   Prior antimicrobial agent use
    II. Prolonged hospitalization
    III. Underdosage of antimicrobial agents

    A. I only
    B. III only
    C. I and II only
    D. II and III only
    E. I, II, and III

5. The sputum sample grows out Pseudomonas aeruginosa. Susceptibilities are as follows:

    Drug MIC breakpoint S/I/R
    Meropenem 0.5 8 S
    Ceftazidime 4 16 S
    Ciprofloxacin 2 4 S
    Piperacillin 128 64 R
    Gentamicin 1 4 S

    On the basis of the above culture and susceptibility data, which regimen is now most appropriate for AS?

    A. Piperacillin plus gentamicin
    B. Ceftazidime plus gentamicin
    C. Meropenem plus gentamicin
    D. Ciprofloxacin plus gentamicin
    E. Ciprofloxacin

6. Two days later, you are on rounds and notice that AS's serum creatinine has increased from 1.2 mg/dL to 2.4 mg/dL. Which of the following statements regarding his antimicrobial therapy are true? (He is currently receiving meropenem 2 g IVPB q 8 h and gentamicin 160 mg IVPB q 12 h.)

    I.   Change regimen to piperacillin plus tobramycin
    II. Consider discontinuation of gentamicin
    III. Recommend that the meropenem dose/interval be adjusted to 1 g q 12 h

    A. I only
    B. III only
    C. I and II only
    D. II and III only
    E. I, II, and III

7. A physician orders ceftazidime 2 g q 8 h for a patient with an Enterobacter spp. nosocomial pneumonia. Susceptibility testing shows that the pathogen is susceptible to ceftazidime. The patient initially responds to therapy but subsequently worsens. What has potentially happened?

    I.   The Enterobacter possesses an inducible beta-lactamase gene (type I beta-lactamase enzyme) that in the presence of a beta-lactam induces this enzyme.
    II. Alteration in DNA gyrase is causing resistance.
    III. Underdosage of the ceftazidime has induced resistance.

    A. I only
    B. III only
    C. I and II only
    D. II and III only
    E. I, II, and III

Case 64

8. Which of the following oral antibiotics could be used to complete therapy for AS as an outpatient?

    A. Oral meropenem
    B. Cefuroxime
    C. Amoxicillin/clavulanate
    D. Ciprofloxacin
    E. Moxifloxacin

9. AS has received 2 weeks of IV therapy for his nosocomial pneumonia. His physician wants to send him home on ciprofloxacin. You are asked to counsel AS on his antibiotic. Other discharge medications include glyburide, theophylline, atorvastatin, terazosin, and enalapril. Which of the following statements would you counsel him about?

    I.   Call your physician if you experience tachycardia, nervousness, tremors, nausea, vomiting, or abdominal pain
    II. Signs and symptoms of hypoglycemia (anxiety, confusion, irritability, tremors, tachycardia, palpitations, and seizures)
    III. Must be taken on an empty stomach

    A. I only
    B. III only
    C. I and II only
    D. II and III only
    E. I, II, and III

10. Which of the following medications/dietary supplements may interfere with the absorption of a quinolone?

    I.   Warfarin
    II. Sucralfate
    III. Ensure

    A. I only
    B. III only
    C. I and II only
    D. II and III only
    E. I, II, and III

Case 65

Patient Name: Theresa Johnson
Address: 567 Waterford Court
Age: 35   **Height:** 5' 6"
Sex: F   **Race:** White
Weight: 60 kg
Allergies: NKDA

Chief Complaint

TJ is a 35-yo woman who presents to the ambulatory clinic this morning with a 2-day history of genital pain.

History of Present Illness

TJ woke up 2 days ago with the pain that she is presenting with today. She was concerned that she may have a UTI and started drinking large quantities of fluids. She took Tylenol 1000 mg every 6 hours for several doses to treat the pain, without relief. Frustrated by the lack of pain resolution with acetaminophen, she presented to the clinic for evaluation. She indicated to the nurse in the clinic on questioning that she has had no symptoms other than the pain.

Past Medical History

TJ was diagnosed with genital herpes 3 years ago. She had two recurrent genital herpes episodes last year and has already had three recurrences during the first 8 months of this year. TJ typically presents to the clinic with each recurrence for treatment. TJ also suffers from occasional GERD and takes famotidine periodically as directed by her physician.

Social History

Divorced; lives alone and has no children

Tobacco use: 1 ppd x 20 years

Alcohol use: 1-2 drinks per day socially on weekends

Drug use: Denied

Family History

Noncontributory

Medication Record

Date	Rx No	Physician	Drug and Strength	Quantity	Sig	Refills
8/17			Tylenol 500 mg		1-2 po q 6 h prn	
6/2	12987	Jones	Acyclovir 400 mg	15	1 po tid	0
4/1	8765	Jones	Acyclovir 400 mg	15	1 po tid	0
3/25	8212	Jones	Pepcid 20 mg	28	1 po bid	1
1/17	3806	Jones	Acyclovir 400 mg	15	1 po tid	0

Review of Systems

Negative except as noted previously

Physical Examination

GEN: WD/WN female in mild to moderate pain

VS: On clinic presentation: BP 118/78 mmHg, HR 68 bpm, RR 16 rpm, T 36.8°C, Wt 60 kg

HEENT: PERRLA, oral cavity without ulcers or lesions

CHEST: Clear to auscultation and percussion

ABD: Soft, nontender

NEURO: Alert and oriented x3

GU: Two shallow ulcers noted on labia

Labs and Diagnostic Tests

Sodium 140 mEq/L	Potassium 4.1 mEq/L
Chloride 102 mEq/L	CO_2 content 26 mEq/L
BUN 14 mg/dL	Serum creatinine 0.8 mg/dL
Glucose 94 mg/dL	Hemoglobin 14.1 g/dL
Hematocrit 42.2%	Platelets 275,000/mm^3

WBC 7100/mm^3 with 64% segs, 1% bands, 30% lymphocytes, 5% monocytes

Genital swab: Tzanck test and culture positive for herpes simplex virus

Diagnosis

Primary:
   1. Recurrent genital herpes simplex episode

Secondary:
   1. History of gastroesophageal reflux disease

Pharmacist Notes and Other Patient Information

6/2 Advised of availability of generic Zovirax.

Case 65

Questions

1. The brand name drug for the equivalent generic antiviral medication that could have been dispensed to TJ is:

    A. Famvir.
    B. Cytovene.
    C. Valtrex.
    D. Zovirax.
    E. Foscavir.

2. Other oral agents that could be effectively used to treat TJ's acute genital HSV episode are:

    I. Oseltamivir.
    II. Foscarnet.
    III. Valacyclovir.

    A. I only
    B. III only
    C. I and II only
    D. II and III only
    E. I, II, and III

3. The primary goal of treatment of recurrent episodes of HSV with acyclovir is which of the following?

    A. Eradication of HSV through cidal effects on the virus
    B. Symptomatic control through inhibition of viral replication
    C. Concomitant prevention of herpes zoster infections
    D. Management of bacterial superinfection caused by virus-induced tissue damage
    E. Prevent acquisition of sexually transmitted diseases other than HSV from an infected partner

4. Which of the following therapies would be appropriate to administer as chronic suppressive therapy to patients who experience six or more recurrent episodes of genital herpes per year?

    I. Acyclovir 400 mg PO bid
    II. Famciclovir 250 mg PO bid
    III. Valacyclovir 1000 mg PO qd

    A. I only
    B. III only
    C. I and II only
    D. II and III only
    E. I, II, and III

5. Which of the following is the active moiety of the prodrug valacyclovir?

    A. Famciclovir
    B. Valacyclovir itself is the active moiety
    C. Acyclovir
    D. Zanamivir
    E. Atazanavir

6. Which of the following acyclovir dosing adjustments would be most appropriate if TJ had pre-existing renal insufficiency with an estimated creatinine clearance of 10 mL/min?

    A. No dosage adjustment is necessary from 400 mg po q 8 h
    B. 800 mg po q 12 h
    C. 200 mg po q 4 h
    D. 1200 mg po q 24 h
    E. 200 mg po q 12 h

7. Had TJ been HIV positive and had severe, disseminated HSV infection, which of the following would be the most appropriate treatment to utilize?

    A. Ganciclovir IV
    B. Acyclovir IV
    C. Foscarnet IV
    D. Acyclovir PO
    E. Ganciclovir PO

8. TJ's most recent sexual partner has just been notified of TJ's HSV diagnosis. What is the best course of action for TJ's partner to take at this time?

    A. See his physician for evaluation of possible HSV infection
    B. No action is necessary at this time
    C. Take at least 3 days of TJ's acyclovir prescription
    D. Receive the chickenpox vaccine
    E. Receive immune globulin

9. Which of the following other STDs should TJ be screened for at this time?

    I. Hepatitis A
    II. HIV
    III. Syphilis

    A. I only
    B. III only
    C. I and II only
    D. II and III only
    E. I, II, and III

Case 65

10. Nonadherence to acyclovir therapy could put TJ at risk for which of the following?

I. Extended duration of symptoms
II. Increased severity of symptoms
III. Acyclovir resistance

A. I only
B. III only
C. I and II only
D. II and III only
E. I, II, and III

Pediatric Therapy

Patient Name: Baby girl Hill
Address: 524 Juniper Street
Age: 0 days   **Height:** 1' 5"
Sex: F   **Race:** White
Weight: 1747 grams
Allergies: NKDA

Chief Complaint

Baby Hill is a 32-week old premature infant admitted to the neonatal intensive care unit immediately after birth to rule out the possibility of sepsis.

History of Present Illness

Baby Hill was born by vaginal delivery at 32 weeks gestation to a 29-yo mother (gravida 4, para 3, spontaneous Ab 1) at 12:45 p.m. today. APGAR's were 6, 8, and 10 at 1, 5, and 10 minutes, respectively. Cord pH was 7.32.

Past Medical History

Maternal history positive for rupture of membranes x20 hours, pregnancy-induced hypertension (beginning 3 weeks ago), and Group B Streptococcus (GBS) positive. Medication use during pregnancy included prenatal vitamins, Zantac, and Tylenol.

Maternal Screen

GBS: pos (no treatment)   RPR: neg

HIV: neg   Hep B: neg

HSV: neg   Chlamydia: neg

Rubella immune

Social History

None

Family History

Will live with Mom, Dad, two sisters (8 and 4 yo) and one brother (2 yo) at home.

Maternal grandmother: HTN

Sister (8 yo): Asthma

Review of Systems

Negative except as previously noted

Physical Examination

GEN: Mottled color, active

VS: T 98.4°F, HR 137 bpm, RR 42 bpm, BP 43/32 rpm, O_2 sat 97% RA, Ht: 17 inches, head circumference 30 cm

HEENT: Anterior fontanelle present, no cleft palate or lip

CHEST: Bilateral breath sounds

CV: RRR, no murmur

ABD: Soft, NTND, positive BS

GU: Normal female genitalia, patent anus

NEURO: Good tone

EXT: 20 Digits, cap refill 4 sec

Labs and Diagnostic Tests

Sodium 139 mEq/L   Potassium 5.2 mEq/L

Chloride 108 mEq/L CO_2 content 25 mEq/L

BUN 14 mg/dL   Creatine 0.8 mg/dL

Glucose 60 mg/dL   Calcium 7.2 mg/dL

Protein 4.2 g/dL   Albumin 2.6 g/dL

Total bili. 4.0 mg/dL   ALP 118 U/L

AST 50 U/L   ALT 13 U/L

WBC 9800/mm^3 with 52 segs, 5 bands, 38 lymphs, and 5 monos

Hgb 15.7 g/dL, Hct 46.3 %, platelets 319,000/mm^3

Blood cx: Pending

CSF cx: Pending

Diagnosis

Primary:

1) Suspected sepsis; GBS infection

2) Prematurity

Medication Record

Ampicillin 175 mg IV q 12 h

Gentamicin 7 mg IV q 24 h

D_{10}W at 10 mL/h

Case 66

Pharmacist Notes and Other Patient Information

Pharmacokinetic monitoring needed

Questions

1. The age of a neonate is defined as:

    A. <1 week of life.
    B. <1 month of life.
    C. <2 months of life.
    D. <6 months of life.
    E. <1 year of life.

2. On initial assessment, Baby Hill has:

    I.   normal hepatic enzymes.
    II. hyperkalemia.
    III. hyperchloremia.

    A. I only
    B. III only
    C. I and II only
    D. II and III only
    E. I, II, and III

3. Which of the following bacteria is a gram negative rod organism that causes early-onset sepsis in the neonate?

    I.   Group B Streptococcus
    II. Listeria monocytogenes
    III. Escherichia coli

    A. I only
    B. III only
    C. I and II only
    D. II and III only
    E. I, II, and III

4. BG Hill is currently being administered _____ mg/kg/d of ampicillin.

    A. 0.1
    B. 0.2
    C. 20
    D. 100
    E. 200

5. Gentamicin levels return for BG Hill. The trough is 1.5 mcg/mL and the peak is 5.8 mcg/mL. How would you adjust her current dose of 7 mg IV q 24 hours?

    A. Increase the dose
    B. Decrease the dose
    C. No change
    D. Increase the interval
    E. Decrease the interval

6. Consideration of discontinuing antibiotics in BG Hill may occur if she shows no signs of illness, feeds well, and cultures are negative for how long?

    A. 12 hours
    B. 24 hours
    C. 48 hours
    D. 72 hours
    E. 5 days

7. Calculate the appropriate maintenance fluid rate for BG Hill at 1 day of age.

    A. 3 mL/h
    B. 6 mL/h
    C. 10 mL/h
    D. 12 mL/h
    E. 15 mL/h

8. Which of the following is NOT a component of the APGAR score?

    A. Color
    B. Heart rate
    C. Temperature
    D. Muscle tone
    E. Reflex irritability

9. Which of the following describes best the mechanism of action(s) of gentamicin?

    I.   Binds to the 30S ribosomal subunit and causes an inhibition of protein synthesis
    II. Binds to the 50S ribosomal subunit and causes an inhibition of protein synthesis
    III. Binds to binding proteins and causes cell wall death

    A. I only
    B. III only
    C. I and II only
    D. II and III only
    E. I, II, and III

10. Ampicillin injection is available in the following dosage form:

    I.   Sodium
    II. Trihydrate
    III. Sulfate

Case 66

A. I only
B. III only
C. I and II only
D. II and III only
E. I, II, and III

Patient Name: George Burke
Address: 4324 Oak Avenue
Age: 8   **Height:** 4' 1"
Sex: M   **Race:** White
Weight: 32 kg
Allergies: NKDA

Chief Complaint

GB is an 8-yo Caucasian male brought to the emergency department for a 2-day history of headache, light-headedness, and fever of 103°F.

History of Present Illness

Three days before developing these symptoms, GB had been at a summer camp in Washington State. He was one of 50 children living dormitory style in a rustic setting in the mountains. While there, he felt fine and appeared healthy.

The day of symptom development (2 days ago), GB went to the emergency department, where he had a CBC and blood culture performed. His WBC was 12,200/mm³ with 81% PMN, 11% bands, and 6% lymphocytes. He was discharged home with a diagnosis of a probable viral infection. He was told to rest, drink plenty of fluids, and take acetaminophen for the fever or aches and pains.

On presentation today, the patient complained of whole body pain, stiff neck, photophobia, and anorexia. He was nauseated and unable to tolerate clear liquids or popsicles. The blood culture that had been drawn 2 days earlier was negative. GB underwent a second complete physical exam including a spinal tap for culture, glucose, and protein. The patient was admitted to the PICU for further evaluation and management. The gram stain of the cerebral spinal fluid today shows gram-positive organisms in chains.

Past Medical History

Tonsillectomy and adenoidectomy 3 years earlier.

Social History

Tobacco use: Denies

Alcohol use: Denies

Caffeine use: 1 can soda/day

Family History

Noncontributory

Review of Systems

Negative except as noted previously

Physical Examination

GEN: Lethargic with shallow respirations, complaining of severe pain in his chest

VS: T 101°F, HR 87 bpm, RR 32 rpm, BP 113/61 mmHg, Wt 32 kg

SKIN: Warm, dry; no lesions, petechiae, or rash

HEENT: Head is normocephalic, atraumatic. Eyes are PERRLA, EOMI. Mouth/throat mucous membranes are pink and moist, no petechiae. Nares are patent. Neck has nuchal rigidity present. Patient refusing to move his neck.

CHEST: Symmetrical, lungs clear to auscultation bilaterally

CV: RRR, NL S_1/S_2, No S_2/S_3 auscultated, no murmurs or rubs, precordium quiet, no pulsus paradoxus

ABD: Soft, nontender, nondistended, NL BS, no hepatosplenomegaly

GU: WNL

NEURO: Moves all extremities slowly; limited by pain

EXT: No CCE; brisk capillary refill

Labs and Diagnostic Tests

(on admission to PICU)

Sodium 137 mEq/L	Potassium 4.1 mEq/L
Chloride 104 mEq/L	CO_2 content 21 mEq/L
BUN 8 mg/dL	Creatinine 0.7 mg/dL
Glucose 120 mg/dL	Phosphorus 2.0 mg/dL
Magnesium 2.0 mg/L	Calcium 8.8 mg/dL
Uric acid 3.4 mg/dL	Cholesterol 137 mg/dL
Iron < 2 mg/dL	Total protein 6.4 g/dL
Albumin 3.7 g/dL	AST 29 IU/L
ALT 33 IU/L	Alk phos 78 IU/L
GGTP 14 IU/L	LDH 100 IU/L
T. bili. 0.3 mg/dL	

WBC 128,000/mm³, polys 75%, bands 14%, lymphs 11%

RBC 26 M/mm³	Hgb 12.1 g/dL
Hct 35.5%	Platelets 103,000/mm³
MCV 83 FL	MCH 28 pgs
MCHC 34.1%	RDW 12.2%

Case 67

Blood culture:

(from ED 2 days before admission) (-).

CSF culture:

24-hour preliminary report Neisseria meningitidis

Coagulation profile:

PT 12 sec, INR 1.04, PTT 28.6 sec, fibrinogen 498 mg/dL, FDP 2-10 µg/mL, ATIII 103%

Urinalysis:

Color yellow, (-) glucose, (-) bilirubin, (-) ketones, specific gravity 1.012, blood trace, pH 5.0, (-) protein, urobilinogen 0.2 mg/dL, (-) nitrite, (-) leukocyte esterase, WBC 0-2/HPF, RBC 0-2/HPF, epith sm/HPF, bact sm/HPF, yeast-bud sm/HPF.

Complement:

CH50 202 units

CSF Fluid Analysis:

Glucose 44 mg/dL	Protein 87 mg/dL
WBC 850/mm^3	RBC 150/mm^3

CXR:

No focal infiltrates, NL heart size and pulmonary vascular markings

 Diagnosis

Primary:

1) Neisseria meningitidis meningitis

 Medication Record

(on admission)

None, immunizations up to date

Hospital course:

The patient was started on IV penicillin G, 250,000 units/kg/d ÷ q 4 h, dexamethasone 1 mg/kg/dose q 6 h x8 doses and ranitidine 2 mg/kg/dose IVP q 8 h. The organism was sensitive to rifampin, ceftriaxone, and penicillin. All subsequent blood cultures and the CSF culture were negative. His family and selected nursing staff were treated with rifampin for prophylaxis. The patient's signs and symptoms of infection resolved quickly and he was discharged from the hospital after 5 days. The discharging resident continued GB on penicillin parenterally then switched to penicillin VK 60 mg/kg/d ÷ q 6 h for 10 days orally and acetaminophen/codeine elixir 1-2 teaspoonfuls q 4-6 h prn pain. The patient was to follow up with his PCP on an outpatient basis.

Medication Administration Records:

1/1, Penicillin 1,335,000 units IV q 4 h, d/c on 1/5

1/1, Dexamethasone 30 mg IVP q 6 h, d/c on 1/3

1/1, Ranitidine 60 mg IVP q 8 h, d/c on 1/5

1/1, Acetaminophen/codeine elixir 12.5 mL po q 4 h prn pain, d/c on 1/5

1/1, Morphine 1-3 mg IVP q 4 h prn pain, d/c on 1/5

Planned Discharge Medications:

Penicillin VK 250 mg po q 6 h x 3 days

Acetaminophen/codeine elixir 2 teaspoonfuls po q 4 h prn pain

 Pharmacist Notes and Other Patient Information

None available

Questions

1. In children older than 5 years of age, which of the following organisms is one of the most common causes of bacterial meningitis?

    A. Group B streptococci (GBS)

    B. Escherichia coli

    C. Streptococcus pneumoniae

    D. Haemophilus influenzae type b (Hib)

    E. Listeria monocytogenes

2. Decadron was prescribed for GB during his course of meningitis. What benefit(s) does Decadron afford to pediatric patients diagnosed with meningitis?

    A. Dexamethasone has anti-infective properties that act synergistically with penicillin to combat infection

    B. Dexamethasone has immunosuppressive properties and you realize should not have been prescribed for GB

    C. Dexamethasone reduces inflammation, thus, decreases the penetration of antibiotic into the CSF

    D. Dexamethasone was prescribed because it has been shown to reduce the incidence of hearing loss sometimes associated with meningitis

    E. Dexamethasone reduces inflammation of the meninges, allowing increased blood flow into the meninges and, thus, better antibiotic penetration

3. A pharmacy technician performs a calculation for preparing the initial course of IV penicillin doses. He calculates 60 mL of penicillin per dose. The penicillin is 50,000 units/mL.

    A. This is correct and the technician is told to prepare the doses STAT

    B. The actual volume of penicillin is 26.7 mL and you instruct the technician to draw up this volume and add to a piggyback

    C. The actual volume of penicillin is 5 mL and you instruct the technician to draw up this volume and add to a piggyback

Case 67

D. The actual volume of penicillin is 16 mL and you instruct the technician to draw up this volume and add to a piggyback

E. The actual volume of penicillin is 2.67 mL and you instruct the technician to draw up this volume and add to a piggyback

4. Penicillin is a broad spectrum antibiotic. It works by:

A. reversibly binding to several enzymes in the cytoplasmic membrane of susceptible bacteria, yielding unstable cell walls.

B. reversibly binding to the 30S ribosomal subunits and the 50S subunits, inhibiting RNA protein synthesis.

C. inhibiting final dephosphorylation step in cell wall synthesis, preventing the mucopeptide incorporation into the growing cell wall.

D. reversibly binding to the 30S ribosomal subunits and the 50S subunits, inhibiting DNA protein synthesis.

E. competitively inhibiting folic acid synthesis from bacterial para-aminobenzoic acid.

5. Vaccination for which of the following organism(s) has decreased the incidence of bacterial meningitis in children?

I. Haemophilis influenzae type b (Hib)
II. Streptococcus pneumoniae
III. Escherichia coli

A. I only
B. III only
C. I and II only
D. II and III only
E. I, II, and III

6. Common signs or symptoms of meningitis in children include all of the following EXCEPT:

A. fever, increased white count, left shift, and pulmonary infiltrates.

B. fever, headache, increased white count, and nuccal rigidity.

C. headache, anorexia, increased white count, and left shift.

D. fever, headache, anorexia, and photophobia.

E: fever, increased white count, and positive Kernig's sign.

7. Who of the following should be administered chemoprophylaxis for meningococcal meningitis:

I. His mother
II. His sister who sleeps in a different room
III. His best friend at camp who shared a room

A. I only
B. III only
C. I and II only
D. II and III only
E. I, II, and III

8. The mother of the patient reads up on meningococcal meningitis and would like to treat her child at home. After 5 days in the hospital, the physicians consider mom's request to send the patient home for the remainder of the treatment. They ask you for your antibiotic recommendation in the home. You answer:

I. Meningitis is serious and you advise against sending the patient home; less serious infections may be safely treated at home, but not meningitis

II. The organism is susceptible to penicillin and the patient is improving, thus, penicillin should be continued, even at home

III. N. meningitis is usually susceptible to ceftriaxone; this antibiotic has good CNS penetration and may be used once daily, making administration in the home more practical

A. I only
B. III only
C. I and II only
D. II and III only
E. I, II, and III

9. Rifampin 640 mg po qd was ordered for close contacts of GB for prophylaxis. You call the resident and state:

A. Would you prefer the patient to get capsules or suspension?

B. Although the dose equals 640 mg, the maximum daily dose is 300 mg

C. Although the dose equals 640 mg, the capsules come as 300 and 600 mg dosed po q day as appropriate

D. Althought the dose equals 640 mg, 300 mg po TID is the optimal prophylaxis dose for Neisseria menigitis

E. Rifampin is not available in an enteral dosage form, only parenteral

10. GB's mother questions you about pain control. She is concerned about the addiction potential of morphine and the codeine in the elixir. You educate mom about proper pain management principles. You conclude with:

A. Patients in pain treated with even larger doses of narcotics for acute pain episodes rarely get addicted and relieving the pain helps her son recover more quickly from the illness

B. No one gets addicted to manufacturer-prepared medications

C. These doses of narcotic are too small for addiction

D. Mom is right to be concerned and you will have them stopped immediately

E. Children should not be treated with morphine because it is too potent; narcotics are for adults only

Patient Name: Baby girl Jones
Address: 102 Thames Street
Age: 7 days   **Height:** 1' 9"
Sex: F   **Race:** African American
Weight: 1.1 kg
Allergies: NKDA

Chief Complaint

Baby Jones is a 28-week gestational age female born to a G_1P_0 36-year-old mother with a history of gestational diabetes and Group B Streptococcus colonization. Developed feeding intolerance 1 week after birth.

History of Present Illness

On Baby Jones' first day of life, parenteral nutrition (PN) was initiated through an umbilical venous catheter (UVC). On day 5 of life she was started on enteral feedings via a nasogastric tube, with a premature formula (24 calories/30 mL). The UVC was removed when enteral feeds were started. On day 7, she was receiving 2 mL/h of enteral feedings in addition to her PN solution. Later that evening she had the following changes:

Increased abdominal girth from 19 to 24 cm

Gastric residuals of 10 mL

Lethargy

An abdominal x-ray showed free air in her abdomen (pneumo-peritoneum). She was diagnosed with necrotizing enterocolitis (NEC). She was started on antibiotics, and she was taken to the operating room for an exploratory laparotomy. It was found that she had extensive disease and required resection of much of her small intestine. She was left with 20 cm of small intestine, and no ilial-cecal valve. A central venous catheter was placed during surgery for access.

Past Medical History

Infant born via emergency cesarean section. Infant's APGAR score was 3 and 5 at 1 and 5 minutes, respectively. At 9 minutes APGAR score was 5. She was immediately intubated in the delivery room and received a dose of surfactant. She was started on dopamine 5 µg/kg/min for hypotension. Over the course of her treatment, it was found she had a patent ductus arteriosus (PDA) and was treated with a course of indomethacin with successful closure of the PDA. She was transitioned from mechanical ventilation on day 5 of life to Vapotherm™.

Social History

Not applicable

Family History

Mother: Healthy, no known health problems, good prenatal care.

Father: Healthy, no known health problems

Review of Systems

Not applicable

Physical Examination

GEN: Small lethargic infant

VS: HR 180 bpm, RR – ventilator, BP 45/25 mmHg, Wt 1.1 Kg, Ht 1' 9", head circumference 20 cm

HEENT: Unremarkable

LUNGS: Ventilated infant

CV: Poor perfusion

GI: Bowel sounds absent, marked abdominal distension

GU: WNL

Labs and Diagnostic Tests

WBC: $8.5 \times 10^3/mm^3$	Hb: 12 g/dL
HCT: 23%	PLT: $68 \times 10^3/mm^3$
Sodium: 132 mEq/L	Potassium: 4 mEq/L
Chloride: 115 mEq/L	CO_2: 20 mEq/L
BUN: 10 mg/dL	Creatine: 0.4 mg/dL
Glucose: 85 mg/dL	Albumin: 3.1 g/dL

Blood and peritoneal cultures: Positive for enterobacter cloacae

Abdominal x-ray: Pneumotosis and pneumoperitoneum

Diagnosis

Primary:

1) Stage III necrotizing enterocolitis requiring parenteral nutrition and antibiotic therapy

Medication Record

Vancomycin 17 mg IV Q24h

Cefotaxime 55 mg IV Q12h

Metronidazole 8 mg IV Q48h

Case 68

NG replacement cc:cc with 0.45 NS and potassium chloride 10 mEq/L

Parenteral nutrition

 Pharmacist Notes and Other Patient Information

None

Questions

1. This infant requires 1.5 x maintenance for her fluids. What would the 24-hour volume be for her?

    A. 110 mL/day
    B. 125 mL/day
    C. 155 mL/day
    D. 165 mL/day
    E. 200 mL/day

2. To initiate PN for this patient, what is the best solution for her first day of therapy?

    A. Protein 0.5 g/kg/day, fat 0.5 g/kg/day, glucose 5 mg/kg/min
    B. Protein 1 g/kg/day, fat 3 g/kg/day, glucose 12 mg/kg/min
    C. Protein 2.5 g/kg/day, fat 1 g/kg/day, glucose 6 mg/kg/min
    D. Protein 3.5 g/kg/day, fat 4 g/kg/day, glucose 10 mg/kg/min
    E. None of the above provide adequate nutrition for the first day of treatment.

3. Baby Jones is now 2 weeks of age on full PN. What would a likely formulation for this infant be?

    A. Protein 0.5 g/kg/day, fat 0.5 g/kg/day, glucose 5 mg/kg/min
    B. Protein 1 g/kg/day, fat 3 g/kg/day, glucose 12 mg/kg/min
    C. Protein 2 g/kg/day, fat 3 g/kg/day, glucose 6 mg/kg/min
    D. Protein 3.5 g/kg/day, fat 4 g/kg/day, glucose 10 mg/kg/min
    E. Protein 7 g/kd/day, fat 3.5 g/kg/day, glucose 18 mg/kg/min

4. How many calories does this infant require for maintenance and growth?

    A. 30 kcal/kg/day
    B. 50 kcal/kg/day
    C. 70 kcal/kg/day
    D. 100 kcal/kg/day
    E. 150 kcal/kg/day

5. What laboratory test would be most useful in determining a patient's tolerance to the intravenous fat emulsion?

    A. Cholesterol
    B. Alpha-1 antitrypsin
    C. Triglyceride
    D. HDL
    E. Alkaline phosphatase

6. Many infants develop metabolic bone disease (Rickett's or osteopenia) while on long-term PN. What laboratory tests might you want to review to assess a patient's risk for developing metabolic bone disease?

    I.   Alkaline phosphatase
    II. Calcium and phosphorus
    III. Alpha-1 antitrypsin

    A. I only
    B. III only
    C. I and II only
    D. II and III only
    E. I, II, and III

7. Infants receiving long-term PN are at risk for which complication(s)?

    I.   Cholestasis
    II. Osteopenia
    III. Selenium deficiency

    A. I only
    B. III only
    C. I and II only
    D. II and III only
    E. I, II, and III

8. What is the optimal ratio of calcium to phosphate that would allow for appropriate growth in a pre-term infant?

    A. 0.5:1 (calcium:phosphate)
    B. 1:1 (calcium:phosphate)
    C. 1:2 (calcium:phosphate)
    D. 1.8:1 (calcium:phosphate)
    E. 10:1 (calcium:phosphate)

9. Which of the following factor(s) influence calcium and phosphate solubility in PN solutions?

    I.   Calcium/phosphate concentrations
    II. pH of the PN solution
    III. Temperature

Case 68

A. I only
B. III only
C. I and II only
D. II and III only
E. I, II, and III

10. In a patient with cholestatic liver disease it may be necessary to hold which of the following trace minerals from the PN formulation?

I. Manganese
II. Copper
III. Chromium

A. I only
B. III only
C. I and II only
D. II and III only
E. I, II, and III

Patient Name: Michael Kelly
Address: 1004 Clark Street
Age: 11 years   **Height:** 4' 9"
Sex: M   **Race:** White
Weight: 52 kg
Allergies: Bactrim (hives)

Chief Complaint

MK is an 11-year-old male who presents with a 1-week history of lethargy, decreased appetite, and petechiae on abdomen and extremities.

History of Present Illness

About 1 week prior to admission, MK started to develop petechiae on his abdomen, which eventually began to spread to his extremities. Patient denied any fever, earache, or headache at that time. Yesterday, the patient vomited in the morning. His emesis was described as non-bloody. The patient has had bowel movements described as normal but denies melena or hematochezia. Patient denies diarrhea or constipation. Patient admits to decreased appetite. For breakfast on the day of admission, he had only one glass of milk. The patient has been lethargic and has been sleeping more than usual. On the day of admission, the patient was brought to the pediatrician's office, where a CBC was done. Based on the results of the CBC, the patient was sent to the emergency department for further work-up and admission.

Past Medical History

The patient has no significant past medical history. Immunizations are up to date.

Social History

Patient lives with both parents. Patient denies any illnesses in the house. He is in the 5th grade and gets Bs and Cs. His development is normal.

Family History

Unremarkable

Review of Systems

Patient is alert and oriented x 3 and is generally in a good mood.

Physical Examination

HT: 146 cm BSA: 1.45 m²

VS: Temp 37.2 °C   Pulse 103   RR 16   BP 115/70

SKIN: Petechiae on abdomen and extremities (diffusely over body); bruising on ankles and bilateral lower extremities; ~ 6-cm ecchymosis over left ankle, smaller over right ankle

HEENT: EOMI, PERRLA, no scleral icterus, conjunctiva pink; TM intact, no fluid behind TM, no exudates; no septal deviation, nasal mucosa pink, no bleeding; no erythema, no gum bleeding, couple petechiae under tongue; neck: supple, no thyromegaly

CHEST: CTA bilaterally

CV: RRR, normal S_1/S_2, no murmur; good capillary refill; equal pulses

ABD: Non-tender, non-distended, + bowel sounds, no hepatosplenomegaly, no masses

GU: Descended testes, anus patent, no fistulas, no adhesions

NEURO: Good reflexes

Labs and Diagnostic Tests

Sodium 140 mEq/L	Potassium 3.53 mEq/L
Chloride 105 mEq/L	CO_2 25 mEq/L
BUN 5 mg/dl	Creatinine 0.6 mg/dL
Glucose 119 mg/dL	Calcium 9.0 mg/dL
Phos 4.1 mg/dL	Magnesium 1.6 mg/dL
Uric acid 8.9 mg/dL	AST 151 units/L
ALT 54 units/L	Alk phos 220 units/L
T. bili. 1.1 mg/dL	D. bili. 0.2 mg/dL
Albumin 3.7 g/dL	WBC 160,000 per mm³
Hemoglobin 9.4 g/dL	Hematocrit 29.1%
Platelets 7000 per mm³	Segs 1%
Lymphocytes 20%	Eosinophils 2%
Blasts 77%	PT 12.9
INR 1.3	PTT 39

Ejection fraction 69%

Lumbar puncture: Findings consistent with precursor B-cell acute lymphoblastic leukemia

Case 69

Diagnosis

Acute lymphoblastic leukemia (ALL)

Medication Record

No medications prior to admission or in the ED

$D_5W/0.45\%$ NaCl with $NaHCO_3$ 40 mEq/L to run at 175 mL/hour (2 x maintenance)

Cefepime 2 g IV q8h (fever of 101°F in ER)

Allopurinol 250 mg PO bid (10 mg/kg/day)

Cytarabine 70 mg IT at time of lumbar puncture

Zofran 8 mg IV 30 minutes prior to chemo, then q4h prn n/v

Vincristine 2 mg IV push x 1 on day 1 of chemo (1.5 mg/m²)

Daunorubicin 36.5 mg IVP x 1 on day 1 of chemo (25 mg/m²)

PEG-asparaginase 3650 units IM x 1 on day 4 of chemo (2500 mg/m²)

Dexamethasone 7.5 mg PO qam and 7 mg PO qpm (10 mg/m²/day) x 14 days

Pharmacist Notes and Other Patient Information

None available

Questions

1. Prior to initiating daunorubicin therapy, the following baseline studies are recommended:

    I.   CBC with differential
    II. Echocardiogram
    III. Liver function tests

    A. I only
    B. III only
    C. I and II only
    D. II and III only
    E. I, II, and III

2. Intrathecal administration of vincristine is:

    A. A relative contraindication
    B. An absolute contraindication
    C. Interchangeable with intravenous vincristine
    D. Contraindicated only in pregnant females
    E. Acceptable with informed, written consent

3. Patients with ALL are usually started on twice or three times weekly regimens of trimethoprim/sulfamethoxazole to provide prophylaxis against Pneumocystis carinii pneumonia. Considering MK's allergy to Bactrim, which of the following medications would be an appropriate alternative to trimethoprim/sulfamethoxazole for this indication?

    I.   Dapsone
    II. Inhaled pentamidine
    III. Daptomycin

    A. I only
    B. III only
    C. I and II only
    D. II and III only
    E. I, II, and III

4. Management of hyperuricemia in leukemic patients may include each of the following EXCEPT:

    A. Hydration with intravenous fluids
    B. Urinary alkalinization with sodium bicarbonate
    C. Allopurinol
    D. Apresoline
    E. Rasburicase

5. Two days after initiation of chemotherapy, MK's lab results reveal the following: potassium 6.7 mEq/L, calcium 5.1mg/dL, phosphorus 14.3 mg/dL, BUN 56 mg/dL, and creatinine 2.3 mg/dL. MK has gone into acute renal failure, most likely secondary to tumor lysis syndrome. Tumor lysis syndrome is an oncologic emergency characterized by severe metabolic derangements, including hyperkalemia, hypocalcemia, hyperphosphatemia, and hyperuricemia. MK is transferred to the PICU for close monitoring and treatment. MK's hyperkalemia may be the most serious manifestation of his tumor lysis syndrome at this point, due to the potential for the development of life-threatening cardiac arrhythmias. Each of the following medications may be appropriate treatments of MK's hyperkalemia EXCEPT:

    A. Sodium polystyrene sulfate 50 g PO or PR
    B. Calcium gluconate 2 g IV
    C. Insulin 5 units IV with dextrose 50% 50-mL IV
    D. Magnesium sulfate 2 g IV
    E. Sodium bicarbonate 50 mEq IV

6. The PICU resident is considering ordering a calcium supplement for MK. She questions you about the different IV calcium salts. Which of the following will you tell the resident about IV calcium supplements?

    A. Calcium chloride contains three times the elemental calcium of calcium gluconate
    B. Calcium gluconate contains twice the elemental calcium of calcium chloride
    C. Calcium chloride and calcium gluconate contain the same amount of elemental calcium

Case 69

D. Oral is better absorbed than IV

E. Parental calcium carbonate provides the highest percent of elemental calcium

7. Which of the following medications that MK is currently receiving will need dosage adjustment in light of his acute renal failure?

I. Cefepime
II. Allopurinol
III. Dexamethasone

A. I only
B. III only
C. I and II only
D. II and III only
E. I, II, and III

8. MK's uric acid level 2 days after initiation of chemotherapy is 8.0, following 3 days of oral allopurinol therapy. The decision is made to change MK's therapy from allopurinol to rasburicase to further reduce his uric acid level. Which of the following is NOT a consideration when administering rasburicase?

A. Hypersensitivity to rasburicase
B. Temperature of blood sample for uric acid measurement
C. G6PD deficiency
D. Renal insufficiency
E. Methemoglobinemia

9. The mechanism(s) of action of rasburicase is best described as:

I. Xanthine oxidase inhibitor
II. Urinary alkalinizer
III. A recombinant form of urate oxidase that catalyzes the enzymatic oxidation of uric acid into allantoin

A. I only
B. III only
C. I and II only
D. II and III only
E. I, II, and III

10. Which of the following would be the most appropriate dose of rasburicase for MK?

A. 7.5 mg IV once daily for up to 5 days
B. 24 mg IV once daily for up to 5 days
C. 15 mg IV once daily for up to 5 days
D. 75 mg IV once daily for up to 5 days
E. 6 mg IV once daily for up to 5 days

Skin Disorders

Patient Name: Sally Jones
Address: 2606 Valley Oak Drive
Age: 19   **Height:** 5' 5"
Sex: F   **Race:** White
Weight: 160 lb
Allergies: NKDA

Chief Complaint

"I'm 19—when will my acne finally go away?"

History of Present Illness

SJ's acne began at age 14 and worsened 1 year later, when she started having periods ("I started to get big pimples then"). Since age 16 she has had big pimples all over her face fairly constantly. She has not had many pimples on her back or chest. Dissatisfied with over-the-counter products, she started Rx therapy about a year ago. She started a new regimen of Sumycin and 5% benzoyl peroxide gel about a month ago. She uses cosmetics marketed as non-comedogenic and washes her face with a product marketed for acne-prone skin. In high school, classmates made fun of her at times, and she believes her acne has made it more difficult getting boyfriends. She told herself to be patient and wait out her teenage years, but the persistence of the acne is starting to worry her, and she is concerned about scarring.

Past Medical History

The patient has been diagnosed with depression and dysmenorrhea within the past 3 years. She had an appendectomy at age 9 but has otherwise never been hospitalized. She sees a counselor periodically but states they "really don't hit it off."

Social History

The patient is a single college student who lives in an apartment with two other girls. She has an "off and on" boyfriend and is occasionally sexually active. She drinks alcohol (2-3 beers at a time) once or twice weekly. She denies using illicit drugs or tobacco.

Family History

The patient's father has high blood pressure and dyslipidemia. Her mother is obese and had a hysterectomy for uterine fibroids. Her younger brother and sister both have acne. The brother also has epilepsy.

Review of Systems

Positive for occasional headaches, use of eye glasses, painful menstrual periods, poor sleeping, and depressed mood. The patient denies shortness of breath, dizziness, nausea or vomiting,

or dry skin. She denies suicidal thoughts or plans. Her last menstrual period was 2 weeks ago.

Physical Examination

VS: BP 116/62 mmHg, HR 78 bpm, RR 14 rpm, T 98.2°F

GEN: Well-developed, overweight young white female with flat affect.

SKIN: Face with multiple papules and pustules, mostly in T-zone, with evidence of excoriation; few lesions on chest and back; no cysts at present; a few small pitted scars on cheeks; no hirsutism.

CV: Regular rate and rhythm; no murmurs, rubs, or gallops.

CHEST: Clear to auscultation and percussion bilaterally; respiration unlabored.

ABD: Soft, nontender, normal active bowel sounds; no organomegaly.

GYN: Normal genitalia, no adnexal tenderness or masses.

Labs and Diagnostic Tests

Na 144 mEq/L	K 4.4 mEq/L
Cl 104 mEq/L	CO_2 24 mEq/L
BUN 11 mg/dL	SCr 0.8 mg/dL
Glucose 84 mg/dL	ALT 11 IU/L
AST 14 IU/L	GGT 24 IU/L
ALP 86 IU/L	Bili 0.6 mg/dL
TC (fasting) 216 mg/dL	LDL-C (fasting) 126 mg/dL
HDL-C (fasting) 50 mg/dL	TG (fasting) 200 mg/dL
Urine pregnancy test negative	

Diagnosis

Primary:

    1. Acne vulgaris, moderate

Secondary:

    1. Depression

    2. Dysmenorrhea

Pharmacist Notes and Other Patient Information

1/6/06 Discussed management of GI adverse effects with Ery-Tab use

8/8/05 Assisted in buying home pregnancy kit

Case 70

Medication Record

Date	Rx No	Physician	Drug and Strength	Quantity	Sig	Refills
2/06			Benzac W 5% gel	60 g	Apply to face bid	2
2/06			Sumycin 500 mg cap	60	1 po bid	1
12/05			Ery-Tab 250 mg tab	60	1 po bid	
5/05			Benzoyl peroxide 2.5% gel	60 g	Apply to face q am	
5/05			Anaprox DS tab	60	1 po bid prn	
2/05			Prozac 20 mg cap	30	1 po qd	

Questions

1. Which products are keratinolytic?

   I. Benzoyl peroxide
   II. Salicylic acid
   III. Lactic acid

   A. I only
   B. III only
   C. I and II only
   D. II and III only
   E. I, II, and III

2. Why are doxycycline or tetracycline preferable to minocycline as initial oral agents for acne vulgaris?

   A. Minocycline has a higher incidence of severe side effects.
   B. Minocycline is less effective than the other two antibiotics.
   C. Minocycline is less well absorbed from the GI tract.
   D. Minocycline needs to be dosed more frequently.
   E. Minocycline has more drug interactions.

3. Which of the following natural products has been used and discussed in the literature for acne?

   A. Grape seed extract
   B. Tea tree oil
   C. Arnica
   D. Flaxseed oil
   E. Feverfew

4. The single most effective medication for the treatment of severe, recalcitrant acne is:

   A. Sumycin.
   B. Ery-Tab.
   C. Retin-A.
   D. Benzoyl peroxide.
   E. Accutane.

5. In addition to using her benzoyl peroxide and tetracycline, SJ should be counseled to:

   A. avoid fatty foods such as fried food and chocolate.
   B. expose acne lesions to sunlight.
   C. use an exfoliating scrub once or twice per week.
   D. use non-comedogenic products if she chooses to wear makeup.
   E. express the contents of comedones using clean hands and sterilized tweezers.

6. When SJ fails to improve adequately on her current regimen, she discusses with her doctor moving on to Accutane. Which of the following labs should be monitored if she does so?

   I. Pregnancy
   II. Cholesterol
   III. Liver function

   A. I only
   B. III only
   C. I and II only
   D. II and III only
   E. I, II, and III

7. Which of the following is/are true for the iPLEDGE program for oral isotretinoin distribution?

   I. Prescribers, drug wholesalers, pharmacies, and patients must all be registered with the program.
   II. Isotretinoin prescriptions can be for no more than a 30-day supply and cannot have any refills.
   III. Pharmacists may only fill isotretinoin prescriptions if they bear the program's yellow sticker (provided to registered prescribers) and are presented within 7 days of the date written.

   A. I only
   B. III only
   C. I and II only
   D. II and III only
   E. I, II, and III

Case 70

8. SJ wants to use hormonal contraception while on Accutane. Her prescriber wants to use a product that is likely to reduce rather than aggravate her acne. Which of the following has FDA approval for treating acne?

   A. Ortho Tri-Cyclen
   B. Alesse
   C. Yasmin
   D. Micronor
   E. Ortho Novum

9. Ery-Tabs are designed to:

   I.   dissolve in the stomach.
   II. release medication slowly over 12 hours.
   III. prevent medication degradation by stomach acid.

   A. I only
   B. III only
   C. I and II only
   D. II and III only
   E. I, II, and III

10. Accutane is usually given 0.5-1 mg/kg/d, divided bid, to a cumulative dose of 120 mg/kg. It is supplied in 10-, 20-, and 40-mg capsules; a generic product is also available in 30-mg capsules. Which of the following regimens would be most appropriate for SJ?

    A. 20 mg po bid x 16 weeks
    B. 20 mg po bid x 21 weeks
    C. 30 mg po bid x 21 weeks
    D. 40 mg po bid x 21 weeks
    E. 80 mg po bid x 16 weeks

Patient Name: Mary Kay Jones
Address: 2927 Glenarm Avenue, Apartment C
Age: 22   **Height:** 5' 8"
Sex: F   **Race:** White
Weight: 116 lb
Allergies: TMP/SMX: rash; codeine: pruritus

Chief Complaint

"How should I treat this burn I got yesterday?"

History of Present Illness

While riding on her boyfriend's motorcycle yesterday, the patient burned her right leg on the exhaust pipe. She applied ice from a drink for about 15 minutes, then continued riding, returning late last night. Before bed, she covered the burn with a gauze pad. This morning she awoke to find the leg more sore and tender to the touch. The gauze was stuck to the burn, so the patient soaked the wound in water to loosen and remove it. She has nothing on the burn now.

Past Medical History

Her history is significant for migraine headache for the past 6 years. She also has had recurrent UTIs. Her last infection progressed to pyelonephritis 6 months ago and required hospitalization and parenteral antibiotics for 2 days.

Social History

The patient is single but engaged to her boyfriend and will be married in 4 months. She is a college student and works part-time as a waitress. She drinks 1-2 beers/day, sometimes 3 beers if out with friends. She does not use tobacco but does smoke marijuana once or twice per week. She does not use any other illicit drugs.

Family History

The patient is adopted and does not know her family history.

Review of Systems

Positive for nonproductive cough, usually associated with work in the smoky restaurant. The patient denies fever, chills, or sweats. She also denies dysuria, frequent urination, or back pain. She denies vaginal discharge. Her last menstrual period was "on time" 3 weeks ago. Her last migraine headache was last month (she averages 3-4 headaches per month).

Physical Examination

VS: BP 108/68 mmHg, HR 88 bpm, RR 20 rpm, T 98.6°F

GEN: Thin, white female in moderate pain.

HEENT: Normal.

CV: Regular rate and rhythm; no murmurs, rubs or gallops.

CHEST: Clear to auscultation and percussion bilaterally.

SKIN: Right inner calf has a 5 x 7.5 cm area of erythema including a 1 x 2 cm bullous area in the center. There is no lymphangitis, pus, or streaking.

EXT: Right knee and ankle appear normal. There is no posterior calf tenderness or pedal edema.

Labs and Diagnostic Tests

None available

Diagnosis

Primary:

     1. Superficial partial-thickness burn, right calf

Secondary:

     1. Migraine headache

     2. History of recurrent urinary tract infections

     3. Contraception

     4. Substance abuse, marijuana

Pharmacist Notes and Other Patient Information

5/27 Discussed possibility of oral contraceptive worsening migraine headache.

Medication Record

Date	Rx No	Physician	Drug and Strength	Quantity	Sig	Refills
2/06			Theragran-M	100	1 po qd	6
2/06			Ortho Tri-Cyclen	28	1 po q am	6
12/05			Imitrex 50 mg	9	1-2 po prn HA	1

Case 71

Questions

1. The pharmacist would have referred MJ to medical care immediately if her burn had been characterized by which of the following signs?

   I. Blanching with pressure
   II. Caused by electric current
   III. White and painless

   A. I only
   B. III only
   C. I and II only
   D. II and III only
   E. I, II, and III

2. MJ must monitor her burn as it heals for signs and symptoms of secondary bacterial infection. Classic signs include all of the following EXCEPT:

   A. increased swelling.
   B. increased or expanding erythema.
   C. increased warmth.
   D. onset of weeping from lesion.
   E. development of streaking from lesion.

3. Tactile and pain sensation is first diminished in burns of which severity?

   A. Superficial
   B. Superficial partial-thickness
   C. Deep partial-thickness
   D. Full thickness
   E. Full thickness with damage to underlying tissue

4. Thin-walled, fluid-filled blisters are the defining characteristic of which type of burns?

   A. Superficial
   B. Superficial partial-thickness
   C. Deep partial thickness
   D. Full thickness
   E. Full thickness with damage to underlying tissue

5. Which of the following is a counterirritant topical analgesic?

   A. Pramoxine
   B. Diphenhydramine
   C. Lidocaine
   D. Allantoin
   E. Menthol

6. The bulla on MJ's calf ruptures, leaving a superficial erosion. The area is sore and pruritic. Which of the following would be the best product for MJ to apply under a protective bandage?

   A. Benadryl Gel
   B. Hydrocortisone 1% cream
   C. Bacitracin Ointment
   D. Gold Bond Cream
   E. Lanacane Cream

7. One burn treatment approach that should be avoided is:

   A. cleansing with water and a mild soap.
   B. cleansing with an alcohol-containing preparation.
   C. application of nonadherent dressing.
   D. use of a skin protectant/lubricant containing cocoa butter.
   E. use of a skin protectant/lubricant containing white petrolatum.

8. Which of the following are potentially fatal complications of severe burns?

   I. Infection
   II. Hypotensive shock
   III. Rhabdomyolysis

   A. I only
   B. III only
   C. I and II only
   D. II and III only
   E. I, II, and III

9. MJ wants to try the following additional therapies. Which are reasonably safe?

   I. Apply ice
   II. Apply aloe
   III. Use over-the-counter ibuprofen

   A. I only
   B. III only
   C. I and II only
   D. II and III only
   E. I, II, and III

10. What healing course and clinical outcome are likeliest for MJ if her burn is appropriately treated?

    A. The burn will heal in 4 days and leave no scar.
    B. The burn will heal in 4 days and leave a slight scar.
    C. The burn will heal in 2 weeks and leave a slight scar.
    D. The burn will heal in 6 weeks and leave a slight scar.
    E. The burn will heal in 6 weeks and leave a significant scar.

Over-the-Counter Medications

Section Editor: Jennifer Ridings Myhra

See all 8 cases for this section on the CD.

Patient Name: Milton Holmes
Address: 4422 Kasey Drive
Age: 56　　　Height: 6' 0"
Sex: M　　　Race: African American
Weight: 205 lb
Allergies: NKDA

Chief Complaint

MH is a 56-yo male who presents to your pharmacy in a grocery store chain on 01/15. He asks you to recommend something for what he thinks is a cold or even the flu. MH does not appear to have watery eyes, nor is he sneezing while he is standing at your counter. However, his nose is quite red and swollen and when he speaks he sounds congested. He tells you that yesterday he started feeling "run down" and he had a sore throat all day. He explains that his symptoms include mild fatigue, a cough that brings up "stuff," a very stuffy nose that prevents him from breathing through his nose and pressure in his head that is causing a severe headache. He says that he has not really been sneezing and his sore throat has gone away already. His temperature was 98.9°F when he took it this morning. He wants you to recommend something to make him feel better.

History of Present Illness

MH states that he had not been feeling bad at all until yesterday, when his sore throat lasted all day and began to make him feel tired. Then he awoke this morning with multiple symptoms that include mild fatigue, chest congestion with a productive cough, nasal congestion and a severe headache. He did not have a temperature when he took it this morning, and his sore throat has subsided. He is concerned that he is coming down with the flu.

Past Medical History

MH was treated 7 years ago for a peptic ulcer that was associated with minor GI bleeding. He has had no recurrences and his history is otherwise unremarkable.

Social History

Tobacco use: none

Alcohol use: 2-3 beers weekly;

Caffeine use: 1 8-ounce cup of coffee daily

Family History

Mother is still living and has diabetes. Father died from injuries sustained in a car accident at age 40.

Review of Systems

Negative except as noted previously.

Physical Examination

GEN: Well-developed adult male with obvious nasal congestion

VS: None available

Labs and Diagnostic Tests

None available

Diagnosis

Primary:

1) Probable rhinovirus infection (cold).

Medication Record

Multiple vitamin with iron daily

Folic acid 400 mcg daily

Pharmacist Notes and Other Patient Information

Most obvious symptoms are the patient's red, swollen nose and his altered voice due to nasal congestion. Also notable are crackling sounds when the patient coughs during consultation.

Questions

1. Which of the following factors supports that MH is likely suffering from a rhinovirus (cold) and not the influenza virus?

   I.　MH's temperature is <100°F
   II.　MH does not have chills or severe myalgias
   III.　MH has a cough

   A.　I only
   B.　III only
   C.　I and II only
   D.　II and III only
   E.　I, II, and III

2. Which of the following factors support that MH is likely suffering from a rhinovirus (cold) and not allergies?

Case 72

I. MH's temperature is <100°F
II. MH has nasal congestion
III. MH has not experienced paroxysmal sneezing or itchy, watery eyes with his other symptoms.

A. I only
B. III only
C. I and II only
D. II and III only
E. I, II, and III

3. Based on the patient's symptoms, which of the following would be appropriate recommendations?

I. Systemic decongestant (sympathomimetic)
II. Analgesic
III. Expectorant

A. I only
B. III only
C. I and II only
D. II and III only
E. I, II, and III

4. Which of the following disease states would have prevented the patient from taking systemic decongestants (sympathomimetics), before consulting his physician?

I. GERD
II. Hypertension
III. BPH

A. I only
B. III only
C. I and II only
D. II and III only
E. I, II, and III

5. Which of the following products is an expectorant?

I. Delsym
II. Actifed
III. Mucinex

A. I only
B. III only
C. I and II only
D. II and III only
E. I, II, and III

6. Which of the following resources would be helpful in identifying the ingredients/generic names for the products.

I. Medline
II. MicroMedex/DrugDex
III. Facts and Comparisons

A. I only
B. III only
C. I and II only
D. II and III only
E. I, II, and III

7. Which of the following long acting cough/cold products is available over the counter?

I. Mucinex
II. Robitussin syrup
III. Tussionex

A. I only
B. III only
C. I and II only
D. II and III only
E. I, II, and III

8. Which of the following non-drug devices would be an appropriate recommendation to relieve MH's symptoms?

I. Humidifier
II. Vaporizer
III. Sitz bath

A. I only
B. III only
C. I and II only
D. II and III only
E. I, II, and III

9. If the patient wanted to use a nasal decongestant spray, which of the following would be appropriate to counsel him about:

A. A product containing oxymetazoline as the active ingredient should be used every 4 to 6 hours.
B. A product containing phenylephrine as the active ingredient should be used every 8 to 10 hours.
C. A product containing xylometazoline as the active ingredient should be used every 10 to 12 hours.
D. Topical decongestants can be used for an indefinate duration, until symptoms subside.
E. Patients with heart disease, hypertension, thyroid disease, diabetes or urinary retention caused by an enlarged prostate should not use a topical decongestant, unless instructed by their physician.

10. Which of the following would be acceptable analgesics for this patient?

I. Ibuprofen
II. Naproxen sodium
III. Acetaminophen

Case 72

A. I only
B. III only
C. I and II only
D. II and III only
E. I, II, and III

Patient Name: Carla Wilson
Address: 2200 East 30th Street
Age: 25   **Height:** 5' 4"
Sex: F   **Race:** Hispanic
Weight: 137 lb
Allergies: NKDA

Chief Complaint

CW is a 25-yo Hispanic female who visits her community pharmacy to drop off a prescription for her urinary tract infection (UTI), and decides to ask for help with other unrelated symptoms she is experiencing. Aside from her UTI symptoms, her chief complaint is burning, itching and watery eyes. Her symptoms started yesterday, the day after she got back from a 3-day sailing trip. CW states that her eyes were actually dry and "gritty" feeling while she was on her sailing trip. But after being home for one day, her symptoms of tearing and itching began. She seeks a recommendation of a nonprescription remedy.

History of Present Illness

CW explains that her symptoms of burning, itching and tearing eyes occurs mainly during the daytime. She states she has been trying to use her contact lens rewetting drops throughout the day for relief of her daytime symptoms, but without success. Her symptoms began the day after she got back from her sailing trip, where she was exposed to very hot and windy conditions for 3 days. CW also mentions she saw the allergy report on the news the night she got home, which stated molds were at record highs. She has not experienced any sneezing or a runny nose, since she takes her Allegra daily. CW would like a recommendation for her current eye symptoms of excessive itching and tearing. She would also like a recommendation for future sailing trips, when she is likely to have the dry and "gritty" symptoms again.

Past Medical History

CW only has the symptoms of burning, itching and watery eyes once or twice yearly. She has visited the doctor for this condition before, and was diagnosed with allergic conjunctivitis. CW only experiences the dry eye symptoms when she sails.

Medication Record

Date	Rx No	Physician	Drug and Strength	Quantity	Sig	Refills
6/1	7212613	Ramirez	Macrobid	14	1 bid	0
6/1	7212614	Ramirez	Phenazopyridine 200 mg	6	1 bid	0
2/5	6551201	Smith	Patanol	5	1 gtt bid prn allergic conjunctivitis	prn
2/5	6551200	Smith	Allegra 180 mg	30	1 qd, prn allergy symptoms	prn

Social History

Tobacco use: none

Alcohol use: occasional mixed drink

Caffeine use: 1 caffeine-containing soft drink daily

Illegal drug use: none

Family History

Mother and father are still living, with no diagnosed health conditions.

Review of Systems

GEN: Well-developed young adult female experiencing burning, itching and watery eyes, which began a few days ago. She experiences dry eye symptoms when she sails. She also has been diagnosed with a urinary tract infection.

Physical Examination

None available

Labs and Diagnostic Tests

None available

Diagnosis

Primary:

    1. Urinary tract infection (UTI)

    2. Allergic conjunctivitis

Pharmacist Notes and Other Patient Information

Patient would like an over the counter recommendation for her eye symptoms. Patient wears soft contact lenses.

Case 73

Questions

1. In which of the following situations would CW need to be referred to her physician for treatment of her eye symptoms?

    I. Eye pain
    II. Mucous discharge
    III. Recent eye trauma and/or eye contact with foreign matter

    A. I only
    B. III only
    C. I and II only
    D. II and III only
    E. I, II, and III

2. Which of the following active ingredients of ophthalmic preparations would address CW's symptoms?

    I. Pheniramine
    II. Antazoline
    III. Methylcellulose

    A. I only
    B. III only
    C. I and II only
    D. II and III only
    E. I, II, and III

3. Which of the following drug products is NOT available on an OTC basis for potential pharmacist recommendation in the treatment of CW's eye symptoms?

    A. Vasocon-A
    B. Visine-A
    C. Opcon-A
    D. Patanol
    E. Naphcon-A

4. Which of the following would be appropriate to counsel the patient concerning her prescription history?

    I. A prescription is on file for olopatadine (Patanol) from four months ago that the physician directed her to use "as needed for allergic conjunctivitis." She could refill this, or use an OTC ophthalmic antihistamine, but not both.
    II. The prescription being filled for phenazopyridine, to treat urinary discomfort associated with her infection, can discolor CW's contact lenses. She should avoid wearing her contacts during and for a few days after taking phenazopyridine.
    III. Her lubricant/rewetting drops will alleviate all of her allergic conjunctivitis symptoms.

    A. I only
    B. III only
    C. I and II only
    D. II and III only
    E. I, II, and III

5. You recommend an eye ointment for CW to use during her sailing trips. Which of the following key points concerning ophthalmic ointments is/are true?

    I. Ophthalmic ointments are primarily recommended to increase the ocular contact time of the instilled product.
    II. Non-medicated ophthalmic ointments can be used for dry eye symptoms.
    III. When using eye ointments, bedtime installation is most appropriate.

    A. I only
    B. III only
    C. I and II only
    D. II and III only
    E. I, II, and III

6. Which of the following are appropriate instructions when couseling a patient on the use of ophthalmic medications in general?

    I. If multiple drop therapy is indicated, it is best for the patient to wait 2 to 5 minutes between drops.
    II. Ophthalmic preparations should not be used past the expiration date, and should be discarded 30 days after opened or the safety seal is broken.
    III. If therapy consists of both eye drops and eye ointment, the ointment should be administered at least 5 to 10 minutes before the drop.

    A. I only
    B. III only
    C. I and II only
    D. II and III only
    E. I, II, and III

7. All of the following can be used as preservatives in ophthalmic preparations EXCEPT:

    A. Thimerosal.
    B. Methylparaben.
    C. Benzalkonium chloride.
    D. Boric acid.
    E. Propylparaben.

8. Which of the following suggestions should help CW avoid experiencing symptoms of dry eyes in the future?

Case 73

    I.   Begin using a lid scrub regularly.

    II.   Avoid overuse of Allegra.

    III. Remind CW that high winds and temperatures can dry out soft contact lenses, further aggrevating dry eye symptoms.

    A.   I only

    B.   III only

    C.   I and II only

    D.   II and III only

    E.   I, II, and III

9. What should CW expect with regards to outcomes with the use of an ophthalmic antihistamine?

    A.   If she does not experience complete resolution of symptoms after 2-3 hours of use, she should call her doctor.

    B.   If she does not experience complete resolution of symptoms afer 2-3 days of use, she should call her doctor.

    C.   If she does not experience complete resolution of symptoms after 2-3 weeks of use, she should call her doctor.

    D.   If she does not experience complete resolution of symptoms after 2-3 months of use, she should call her doctor.

    E.   She should wait for her doctor to call her, as they will routinely check on patients a few days following their office visit.

10. Which of the following would be appropriate when counseling CW about the proper administration of any medicated eye drops?

    I.   Try not to touch the tip of the dropper to the eye, with fingers or any other surface.

    II.   Administer drops while tilting head back, in a pouch created by pulling down the lower eye lid with the index finger.

    III. It is okay to administer eye drops while wearing soft contact lenses.

    A.   I only

    B.   III only

    C.   I and II only

    D.   II and III only

    E.   I, II, and III

Patient Name: Nell Basinger
Address: 805 W. 6th Street
Age: 47   **Height:** 5' 2"
Sex: F   **Race:** White
Weight: 110
Allergies: NKDA

Chief Complaint

"I am experiencing vaginal dryness, and pain during intercourse because of it."

History of Present Illness

NB is a 47-yo female who presents to the pharmacy complaining of vaginal dryness for the past 4 months. Recently, she has begun experiencing pain during intercourse due to the dryness. Her last natural menstrual period was 2 weeks ago. She is generally in good health, and exercises three times weekly.

Past Medical History

Hyperlipidemia, presently controlled by diet

Social History

Alcohol use: 1-2 drinks/week

Tobacco use: none

Occupation: Attorney

Married, with 2 teenage children

Family History

Mother is currently being treated for asthma and osteoporosis.

Father has hyperlipidemia.

Review of Systems

Otherwise negative except for occasional tension headaches due to job-related stress. Headaches are relieved by acetaminophen or ibuprofen. Patient denies any recent changes in bowel habits, weight or appetite.

Medication Record

Prescription and OTC

Date	Rx No	Physician	Drug and Strength	Quantity	Sig	Refills
10/15			Calcium carb 500 mg	100	1 po qd	
10/15			Multivitamin	100	1 po qd	

Physical Examination

VS: BP 120/60 mmHg, HR 65 bpm, Temperature 98.6°F

Pelvic: No tenderness or masses (self-reported by patient)

Labs and Diagnostic Tests

Total cholesterol 200 mg/dL

Diagnosis

Primary:

1. Atrophic vaginitis

Pharmacist Notes and Other Patient Information

None available.

Questions

1. Which of the following factors could be contributing to the patient's recent vaginal dryness?

    I. The patient is perimenopausal.

    II. The patient is stressed and/or fatigued.

    III. The patient and her husband are using nonlubricated condoms for birth control.

    A. I only

    B. III only

    C. I and II only

    D. II and III only

    E. I, II, and III

2. Which of the following would NOT be an appropriate treatment option for vaginal dryness?

    A. Astroglide (glycerin, propylene glycol)

    B. Replens Gel (glycerin, mineral oil)

    C. Lubrin Suppositories (caprylic/capric triglyceride, glycerin)

    D. Massengill Disposable Douche (purified water, sodium citrate, citric acid, vinegar)

    E. H-R Lubricating Jelly (hydroxypropyl methylcellulose)

Case 74

3. How often should a vaginal lubricant be used?

    A. As often as needed
    B. Prior to intercourse only
    C. Once daily at bedtime
    D. Once daily in the morning
    E. Twice daily in the morning and at bedtime

4. If the patient uses a vaginal lubricant and sees no improvement after 2 weeks, what would be the next appropriate step?

    I. Refer to a physician for oral estrogen
    II. Refer to a physician for a vaginal estrogen product
    III. Switch lubrication products

    A. I only
    B. III only
    C. I and II only
    D. II and III only
    E. I, II, and III

5. What other recommendation could you make to the patient to help improve vaginal lubrication?

    A. Try a petroleum based lubricant such as petroleum jelly
    B. Regular sexual activity
    C. Baths instead of showers
    D. Regular exercise
    E. Sitz bath daily

6. NB has been using a non-lubricated latex condom for birth control. Which of the following would be an appropriate lubricant for use with the latex condom?

    A. Mineral oil
    B. Miconazole vaginal cream
    C. Petroleum jelly
    D. Glycerin
    E. Baby oil

7. NB is interested in other birth control options. Which of the following recommendations would you provide in private consultation with this patient?

    I. Female condom
    II. Sponge
    III. Lubricated latex condom

    A. I only
    B. III only
    C. I and II only
    D. II and III only
    E. I, II, and III

8. If NB chooses the sponge, what counseling information would NOT be appropriate regarding the proper use of a contraceptive sponge?

    A. The sponge must be left in place for at least 6 to 8 hours after intercourse.
    B. The sponge can be left in place for up to 24 hours.
    C. The sponge can be inserted up to 24 hours prior to intercourse.
    D. The sponge should be inserted at least 15 minutes prior to intercourse.
    E. The sponge can be removed by pulling on the loop attached to the sponge.

9. Which of the following vaginal lubricants does not contain a spermicide?

    A. Ortho Options Delfen Foam
    B. K-Y Plus Lubricating Gel
    C. Encare Vaginal Inserts
    D. VCF Vaginal Film
    E. Astroglide

10. NB tries the sponge and does not like it. She comes in requesting information on the female condom. Which of the following would be appropriate counseling points for the female condom?

    I. It can be reused, but should be inspected for tears each time before use.
    II. It can be combined with a male latex condom to ensure more effective birth control.
    III. Additional lubrication can be added during intercourse without removing the condom.

    A. I only
    B. III only
    C. I and II only
    D. II and III only
    E. I, II, and III

Case 75

Patient Name: Danielle Davidson
Address: 100 S. Terry Drive
Age: 26   **Height:** 5' 8"
Sex: F   **Race:** White
Weight: 130
Allergies: No known drug allergies

Chief Complaint

DD is a 26-yo female who presents to the pharmacy with a scabbed lesion on the top right-hand side of her upper lip. DD is otherwise healthy. She has recently returned from a week-long Caribbean vacation.

History of Present Illness

The lesion began forming on day 6 of her vacation. She remembers feeling a tingling or itching a day or so prior to the pustule forming. She remembers having similar lesions appear in her teens, but she cannot remember what her mother used to treat them or what triggered them to occur.

Past Medical History

Patient has asthma that is controlled with an albuterol inhaler used prn.

Social History

Patient works as an accountant, and has had the same job for the past 4 years. She is single. She denies using illegal drugs or tobacco. She drinks alcohol occasionally at social functions, but limits her consumption to two beverages.

Family History

Father has hypertension and history of PUD.

Mother has asthma.

Review of Systems

Appearance of lesion on upper lip.

LMP: 2 weeks previously

Medication Record

Date	Rx No	Physician	Drug and Strength	Quantity	Sig	Refills
7/8	892217	Camden	Ovcon-35	1	1 po qd	prn
8/9	97217	Mock	Albuterol inhaler	1	1-2 puffs po q 4-6 h prn SOB	prn

Physical Examination

GEN: Healthy female with lesion on upper lip.

VS: BP 120/60 mmHg, HR 80 bpm, T 37°C, Wt 59 kg

Labs and Diagnostic Tests

None available

Diagnosis

Primary: Herpes simplex labialis

Pharmacist Notes and Other Patient Information

None available

Questions

1. What is the likely cause of DD's fever blister?
   A. Stressful job
   B. Sharing a straw with a friend
   C. Excessive sun exposure
   D. History of chicken pox
   E. None of the above

2. Which of the following would be an appropriate recommendation for treating DD's fever blister?
   I. Abreva Cold Sore Treatment (Docosanol 10%)
   II. Anbesol Cold Sore Therapy (White petrolatum 64.9%, benzocaine 20%, camphor 3%, allantoin 1%)
   III. Zilactin-L Cold Sore Liquid (Lidocaine 2.5%)

   A. I only
   B. III only
   C. I and II only
   D. II and III only
   E. I, II, and III

3. If you choose to have the patient use docosanol, how would you tell the patient to use the medication?

Case 75

A. Twice daily for up to 10 days
B. Three times daily for up to 14 days
C. Four times daily for up to 7 days
D. Five times daily for up to 10 days
E. Six times daily for upto 14 days

4. When counseling DD, which of the following statements would be appropriate for her to prevent future outbreaks?

   I. The patient should regularly use a lip balm that contains sunscreen.
   II. The patient should wear a hat when in the sun to further protect the face.
   III. The patient should avoid excessive sun exposure.

   A. I only
   B. III only
   C. I and II only
   D. II and III only
   E. I, II, and III

5. When selecting a lip balm with sunscreen, DD should look for a minimum SPF of:

   A. 4.
   B. 8.
   C. 15.
   D. 30.
   E. 45.

6. DD returns to the pharmacy the next day reporting that the lesion has "changed." On inspection you notice that the lesion appears to be infected. What would you recommend the patient do now?

   A. Apply hydrocortisone 1% cream/ointment to the lesion three times daily.
   B. Remove the scab and express the puss.
   C. Apply petroleum jelly to the lesion four times daily.
   D. Apply a triple antibiotic cream/ointment to the lesion three to four times daily.
   E. Refer the patient to a physician.

7. DD returns to the pharmacy in January complaining of something bothering her knees. Upon physical inspection, you notice red plaques with white scales that have formed on both knees. The patient does not report any changes in her health, diet, or exercise regimen. The patient states that the lesions started as small blister-like spots that grew into each other, and she is concerned that this is the same type lesion that she had on her lip previously. What is DD suffering from?

A. Seborrheic dermatitis
B. Contact dermatitis
C. Allergic contact dermatitis
D. Prickly heat
E. Psoriasis

8. Which of the following would be appropriate recommendations for DD?

   I. A topical emollient
   II. A lubricating bath product
   III. Topical hydrocortisone

   A. I only
   B. III only
   C. I and II only
   D. II and III only
   E. I, II, and III

9. Which of the following ingredients may be used to treat psoriasis?

   I. Pyrithione zinc
   II. Coal tar
   III. Salicylic acid

   A. I only
   B. III only
   C. I and II only
   D. II and III only
   E. I, II, and III

10. DD has followed your previous recommendation of topical emollient, lubricating bath product, and topical hydrocortisone. The symptoms have not resolved after 7 days of self-treatment. What would you recommend the patient do next?

    A. Coal tar applied topically at bedtime and removed with shower in morning
    B. Exposure to UV light
    C. Salicylic acid preceded by soaking the area in warm water for 15 minutes
    D. Continue treatment regimen for another 7 days
    E. Refer to a dermatologist

Federal Law Review

Jesse Vivian

Compounding & Calculations Review

Robert O. Williams, Jason M. Vaughn

Federal Law Review

Background

A majority of states and jurisdictions assess the pharmacy law competencies of individuals applying for a pharmacist license through administration of the National Association of Boards of Pharmacy's (NABP) Multistate Pharmacy Jurisprudence Examination™ (MPJE™). The MPJE uses questions that are applicable to all jurisdictions through the federal laws but also tailors questions to the individual states and territories. The states that do not administer the MPJE use examinations that are developed by each individual state. However, even these examinations almost always include questions dealing with federal laws, especially controlled substances. As such, no matter where the exam is taken, licensure applicants must be proficient in both state and federal laws pertaining to pharmacy. In any event, candidates must take a separate law exam for each state in which they are seeking licensure.

License applicants should consult the competency statements provided by NABP with the MPJE materials as a starting point for determining which subjects should be studied. This advice applies to candidates in non-MPJE states as well, because the subject matter of pharmacy law is similar in all jurisdictions. The MPJE competency statements and other study tools may be accessed at the NABP Web site: http://www.nabp.net. There is a wealth of information about the examination located there and applicants should take advantage of those materials.

The exam consists of 90 multiple choice questions; however, 30 of those questions will not be counted for the purpose of calculating your score. These "pre-test" questions are dispersed throughout the examination and there is no way that candidates can tell which questions are counted and which ones are not. Candidates will be given 2 hours to complete the exam. If a candidate answers fewer than 77 questions, the exam will not be scored. Candidates should try to answer all 90 questions because there is a penalty for not answering questions. No two exams are the same because there is a large block of test questions. The difficulty of subsequent questions depends on whether or not the prior question was answered correctly. Candidates will not know whether a question was answered correctly while taking the exam or afterwards because only scores are reported. The minimum passing score is 75.

Unlike the NAPLEX exam, scores for the MJPE are not transferable between the states or jurisdictions that use the MPJE because the MPJE is uniquely tailored for each state.

The law exam is administered as a "computer adaptive" format. This means that a candidate cannot go back and forth between questions and change an answer after the question is finished. This testing format is very different from traditional paper and pencil exams commonly used in academic settings. Please consult the NABP materials for further explanation of the test-taking procedures.

It is also important to know the competencies the MJPE is attempting to assess. In its Registration Bulletin, the NABP states: "The MPJE Competency Statements serve as a blueprint of the topics covered on the examination. They offer important information about the knowledge, judgment, and skills you are expected to demonstrate while taking the MPJE. A strong understanding of the Competency Statements will aid you in your preparation to take the examination."

The following competency statements and weights are from the 2006 NABP Registration Bulletin for the NAPLEX/MJPE.

Area 1. Pharmacy Practice (approximately 78% of test)

1.01 Identify the legal responsibilities of the pharmacist and other pharmacy personnel.

1.02 Identify the requirements for the acquisition and distribution of pharmaceutical products.

1.03 Identify the legal requirements that must be observed in the issuance of a prescription/drug order.

1.04 Identify the procedures necessary to properly dispense a pharmaceutical product, including controlled substances, pursuant to a prescription/drug order.

1.05 Identify the conditions for making an offer to counsel or appropriately counsel patients, including the requirements for documentation.

1.06 Identify the requirements for the distribution and/or dispensing of prescription and/or non-prescription pharmaceutical products, including controlled substances.

1.07 Identify the proper procedures for keeping records of information related to pharmaceutical products, including requirements for protecting patient confidentiality.

Area 2. Licensure, Registration, Certification, and Operational Requirements (approximately 17% of test)

2.01 Identify the qualifications, application procedure, necessary examinations, and internship requirements for licensure, registration, or certification of individuals engaged in the manufacture, storage, distribution, and/or dispensing of pharmaceutical products (prescription and nonprescription).

2.02 Identify the requirements and application procedure for the registration, licensure, certification, or permitting of a practice setting or business entity.

2.03 Identify the operational requirements for the registration, licensure, certification, or permitting of a practice setting (e.g., space, equipment, advertising and signage, automated equipment, storage, and security).

Area 3. Regulatory Structure and Terms (approximately 5% of test)

3.01 Identify the purpose of, and the terms and conditions found in, the laws and rules that regulate or affect the manufacture, storage, distribution, and dispensing of pharmaceutical products (prescription and nonprescription), including controlled substances.

3.02 Identify the authority, responsibilities, and operation of the agencies or entities that enforce the laws and rules that regulate or affect the manufacture, storage, distribution, and dispensing of pharmaceutical products (prescription and nonprescription), including controlled substances.

This Heading will discuss topics generally associated with competencies addressed by the MPJE and other common sources of pharmacy law evaluations. In terms of the competency statements listed above, the majority of the materials presented here will focus on Area 1 because many of these topics are the subject of federal regulation. Areas 2 and 3 are governed primarily by state laws. Only a few of the most common issues addressed by state laws are considered. Because there are many variations in state laws, you will need to consult legal resources tailored to the particular state in which you seek your licensure.

In adopting this approach, we presume that readers have already completed a course dealing with pharmacy law issues and are familiar with the basic methods used to regulate pharmacy practice. We also presume that readers know the basic terminology pertaining to pharmacy law as well as the procedures used to adopt and enforce pharmacy regulations. You should consult basic pharmacy law textbooks when you need more detailed information other than what is provided here. NABP recommends using reference materials such as "Facts and Comparisons, Pharmacy Law Digest, the United States Pharmacopeia Dispensing Information, or Approved Drug Products and Legal Requirements, which contain federal statutes and regulations applicable to the several states." NABP also suggests that additional information may also be obtained from the state board of pharmacy where you are seeking licensure.

In analyzing any legal question, keep in mind that the regulation of drugs and many aspects of pharmacy practice are subject of both state and federal laws. Because of this concurrent (duel) jurisdiction, there may be significant differences between the laws insofar as the obligations of a pharmacist are concerned. Usually, pharmacists will follow the stricter law, i.e., the law requiring a higher level of behavior. For example, federal law requires that pharmacies maintain some controlled substances records for 2 years; many states require pharmacies to keep these same records for 5 years. In those locations, the pharmacy would have to adhere to the longer period for maintaining these documents.

It is also useful to remember that there are differences in the organizational demands and goals of the various agencies that regulate drugs. The Food and Drug Administration (FDA), a section within the Health and Human services Department is charged with determining if drugs are safe and effective and whether they should be available with or without a prescription. It is staffed by health care practitioners that approach drug quality and safety from a scientific point of view. The Drug Enforcement Agency (DEA), on the other hand, is primarily concerned with whether a substance (remember this agency deals with things that are not necessarily drugs) is subject to abuse or capable of causing physical or emotional addiction. Instead of a scientific approach, this agency uses a police mentality to make its determinations. In most states a Board of Pharmacy or a similar agency regulates all aspects of drugs, controlled substances and the practice of pharmacy.

It may also be useful to think of federal laws as those that apply to drugs, such as their manufacture, labeling and distribution while state laws apply primarily to the practice of pharmacy, i.e., what a pharmacist does. This is, of course, a simplistic explanation of a complex set of interactive laws. But it is a useful tool, like keeping in mind the differences between the trees and a forest.

Definitions, Abbreviations, and Explanations

Think of studying pharmacy law as learning a new language. Understanding words and phrases in a foreign language requires knowledge of how those words and terms are defined. In studying pharmacy law, it is most helpful to start with common legal definitions. For example knowing the difference between a "drug," a "food," a "dietary supplement," and a "cosmetic" will determine which records, if any, a pharmacist must keep or what labels must be provided when "distributing" or "dispensing" these various "articles." It is also important to know what the terms "label" and "labeling" mean. Likewise, it is helpful to know which activities are encompassed in the legal notion of the "practice of pharmacy" in order to understand what is meant by a statute that contains a statement such as "No one is allowed to engage in the practice of

pharmacy unless properly licensed." Equally important, it is necessary to understand what "delegation" means to determine what acts, tasks, or functions normally associated with the practice of pharmacy may be delegated by a pharmacist to non-pharmacist supportive personnel including pharmacy interns and technicians. Some of these terms, such as "drug" and "food," are defined primarily by federal laws like the Food Drug and Cosmetic Act (FDCA). Others, such as the "practice of pharmacy," will be determined by state law. It is also important to understand the context might change the definitions of these words or phrases. For example when one refers to a "label" the content included thereon will differ if the term is used in connection with a manufacturer's label, the pharmacy's dispensing label or a patient-package label.

Another useful review activity is to consider common abbreviations associated with pharmacy laws. Knowing what NDA, ANDA, SNDA, DEA, DESI, FDA, USP/NF, and similar abbreviations stand for may make studying much easier. Recognize that the context in which these abbreviations are used may also change the meaning. For example an NDA might refer to a "new drug application" or a "new drug approval" depending on the status a drug is in during an FDA review.

Obviously, a review Heading of this size cannot list definitions and abbreviations for all key terms from all jurisdictions. Furthermore, it is important to note that several of these terms may have additional or different definitions under other federal or state laws. Some of the more important terms and abbreviations (in alphabetical order) associated with federal laws include:

Adulterate: A drug is deemed to be adulterated when it is produced under conditions that are not sanitary. Any drug produced under conditions that violate the CGMPs (discussed below) will be deemed adulterated. Drugs that are listed in any of the official compendia (e.g., USP/NF, defined further below) but fail to meet the purity or strength standards established by the compendia will also be deemed adulterated. Students sometimes mix up the concepts of adulteration and misbranding (see below). Adulteration deals with the quality of the drug itself. Misbranding deals with the packaging and labeling of the drug. Note that drugs may be both adulterated and misbranded under certain conditions.

Adequate directions for use: directions under which the layman can use a drug safely and for the purposes for which it is intended. All OTC drugs must bear a label containing adequate directions for use. For Rx-only drugs, the manufacturer or distributor's labeling must include adequate directions for use up and until drugs are dispensed pursuant to a prescription when the labeling requirements change. The directions must include a statement of all conditions, purposes, or uses for which such drug is intended, quantity of dose, frequency of administration, duration of use, time of administration (in relation to time of meals, time of onset of symptoms, or other time factors), route or method of administration and preparation for use (shaking, dilution, adjustment of temperature, or, other manipulation or process).

ANDA: Abbreviated New Drug Approval (or Application). This is the process by which a generic manufacturer of a drug already on the market with an NDA obtained by the innovator company obtains pre-market approval from the FDA. In order to have an application for an ANDA approved, the applicant must prove that the generic active drug component is the exact same chemical entity as and is bioequivalent to the innovator product. The generic company is not required to submit safety and efficacy data because that evidence is already on file from the innovator company.

CGMP (or GMP): Current Good Manufacturing Practices (or just Good Manufacturing Practices). These are FDA regulations that dictate the conditions under which all drugs are produced in the United States. This includes drugs that are exempt from NDA requirements for safety and efficacy data under the grandfather clauses of the FDCA. See NDA (below) for a discussion of the grandfather clause. In other words all drugs manufactured in the U.S. or for importation into the U.S. must be manufactured under the CGMP standards irrespective of whether they are grandfathered or if they are OTC drugs or Rx-only drugs.

Cosmetic: Something that is intended to be rubbed, poured, sprinkled, sprayed on, introduced into, or applied to the human body for purposes of cleaning, beautifying, or promoting human attractiveness. Soap is excluded from the definition.

DEA: Drug Enforcement Administration. This is a division of the Department of Justice. It is responsible for administering and enforcing the Controlled Substances Act.

DESI: In 1968 the FDA established the Drug Efficacy Study Implementation program to implement recommendations of the National Academy of Sciences investigation of effectiveness of new drugs that were marketed between 1938 and 1962. Recall that drugs on the market before 1938 were exempted from having to prove they are safe. Drugs put on the market after 1938 had to obtain the pre-market approval of the FDA through the NDA process. The efficacy requirement did not go into effect until 1962 after which manufacturers had to prove that new drugs were both safe and effective. For drugs put on the market between 1938 and 1962, manufacturers had to only prove there drugs were safe. The DESI program was established to provide a mechanism for the federal government to establish evidence as to whether or not these groups of drugs were also efficacious for intended purposes.

Dietary supplement: An item other than tobacco that is intended to supplement the diet and contains a vitamin, mineral, herb or other botanical ingredient, or an amino acid, or is a dietary substance taken by humans to supplement total dietary intake. The definition also includes many other items that are not likely the topic of license exams.

Dispense: The act of a pharmacist preparing a medication for a patient pursuant to a prescription issued by a licensed practitioner and delivery of that medication to the patient or a patient caregiver.

Distribute: In pharmacy this term means the act of transferring a drug by means other than dispensing between individuals or persons who are licensed or registered to handle the drug. For example, a physician might wish to purchase an office supply of a prescription-only medication directly from a pharmacy. The act of taking the drug out of the pharmacy's inventory and selling it to a physician's office constitutes distribution, not dispensing.

Drug: An item listed in the United States Pharmacopeia/National Formulary (USP/NF, see below) or the Homeopathic Pharmacopeia of the United States, an item intended for use in the diagnosis, cure, mitigation, treatment or prevention of disease in humans or other animals, an item (other than food) intended to affect the structure or function of humans or other animals. This includes components of any of these listed items.

FDA: Food and Drug Administration. This is a division of the Department of Health and Human Services (HHS) responsible for administering and enforcing the FDCA and its amendments. Note that the FDA has jurisdiction over the distribution of food, drugs, and cosmetics in interstate commerce. It has limited authority over dietary supplements. More importantly, the FDA has authority to regulate the manufacture, research, labeling, and distribution of all drugs including those available over the counter (OTC) and by prescription only (federal legend drugs). It also has authority to regulate the marketing of prescription-only drugs. The

FTC (Federal Trade Commission, see below) regulates most of the advertising claims for OTC drugs and several aspects of the advertising of dietary supplements.

FDCA (sometimes abbreviated in other texts as "FD&CA"): The Food Drug and Cosmetic Act. This law, originally enacted in 1938, has been amended several times over the years. References to the FDCA may be to the whole Act, as amended, or may be only to portions of the Act or specific Amendments. For example, as explained in more detail below, the PDMA amended the Act in 1987 and affected the distribution of prescription-only drugs and drug samples. The Food and Drug Administration Modernization Act (FDAMA) was adopted in 1997 as an amendment to the FDCA and affects many FDA activities. Readers should take care in understanding the context under which references are made to any of these acts and amendments so as to avoid confusion.

Food: An item that is used for food or drink in humans and other animals. Chewing gum is always a food. Note that gum may be used as a drug delivery device as with nicotine gum but the gum itself is still a food.

FTC: Federal Trade Commission. This agency has authority to investigate and prevent unfair trade practices including false and misleading advertising of OTC drugs and dietary supplements. For all intents and purposes, the FTC does not regulate the advertising or promotion of prescription-only drugs; this function is performed by the FDA.

Grandfather: This term, in law, does not refer to the kindly old gentleman that gave you candy and money when your parents were not looking. Instead, when it comes to use in context with the FDCA, it is used to denote drugs that were on the market before 1938 when the "new drug approval" (NDA) process was adopted to require manufacturers to get pre-market approval from the FDA by showing that the drug is safe for its intended purposes. The "grandfather" provision exempts pre-1938 drugs from the NDA requirement. Had this provision not been written into the law there would have been a great deal of protest from manufacturers who were allowed to market their pre-1938 drugs without very much government regulation. This probably would be found in violation of the United States Constitution's prohibition about enacting "ex post facto" laws. It is very unlikely that the MPJE would ever ask about anything so esoteric as ex post facto laws.

GRAS: a term used by the FDA for a vast variety of things that it regulates when those things are Generally Recognized as Safe.

IND: Investigational New Drug. Whenever the maker of a new drug wishes to begin human testing, in order to assemble evidence that the drug is safe and effective, the company files an IND application with the FDA. The IND application must disclose safety and efficacy data collected in animals and describe how the drug will be tested using human volunteers. An IND application is required when the maker of a drug on the market with an NDA wishes to test the drug in humans for uses not contemplated in the original NDA application. Usually the applicant is required to perform three categories of human clinical testing beginning with small-scale testing on a few individuals and concluding with full-scale clinical research with multiple subjects.

Label: Written or printed material on the immediate container of an item such as a drug. In pharmacy practice, this usually means the written matter that appears on the outside of a commercial or pharmacy bottle containing drugs.

Labeling: Includes labels and any other written material on or accompanying an item. In pharmacy, this means the manufacturer's package insert and anything else that might accompany a drug. It also includes patient package inserts for the few drugs (e.g., oral contraceptives and estrogen products) that require them. The FDA must approve the content and appearance of all labels and labeling. Drugs that have improper labels or labeling are considered misbranded.

Misbrand: A drug is considered misbranded when the labeling is false or misleading or when a label that is required by law is not provided. Drugs that are packaged without conforming to the child-resistant safety restrictions established by the Poison Prevention Packaging Act, PPPA (discussed below) are also considered misbranded.

NDA: New Drug Approval or New Drug Application. A manufacturer or distributor that wishes to introduce a new drug must obtain approval of its application before the drug may be sold (i.e., pre-market approval) in this country. In order to obtain an NDA, the applicant must prove that the drug is both safe and effective for its intended purpose. Evidence is gathered from testing the drugs in humans. Before human testing may begin, the applicant must obtain an IND (discussed previously). Note that there are a few drugs on the market today that do not have an NDA. These drugs were on the market before the FDCA became effective in 1938. These drugs were allowed to remain on the market under a grandfather clause in the Act that exempted them from the NDA process for pre-market approval. As such, there is no evidence on file at the FDA that these drugs are safe. Multiple years of experience with the use of these few drugs has demonstrated that they are, in fact, safe when used as intended.

New Drug: Any drug that has not previously been marketed in the United States and is not generally recognized as safe and effective by qualified experts under conditions for use specified in the labeling of the drug. A new drug may be created from an existing FDA approved drug if there are any changes in the dosage form, labeling claims, or indications or other significant changes in the marketing of the drug.

SNDA: Supplemental New Drug Approval (or Application). When the maker of a drug already on the market with an NDA wishes to make new claims for the drug it must seek approval from the FDA to change the approved labeling. This is done through the SNDA process whereby the applicant provides evidence that the drug is safe and effective for the newly claimed uses.

USP/NF: The United States Pharmacopeia–National Formulary is a book of pharmacopeial standards that contains standards for medicines, dosage forms, drug substances, excipients, medical devices, and dietary supplements. Drugs that do not conform to these compendial standards may be deemed adulterated, misbranded or both.

The FD&CA

The FDCA

There are only a few historical facts that pharmacists need to know about regulations of drugs at the federal level. While the MPJE does not ask questions about when an amendment to the FDCA was passed into law or what the popular name of an amendment is, it may be easier to understand current regulations if a few drug law developments are kept in mind. There is one exception: know that the FDCA became law in 1938. This date is critical to determine which laws apply to specific drugs. For example, not every drug on the market in the United States has been proven safe and effective for its intended use. This is because drugs that were on the market before the original FDCA was enacted in 1938 were "grandfathered" from the mandates of the then new law. However, any drug placed on the market after 1938 must be proven to be safe when used

according to the labeled directions. This law also instituted the NDA process mandating that a drug manufacturer obtain pre-market approval from the FDA before offering a drug for sale. As explained below, it was a later amendment to the FDCA that added the requirement that manufacturers also must prove that a drug is efficacious for its intended purpose.

The FDCA was amended in 1951 by the "Durham-Humphrey Act" to establish two classes of drugs. OTC drugs are those that are considered safe to use according to the labeled directions. OTC labeling must include "adequate directions for use" rendering them safe to use without further medical directions. Drugs that are not safe for use without medical direction are limited to sale to a patient only pursuant to a prescription issued by someone who is allowed to prescribe under state law. (Note that federal law defers to the states for determining who is allowed to prescribe.) These items are known as "prescription only" or "federal legend" drugs. Up until very recently, the commercial container from the manufacturer or distributor of these drugs had to bear a label stating, "Caution: Federal law prohibits dispensing without a prescription." This phrase was called the "federal legend." The Food and Drug Administration Modernization Act of 1997 (FDAMA) amended this mandate; now federal legend drugs must be labeled, at a minimum, with the designation "Rx Only." In effect, this amendment changed the content of the "federal legend" to "Rx Only."

Federal legend drugs are exempt from the "adequate directions for use" labeling requirements because they are otherwise properly labeled when they are dispensed pursuant to a prescription. Under federal law, a pharmacy label of a dispensed prescription must contain the name of the prescriber, the serial number (more commonly known as the prescription number), the name and address of the dispensing pharmacy, and the date the prescription was originally written, dispensed, or most recently refilled. This amendment also provides that federal legend drugs may be refilled according to the prescriber's directions. In addition, the name of the patient and any directions for use, including precautions must also appear on the pharmacy label if this information appears on the prescription. In other words, the patient's name and directions for use are not always required on the pharmacy label of a prescribed drug under federal law. It is important to note that this provision applies only to federal-legend non-controlled substances. As discussed below, labeling requirements for prescription-legend controlled drugs that are dispensed from a pharmacy do require this information. Be aware, however, that every state has additional labeling requirements for dispensed medications. In addition to the patient's name and directions for use, the vast majority of states also require the drug name to appear unless there are special circumstances. If questions arise as to the labeling mandates for a dispensed drug, responses should include considerations for both state and federal law.

The "Kefauver-Harris Amendment of 1962" (also called the "Drug Efficacy Amendment") added a section to the FDCA to mandate that manufacturers of drugs submit proof that a new drug is effective in addition to being safe, as mandated in the original 1938 Act. After implementation of this Amendment, manufacturers had to prove that new drugs are both safe and effective. Drugs placed on the market between 1938 and 1962 must also be shown to be effective; however, for this category of drugs, the FDA established the "Drug Efficacy Study Implementation" (DESI) program. Most, if not all, drugs subject to the DESI program have been removed from the market where evidence is not available to substantiate that they are effective.

This amendment also established the CGMPs that specify the conditions under which all drugs made in the United States must be produced. Note that the CGMPs apply to all drugs, both OTC and prescription-only and irrespective of when introduced to the market in the United States. In other words, a "grandfathered" drug, not subject to the NDA pre-market approval and safety requirements, is nevertheless subject to the CGMPs. This Act also gave the FDA authority to regulate prescription drug advertising. Keep in mind that the FTC has authority to regulate the advertising of OTC drugs. Under this scheme, the FDA regulates the labeling of all drugs, but a jurisdictional division exists between these classes of drugs insofar as advertising is concerned.

The FDCA was amended again in 1984 by the "Drug Price Competition and Patent Term Restoration Act" (also known as the "Waxman-Hatch Amendment") to exempt generic drug manufacturers or distributors from having to submit original safety and efficacy evidence for drugs already subject to an NDA from the innovator manufacturer. The generic company must prove that the generic drug is bioequivalent to the innovator drug. Successful applicants are awarded approval of an ANDA from the FDA. This event gave rise to the FDA's practice of rating the equivalency of drugs that are listed in the so called "Orange Book," which is formally known as the "Approved Drug Products with Therapeutic Equivalence Evaluations. The online version is often referred to as the "Electronic Orange Book" (http://www.fda.gov/cder/ob/default.htm). For applicants living in jurisdictions that use the Orange Book as a guide for pharmacists in making "generic substitution" (also called "drug product selection" or "DPS") decisions, it is important to recall that drugs in the listings with a designation in the first letter or the equivalency rating (the FDA assigns two alphabetical letters for each listed drug) as an "A" are deemed to be equivalent with the innovator companies product. If the first letter is a "B," the FDA considers the generic drug to NOT be equivalent with that of the innovator company.

It is important to know that not all generic and innovator drugs are listed in the Orange Book. Only those that have an existing NDA are listed. Drugs that were "grandfathered" from the safety evidence requirement of the 1938 act are not included in the Orange Book even though there may be generic products available. Note also that some states use the Orange Book as a reference for drug product selection or generic substitution activities as well as for formulary development.

The "Prescription Drug Marketing Act (PDMA) of 1987" amended the FDCA to implement controls on the distribution of prescription drugs, prescription drug samples, and prescription drug coupons. The PDMA prohibits drug manufacturers and their representatives from distributing drug samples to physicians unless the physician makes a request in writing. Under federal law, hospital pharmacies may receive and maintain drug samples for and on behalf of prescribers when the prescriber has made a proper request. Community pharmacies are not allowed to have any drug samples in stock or on hand. The PDMA also prohibits, with a few rare exceptions, manufacturers and distributors from importing drugs into the United States after drugs have been exported. The sale of coupons for federal legend drugs is also prohibited under this Act.

Another important amendment to the FDCA is the Dietary Supplement Health and Education Act of 1994. This act often referred to as the DSHEA law carves out a regulatory scheme for dietary supplements separate and apart from drug regulation. The act severely limits the FDA from having jurisdiction to regulate many aspects of the marketing of dietary supplements. Instead, the FTC monitors advertising for dietary supplements to ensure that no false or misleading claims are made by the manufacturers or distributors. Effects of the DSHEA law are discussed in more detail in the section dealing with distinguishing between food, dietary supplements, cosmetics and drugs.

Another amendment to the FDCA is the "Food and Drug Administration Modernization Act (FDAMA) of 1997." This act has far-reaching effects on how the FDA conducts its mandates for overseeing the marketing and distribution of drugs. As mentioned above, this is the Act that changed the traditional federal legend that has to appear on the manufacturer or distributor labels of drugs that are restricted to distribution pursuant to a prescription; following implementation, the drugs must bear a label that, at a minimum, states "Rx Only." This Act also eliminated the need for a warning label on certain habit-forming drugs. It also specifies that drugs and drug products compounded by pharmacists are exempt from FDA regulation under specified circumstances. This provision was included because the FDA had, in a few instances, attempted to restrict pharmacist compounding on the notion that the compounded product was a new drug subject to NDA and CGMP requirements. The United States Supreme Court ruled in 2002 that the FDAMA statute that restricts compounding to pharmacies that do not solicit or advertise this service is unconstitutional. Further discussion of the implications of this decision is addressed below in the section entitled "Compounding Prescription Drugs."

There have been numerous other amendments to the FDCA over the years. The above descriptions only highlight some of the more important provisions that pharmacist licensure candidates should be aware of.

Distinguishing between Foods, Dietary Supplements, Cosmetics, and Drugs

In the language of the FDCA, the things we put on, into or around us are "articles" that fall into four distinct classifications: food, dietary supplements, cosmetics or drugs. The key to understanding whether an article falls into one or another of the named categories is to focus on the intent of the manufacturer or marketer of the item. Intent is most often determined by looking at claims that are made for the item. For example, if the manufacturer of a cereal that contains naturally occurring oat-bran advertises that this cereal builds strong bones, then the cereal would likely be classified as just a food. If that manufacturer advertises that this product helps control cholesterol, it might be viewed as either a food or a dietary supplement. But if that manufacturer advertises the cereal will prevent heart attacks by lowering cholesterol levels, the FDA may view this claim as one for prevention of a disease and, therefore, deem this to be a drug claim.

There are serious ramifications in classifying an item as a drug or one of the other categories. If an item is a drug, it is subject to the whole array of FDA regulations including the need for a pre-market NDA approval, proof that the drug is safe and effective, is manufactured by an FDA registered manufacturer in accordance with the CGMPs, and that its labeling is proper and approved by the FDA. If the drug may be sold without a prescription, it must be labeled with "adequate directions for use" and packaged in accordance with federal anti-tamper proof and child-resistant regulations. Additional storage and labeling mandates apply to prescription drugs dispensed by a pharmacist. If the drug is packaged with the labeling required by the FDA for Rx-only drugs, the pharmacy label will replace the adequate directions for use requirement. A pharmacist who sells any drug, OTC or Rx-only, that does not comply with all legal mandates is subject to severe disciplinary sanctions including criminal prosecution. Improperly labeled drugs will be deemed misbranded under the FDCA. Drugs produced in violation of the CGMPs are considered adulterated under the federal law.

In comparison to drugs, cosmetics are subject to very few regulations. Foods and food supplements are subject to some labeling and packaging requirements at both the state and federal levels. However, with rare exceptions, pharmacists need not be concerned with these regulations. Perhaps the more difficult distinction, in terms of regulations, involves dietary supplements and claims made for their usefulness. There is a fine, and often vague, line between a claim for a dietary supplement and a claim that would cause such an item to be classified as a drug. While readers should be aware of these issues, it is unlikely that detailed questions would appear on a licensure exam because so many questions are unsettled and controversial. Readers should, however, recognize that dietary supplements, a classification that includes vitamins, herbs, botanicals, and anything else intended to supplement the diet, are exempt from most FDA scrutiny, including the need for an NDA and compliance with the CGMPs. Regulations adopted by the FDA do attempt to define what kinds of labeling and other claims will render a dietary supplement to be considered a drug. The FTC does review claims made for dietary supplements to make sure the claims are truthful and not misleading.

The 1994 DSHEA law establishes dietary supplements as a category distinct and separate from foods or drugs. Unlike drugs that must be pre-approved for the United States market by the FDA, DSHEA shifts the burden of proof to the FDA to prove a dietary supplement put on the market in the United States by a manufacturer or distributor is not safe before the FDA can take the item off of the market.

The most controversial part of the DSHEA law is its permission for dietary supplement makers to make certain function-structure claims for their products. It is often difficult to tell whether a manufacturer or distributor of a product is making a claim that the product does something to cure, treat or mitigate a disease (which would classify the product as a drug) or is merely making a claim that the product will enhance nutrition (which would result in a dietary supplement categorization for the product). When a dietary supplement manufacturer makes a function-structure claim on the labeling of the product, the label must also carry a disclaimer stating: "This statement has not been evaluated by the Food and Drug Administration. This product is not intended to diagnose, treat, cure or prevent disease." The manufacturer or distributor of a product must notify the FDA of its actions within 30 days of putting the product on the market in the United States. Presumably, the 30 day notification requirement would give the FDA time to amass evidence that the product is unsafe or not effective for the claimed purpose.

While it is not likely that the MPJE would ask questions of a pharmacist licensure applicant, there is a fifth category of articles regulated to some extent by the FDA. Veterinary Pharmaceuticals, that are drugs intended for animals other than humans must also meet safety and efficacy standards.

Poison Prevention Packaging Act (PPPA)

The PPPA requires that all oral drugs intended for use in humans be placed in "special packaging" that is "child-resistant" as described in regulations adopted by the Consumer Products Safety Commission (CPSC). The intent of these laws is to prevent the poisoning of young children from common household products including most drugs. In community pharmacy practice, this means that oral dosage forms of dispensed drugs must be delivered to the patient (or caregiver) with child-resistant safety caps irrespective of whether the drug is intended for adult or pediatric patients and irrespective of whether or not there are children present in the patient's home.

Note that these regulations are mandated separate and apart from FDA packaging and labeling requirements. However, the FDA does consider drugs sold in packaging that does not conform to PPPA requirements to be misbranded. The poison prevention act does not apply to drugs dispensed to institutional or hospital patients.

A prescriber or patient may request that child-resistant packaging not be used. It is important to note that while the request does not have to be in writing under the PPPA, pharmacists should always note the request for non-child-resistant packaging has been made on the prescription or in the patient profile record.

There are 17 drug and drug categories that are expressly exempted from the mandates of this law. Pharmacist licensure applicants should know the drugs and drug categories that are exempted from the child-resistant packaging regulations. Only the most common are listed here: sublingual dosage forms of nitroglycerin, sublingual and chewable forms of isosorbide dinitrate in 10-mg or less strengths, progesterone or estrogen oral contraceptives dispensed in packages for cyclical administration, sodium fluoride when sold in containers with 264 mg or less per package, prednisone tablets in packages containing no more than 105 mg, conjugated estrogen tablets in packages of no more than 32 mg, and erythromycin ethylsuccinate tablets in packages containing 16 g or less of erythromycin. Readers should consult pharmacy law texts for a listing of drugs exempt from this law. Note that the exceptions are narrowly construed. For example, the exception applies to sublingual nitroglycerin tablets, not to any other forms. Note also that the Act applies only to oral dosage forms of drugs. Therefore, creams, pastes, injectables, and patches are not covered by this law.

The law also prohibits reusing child-resistant packaging; glass containers may be reused only if a new safety closure is provided at the time the glass container is reused. In practical terms, this means, for the most part, that pharmacists cannot reuse patient vials for oral prescription drugs that are refilled. Essentially, commercial containers of federal legend drugs distributed to a pharmacy do not have to contain child-resistant closures. Exceptions exist when the commercial container is intended to be relabeled by a pharmacy and sold or otherwise transferred directly to a patient; in these cases, the commercial container must include child-resistant packaging.

Note also that the Act applies to OTC drugs. Regulations allow manufacturers and distributors of OTC drugs to package one size of a product that does not conform to the child-resistant requirement as long as the label clearly states that the product is not in child-resistant packaging.

Anti-Tampering Act

Tamper-resistant packaging is required for many consumer products, including most OTC drugs, cosmetics, and medical devices. Contact lens solutions and lubricants are also subject to these restrictions. Dentifrices, dermatological products, lozenges, and insulin are exempted from the regulations. Prescription drugs dispensed from a pharmacy are also exempted.

Tampering is defined as an intentional act of altering a product to make objectionable and unauthorized changes. Anyone charged with tampering with a product is subject to criminal charges.

Three federal agencies have jurisdiction to enforce anti-tampering regulations. The Federal Bureau of Investigation (FBI), the United States Department of Agriculture and the FDA each have authority to regulate products that must be marketed with these preventative measures. The FDA regulation applicable to OTC drugs requires a statement on the label indicating that it is packaged with tamper-resistant materials.

Other Packaging Requirements

Commercial containers of drugs must meet federal standards for maintaining the integrity of the drugs during distribution throughout the marketing chain. For all federal legend drugs, manufacturers' labeling (package insert) must contain a statement indicating to a pharmacist what kind of container a particular drug should be dispensed in to maintain its identity, strength, and purity. For the most part, the FDA regulations defer to standards established by the USP/NF for determining adequate container standards. Drugs that are not packaged in accordance with these standards are considered misbranded.

Drug Recalls

Although the FDA does not have inherent authority to order a drug manufacturer or distributor to remove an adulterated or misbranded drug from the market, the FDCA prescribes the procedures followed by the FDA to obtain court-ordered recalls or seizures. Of course, a company may voluntarily engage in a product recall if it believes that a product is adulterated or misbranded. The law establishes three categories of recalls designed to alert practitioners and the public as to the level of concern that ought to be raised about the recall. A Class I recall indicates that there is reason to believe use of the drug will cause serious adverse health consequences or even death. A Class II recall means that use of the drug may cause medically reversible consequences but the likelihood of serious adverse results is remote. A Class III recall means that use of a drug will not likely cause adverse health reactions. The manufacturer or distributor of a recalled drug is responsible for notifying the organizations that received the drug. The FDA is responsible for notifying the public about drug recalls.

Some students of pharmacy law confuse the class of drug recall with controlled substances schedules due to the similarities in the numbering system. A simple way to recall the order of severity of a drug recall follows the kind of categorization for controlled substances. A schedule I controlled substance has the highest level of concern because of the addiction potential of a drug in this class. A class I drug recall is the one where serious harm or death might result. As the numbers increase the level of severity in both groups goes down.

Omnibus Budget Reconciliation Act of 1990 (OBRA-90)

The federal laws discussed up to this point generally deal with the manufacturing, packaging, and labeling of drugs and do not directly impact the practice of pharmacy as such. This is partly because the federal government does not have direct authority to regulate pharmacy practice. This right is, at least theoretically, reserved to the states. The law, commonly known as OBRA-90, is somewhat of an exception to this notion because it does mandate certain actions by pharmacists when dispensing drugs to certain patients. This law has much more impact because the vast majority of states have enacted provisions to make the OBRA-90 requirements apply to all patients. Readers will have to take care to determine the specific laws in the states where licensure is sought. Although it is unlikely to be a question on the MJPE, be aware that OBRA-90 did not take effect until 1993.

OBRA-90, insofar as outpatient pharmacy practice is concerned, requires that pharmacies which participate in Medicaid reimbursement programs perform a drug utilization review before dispensing a drug to a Medicaid-eligible patient. This review requires that a pharmacist make an attempt to obtain and maintain a medication history of the patient and determine that a prescribed drug is both necessary and appropriate for the patient before the drug is dispensed. The pharmacist must also be available to counsel a patient on the proper administration of the drug, its common adverse effects, how to monitor the drug's use and effectiveness and on proper storage techniques. An offer to counsel may be made by someone other than a pharmacist but the counseling itself must be performed by a pharmacist if the offer is accepted.

As noted, OBRA-90 applies only to outpatient drugs dispensed to Medicaid-eligible recipients. Congress has authority to regulate pharmacy practice to this limited extent because the federal government pays a portion of the Medicaid drug benefit. Medicaid programs are administered by each state but the states are allowed to seek reimbursement from the federal government for approximately 50% of the costs of drugs paid to pharmacies by the state. At the federal level, Medicaid is administered by the Centers for Medicare & Medicaid Services (http://cms.hhs.gov) (formerly known as the Health Care Financing Administration [HCFA]), which is a division within Health and Human Services. OBRA-90 sets forth the conditions that must be met by the state to be eligible for this reimbursement. As a result, every state has enacted some type of law to implement OBRA-90 mandates. However, very few states restricted the OBRA-90 provisions to just Medicaid patients. Instead, nearly every state has, in one form or another, made the drug utilization review process applicable to all patients. In other words, the duty of a pharmacist to offer to counsel all patients on drug use is almost standard across the country. MPJE candidates should consult the laws in the state where pharmacist licensure is sought.

Compounding Prescription Drugs

The FDAMA amendments to the FDCA (discussed in the FDCA section, above) contain restrictions on when pharmacists are allowed to compound prescription drugs. Basically, the statute permits pharmacists to compound drugs pursuant to valid prescriptions so long as the pharmacy does not solicit compounded prescriptions or advertise to the health care community or the general public that it performs compounding services. While the history underlying this policy is interesting, it is not likely to be the subject of licensure examination questions. Nevertheless it is important for applicants to understand that the United States Supreme Court struck down the entire compounding statute as an unconstitutional restriction on freedom of speech. The decision in Thompson vs. Western States Medical Center was released in 2002. In a close 5-4 decision, the majority of the members on the Court ruled that the restriction on advertising violated the first amendment because the government failed to articulate why a ban on advertising was necessary in order to prevent manufacturing under the guise of compounding and because the government went too far in its restriction of advertising of compounded products.

It should be understood that before the FDAMA amendments went into effect, pharmacists always enjoyed the right to compound drugs for individual patients. The Supreme Court decision, in essence, returns the pharmacy compounding rules to where they were before FDAMA went into law. The FDA, however, issued internal guidelines for FDA Field Offices to use in trying to determine whether a pharmacy has crossed the line between accepted compounding practices and entered into the drug manufacturing role.

Suffice it to say, for examination purposes, that pharmacists may legally compound drugs pursuant to a prescription for an individual patient. The resulting compounded drug product will not be characterized as an unapproved new drug by the FDA under normal circumstances.

Privacy Considerations

Confidentiality of patient records and information is regulated at both the state and federal level. The traditional methods of protecting individual's privacy concerns are governed primarily by state laws. The approach of the states varies greatly from simple statements like, "Prescription records are not public records" (perhaps the lowest forms of protection) all the way up to "Prescription information and the information learned by a pharmacist in the course of serving a patient are privileged." Because there is such a diverse set of state laws, MJPE applicants are directed to state laws in the state where pharmacist licensure is being sought.

At the federal level, there is a fairly new set of laws affecting privacy rights. The Health Insurance Portability and Accountability Act of 1996 (HIPAA) required the Health and Human Services Department (HHS) to adopt regulations affecting the confidentiality of patient information. Even though the law was adopted in 1996, its provisions were not fully enacted until 2004.

The essential point to remember is that providers, including pharmacists and pharmacies, must obtain their patients' consent for uses and disclosures of "protected health information" (PHI) about the patient to carry out "treatment, payment, or health care operations" (TPO). Use of PHI beyond basic TPO requires additional patient authorization. Health care providers must have a documented privacy procedure in place. Each health care organization must train employees so that they understand the privacy procedures and there must be at least one designated individual responsible for seeing that the privacy procedures are adopted and followed.

Providers must also detail security measures for patient records containing individually identifiable health information with a goal of preventing access by those who have no express need for access.

The privacy rules apply to all business associates of providers. For example, a third party hired by a pharmacy to administer prescription claims or process bills would also have to adhere to the same rigid standards applicable to the pharmacy personnel.

Controlled Substances Laws

Study Tips

Significant portions of the MPJE are devoted to assessing licensure candidates' knowledge of both federal and state controlled substances laws. This is because pharmacists spend significant time complying with the laws regulating the ordering, delivery, storage, recordkeeping, and dispensing of these drugs. It is important to note at the outset that the state and federal governments share concurrent jurisdiction over the regulation of controlled substances. This means that at least two sets of laws need to be considered with reference to controlled substances.

While controlled substances laws have been in place for several years, there are a number of changes that must be taken into account. The DEA published a revised version of The Pharmacist's Manual in 2004. At the time of printing this text, the most current edition of the Manual is available online at:

www.deadiversion.usdoj.gov/pubs/manuals/pharm2/index.htm

Do not use any printed or online versions of The Pharmacists

Manual prior to the eighth edition as a study reference. If a newer edition of the Manual is published, use the then current version in preparation for the MPJE.

There was one development as of August 2005 that had not been incorporated into the Manual at the time this manuscript was submitted for publication dealing with the DEA's newly adopted Controlled Substances Ordering System (CSOS). This new ordering system is discussed in the "Distributions of Controlled Substances" section below. The online reference for the CSOS is:

www.deaecom.gov/csosmain.html

It cannot be overemphasized that studying from The Pharmacist's Manual will greatly improve the chance of success in taking the MJPE. This document has been the source of many questions that appear on the examination. Pay attention to the details. By way of example, knowing which DEA form is used for what purpose will be worth points. This controlled substances law review section was compiled from information found in The Pharmacist's Manual and other information dealing with the DEA as well as the Controlled Substances statutes and regulations.

Many states have adopted modifications that take into account newer practice settings such as group homes and assisted living arrangements and newer technologies such as the internet, online prescribing and electronic signatures. Because of this, it is important for applicants to recognize that some laws may have changed since taking a pharmacy law course in school.

One of the most common issues that students raise is whether they will be asked questions about which drugs are designated as controlled substances and which schedule a drug is placed in. The answer is that the states take a wide variety of approaches to assessing a candidate's knowledge about these topics. The best advice is that all candidates should know the controlled substance status of the most commonly prescribed and dispensed controlled substances and non-controlled drugs. There are several lists of commonly prescribed drugs online. Try to find a list tailored to the state in which licensure is being sought.

The other important piece of advice is to pay attention to drugs that may be placed in different schedules by the DEA as compared with the state agency that regulates these drugs. In some cases, a state will place a drug into a higher classification at the state level compared to the schedule it is assigned by the DEA. For example, pentazocine (Talwin) is a Schedule 4 controlled substance under DEA regulations. In Michigan, however, it is classified as a Schedule 3 controlled substance. Another point of departure between state and federal laws is that some states will designate a drug as a controlled substance when the DEA has not put the drug into any schedule. The last issue to consider deals with drugs designated as OTC Schedule 5 drugs under federal law. Some states have elected to make the medication available only by prescription.

Historical Background

While it is highly unlikely that questions would appear on the MJPE about the history of Controlled Substances regulation, preparation for the exam might be easier if just a few historical developments are kept in mind. Congress adopted the federal Controlled Substances Act (CSA) in 1970. The CSA repealed many of the earlier laws and adopted a comprehensive approach to preventing drug abuse. The CSA is sometimes referred to as Title 2 of the Comprehensive Drug Abuse Prevention and Control Act of 1970. The provisions of Title 2 of that Act directly affect pharmacy practice and contain the laws most familiar to pharmacists.

At the time that the CSA was enacted, the FDA was given authority to make the scientific and medical findings that determined whether a drug would be controlled and, if so, how it would be scheduled. That authority changed over time. In 1973, the Drug Enforcement Administration (DEA) was created in the Department of Justice (DOJ), and the Bureau of Narcotics and Dangerous Drugs (BNDD), the agency that had responsibility over these drugs, was abolished. While most current laws have eliminated reference to the BNDD, a few still exist. Where a reference in state or federal law is made to the BNDD, it should be understood to mean the DEA as the successor federal agency. By 1986, the FDA's role in scheduling drugs was eliminated for the most part and the DEA assumed this authority. The DEA is now the organization that has primary responsibility for promulgating the regulations that implement, interpret, and enforce the CSA. As the head of the Department of Justice, the United States Attorney General is responsible for the DEA operations. The DEA Director reports to the Attorney General.

Goals and Objectives of the CSA

Prevention of drug abuse is one of the CSA's main goals. It attempts to accomplish this objective in several ways. Record-keeping mandates for manufacturers, distributors, prescribers, and dispensers of controlled substances are designed to reduce the diversion of drugs from the legitimate course of commerce into illegal markets. One of the major impacts of the CSA is the establishment of a "closed" system of distribution that regulates controlled substances from the moment of initial manufacture or harvest until they reach the hands of the "ultimate user." An ultimate user is a person who lawfully obtains and possesses a controlled substance for his or her own use or use by a member (including an animal) of his or her household. No one is permitted to obtain or possess a controlled substance unless authorized under the provisions of the CSA. Another method of limiting drug diversion is through the requirement of federal registration of persons who handle controlled substances. As used in this law, the term "person" means both individuals and any legally recognized entity including corporations, partnerships, etc. The registration mandate is discussed in detail below.

Concurrent Jurisdiction

Controlled substances are regulated by both federal and state law. Many state laws require additional or different steps than those demanded by federal laws. For example, federal law mandates that a pharmacy maintain controlled substances records, including prescriptions, for a minimum of 2 years. Many states require a pharmacy to maintain all prescription records for a minimum of 5 years from the date the prescription was filled or last refilled. Using the rule that the stricter law controls, in this instance the pharmacy would have to keep the prescriptions on file for the longer period.

Regulatory Authority

From a Constitutional standpoint, the federal government exerts jurisdiction over controlled substances under the "interstate commerce" clause on the presumed notion that these products will cross between state lines at some point in time. The Attorney General of the United States has the primary authority to enforce the CSA. As head of the DOJ, the Attorney General determines which substances will be controlled and which schedule the substance will be placed in. The Attorney General also determines whether violations of the CSA and DEA regulations may have occurred and whether to seek penalties through the federal court system.

The CSA has been amended many times and the DEA has been given expanded authority. For example, in 1990, the DEA was given authority to regulate anabolic steroids. The agency also regulates precursor chemicals that may be used in producing controlled substances, machinery used in controlled substances manufacturing, and controlled substance analogues.

Schedules

The CSA regulates drugs and other substances by placing affected chemical entities into a hierarchy of five schedules that vary depending on the abuse and dependence-producing potential of an individual substance. It is significant that not all of the substances regulated under the CSA are drugs. By definition, schedule 1 controlled substances do not have any accepted medical use in the United States and should not properly be referred to as drugs. Nevertheless, it is common to refer to all controlled substances as drugs, and that convention is followed here.

The listing of the various controlled substances in each of the five schedules was initially established by the CSA. The Attorney General, not the DEA director, is given authority to modify the substances in each schedule by adding, deleting, or rescheduling the substances. The schedules are updated and republished on an annual basis. The lists of which drugs are controlled and which schedule each controlled drug is placed in are available from a variety of sources. License applicants are presumed to know the schedule that the common controlled drugs are placed in. States may also place drugs into schedules established by the individual states. For the most part, the state schedules will track the federal schedule. However, there may be some differences making it worthwhile for license applicants to check the law of the state where a license is sought. It should also be useful to review the criteria for placing a substance into a particular schedule.

Schedule 1

(C-I): The drugs and other substances in this schedule are those that have (a) a high potential for abuse; (b) no current accepted medical use in the United States; or (c) there is a lack of accepted safety for use under medical supervision.

Pharmacies, other than those in facilities that are registered for investigative or research uses, should not have any Schedule 1 controlled substances in inventory. Further, physicians are not authorized to prescribe Schedule 1 controlled substances unless registered to perform investigations or do research under approved protocols. Most of the controlled substance analogues of drugs in other schedules, sometimes called "designer drugs," are classified as Schedule 1 controlled substances. Examples of substances classified in Schedule include heroin, LSD, marijuana, and MDMA (ecstasy).

Schedule 2

(C-II): To be placed in this schedule, the drug or other substance must be determined to (a) have a high potential for abuse; (b) have a currently accepted medical use in treatment in the United States or a currently accepted use with severe restrictions; and (c) abuse may lead to severe psychological or physical dependence.

Schedule 1 and 2 drugs are subject to annual production quotas established by the DEA. The amount of any given drug subject to this regulation that may be manufactured and distributed is determined each year by medical usage in prior years as measured by studies conducted by the HHS. The quotas are revised once annually.

Some examples of Schedule 2 narcotics include morphine, codeine, hydrocodone, and opium, hydromorphone (Dilaudid), methadone (Dolophine), meperidine (Demerol), oxycodone (Percodan) and fentanyl (Sublimaze). Some examples of Schedule 2 stimulants include amphetamine (Dexedrine), (Adderall), methamphetamine (Desoxyn) and methylphenidate (Ritalin). Other Schedule 2 substances include cocaine, amobarbital, glutethimide, pentobarbital and secobarbital.

Schedule 3

(C-III): In order to be placed in this schedule, a drug or other substance must have (a) less potential for abuse than substances in Schedule 1 or 2; (b) a currently accepted medical use for treatment in the United States; and (c) a moderate or low physical or high psychological dependence potential when abused. Some examples of Schedule 3 narcotics include products containing less than 15 milligrams of hydrocodone per dosage unit (i.e., Vicodin, Lorcet, Tussionex, and products containing not more than 90 milligrams of codeine per dosage unit (i.e., codeine with acetaminophen, aspirin or ibuprofen). Other Schedule 3 substances include anabolic steroids, benzphetamine (Didrex), phendimetrazine, buprenorphine (Buprenex) and any compound, mixture, preparation or suppository dosage form containing amobarbital, secobarbital, pentobarbital, dronabinol (Marinol) or ketamine.

Schedule 4

(C-IV): Drugs or other substances in this schedule have (a) a low potential for abuse relative to substances in Schedule 3; (b) a currently accepted use for treatment in the United States; and (c) a limited physical or psychological dependence potential when abused relative to substances in Schedule 3. Schedule 4 drugs include the benzodiazepines: alprazolam (Xanax), clonazepam (Klonopin), clorazepate (Tranxene), diazepam (Valium), flurazepam (Dalmane), halazepam (Paxipam), lorazepam (Ativan), midazolam (Versed), oxazepam (Serax), prazepam (Verstran), temazepam (Restoril), triazolam (Halcion), and quazepam (Doral). Other Schedule 4 substances include barbital, phenobarbital, chloral hydrate, ethchlorvynol (Placidyl), ethinamate, meprobamate, paraldehyde, methohexital, phentermine, diethylpropion, pemoline (Cyler), mazindol (Sanorex), and sibutramine (Meridia).

Schedule 5

(C-V): Drugs or other substances in this schedule must have been determined to (a) have a low, but still very real, potential for abuse relative to substances in Schedule 4; (b) have a currently accepted use for treatment in the United States; and (c) lead to a limited physical or psychological dependence potential when abused relative to the substances listed in Schedule 4. Some examples are cough preparations containing not more than 200 milligrams of codeine per 100 milliliters or per 100 grams (Robitussin AC), Phenergan with codeine).

OTC Schedule 5

It is noteworthy that there are some drugs on the market that are Schedule 5 controlled substances but do not require a prescription. Most of these are either codeine-based cough syrups or paregoric-based anti-diarrheals. This seemingly peculiar inconsistency exists because the FDA, which is part of the HHS, makes the determination as to whether a drug will be available on a prescription-only basis or available without a prescription as an OTC drug. The FDA uses scientific and medical data to make its decisions on the availability and access of drugs. Safety and efficacy are the primary concerns of the FDA. The DEA, which is a totally unrelated government agency, determines whether a substance or drug will be designated as a controlled substance. In addressing this decision, the DEA behaves more like a police agency that is concerned with crime prevention and prosecution of criminal activity. The DEA uses abuse potential and concerns over diversion as the primary factors in making decisions on the control and scheduling of drugs and other substances. In this respect, the jurisdiction of the agencies is separate and does not overlap. As far as Schedule 5 OTC drugs are concerned, the FDA has determined that they are safe and effective for use without the need of medical supervision, while the DEA has concluded that they have a potential, albeit small, for abuse.

Exempt Narcotics

Schedule 5 OTC drugs in the past were referred to as "exempt narcotics." This archaic but still common term dates back to an exemption from taxation for "Class X" drugs under the 1914 Harrison Narcotic Act. Take care to note how the state where the applicant is seeking licensure regulates non-prescription schedule 5 drugs. Usually, these preparations are available only in a state licensed-DEA registered pharmacy and the pharmacist who sells these medications must keep a record of sales by filling out information about the purchaser and the date of the sale.

Sale of Controlled Substances without a Prescription

It may seem odd upon first consideration that the DEA regulations would permit a retail-based pharmacist to dispense a schedule 2, 3, 4 or 5 controlled substance without a prescription if it has not been designated as a prescription-only substance by the FDA or under the applicable state law and the following procedures are followed:

1. The sale is made by a pharmacist, not by a non-pharmacist employee, even if under the direct supervision of a pharmacist. However, after the pharmacist has fulfilled professional and legal responsibilities, the actual cash, credit transaction or delivery may be completed by a non-pharmacist.

2. The pharmacist must use professional judgment to ensure the medical necessity of the need for the product.

3. Not more than 240 mL or not more than 48 solid dosage units of any substance containing opium, not more than 120 mL (4 fluid ounces), or not more than 24 solid dosage units of any other controlled substance, may be distributed at retail to the same purchaser in any given 48-hour period without a valid prescription.

4. The purchaser is at least 18 years of age.

5. The pharmacist must obtain suitable identification, including proof of age, where appropriate if the pharmacist is not familiar with the purchaser.

6. A bound record book must be maintained containing the name and address of the purchaser, name and quantity of controlled substance purchased, date of each sale, and initials of the dispensing pharmacist. This record book must be maintained for a period of two years from the date of the last transaction and it must be made available for inspection and copying.

Chemical Control Requirements

In recent years, the DEA has recognized that some OTC drug products contain chemical precursors of controlled substances. For example, pseudoephedrine (Sudafed) can be converted to methamphetamine with rudimentary chemical procedures. Ephedrine and phenylpropanolamine are also commonly involved in the clandestine manufacture of controlled substances. These precursors have garnered the attention of regulators at both the state and federal levels. MPJE applicants should review the laws in the states where pharmacist licensure is sought to determine the current regulations for these products.

Persons who handle controlled chemicals need to register with the DEA. Community pharmacies that are registered to receive and dispense controlled substances do not have to register a second time to also carry the affected chemicals unless the pharmacy also engages in the wholesale distribution of the chemicals. DEA Form 510 is used to register as a chemical distributor.

Registration

Most persons (recall that this means both individuals and legal entities including corporations and partnerships) who handle controlled substances must be registered with the DEA unless specifically exempted from federal registration. Manufacturers and distributors of controlled substance drugs are usually required to register on an annual basis. Pharmacies and prescribers (both are often referred to as dispensers or practitioners in the regulations) usually are required to register once every 3 years.

Pharmacists (with the exception of sole proprietorships), pharmacy interns, technicians, and other agents or employees of a properly registered pharmacy do not have to register independently of the pharmacy. These individuals may handle controlled substances without registration so long as they do so while acting in the usual course of business and within the scope of their employment or agency relationship.

This same kind of exemption applies to most other DEA registrants. As such, the employees of manufacturers and distributors need not apply for registration and do not violate the law when possessing controlled substances in the course of their employment. Military officials, including Public Health Service employees, law enforcement agents, and civil defense workers are also exempted from registration so long as their employment situation requires them to handle controlled substances.

Medical students and residents associated with medical institutions including hospitals need not obtain a DEA registration as long as they are working under the supervision of a registered physician and the institution is registered. Physician's assistants and nurse practitioners (or nurse clinicians) must register as midlevel practitioners in almost all situations.

Separate registrations are required for each individual site where controlled substances are stored or dispensed. Each pharmacy must have its own separate registration and DEA number even if a single corporate entity operates several pharmacies. Thus, if a chain-store owns 100 pharmacies each operating at a separate street address, 100 separate registrations must be obtained. If a hospital or other health care facility operates more than one pharmacy at several satellites within the facility only a single registration is necessary so long as the facility operates from a single street address. However, if that same facility operates hospital and several clinic pharmacies at different locations, multiple registrations will be required.

Separate registrations are also required for multiple activities even if they occur at the same location. For example, a large health care facility may manufacture, distribute, and dispense controlled substances. Each activity requires a separate registration. If research is also conducted at the facility, an additional registration is necessary.

A pharmacy applies for a DEA registration on DEA form 224 which is available online in the Pharmacist's Manual, and may be obtained from any DEA Field Office, or at the DEA Headquarters in Washington DC. Once the registration certificate is issued to the pharmacy, it must be kept on file in the pharmacy and made available for inspection upon request. The DEA should send the pharmacy an application for renewal 45 days before the end of the three year registration period. If the pharmacy does not receive the renewal registration by 30 days before its expiration date, the pharmacy will have to request a renewal form. Renewal requests are made on DEA Form 224a. Corporation or other forms of ownership that operate pharmacies at multiple locations use DEA Form 224.

The DEA requires a pharmacy engaged in co-op buying of controlled substances to also register as a distributor. As a distributor, a pharmacy must meet distributor (wholesaler) security and recordkeeping requirements.

If a DEA registered pharmacy moves locations or the postal address of the pharmacy changes, the pharmacy is responsible for submitting a written request for a new registration certificate from the DEA before the change occurs. The request should be made to the local DEA Field Office. Once the new location is noted by the DEA it will issue new DEA Form 222 (if the pharmacy is still using hardcopy forms to order Schedule 2 controlled substances).

A DEA registration may be suspended or revoked, or an application for renewal or for a change in location may be denied if the DEA has reason to believe the registrant is involved in the diversion of controlled substances from legitimate channels into illegal markets. Decisions resulting in the suspension, revocation or denial of renewals or change of locations are made by the Attorney General of the United States. The grounds for making these adverse decisions include false statements made by applicants, conviction of the applicant of a felony related to the use of controlled substances or controlled chemicals, revocation, suspension, or denial of a state-issued controlled substance or pharmacy license, exclusion from the Medicaid or Medicare programs and performing an act which would render continuance of a DEA registration "inconsistent with the public interest."

The "inconsistent with the public interest" standard requires the US Attorney General to take into account specific factors including:

1. The recommendation of the appropriate state licensing board or professional disciplinary authority;

2. The applicant's experience in dispensing or conducting research with respect to controlled substances;

3. The applicant's conviction record under federal or state laws relating to the manufacture, distribution or dispensing of controlled substances;

4. Compliance with applicable state, federal or local laws relating to controlled substances; and

5. Such other conduct which may threaten the public health and safety.

If a DEA registered pharmacy discontinues doing business or transfers ownership to another legal entity, the pharmacy is obligated to notify the nearest DEA Field Office in writing in advance of the termination or transfer. The pharmacy is required to return any unused DEA Form 222s with the word "VOID" written on each one. The notification must indicate where the controlled substances inventory and records will be located after the termination or transfer and how they were transferred or destroyed. Even though the pharmacy may be closing, the pharmacist-in-charge must make arrangements to have the records kept available for inspection up until 2 years after the final controlled substance transaction occurred.

If the pharmacy is being transferred to a different owner, the registered pharmacy is obligated to inform the nearest DEA Field Office of the change at least 14 days prior to the change. The notice must include:

1. The name, address, registration number of the registrant discontinuing business;

2. The name, address, registration number of the registrant acquiring the pharmacy;

3. Whether the business activities will be continued at the location registered by the current business owner or moved to

another location. If the latter, give the address of the new location.

4. The date on which the controlled substances will be transferred to the person acquiring the pharmacy.

A complete and final controlled substances inventory must be conducted on the day the pharmacy is terminated or ownership is transferred and, if a transfer is involved, both the seller and the buyer should each keep a copy of the inventory for at least 2 years from the date the inventory was performed.

Electronic Prescribing and Communications

In June 2000 the Electronic Signatures in Global and National Commerce Act (E-Sign) was adopted into law. While the law is general in nature, it has the potential to have significant impact on the way the practice of pharmacy is conducted. In its most basic form, this law applies to all transactions and permits electronic signatures to have the same validity as traditional ink and paper signatures for purposes of binding agreements. The law specifically bars state and federal agencies from mandating or recognizing only hardcopy signatures. It also indicates that any state or federal law that mandates traditional hardcopy signatures to be preempted. The other part of this law applies to recordkeeping procedures and states that electronic copies of records must be given the same accord as traditional paper-based records.

There is a provision that will permit a federal agency that can prove electronic signatures or records will create a "substantial" hardship can still mandate traditional signatures and records. At the time of writing this text, the DEA had not presented any materials to suggest that electronic signatures or records pertaining to the prescribing or dispensing of controlled substances drugs would cause a substantial hardship.

At the time this manuscript was being prepared, a majority of states have adopted laws implementing electronic signatures and recordkeeping provisions. However, to date, the DEA had not yet authorized electronic prescribing or transmittal of information for controlled substances prescriptions in anything other than traditional hospital-based pharmacy practices. The DEA has had test projects going on for several years. It is expected that the DEA will develop electronic prescribing standards soon and readers are urged to check both state and federal laws on the validity and scope of activities related to electronic communications in pharmacy practice before sitting for the MJPE test.

Classifications of Pharmacies and Special Provisions for Unique Practices

Traditionally, the DEA only recognized two kinds of pharmacies: the typical community "retail" pharmacy and the "institutional" or hospital-based pharmacy. Over time, the DEA started to accept that there are different sets of considerations that need to be made for long-term nursing homes. In DEA language, these institutions are known as "Long Term Care Facilities" (LTCFs). The DEA has not yet recognized pharmacy services to senior citizen independent living situations or assisted living institutions as anything other than community based pharmacy. In one of the more recent developments, the DEA has developed rules for "central fill pharmacies" as described below. There are also some regulations pharmacists should know about using controlled substances in drug addition and rehabilitation clinics.

LTCFs

Nursing homes, retirement care, mental health care, or other facilities or institutions which provide extended health care to resident patients are deemed to be Long Term Care Facilities

(LTCFs) by the DEA. Despite the fact that these institutions are not routinely registered with the DEA, they do maintain inventories of controlled substances, usually in the form of medications dispensed by an outside pharmacy directly to the patients but held at nursing stations for administration by LTCF personnel. When patients of these institutions are discharged or expire, or there is a change in the medications of patients, the LTCF may need to dispose of controlled substances it was holding for the patients. The DEA advises operators of these facilities and pharmacists who dispense medications to patients to follow state laws with respect to handling controlled substances no longer needed for a patient or to contact the nearest DEA Field Office for instructions on how to proceed.

There are some exceptions for transmitting Schedule 2 drugs for patients in LTCFs. See the discussion in Prescription Formats and Transmittals, below. The DEA has also issued guidelines for states to use in formulation rules for emergency kits in LTCFs.

Internet Pharmacies

Internet commerce has presented a number of challenges to the DEA because the majority of its experience and requirements deal with traditional community and hospital-based pharmacy practices. The potential for drug diversion and need for new, innovative solutions takes on global proportions. In what will likely be the first of many attempts by the DEA to regulate controlled substance dispensing and distribution with this newer technology, the DEA issued some regulations addressed to pharmacies that pursue internet opportunities.

As with all pharmacies, those that wish to use the internet must be registered with the DEA at the pharmacy's physical location where controlled substances will be held in inventory if it plans on doing any controlled substances dispensing or distributing. There is no need to register the internet homepage or internet ownership information. The pharmacy must also be licensed by the state in which the pharmacy is physically located and, if required, in those states where it does business. In most cases this means that if the pharmacy located in state X sends prescriptions ordered on the internet to state Y, it would have to have the appropriate licenses from both state X and state Y, in addition to being registered with the DEA. All of the other DEA regulations apply to the internet pharmacy as would apply to any retail pharmacy.

Note that the regulations for delivering drugs, including controlled substances by the United States Postal Services are discussed in the Mailing Prescription Drugs section of this section.

Narcotic Treatment Programs

Congress adopted laws specifically geared for the use of controlled substances in the treatment of addicted patients seeking rehabilitation. The laws deal with two different treatment programs. One is for "maintenance" treatments, usually in Methadone Clinics, and the other is for "detoxification." Operators of either type of program must register with the DEA using DEA Form 363. The registrant will only be approved to use the narcotics listed on the form in treatment programs. Controlled substances cannot be used for any purpose other than maintenance or detoxification unless the practitioner who operates the program is also registered for "normal" practices associated with controlled substances.

While the DEA has adopted regulations governing these programs, there is also a widely divergent set of regulations adopted by state agencies having jurisdiction over these treatment modalities. Regardless of these differences, Narcotic Treatment Programs must use DEA Form 222 for all transactions involving Schedule 2 drugs; presumably the new electronic CSOS system will replace the need for use of the hardcopy forms once it is implemented. See, www.deaecom.gov/csosmain.html.

Methadone

In addition to the use of methadone in narcotic maintenance programs, methadone is used as an analgesic to treat severe forms of pain. This raises concerns when methadone is used to treat pain in an individual who is also a narcotic addict. With one exception, the DEA has taken the position that practitioners who are not registered as operating a narcotic maintenance program cannot prescribe methadone to an addicted patient under the guise of treating pain. The exception occurs when a practitioner who is not part of a narcotic treatment facility prescribes methadone to a narcotic addict experiencing withdrawal while waiting to get into a treatment program. The methadone used in this manner is limited to a maximum three day supply under DEA regulations. There are some states that do not permit this practice.

Narcotics for Patients with Terminal Illnesses or Intractable Pain

The DEA recognizes that the use of narcotics for treatment of patients with intractable pain or pain associated with a terminal illness is effective, appropriate and legitimate. The regulations require that prescriptions for controlled substances be issued for legitimate medical purposes by a practitioner (i.e., an individual authorized under state law to issue a controlled substances prescription) who is acting in the course of medical practice. The DEA has stated that pharmacists should not be concerned when dispensing controlled substances so long as they act with "good faith" when evaluating the legitimacy or appropriateness of a controlled substance prescription. While inappropriate use of narcotics is not acceptable, the DEA does acknowledge that appropriate narcotic drug use will often be accompanied by drug tolerance and physical dependence in individuals who have the need for high doses or prolonged treatment. The DEA has specifically stated that pharmacists receiving prescriptions for high strengths or large quantities of controlled substances for a individual patient should not fear DEA sanctions because "the quantity of drugs prescribed and frequency of prescriptions filled alone are not indicators of fraud or improper prescribing."

Medical Missions and Humanitarian Charitable Solicitations

In order for practitioners to hand carry controlled substances overseas, while providing charitable medical, dental or veterinary treatment in foreign countries. They must obtain approval from the DEA and the appropriate authority in the foreign country. In these situations, practitioners should allow at least 30 days to obtain the necessary approvals from a local DEA Field Office. If a pharmacy is asked to donate controlled substances, the pharmacist should contact the state agency that regulates controlled substances and the DEA Field Office for information on how to proceed.

Central Fill Pharmacies

In recent years the DEA has acknowledged that new technologies and differing market needs have developed so that there are more ways of delivering pharmacy services than the traditional retail and hospital settings. One of these developments has given rise to the concept of a "central fill pharmacy." The DEA describes a central fill pharmacy as one that "fills prescriptions for controlled substances on behalf of retail pharmacies with which central fill pharmacies have a contractual agreement to provide such services or with which the pharmacies share a common owner". In this scenario a retail pharmacy receives a prescription from a patient and transmits it to second pharmacy where the prescription

medicine is prepared and delivered to the first retail pharmacy for dispensing to the patient.

In this kind of arrangement, records must be maintained by both the central fill pharmacy and the retail pharmacy that completely reflect the disposition of all controlled substance prescriptions dispensed. Central fill pharmacies, in essence, must comply with the same security requirements applicable to retail pharmacies. Note that retail pharmacies that also perform central fill activities may do so without a separate DEA registration, separate inventories, or separate records.

Central fill pharmacies are permitted to prepare both initial and refill prescriptions, subject to all applicable state and federal regulations. Both the central fill pharmacy and the retail pharmacy share responsibility for determining the validity of a controlled substance prescription. The procedures developed by the DEA for central fill pharmacies apply to all controlled substances prescriptions in Schedules 2 through 5.

For reasons that are not clear, the DEA does not permit a central fill pharmacy to accept prescriptions from or deliver medications directly to patients by use of the mail. This seems odd given that patients may obtain controlled substance medication from a regular mail order pharmacy. The distinction between a mail order pharmacy and a central fill pharmacy may not make much logical sense but this is the way the DEA has indicated it will treat central fill pharmacies.

There are two ways for a retail pharmacy to submit prescriptions to a central fill pharmacy. The first is to permit faxed prescriptions between the entities. In this situation, the retail pharmacy keeps the original prescription and the central fill pharmacy uses the faxed prescription as its record of dispensing. All records must be retained in a readily retrievable manner. Interestingly, the DEA does allow the prescription information to be transmitted electronically through the internet.

MPJE candidates should check the state laws in the state where licensure is sought to determine if state law permits central fill pharmacies. Many states have been adopting standards that follow the model described by the DEA. Other states have not done so or have unique variations.

Destruction or Transfer of Controlled Substances

When a pharmacy goes out of business, it may transfer its inventory of controlled substances to another pharmacy as described above. It may also transfer the drugs to a DEA registered distributor or back to a DEA registered manufacturer that is also registered by the DEA to destroy controlled substances. This process is known in DEA terms as "reverse distribution." Records detailing the transfer or destruction must be kept by the pharmacy owner for 2 years after the transfer or destruction, or longer if required by the laws of an individual state.

To transfer Schedule 2 substances, the receiving registrant must issue a DEA Form-222, to the registrant transferring the drugs. This procedure may change with the advent of the paperless Controlled Substances Ordering System (CSOS). MPJE candidates should check the status of the CSOS at the time the examination is taken.

When Schedule 2 through 5 controlled substances are transferred, the transaction must be recorded in writing to show the drug name, dosage form, strength, quantity and date transferred. The document must include the names, addresses and DEA registration numbers of the parties involved in the transfer of the controlled substances.

If the pharmacy going out of business is transferring its controlled substances back to a distributor or manufacturer, the pharmacy must maintain a written record showing:

1. The date of the transaction.

2. The name, strength, form and quantity of the controlled substance.

3. The supplier's or manufacturer's name, address, and, if known, registration number.

4. DEA Form-222 will be the official record for the transfer of Schedule 2 substances.

If the transfer is to a reverse distributor registered to dispose of controlled substances, the pharmacy is permitted to forward its controlled substances to DEA-registered reverse distributors who handle the disposal of drugs.

Destruction of Controlled Substances

The DEA asks that any pharmacy having controlled substances it needs to destroy because they have expired, or become adulterated or misbranded to notify the local DEA Field Office for disposal instructions. There is no provision in the law for transferring drugs that should be destroyed between a pharmacy and the DEA. Once each calendar year, a pharmacy may request permission from the DEA to destroy controlled substances using DEA Form 41. All drugs proposed to be destroyed must be listed on the Form together with the proposed date and method of destruction. Written notice to the DEA must also contain the names of at least two witnesses who will observe the destruction. Appropriate witnesses include a licensed physician, pharmacist, mid-level practitioner, nurse, or a state or local law enforcement officer.

Both the DEA Form and the written notice must be received by the nearest DEA Diversion Field Office at least 14 days prior to the proposed destruction date. After reviewing all available information, the DEA Field Office should notify the pharmacy in writing of its decision. Once the controlled substances have been destroyed, signed copies of the DEA Form-41 must be forwarded to DEA. It should be noted that this prior notification procedure need not be followed if an authorized member of a state law enforcement authority or regulatory agency witnesses the destruction. However, DEA Form 41 must still be filled out be the pharmacy and sent to the local DEA Field Office. Although not necessarily covered in the DEA regulations, the DEA suggests that pharmacists contact local environmental authorities prior to implementing the proposed method of destruction to ascertain that hazards are not associated with the destruction.

It should be noted that there is a procedure whereby the DEA will provide a "Blanket Authorization" for Destruction of Controlled Substances" on a very limited basis to registrants who are associated with hospitals, clinics or other registrants having to dispose of used needles, syringes or other injectable objects only. The DEA states that "this limited exception is granted because of the probability that those objects have been contaminated by hazardous bodily fluids." A pharmacist practicing in these kinds of environments should contact their local DEA Field Office for information about how to request such an authorization. DEA will evaluate requests for a blanket authorization.

If a pharmacy removes controlled substances from the regular inventory because the drugs are damaged, defective, adulterated or misbranded, the drugs must be inventoried and the records maintained with the other controlled substances records. The document must include the following:

1. The inventory date.

2. The drug name.

3. The drug strength.

4. The drug form (e.g., tablet, capsule, etc.).

5. The total quantity or total number of units/volume.

6. The reason why the substance is being maintained.

7. Whether substance is capable of being used in the manufacture of any controlled substance in finished form.

Labeling

Commercial containers (from a manufacturer or distributor) of controlled drugs must bear a label containing a specific symbol indicating the schedule that the drug has been placed in (e.g., C-II or CII). The symbol must be prominent and easily identifiable. There are some exceptions, such as the circumstance that the container is too small to display the symbol or that the container is being used in the course of blinded drug research protocols.

For controlled substances that are dispensed pursuant to a prescription, the prescription label must contain (a) the name and address of the pharmacy (or dispenser); (b) the patient's name; (c) a prescription serial number; (d) the date that the medication is dispensed; (e) the prescriber's name; (f) directions for use; and (g) cautionary statements, if any are required by the prescription or other laws. Schedule 2, 3, and 4 prescription labels must also contain the federal transfer warning statement. This statement must include these specific words: Federal law prohibits the transfer of this drug to any person other that the patient for whom it was prescribed. Take specific notice that this transfer warning is not required on a Schedule 5 prescription label. These labeling requirements do not apply to drugs that are dispensed for or to patients who are admitted to a health care facility such as a hospital or nursing home if the drugs are to be administered on site. The DEA regulations do not recognize group homes for the physically or mentally disabled or assisted living homes. In these situations a pharmacist would label prescription drugs dispensed to residents of these facilities as for any other community-based patient.

There are almost as many variations in prescription drug labeling laws for controlled substances at the state level as there are states and territories. Reference must be made to individual state laws to determine what information must appear on the pharmacy label.

Security

Most practitioners are required to store all controlled substances in a "securely locked, substantially constructed cabinet." The DEA, however, allows some flexibility in how controlled substances are stored in a pharmacy and registered institutions. In these facilities, scheduled drugs may either be stored in an appropriate locked cabinet or be dispersed throughout the stock of non-controlled drugs in a manner calculated to obstruct theft or diversion or a combination of both options may be used. For example, many pharmacies will lock Schedule 2 drugs in a cabinet or drawer and disperse Schedule 3, 4, and 5 drugs throughout the pharmacy inventory. Although not required by the CSA statutes of DEA regulations, the DEA does recommend that pharmacies use a security alarm to deter thefts.

In recognition of the fact that DEA registered pharmacies and other registrants can be the target of thefts, armed robberies, violence and even death, Congress passed the Controlled Substance Registrant Protection Act of 1984 (CSRP). A federal investigation of thefts and robberies is mandated when controlled substances valued at $500.00 or more are lost, a registrant or other person is killed or suffers significant bodily injury during a robbery or theft of controlled substances or a crime occurs or is planned involving the interstate transport of controlled substances. Breach of this law could result in federal criminal charges and punishment includes fines, imprisonment in a federal penitentiary and the death penalty if a murder occurs during a controlled substances robbery.

Prescriptions

Under the CSA, a prescription is just one of the means of moving a controlled substance drug from the inventory of a practitioner (i.e., a physician or a pharmacy) into the hands of a patient. This is the primary method of authorizing an ultimate user to obtain controlled substances in the community setting. Patients may also receive controlled substances without prescriptions when a drug is administered directly to a patient, when it is dispensed to a nursing unit for administration to a patient in a hospital, or when it is transferred directly from a physician to a patient for later use outside the physician's presence.

Pharmacists are considered "gatekeepers" when it comes to determining the validity of prescriptions. By authorizing pharmacists to dispense controlled substances only pursuant to legitimate prescriptions, the DEA attempts to minimize the diversion of controlled substances from legal markets into the hands of illegitimate users, sellers, and abusers. Understanding the regulations and duties imposed on pharmacists should help control drug diversion while insuring that legitimate and needy patients have access to necessary and appropriate drug treatments.

Purpose

A prescription for a controlled substance must be issued by a qualified prescriber and for a "legitimate medical purpose." Under the DEA regulations, an order (also referred to as a "purported prescription") for a controlled substance may not necessarily be a prescription even if that order is issued by an authorized prescriber. This means that a pharmacist must make a determination as to whether a controlled substance prescription is issued for a valid purpose before medication is dispensed. The appearance of an order, while an important factor, is not determinative of whether or not the order is in fact a prescription. An order might appear to be proper in that it contains all the information necessary to constitute a prescription. It may be issued by an authorized prescriber (see Scope of Practice, below). It may even contain a valid DEA number. But the order is still not valid unless it is issued for a recognized medical use. While the prescriber may have responsibility for prescribing controlled substances for proper purposes, pharmacists also have a "corresponding responsibility" to determine the legitimacy of an order before controlled substances are dispensed.

Validity

There is no single acid test or bright line determinant for assessing the validity of any one prescription. Instead, a list of factors must be considered in making a professional judgment as to whether a controlled substance order should be filled. The DEA suggests that prescribers who write large numbers of controlled substance prescriptions or write for large quantities relative to other prescribers in the area should be suspect. Issuance of prescriptions for antagonistic drugs (depressants and stimulants) at the same time may be another cause for concern. Patterns of patients who appear frequently in the pharmacy with new controlled substance prescriptions or return for refills too soon suggests a problem may be occurring. Patients who present prescriptions in the names of other people or from multiple physicians could be involved in drug diversion. A number of patients appearing in the pharmacy within a short period of time with similar prescriptions from the same prescriber also ought to send up a red flag. A large number of

"strangers," people who have never been patients in the pharmacy before, who show up at the same time with controlled substance prescriptions from the same prescriber may be another factor to consider. A dramatic increase in the controlled substances inventory could be another sign that the pharmacy is being targeted by drug abusers.

Scope of Practice

The only individuals who are authorized to issue controlled substances prescriptions are those who are licensed by a state to prescribe controlled substances and who are either registered with the DEA or exempted from registration. State laws vary considerably on which practitioners are allowed to prescribe controlled substances. Prescribing is also limited by the scope of a practitioner's license. For example, a state licensed medical doctor may be able to prescribe just about any controlled substance to treat a human disease. A dentist, however, is limited to prescribing controlled substances for treatment of conditions relating to the oral cavity and its supporting structures. Veterinarians are allowed to prescribe controlled substances for animals in most states but a controlled substance prescription from a veterinarian for a human would not be valid. Some states also allow midlevel practitioners to prescribe controlled substances.

Verification

When a pharmacist is presented with a controlled substance prescription or an order that purports to be a prescription, the validity of the prescription should be verified. Knowledge of the prescriber and his or her prescribing habits is perhaps the most efficient means of verification. Validation of the prescriber's DEA registration number is important. A mathematical check should be performed to determine if the number is valid.

Recall that a DEA registration is usually composed of two letters followed by seven digits, the last of which is a "check" number. If the DEA number on a prescription, for example, showed AB1234563, the prescriber's last name should begin with a "B." The formula for determining the validly of the check number is to add the first, third and fifth digits and note the last number of that addition. Then add the second, fourth and sixth numbers and multiply that product by 2. Take the last number in that calculation and add it to the number saved in the first equation. The last number in the product of this equation should be the same as the seventh digit in the DEA registration number. Using the number in the example above the calculation would look like this:

$$1 + 3 + 5 = 9$$

$$2 + 4 + 6 = 12 \times 2 = 24$$

Then add 9 + 4 to equal 13.

The last digit, 3, should be the same as the last digit of the registration number. Candidates taking the MPJE are expected to know this equation. In practice, if the math is too cumbersome, there are online sites that will do the math and indicate whether the check digit number is valid. For example see: http://www.msspnexus.com/msspn_dea.asp. There are some variations including how the number is expressed if the first character in a registrant' name is a number, e.g., 123 Pharmacy Corp. See the pharmacist's Manual for determining the validity of a registration number in these situations.

Prescription Formats and Transmittals

With the exception of emergency situations, Schedule 2 prescriptions must be in writing and signed by the prescriber. A prescriber may transmit a Schedule 2 prescription to a pharmacy via a facsimile machine (fax) provided that the pharmacist is presented with the original written and signed prescription before the medication is dispensed in normal situations. License applicants and pharmacists should consult state laws to determine whether this provision applies in their particular state. State laws may also dictate that a particular prescription form must be used.

In an emergency situation the pharmacy may receive an oral order or an order transmitted by fax from the prescriber for a Schedule 2 drug but an original written and signed prescription (i.e., a hard-copy backup) must be transmitted to the pharmacy within 7 days of the oral order. Under earlier regulations, the prescriber had to transmit the written prescription to the pharmacy within 72 hours. This extension of time was intended to ease the burden of pharmacists involved with dispensing to long-term care patients or those who receive Schedule 2 drugs for home-hospice care. The backup must contain the statement "Authorization for Emergency Dispensing" and contain the date of the oral order. If the backup is mailed to the pharmacy it must be postmarked within the 7 day period. When received, the pharmacist must attach the backup to the original orally or fax transmitted form and file the documentation with the other Schedule 2 prescriptions. Other provisions allow for fax transmittals of Schedule 2 prescriptions without backup written copies for patients residing in qualified institutions.

The regulations also permit the use of fax transmittals for drugs listed in Schedules 3, 4, and 5. As such, prescriptions for drugs listed in these schedules may now be written, orally transmitted or sent to the pharmacy via a fax machine. Again, state laws should be consulted to determine if there are any restrictions or modifications regarding the transmittal of controlled substance prescriptions.

A controlled substance prescription, if written, must be signed on the date issued; predated and postdated prescriptions are not valid. For Schedule 2 drugs, the prescription must be written in ink, indelible pencil or typewritten and manually signed by the prescriber. Prescriptions may be prepared by a secretary or agent of the prescriber but the prescriber remains responsible for compliance with the legal requirements for issuing the prescription. Pharmacists also have a corresponding responsibility to insure the prescription contains all necessary information and conforms to the legal mandates. Secretaries and agents of a prescriber are permitted to communicate controlled substance prescriptions and refills to a pharmacy but only the authorized prescriber is permitted to actually prescribe.

Refills and Prescription Transfers

Unlike Schedule 2 drugs, which cannot be refilled, Schedule 3, 4, and 5 drugs may be refilled if authorized by the prescriber. Schedule 3 and 4 drugs may be refilled up to a maximum of five times within 6 months from the date of issuance. Schedule 5 prescriptions may be refilled as authorized up to the amount allowed under state law (frequently up to one year measured from the date the prescription was issued, not from the date the prescription was first filled). Schedule 2 drugs may be partially filled, giving the effective appearance of a refill, under limited circumstances such as in a long-term care facility or in the rendering of hospice services.

Where refills are permitted, transfers of controlled substance prescriptions between different pharmacies are allowed one time only. However, additional transfers between pharmacies that share an electronic real-time database of prescription information are permitted. In other words, there is a distinction between transfers between individually owned pharmacies and those that may share a common ownership such as a chain-store. In this later situation, transfers are allowed up to the maximum number of refills authorized by the prescriber. The information that must be captured in making a transfer of this type is specific and detailed. License applicants and pharmacists should review state law and employer policies before attempting to transfer controlled substance prescriptions.

When a prescription for any controlled substance in Schedule 3, 4 or 5 is refilled, the dispensing pharmacist's initials, the date the prescription was refilled, and the amount of drug dispensed on the refill must be recorded on the back of the prescription or, if the pharmacy uses computerized records, in accordance with the rules for using computerized records discussed under the Record Keeping section below. If the pharmacist only initials and dates the back of the prescription, it will be assumed that the full amount of the drug called for on the front of the prescription was dispensed on a refill.

Distributions of Controlled Substances

A clear distinction should be made between dispensing activities and controlled substances distributions because the record-keeping requirements are very different. Dispensing is the act of delivering a controlled substance to an ultimate user based on a legitimate prescription order. Distribution, on the other hand, is the delivery of a controlled substance to a person by means other than dispensing or administering. Distribution is the transactional method by which a pharmacy transmits or delivers controlled substances to another pharmacy, a wholesale distributor, or a prescriber or another entity that is registered with the DEA and has the right to possess controlled substances. The DEA has a regulation that permits a pharmacy to distribute up to 5% of its annual dispensed controlled substances before a distributor license will be required.

A prescription cannot be used by prescribers to obtain office supplies of controlled substances for the purpose of dispensing drugs directly to patients. DEA Order Form 222 must be used to distribute Schedule 2 drugs from a pharmacy to a practitioner. An invoice should be used to distribute Schedule 3, 4, and 5 drugs from a pharmacy to a practitioner.

Up until September 2005, when a pharmacy ordered Schedule 2 controlled substances from a manufacturer or wholesale distributor, it had to use the 3 part DEA Order Form 222. Under federal law, the registrant had to sign the form or designate authority to sign it to another responsible individual using a "power of attorney" This is a legal document that must be signed by the registrant that gives the designated individual the power to sign the form on behalf of the registrant. The document has to be kept on file with the order forms and is subject to inspection by the DEA. Pharmacists should exercise extreme caution in giving someone else the power of attorney to order controlled substances. Because this power can be abused, many state laws place limitations on who may sign the DEA form. The DEA now permits registrants to use the "Paperless Controlled Substances Ordering System (CSOS)" which provides an alternative to using the hardcopy Form 222 to purchase Schedule 2 controlled substances. See, http://www.deaecom.gov/csosmain.html as discussed above in the Study Tips and Narcotic Treatment Programs sections.

Record Keeping

Under the CSA, one of the major responsibilities of pharmacies is to keep accurate and detailed records of activities relating to controlled substances. As with dispensing activities, there is a wide variation between the states in record-keeping mandates that must be followed in addition to the federal requirements.

The DEA requires that all controlled substances records be maintained in the registered pharmacy for a minimum period of 2 years dating from the last transaction pertinent to a particular record. For example, if a Schedule 4 controlled substance prescription is authorized for up to five refills and the patient orders the last refill before the end of the six months since the prescription was issued, the pharmacy would have to maintain the prescription for at least two years after the date of the last refill.

All records dealing with controlled substances must be maintained in "readily retrievable" manner in the pharmacy. This term means controlled substances records kept in some form of computer database storage must be retrievable separate from all other records.

In terms of specific records, the DEA mandates pharmacies maintain the following documents in a readily retrievable fashion:

1. Official Order Forms (DEA Form-222);

2. Power of Attorney authorization to sign Order Forms;

3. Receipts and invoices for Schedule 3, 4 and 5 controlled substances as well as registered chemicals, if any;

4. All inventory records of controlled substances, including the initial and biennial inventories;

5. Records of controlled substances distributed or dispensed (i.e., prescriptions) and threshold amounts of List I chemicals distributed;

6. Report of Theft or Loss (DEA Form-106);

7. Inventory of Drugs Surrendered for Disposal (DEA Form-41);

8. Records of transfers of controlled substances between pharmacies; and

9. DEA registration certificate.

For entities that own two or more DEA registered pharmacies, there is a provision for "central recordkeeping." Shipping and financial records may be stored at a headquarters or offices of the organization if it notifies the nearest DEA Field Office of the intent to do so. Once 14 days have passed after issuing this notice the organization may start keeping these records at the intended location unless the DEA informs the organization that permission to store required records at the intended place is denied.

Computerized Records

A DEA registered pharmacy may use either manual records on hardcopy or computerized records for keeping track of refills for controlled substances prescriptions. It cannot use one method some of the time and the other on different occasions. It must choose one or the other. State law should also be consulted to determine if there are any other requirements for computerized pharmacy data.

Any computer system utilized must provide a mechanism for accessing the original prescription information. At a minimum the original prescription number, date the prescription was issued, the name and home address of the patient, the prescribers name, address and DEA registration number, the name, dosage form, quantity dispensed and strength of the drug dispensed and number of refills authorized, if any, must be available on the computer. The database must also have refill information available. Computerized records must provide for a backup method in case there is a problem with retaining original information in the system.

If the system utilized by the pharmacy permits printouts of the daily controlled substances dispensing activities, a pharmacist must verify the accuracy of the printout information be signing and dating the document. This printout must be available within 72 hours of the date any refills were recorded.

If the system does not permit printouts as described above, the pharmacy must keep a bound record book that a pharmacist must sign and date showing that the refill records were reviewed and are accurate. All systems are required to have the capacity to print refill data that includes the prescribers name, amount dispensed on the refill, the refill dispensing date, identification of the pharmacist (name or initials) and the prescription number. If the entity that owns the pharmacy is permitted to maintain records at a central office such as a headquarters, the refill records must be made available in the pharmacy within 48 hours upon request.

Inventories

Pharmacies are required to maintain a current and complete record of controlled substances inventories and perform an audit of these drugs every 2 years. The required date that the inventory is performed was altered somewhat under the 1997 amendments to the DEA regulations. Now the biennial inventory may be taken anytime within 2 years of the prior inventory. Inventory records for Schedule 2 drugs (and Schedule 1 drugs in the rare event that a pharmacy has any) must be maintained separate and apart from all other records. Schedule 3, 4, and 5 inventory records must also be maintained separate and apart from all other records or maintained in a format that they will be readily retrievable from the ordinary records of the pharmacy. No special form is required for inventory records. However, all records must be written, typewritten, or printed. The name of the drug, its dosage form (i.e., 10-mg capsule), the size of the commercial container (i.e., 100 tablets) and the number of commercial units on hand must be recorded. For open stock containers of Schedule 2 drugs, an exact count of the drugs on hand is required. For open stock of Schedule 3, 4, and 5 drugs, an estimate of the amount on hand is permitted unless the container holds more than 1000 units in which case an exact count is necessary. All inventories, records of purchases, executed order forms (DEA Order Form 222), prescriptions, and distribution records must be kept on file at the pharmacy for a minimum of 2 years.

Prescription Records

Schedule 2 prescriptions must be maintained in a separate file. Similarly, Schedule 3, 4, and 5 prescription records must be maintained separate and apart from all other prescriptions or maintained in a manner that allows them to be readily retrieved from all other prescriptions. There are, however, options available for filing Schedule 3, 4, and 5 prescriptions. If separate prescription files are not kept for prescriptions in these schedules, the prescriptions may be mixed in with the Schedule 2 prescriptions or, mixed in with the non-controlled prescriptions; in either of these options, the Schedule 3, 4, and 5 must be stamped with red ink on the face of the prescription in the lower right hand corner with the letter "C" no less than 1 inch high. Another option is available for pharmacies that utilize automatic data processing (ADP) systems or some other form of electronic record keeping. As in the prior option, Schedule 3, 4, and 5 prescriptions may be mixed in with either the Schedule 2 prescriptions or the non-controlled prescriptions. The red "C" stamp requirement is waived as long as the ADP or other system permits identification of the prescriptions by serial number and retrieval by prescriber name, patient name, drug name, and date dispensed. In addition, records have to be kept of the number of units or volume of scheduled drugs that are dispensed, including the name and address of the person to whom it was dispensed, the date of dispensing, the number of units or volume dispensed, and the written or typewritten name or initials of the pharmacist who dispensed or administered the drug. State laws vary on these procedures and may require other alternatives.

Distribution Records

The kind of information that must be recorded by a pharmacy when it receives controlled substances is complex. For each controlled substance distributed to a pharmacy, a record must be kept of the name of the drug, its finished dosage form (e.g., 10-milligram tablet or 10-milligram concentration per fluid ounce or milliliter) and the number of units or volume of finished form in each commercial container (e.g., 100-tablet bottle or 3-milliliter vial), the number of commercial containers acquired from other persons, including the date of and number of units and/or commercial containers in each acquisition to inventory and the name, address, and registration number of the person from whom the units were acquired. If a pharmacy distributes (as opposed to dispenses) controlled substances to other registrants, the number of commercial containers distributed, including the date of and number of containers in each reduction from inventory, and the name, address, and registration number of the person to whom the containers were distributed must be recorded. The pharmacy must also record the number of units of finished forms and/or commercial containers distributed or disposed of in any other manner, such as destruction, including the date and manner of distribution or disposal, the name, address, and, if applicable, the registration number of the person to whom distributed, and the quantity in finished form distributed or disposed.

Location of Records

Prescriptions, completed inventories, and executed order forms (DEA Order Form 222) must be kept in the pharmacy where the prescription was originally filled for at least 2 years from the date the drugs were last dispensed. All controlled substance prescriptions and records maintained in the pharmacy are subject to inspection by DEA officers. Pharmacies may keep financial and shipping records, such as invoices and packing slips, at a central location like a chain store headquarters. Special permission to store the other records at a central location may be available in limited circumstances.

Employment Disqualifications and Requests for Waivers

The DEA prohibits pharmacies with controlled substances available from employing anyone with access to those controlled substances who has been convicted of a felony relating to controlled substances, or who, at any time, has had an application for DEA registration denied, revoked, or surrendered "for cause." This term is defined to mean "surrendering a registration in lieu of, or as a consequence of, any federal or state administrative, civil or criminal action resulting from an investigation of the individual's handling of controlled substances." While there is a procedure that permits pharmacies to apply for a waiver of this provision, permission is rarely granted.

Reporting Controlled Substance Theft or Loss

Upon discovery of a significant loss or theft of controlled substances a DEA registered pharmacy must immediately notify the local DEA Field Office and the local police authority by telephone, facsimile or by a brief written message explaining the circumstances. There is no bright line test of how "significant" the loss or theft must be. Pharmacists should judge the situation in the context of the amount of theft or loss as compared to the general controlled substances inventory. Missing six or seven phenobarbital pills is not significant. Loss of a whole unopened bottle of 500 Valium tablets is definitely significant. The DEA asks pharmacists to err on the side of caution and report losses when not sure of whether or not the loss should be considered significant. Some factors to consider suggested by the DEA for determining significant loss include:

1. The schedule of the missing items.

2. The abuse potential of the missing items.

3. The abuse potential in your area of the missing substance.

4. The quantity missing (one tablet vs. one bottle or container).

5. Is this the first time this loss has occurred? Has a similar loss occurred before?

6. Was this loss reported to local law enforcement authorities?

In addition to the immediate notification requirement, a pharmacy must also complete DEA Form 106 and send it to the local DEA Field Office. Most states also require pharmacies to send a copy of this form to the state Board of Pharmacy or the agency that oversees pharmacy licensure. In any event, the pharmacy must also keep a copy of the Form 106 with its own controlled substances records for use if a controlled substances audit is performed. The Form 106 must also be made available for inspection upon request. Information on this form is to include the circumstances of the loss and theft and the quantity and names of the controlled substances involved. At a minimum the DEA Form 106 must include:

1. Name and address of the pharmacy

2. DEA registration number

3. Date of theft (or date that the theft was discovered).

4. Name and telephone number of local police department notified

5. Type of theft (night break in, armed robbery, etc.)

6. Listing of symbols or cost code used by pharmacy in marking containers (if any)

7. Listing of controlled substances missing from theft or significant loss

If a pharmacy reports a theft or loss of controlled substances to the DEA and later discovers after an investigation that no loss or theft actually occurred (e.g., the missing bottle of 500 Valium tablets was found to have been accidentally thrown out and recovered from the trash), the DEA does not require that the reporting form be filed. However, the DEA should be given written notice of the circumstances as to why the pharmacy is not completing Form 106. The state agency and local police should also be informed.

Breakage/Spillage

The DEA does not consider that incidental breakage, damaged goods received in transit or spillage of controlled substances as a "loss" that must be reported. When these kinds of incidents occur, the method discussed above for reverse transfer or destruction of controlled substance should be followed. Note the action taken in the controlled substances records in case an audit is performed. DEA Form 41 should be used to make a record of the circumstances involved.

Penalties

Penalties for violation of the CSA and DEA regulations may be very severe. Many provisions require intent to violate or knowledge of an infraction of the CSA. There are other provisions, however, including many of the record-keeping mandates applied to pharmacists that impose a strict liability type of penalty where knowledge or intent are not considered. Both civil fines and criminal sanctions are possible. In addition, states may also impose penalties for controlled substance violations. Revocation of the federal registration and suspension or revocation of any state issued controlled substance licenses or registrations may also be administratively imposed. Penalties are not exclusive to any one jurisdictional body. In other words, the same act of wrongdoing could result in federal civil and/or criminal penalties, and state criminal and/or civil penalties and administrative sanctions against federal and state registrations and licenses. Put still another way, the prohibitions against double jeopardy in the United States Constitution do not apply to health care licensees who violate the multiple requirements of controlled substances laws. This means that one offending activity may result in multiple penalties. Therefore, it is in the best interest of pharmacists to know and follow the controlled substances laws.

Intentional or Knowledgeable Penalties

Pharmacists who knowingly dispense controlled substances based on orders that are not valid are subject to significant penalties. Imprisonment of up to four years and fines as high as $30,000 may be imposed for each violation. The knowledge requirement may be implied by the circumstances. Deliberate ignorance of objectively determined facts that should indicate that a prescription has been forged, altered, or issued for a non-legitimate medical purpose will expose the dispensing pharmacist to criminal penalties. In other words, the "ostrich defense," i.e., figuratively sticking one's head in the sand to ignore objectively verifiable facts, does not work in the pharmacist' favor. Studied avoidance of realities and circumstances may be used as evidence to create an inference that the pharmacist knew or should have known that a purported prescription was not legitimate.

Record-Keeping Penalties

The penalties for failure to keep records as mandated by the CSA and DEA regulations include monetary fines, loss of registration and criminal sanctions. A pharmacy that is charged with a record-keeping violation may be subject to a civil penalty of $25,000 for each violation. Imprisonment is also possible for intentional record-keeping violations. However, for civil charges to apply, no knowledge or intent is needed. In other words, pharmacists and pharmacies are strictly liable for record-keeping violations. Innocent errors, mistakes, and negligent inadvertence to details could still lead to significant penalties under the applicable laws.

Applicants should be aware of all state laws in their jurisdictions that may modify the rules discussed above. Also see the State Pharmacy Practice Laws section below.

Mailing Drugs

Mailing Drugs

Ever since 1994, pharmacists may send nearly all OTC and prescription-only drugs to patients using the United States Postal Service (USPS), an agency of the federal government. The postal regulations still prohibit the mailing of abortive drugs or devices and the unsolicited mailing of contraceptives. About the only other special alert pharmacists should be aware of is that postal service bans mailing of powders that might be able to escape from their containers; however, if the powder is packed in leak-proof receptacles or sealed in durable, leak-proof outer containers they can be mailed. There are also provisions for shipping chemicals but they do not apply to pharmaceutical products.

The DEA's Pharmacist's Manual contains pertinent information about the mailing of controlled substances. Basically these are the same as those for non-controlled substances. The USPS regulations permit mailing any controlled substances, provided that they are not "outwardly dangerous or of their own force could cause injury to a person's life or health." In addition, the pharmacy packaging of the controlled substance must be properly labeled with all of the information the DEA mandates for dispensed medications including the name and address of the pharmacy. The visible outer wrapper should be securely wrapped in plain paper and should not have any indication as to the contents of the package.

Pharmacists are prohibited from shipping or delivering controlled substances dispensed pursuant to a valid prescription to a different country without authorization. This activity is deemed by the FDA to be drug exporting and is not permitted unless the pharmacy has a DEA exporter registration.

Private carriers like United Parcel Service (UPS), and DHL Worldwide Express have their own rules and regulations about the products they will accept for delivery. The policies of private carriers are beyond the scope of this review.

State Pharmacy Practice Laws

Every state has legislation that regulates the profession of pharmacy. Even so, there is a great deal of variation in state laws pertaining to pharmacy practice. The laws of each state for which licensure candidates will be taking the pharmacy law exam should be reviewed individually. There are some general issues addressed by nearly all states. The NABP Survey of Pharmacy Law provides lists of the common issues and how they are addressed in each state. Some of the items that should be reviewed include:

1. The minimum education, training, and experiential qualifications which license applicants must satisfy at the time of examination or registration.

2. The authority, makeup, and duties of the agency, usually known as the State Board of Pharmacy, charged with enforcement and administration of the pharmacy laws.

3. How licenses or other permits to engage in the practice of pharmacy are granted and renewed and for what period of time.

4. The conditions under which licenses or registrations to engage in the practice of pharmacy may be restricted, canceled, or revoked.

5. The activities included in the scope of pharmacy practice and what duties might be delegated to non-pharmacists.

6. The individual who is responsible for compliance with state and federal pharmacy laws.

7. Whether continuing education is necessary for maintaining a pharmacist license and what those requirements include.

8. What kinds of labels, labeling, and record keeping are required for controlled and non-controlled prescription drugs dispensed in a pharmacy.

9. Whether there are any special rules that distinguish how pharmacy is practiced in community (retail) settings vs. an institutional (hospital) setting.

10. Whether the state participates in "reciprocal" registration with other states and, if so, what conditions have to be satisfied before reciprocating.

11. Who is qualified to prescribe drugs and the conditions that must be met before a prescription is dispensed.

12. Whether the state has any laws regarding drug product selection, generic substitution, therapeutic substitution, or formularies.

13. Whether licensure, registration or certification is required for pharmacy technicians and/or educational requirements for personnel who assist a pharmacist.

There are, of course, numerous other issues such as nuclear pharmacy regulations, prescription drug compounding, and third-party benefits laws that are too long and complex for a law review of this type. The above list is only a suggestion to help license applicants get started on studying for a pharmacy law examination.

On a broad scale, one of the more common issues confronted under state laws deals with the scope of pharmacy practice. Activities that are normally associated with the practice of pharmacy include evaluation and interpretation of a prescription, selecting a drug product to be dispensed pursuant to a prescription, preparation of the patient label and performing a drug utilization review to determine that a prescription medication is necessary and appropriate for a patient. Patient counseling on the proper use and storage of medications is usually included in the scope of pharmacy. In contrast, pharmacists rarely are assigned duties to make physical assessments of patients while engaging in the practice of pharmacy. Most state laws also make provisions for assigning responsibility for compliance with state and federal pharmacy laws to a pharmacist-in-charge or a pharmacist on duty. In addition, a corporate officer or other designated corporate employee may be designated as one of the responsible parties when the pharmacy is owned and operated as a corporation.

Questions

1. Under which of the following circumstances may a drug manufacturer's representative legally distribute a federal legend drug sample?

   A. When requested by a community pharmacist.
   B. When requested by a hospital pharmacist.
   C. When requested in writing by a prescriber.
   D. All the time.
   E. When requested by an community-based mental health pharmacist.

2. A DEA registration is NOT required for an individual who is legally recognized as a prescriber and is a:

   A. doctor of medicine practicing as a family physician.
   B. physician's assistant working in a hospital.
   C. medical resident employed by a teaching and research hospital.
   D. doctor of osteopathic medicine and surgery specializing in psychiatry.
   E. nurse clinician (nurse-practitioner).

3. The pharmacist who is charged with responsibility for compliance with state and federal pharmacy laws is most often designated as the:

   A. chief operating officer.
   B. pharmacist-in-charge.
   C. pharmacy manager.
   D. responsible pharmacist.
   E. Pharmacy District Manager.

4. Which of the following activities is NOT usually associated with the practice of pharmacy?

   A. Selecting a specific drug product to be dispensed pursuant to a prescription.
   B. Monitoring a patient's drug therapy and use.
   C. Making a physical assessment of the patient.
   D. Counseling a patient on the safe use and storage of prescription medications.
   E. Interpreting and evaluating a prescription.

5. Which of the following institutions or individuals is NOT ordinarily required to obtain a registration from the DEA before handling controlled substances?

   A. A hospital
   B. A staff physician performing research with controlled substances at a medical teaching hospital
   C. A community pharmacy owned by a chain store corporation
   D. A pharmacist employed by a hospital or community pharmacy
   E. A nursing home

6. Assume that a podiatrist asks a community pharmacist to sell a 1-month supply of a prescription-only oral contraceptive for his wife, who also happens to be his office manager, using the podiatrist's prescription. Which of the following responses by the pharmacist are lawful?

   A. Have the podiatrist write a prescription and dispense it as ordered.
   B. Decline the request because it is beyond the scope of practice of the podiatrist to prescribe oral contraceptives.
   C. Sell the oral contraceptives to the podiatrist as an office supply, using a pharmacy invoice to record the transaction.
   D. Sell the podiatrist a 2- or 3-day supply as a professional courtesy and tell him that this is a one-time favor.
   E. Dispense the oral contraceptive as written and make a call to the state podiatry board.

7. Which of the following statements regarding patient counseling about drugs is TRUE?

   A. All state laws require a pharmacist to counsel patients on all prescription drugs including refills.
   B. Any individual designated to work in a pharmacy department may provide counseling about prescription drug use.
   C. A pharmacist may counsel any patient about the use of OTC and prescription-only drugs at any time the pharmacist believes counseling is necessary and appropriate.
   D. Licensed pharmacy interns may counsel patients about prescription drug use without the supervision or presence of a pharmacist.
   E. Pharmacies employing the United States Postal Service to provide prescription drugs are exempt from all counseling requirements as long as written information about the drug is provided.

8. Pharmacies are licensed or registered to engage in the practice of pharmacy by which one of the following administrative agencies?

A. Centers for Medicare and Medicaid Services (CMS)

B. The Joint Commission on Accreditation of Healthcare Organizations™ (JCAHO ®)

C. Department of Health and Human Services (DHHS)

D. The State Board of Pharmacy or its equivalent and the Drug Enforcement Administration (DEA)

E. The Food and Drug Administration (FDA)

9. If a drug is placed in a schedule that is regulated by the Drug Enforcement Administration, that drug is classified as a:

A. controlled substance.

B. federal legend.

C. sample.

D. generic.

E. investigational new drug (IND).

10. On June 1, 2007 a medical doctor legitimately issues a prescription for #35 Darvon, a prescription-only C-IV controlled substance to a patient with directions to take one dose every 4-6 hours as needed for migraine. The prescription indicates that it may be refilled six (6) times. The patient has the prescription filled at First Community Pharmacy on June 1, 2007. The patient returns to that pharmacy on July 1, 2007 and obtains a refill. On August 1, 2007 the patient goes to ABC Retail Pharmacy, an independent pharmacy not affiliated in any way with First Community Pharmacy, and asks that the prescription be transferred and refilled. The prescription is filled and dispensed at ABC Retail Pharmacy on August 1, 2007. The patient returns to ABC pharmacy on September 1, 2007, again on October 1, 2007 and again on November 1, 2007 and obtains refills of the prescription on each day.

Under federal law, how long must First Community Pharmacy maintain the prescription in its records?

A. Until at least June 30, 2009

B. Until at least June 30, 2008

C. Until at least November 1, 2009

D. Until at least November 1, 2008

E. Until the pharmacy is either closed or transferred to a new owner

11. On June 1, 2007, a medical doctor legitimately issues a prescription for #35 Darvon, a prescription-only C-IV controlled substance to a patient with directions to take one dose every 4-6 hours as needed for migraine. The prescription indicates that it may be refilled six (6) times. The patient has the prescription filled at First Community Pharmacy on June 1, 2007. The patient returns to that pharmacy on July 1, 2007 and obtains a refill. On August 1, 2007, the patient goes to ABC Retail Pharmacy, an independent pharmacy not affiliated in any way with First Community Pharmacy, and asks that the prescription be transferred and refilled. The prescription is filled and dispensed at ABC Retail Pharmacy on August 1, 2007. The patient returns to ABC pharmacy on September 1, 2007, again on October 1, 2007, and again on November 1, 2007, and obtains refills of the prescription on each day.

Under federal law, how long is ABC Retail Pharmacy required to maintain the prescription in its records?

A. Until at least October 31, 2009

B. Until at least May 31, 2009

C. Until at least October 31, 2009

D. Until at least December 31, 2009

E. Until the pharmacy is either closed or transferred to a new owner

12. On June 1, 2007, a medical doctor legitimately issues a prescription for #35 Darvon, a prescription-only C-IV controlled substance to a patient with directions to take one dose every 4-6 hours as needed for migraine. The prescription indicates that it may be refilled six (6) times. The patient has the prescription filled at First Community Pharmacy on June 1, 2007. The patient returns to that pharmacy on July 1, 2007 and obtains a refill. On August 1, 2007, the patient goes to ABC Retail Pharmacy, an independent pharmacy not affiliated in any way with First Community Pharmacy, and asks that the prescription be transferred and refilled. The prescription is filled and dispensed at ABC Retail Pharmacy on August 1, 2007. The patient returns to ABC pharmacy on September 1, 2007, again on October 1, 2007, and again on November 1, 2007, and obtains refills of the prescription on each day.

In addition to the above facts the patient returns to ABC Retail Pharmacy on December 2, 2007, and asks for another refill. What is the pharmacist legally required to do?

A. Dispense the refill because the prescription is still valid.

B. Refuse to dispense the refill because the legal limit on the number of refills allowed would be exceeded.

C. Transfer the prescription back to First Community Pharmacy so that the patient may obtain the remaining refill called for in the original prescription.

D. Inform the local DEA office that the patient is attempting to obtain controlled substances on an illegally issued prescription.

E. Give the prescription order to the patient and ask that additional refills be obtained from a different pharmacy.

13. A hospital-based pharmacy is legally permitted to provide a limited quantity of controlled substances medications that are not under the control of a pharmacist to:

A. an emergency-room supply cabinet that is secured under a protocol approved by the pharmacy director.

B. an unsecured cabinet in a nursing station.

C. a stockroom in the hospital basement.

D. an automobile owned and operated by the hospital for transferring patients between the hospital and off-site clinics.

E. a supply cabinet located just outside the pharmacy.

14. In most states, the Board of Pharmacy or equivalent administrative agency issues controlled substances licenses to:

A. pharmacies.
B. pharmacists.
C. physicians.
D. authorized prescribers.
E. all of the above.

15. Which federal agency determines whether drugs are safe and effective for intended uses?

A. FDA
B. DEA
C. DHHS
D. CMS
E. BNDD

16. Which federal agency determines whether drugs should be designated as controlled substances?

A. FDA
B. DEA
C. DHHS
D. CMS
E. BNDD

17. Which governmental agencies have authority to regulate controlled substances?

A. The federal government exclusively
B. State governments exclusively
C. The World Trade Federation
D. State and federal governments concurrently
E. Local municipalities only

18. Who determines which schedule a drug designated as a controlled substance will be placed in?

A. The President of the United States
B. The FDA Commissioner
C. The US Attorney General
D. The Secretary of Health and Human Services
E. The Speaker of the House of Representatives

19. Who is required to register with the DEA?

A. All pharmacies that dispense controlled substances
B. All pharmacists who dispense controlled substances
C. All licensed pharmacy interns while working in a pharmacy that dispenses controlled substances
D. All employees of drug manufacturers that produce controlled substances
E. All police officers who might encounter controlled substances while on duty

20. Which of the following categories of drugs must be labeled with the federal transfer warning when dispensed from a community pharmacy?

I. Schedule 2 controlled substances
II. Schedule 3 and 4 controlled substances
III. Schedule 5 controlled substances

A. I only
B. III only
C. I and II only
D. II and III only
E. I, II, and III

21. How are controlled substances to be stocked in a pharmacy?

A. In a locked cabinet in the pharmacy
B. Dispersed throughout the inventory of non-controlled drugs in the pharmacy
C. In a separate storage room away from the pharmacy
D. In a safe that is accessible only by the pharmacist-in-charge
E. Either choice A and B or a combination of both.

22. What is a "purported prescription"?

A. An order for a controlled substance that has not been issued for a legitimate medical purpose.
B. An order for a controlled substance from a prescriber that has not yet been verified by a pharmacist.
C. A legitimately prescribed controlled substance order that was communicated to a pharmacist by the prescriber's agent.
D. A legitimately prescribed controlled substance order issued by a midlevel practitioner.
E. An order for a controlled substance issued by a prescriber whose practice is located in a state other than where the pharmacy is located.

23. How many times may a Schedule 5 drug be refilled according to federal law?

A. Five times in a 6-month period
B. Twelve times in a 12-month period
C. For a maximum of 2 years
D. As authorized by the prescriber
E. Schedule 5 drugs cannot be refilled

24. Under federal law, how many times may a prescription for a refillable controlled substance be transferred between different (unrelated) pharmacies?

A. As often as the patient and the prescriber agree
B. A maximum of 3 times
C. A maximum of 2 times
D. One time only
E. Never

25. Under federal law, how many times may a prescription for a refillable controlled substance be transferred between commonly owned pharmacies that share an electronic real-time database of prescription files?

A. As often as the patient and the prescriber agree
B. A maximum of three times
C. One time only
D. As many times as the prescription is legally refillable
E. Never

26. According to federal law how does a prescriber obtain a supply of Schedule 2 controlled substance drugs from a pharmacy for use in the prescriber's office?

A. The supply is obtained by using one of the prescriber's prescriptions marked "For Office Use" in the space designated for a patient's name.

B. The supply is obtained by using a DEA Form 222.

C. The supply is obtained by using a DEA Form 106.

D. The supply is obtained by having the pharmacist record the transaction on a pharmacy invoice that is kept with the other Schedule 2 controlled substances records.

E. This practice is not permitted. The prescriber must obtain the drugs from a wholesale distributor of the manufacturer.

27. According to federal law, how does a prescriber obtain a supply of Schedule 3 or 4 controlled substance drugs from a pharmacy for use in the prescriber's office?

A. The supply is obtained by using one of the prescriber's prescriptions marked "For Office Use" in the space designated for a patient's name and the document is filed in the pharmacy with its Schedule 3 and 4 controlled substances prescriptions.

B. The supply is obtained by using a DEA Form 222 or the online CSOS.

C. The supply is obtained by using a DEA Form 106.

D. The supply is obtained by having the pharmacist record the transaction on a pharmacy invoice that is kept with the other Schedule 3 and 4 controlled substances records.

E. This practice is not permitted. The prescriber must obtain the drugs from a wholesale distributor of the manufacturer.

28. How often does federal law require a pharmacy to perform a controlled substance inventory?

A. Monthly

B. Once every year

C. Every 2 years

D. Every 3 years

E. Every 4 years

29. According to federal law, how long does a pharmacy have to keep prescriptions, invoices, and inventory records for Schedule 2 drugs?

A. 1 year

B. 2 years

C. 3 years

D. 5 years

E. Until the pharmacy is closed or transferred to a new owner

30. If the DEA believes that a pharmacy has knowingly violated the controlled substances laws, it may proceed against the pharmacy by:

A. seeking criminal penalties.

B. seeking civil penalties.

C. seeking to have the pharmacy's DEA registration revoked.

D. seeking to have the pharmacy's DEA registration suspended.

E. seeking any and all of the above sanctions.

Compounding and Calculations Review

Compounding

Pharmaceutical Solid Dosage Forms

Important Terms

Hygroscopic – readily absorbing moisture from the atmosphere

Deliquescent – liquefying upon contact with the air; capable of attracting moisture from the atmosphere and becoming liquid

Efflorescent – will give off moisture or attract moisture, depending on the vapor pressure difference between the atmosphere and the powder

Geometric dilution – a mixing technique used to incorporate potent drugs or small quantities of powders in which equal volumes of drug and diluent are blended so as to ensure homogeneous mixing

Trituration – the process of grinding a drug in a mortar and pestle to reduce the particle size

Levigation – the formation of a paste by wetting a powder with a levigating agent and reducing the particle size of the powder

Eutectic – solid substances that when mixed together reduce the melting point of each solid and cause liquid formation

Comminution – the term describing the reduction in particle size of a powder

Levigating agent – a dispersing agent used to wet powders for their incorporation into semisolid or suspension dosage forms.

Powders

Description of delivery system

Powders are homogeneous mixtures of finely divided drug and excipient combinations. They can be manufactured for both oral and topical uses. They are typically dispensed in dry form, but they may require the addition of a liquid, such as water, or food. Powders can be compounded into bulk products or into divided powders for unit-dose dispensing. Dry powders are typically not preferred by patients because of confusion with the method of administration and bitter or unpleasant tasting drugs or excipients. Also, the difficulty associated with protecting some powders from degradation, such as hygroscopic or deliquescent powders can make it difficult for pharmacists to find a suitable package for dispensing. The powder components must be homogeneously mixed, meaning the pharmacist must use the technique of geometric dilution when compounding such prescriptions. Also, the components of the powder must be appropriately sized (e.g., micronized). The USP/NF defines particle sizes as very coarse, coarse, moderately coarse, fine, and very fine. This is determined by the proportion of powder that is able to pass through a sieve of a defined size. Methods used to decrease the particle size of different powders are collectively termed comminution. Pharmacists compounding a powder or other dosage forms that include powders may need to decrease the particle size in order to have a uniform distribution of smaller diameter particles. The particle size is important because it can prevent segregation and is also important in the dissolution of oral powders. Trituration can be accomplished with a mortar and pestle, typically of the porcelain type, which has a coarser contact surface suitable for comminution. Powders used in ointments or suspensions are typically wetted with a levigating agent, such as propylene glycol, in order to form a paste prior to spatulation with the ointment base or for diluting. When blending powders, geometric dilution should be employed and can be accomplished by spatulation or using a glass mortar and pestle.

Interpreting the prescription order

Prescriptions for powders should include the intended use and ingredients for compounding. The prescription will typically call for the blending of powders, usually a drug and diluent mixture. Latin terms are usually employed to instruct the pharmacist on manufacturing procedure and dispensing instructions.

Calculating the prescription

For most powders, the ingredients will be listed as % w/w or total weight of each substance. When calculating the amount and proportion of each ingredient, it is important to remember the basics of pharmaceutical calculations in order to ensure

Compounding and Calculations Review

proper compounding and dispensing. When powders are needed in amounts less than the smallest amount weighable, the aliquot method should be used to ensure accurate weighing (see the Calculations section for further assistance).

Compounding the product

Powders can be compounded by two well-known techniques. First, the method of spatulation involves the use of a pill tile or ointment slab to mix the powders. The drug and other excipients are mixed geometrically with the diluent using a spatula. This method is tedious, time-consuming, and does not result in a high degree of homogeneity compared to other techniques. Second, the pharmacist uses the mortar and pestle method most often to mix powders. The drug is admixed with the excipients by geometric dilution in the mortar by stirring or grinding the powders together using the pestle. This method is less time-consuming and shows a higher degree of homogeneity compared to the spatulation method.

Capsules

Description of delivery system

Capsules comprise enclosure of a substance, typically a powder, within a capsule shell. The outer shell is generally made from some type of gelatin, but for patients refusing gelatin capsules, there are other alternatives available (e.g., HPMC, starch). Gelatin capsules are composed of hard or soft gelatin but, for compounding purposes, hard gelatin capsules are typically used. Because most capsules are intended for oral use, the size of the capsule becomes important when compounding such prescriptions. Capsule sizes range from the largest (#000) to the smallest size (#5), which can hold 1000 or 100 mg of aspirin, respectively (Table 1).

Table 1. Approximate capacity of empty gelatin capsules in grams

No.	000	00	0	1	2	3	4	5
Quinine Sulfate	0.65	0.40	0.32	0.25	0.20	0.15	0.10	0.06
Aspirin	1.00	0.65	0.50	0.32	0.25	0.20	0.15	0.10
Na Pentobarbital	1.10	0.80	0.57	0.42	0.32	0.24	0.17	0.11
Powdered Lactose	1.20	0.85	0.60	0.45	0.35	0.27	0.19	0.12
Na Bicarbonate	1.50	1.00	0.70	0.52	0.40	0.32	0.25	0.15

When compounding prescriptions for specific patients, age and ability to swallow certain size capsules become important factors, as well as the amount of powder needed for each capsule. The size of the capsule determines the total amount of powder (diluent and drug) that can be encapsulated and the drug concentration within the diluent must be calculated accordingly. Filling the capsule shells is performed by various techniques, including the punch method or commercially available machines for the manufacture of capsules on a small scale. Compounded capsules should be dispensed and stored in appropriate child-resistant, tight, light-resistant containers.

Interpreting the prescription order

A prescription order will contain the number of capsules and the amount of drug per capsule, and may or may not give the capsule size to use. The pharmacist should use his or her professional judgment to choose the capsule size based on the patient's age, health status, and ability to swallow solid objects. Generally, the smallest capsule that will hold the desired amount of drug is used. The directions will be in abbreviations, as are most prescription orders, and must be translated into directions appropriate for the patient. The amount of powder in each capsule and the relative concentrations of drug in each capsule must be calculated. The pharmacist must be aware of compatibility of the drug with the excipients when compounding tablets, and should use available resources, such as the United States Pharmacopoeia, journal literature, or the Merck Index, to confirm that the ingredients are compatible.

Calculating the prescription

If the prescription order calls for eight capsules that contain 30 mg of pseudoephedrine HCl, the total amount of powder required to fill eight capsules should be calculated. When using the punch method, a two-capsule overage is recommended in order to ensure that sufficient powder is available to yield the correct number of capsules. So in this example, the calculation would be for 10 capsules. If a #2 capsule shell is used and the diluent is lactose, the total weight of powder per capsule is 350 mg (Table 1). So the total weight of powder required for 10 capsules is 3500 mg or 3.5 g. The amount of pseudoephedrine HCl is 10 x 30 mg = 300 mg. By subtracting the 300 mg from the total of 3500 of pseudoephedrine HCL the pharmacist calculates the quantity of lactose required for the prescription (3500 mg - 300 mg = 3200 mg lactose).

Compounding the product

Compounding a capsule using the punch method is typically done for smaller quantities, due to the enormous amount of time required to precisely fill the proper weight into each capsule shell. Commercial equipment is available for compounding of capsules on a slightly

Compounding and Calculations Review

larger scale, ranging from manual to fully automated. To compound the prescription order using the punch method, the pharmacist must first calculate and weigh out the appropriate amounts of drug and diluents to deliver the desired amount of drug in each capsule. The drug should be mixed by geometric dilution with the diluent using spatulation or using a glass mortar and pestle. Once the powders are thoroughly mixed to make a homogeneous dispersion, the powder should be positioned in a cone shape in the center of a glass pill tile. Gloves should be worn in order to prevent finger printing onto the outer shell walls. Prior to compounding, the empty capsule is weighed and subtracted from the final weight when determining the amount of powder in each capsule or the scale should be zeroed with an empty capsule. The first capsule shell should be opened and the body, which is the narrow half that fits inside the cap, should be removed. Now, with the filling half (body) in hand, place a small amount of powder into the body by dragging it horizontally across the glass pill tile. Then, in a smooth motion, invert the capsule shell and punch it into the powder cone. This will cause the powder to pack tightly into the capsule body. Each capsule (body and cap rejoined) should be weighed after each fill and adjusted to the desired weight by the removal or addition of powder. This procedure should be followed for each capsule in the prescription order.

Tablets

Description of delivery system

Tablets are solid dosage forms prepared by the compression of powders using a tablet press or small-scale press. The formulation is designed to fulfill certain characteristics that improve bioavailability and patient compliance. Tablet hardness, disintegration time, friability, taste, color, stability, and size are all attributes of a tablet that must be optimized during the formulation process. Most pharmacies do not manufacture tablets on such a small scale. However, some compounding pharmacies do have the capability to manufacture tablets and should have formulations available that are optimized based on tablet properties. The choice of tablets over capsules would be one of judgment based on the patient's use of this medication, such as effervescent or chewable tablets, or as will be discussed further, the manufacture of lozenges and troches using a tablet press.

Interpreting the prescription order

The prescription order for tablets presented by the patient includes the ingredients and the number of tablets to be dispensed. It is important when making tablets that the ingredients used be physically and chemically compatible. The pharmacist must be aware of compatibility of the drug with the excipients when compounding tablets, and should use available resources to confirm that the ingredients are compatible.

Calculating the prescription

The process for calculating prescription orders for tablets is similar to that used for capsules. The number of tablets and the weight of each tablet should be multiplied to get the total quantity of powder needed. An overage amount should be added to ensure that sufficient powder is available for the prescription order. The concentration of drug in each tablet must be equal and precise. Because the tablet dimensions, size, and fill amount will vary according to the tooling and equipment, the tablet weight must be calculated for the specific apparatus used.

Compounding the product

The drug should be mixed by geometric dilution with the diluent and other ingredients such that it is homogenously mixed. Then powder is loaded into the tableting machine and compressed to form the tablets. The compression force used affects the hardness of the tablet, which in turn affects the disintegration and dissolution properties of the tablet. The pharmacist should be aware of this and should consult the available literature to ensure proper tableting technique.

Troches and Lozenges

Description of delivery system

Lozenges, which are synonymous with troches, are tablet-shaped solid dosage forms that are held in the oral cavity and allowed to slowly dissolve. They can be used to deliver topical antifungals to the mouth, or as a method to deliver systemic medications, such as hormones. Lozenges can be made by direct compression on a tablet press or by melting the components and adding them to a mold. The latter method is most useful to a compounding pharmacist, due to the lack of equipment for manufacturing tablets in most pharmacies. When melting pharmaceuticals, the pharmacist should be aware of the effect elevated temperatures have on drug stability.

Interpreting the prescription order

Prescriptions for lozenges include the ingredients (drug and excipients) and the number of lozenges to be made. The actual carrier or dissolving ingredient (e.g., sorbitol) used may vary and the choice is usually made by the pharmacist. The decision for this should be made based on literature citations or on previous formulations. If the drug being compounded is known to be bitter, a taste modifier should be added to improve patient compliance.

Compounding and Calculations Review

Calculating the prescription

The calculations involved are the same as discussed for capsules and tablets. However, rather than being based on the capsule or tablet, calculations are usually based on the size of the mold used for compounding.

Compounding the product

Lozenges or troches can be manufactured by the tableting method or by melting the ingredients together and pouring them into a mold. The tableting method is advantageous for heat labile drugs and for large-scale production. For most pharmacies, the melting technique is more convenient. The diluent, which is the carrier in this case, is melted to a molten state at which time the drug and other excipients are added and mixed. The molten mixture of drug and excipients are then poured into lozenge molds, which are similar to suppository molds, and then allowed to cool to room temperature to form the hardened final molded product.

Pharmaceutical Liquids

Important Terms

Solution – a liquid preparation containing one or more chemical substances molecularly dissolved in a suitable solvent or mixture of mutually miscible solvents

Suspension – a system consisting of a solid dispersed in a liquid, in which the particles are typically larger than 5 microns

Agglomeration – the clumping of particles in air or liquid medium as an attempt to increase particle size and decrease the surface free energy

Aseptic – free of pathogenic microorganisms

Solubility – the amount of substance that can be dissolved in a given amount of solvent

Solutions

Description of delivery system

A solution is a liquid preparation containing one or more chemical substances dissolved in a suitable solvent or mixture of mutually miscible solvents. Solutions can be used for oral, topical, and parenteral administration. Depending on the composition, solutions may be classified as syrups, elixirs, aromatic waters, tinctures, or fluid extracts. A syrup typically contains sucrose as a sweetening agent, the most common being Syrup NF which is 85% (w/v) sucrose solution. Elixirs contain various amounts of ethanol as a cosolvent, whereas aromatic waters contain aromatic compounds with or without alcohol (also known as spirits). Solutions that are made from drugs extracted from plants or other substances are termed tinctures or fluid extracts. When a solid or liquid is dissolved into another liquid, the solubility of the substance must be considered. If the level of material added to the solution exceeds the solubility, the substance may precipitate to form a suspension or phase separate in the case of liquid-in-liquid solutions.

Specialty excipients for compounding

Liquid Vehicle	Composition	pH	Alcohol Content (%)
Aromatic Elixir NF	Essential oils, syrup, alcohol, purified water	5.5-6.0	21-23
Compound Benzaldehyde Elixir NF	Benzaldehyde, flavoring, alcohol, purified water	6.0	0
Peppermint Water NF	Peppermint oil, purified water	-	0
Sorbitol Solution USP	65% D-sorbitol, purified water	-	0
Suspension Structured Vehicle NF	Potassium sorbate, xanthan gum, anhydrous citric acid, sucrose, purified water	-	0
Sugar-Free Suspension Structured Vehicle NF	Xanthan gum, saccharin sodium, potassium sorbate, citric acid, sorbitol, manitol, glycerin, purified water	-	0
Syrup NF	85% sucrose, purified water	-	0
Xanthan Gum Solution NF	Xanthan gum, methylparaben, propylparaben, purified water	-	0
Acacia Syrup	Acacia, sodium benzoate, vanilla tincture, sucrose, purified water	5.0	0

Compounding and Calculations Review

Liquid Vehicle	Composition	pH	Alcohol Content (%)
Cherry Syrup	Cherry juice, sucrose, alcohol, purified water	3.5-4.0	1-2
Citric Acid Syrup	Citric acid, syrup, lemon tincture	-	<1
Cocoa Syrup	Cocoa, sucrose, liquid glucose, glycerin, sodium chloride, vanillin, sodium benzoate, purified water	-	0
Raspberry Syrup	Raspberry juice, sucrose, alcohol, purified water	3.0	1-2
Tolu Syrup	Tolu balsam tincture, magnesium carbonate, sucrose, purified water	5.5	2-4
Wild Cherry Syrup	Wild cherry powder, sucrose, glycerin, alcohol, purified water	4.5	1-2
Ora-Sweet Syrup Vehicle	Citrus-berry flavoring, glycerin, sorbitol, sucrose, sodium phosphate, citric acid, potassium sorbate, methylparaben, purified water	4.0-4.5	0
Ora-Sweet SF Syrup Vehicle	Citrus-berry flavoring, glycerin, sorbitol, sodium saccharin, Xanthan gum, glycerin, sodium phosphate, citric acid, potassium sorbate, methylparaben, purified water	4.0-4.4	0

Interpreting the prescription order

Determination of the type of liquid desired by the physician is the first step in interpreting prescription orders for liquids. The components of the solution should be listed as % w/v, % v/v or g/mL. Depending on the availability of solubility data for the ingredients, it should be determined whether the liquid that is made will be a solution or a suspension, each of which have different properties and dispensing instructions. As previously stated, if the concentration of an ingredient is above the solubility, it will precipitate to form a suspension.

Calculating the prescription

The calculations used to compound solutions involve converting directions, given in parts or in percents, into the actual amount needed for the prescription. Compounding directions typically give the amounts needed for an arbitrary volume, which may be different from the actual amount directed to be dispensed. The pharmacist must convert (reduce or enlarge) the amount needed for the prescription from the amount specified in the directions. This can involve proportions or if the quantity is given in a percentage, it can be calculated directly. Any stock solutions used must be accounted for in the final volume calculations. For example, if the prescription called for 1 gram of lidocaine HCl and a stock solution containing lidocaine HCL 100 mg/mL was available, then the pharmacist would need to account for and remove the 10-mL volume containing the lidocaine HCl from the water used to fill to the final volume.

Compounding the product

When compounding a solution, the drug particles must be dissolved in a suitable solvent for the application in which it will be used. Solutions containing high alcoholic components should not be used for oral administration. Also, the solubility of the ingredients should be taken into account when choosing the solvent. The components should be mixed with the solvent in a beaker or mortar, and, in some cases, filtered prior to dispensing in order to prevent particulate material from being incorporated into the final preparation.

Suspensions

Description of delivery system

Suspensions are liquid dosage forms that contain solid materials dispersed in a liquid vehicle. Suspensions are useful for chemically unstable drugs. This type of delivery system allows for the administration of medicines that are unstable in solution, as well as to patients unable to take solid dosage forms. Also, the dose of drug can be precisely titrated to deliver the required amount. Pediatric patients as well as the elderly benefit from this type of delivery system. Poor tasting or bitter compounds are more difficult to formulate into a suspension, but the problem can be overcome by the addition of a taste modifier. The suspension should be formulated to prevent agglomeration and caking (formation of a solid pellet at the base of the container) of the suspended drug particles.

Compounding and Calculations Review

Interpreting the prescription order

A prescription order for a suspension will contain the desired ingredients (drug, excipients, and taste modifier) that should be added to the suspension formulation. Typically, the pharmacist is required to formulate a commercially available solid dosage form (e.g., tablet or capsule) into a suspension. The pharmacist must exercise caution to choose ingredients that are known to be compatible with the drug substance. If unsure, the pharmacist must consult the literature or other sources for stability and compatibility information (e.g., USP, Merck Index, journal literature).

Calculating the prescription

The prescription is calculated based on the total volume of the prescription. If commercially available tablets are used, the volume used should be proportional to the number of tablets used. For example, if tablets containing 5 mg of active drugs are available and the prescription asks for 1 mg/mL, the volume used should be in multiples of 5 mL, since it would take one whole tablet for every 5 mL. Partially divided tablets should not be used, since it is unknown what the actual quantity of drug is in each subdivided part of the tablet.

Compounding the product

Following the selection of an appropriate suspension formulation and completion of the calculations, the pharmacist can begin to combine and mix the ingredients to make the suspension. This is typically done using a mortar and pestle to disperse and thoroughly mix the ingredients. First, the powder or tablets (pulverized first in a ceramic mortar) should be added to the mortar and pestle and wetted with a levigating agent, such as propylene glycol. The suspending agent along with the liquid vehicle (usually water or flavored syrup) is added and mixed with the solid ingredients. The suspension is poured into the dispensing container and the mortar and pestle is rinsed with a portion of the water in order to ensure complete mass transfer of the drug substance. The suspension is brought to volume with the liquid vehicle.

Sterile Solutions

Description of delivery system

Sterile solutions are used for injectable, ophthalmic and nasal/pulmonary delivery of drug substances. Solutions for intravenous administration must be in solution, while intramuscular, subcutaneous, ophthalmic, and nasal/pulmonary preparations can be administered as either a suspension or solution. When compounding prescriptions, it is difficult to prepare sterile suspensions because of the sterile filtering step that is required to make the preparation sterile that will collect the suspension particles on the filter membrane. Suspensions are reserved for pre-manufactured products that are reconstituted by the pharmacist. Sterile compounding is performed using a laminar flow hood or other suitable equipment to ensure an aseptic environment. The tonicity of the preparation is important when manufacturing injectable, ophthalmic and nasal/pulmonary preparations. If the tonicity is different from physiologic osmolarity, the patient may experience tissue irritation and pain at the site of administration. Therefore, the pharmacist must calculate the tonicity of the preparation and compare it to physiological parameters. Preservatives are used to maintain sterility of the preparation over the expected shelf life. Single-dose preparations do not necessarily require preservatives, but multiple-dose preparations must contain a preservative system. To ensure sterility and to prevent particulate matter within the sterile preparation, the final solution should be filtered through a 0.22-μm sterilizing filter using aseptic processing techniques.

Interpreting the prescription order

The mode of administration will determine whether the preparation should be sterile. Like other solutions, the concentration of ingredients is listed as parts or percentages and must be converted to the actual amounts for the prescribed preparation volume.

Calculating the prescription

The calculations involved for sterile solutions are similar to nonsterile solution calculations. However, injectable or ophthalmic preparations should be formulated at a pH and osmolarity similar to those of the biological fluids which they contact.

Compounding the product

Sterile preparations should be compounded in an approved aseptic environment, preferably in a laminar flow hood. The pharmacist should be trained in aseptic techniques and should be aware of the potential for contamination. Compounding of sterile solutions is similar to nonsterile solutions.

Compounding and Calculations Review

Topical Pharmaceutical Delivery Systems

Ointments

Description of delivery system

Ointments are semisolid preparations consisting of an ointment base with or without the incorporation of a medication. Nonmedicated ointments are often used as protectants, emollients, or lubricants.

Specialty excipients for compounding

Hydrocarbon bases

Hydrocarbon bases, also known as oleaginous bases, have an emollient effect when placed on the skin. They prevent the escape of moisture and because they are hydrophobic in nature, they are difficult to wash from the skin using water. Typically, mineral oil is used as a levigating agent when powdered substances are incorporated into hydrocarbon bases.

Petrolatum, USP, is a purified mixture of semisolid hydrocarbons. It may vary in color from yellowish to light amber and melts between 38°C and 60°C. This product is also known as yellow petrolatum or petroleum jelly.

White petrolatum, USP, has the same composition as petrolatum, USP, but has been decolorized. It has the same chemical attributes and melts within the same range as petrolatum, USP.

Yellow ointment, USP, is a combination of yellow wax and petrolatum, USP. To make 1000 g of this ointment, 50 g of yellow wax is melted and mixed with 950 g of petrolatum, USP to make a uniform mixture.

White ointment, USP, is similar to yellow ointment, USP, but is made from white wax (decolorized yellow wax) and white petrolatum, USP.

Absorption bases

Absorption bases are water-in-oil emulsions that permit the incorporation of aqueous solutions into the base. They are not easily washed from the skin with water because the continuous or external phase is oleaginous and they possess less significant emollient characteristics than hydrocarbon bases. Absorption bases act as adjuncts for the incorporation of aqueous solutions into hydrocarbon bases, synonymous with a co-solvent system. Examples of absorption bases include hydrophilic petrolatum and lanolin, USP.

Water-removable bases

Water-removable bases are oil-in-water emulsions that are easily washed from the skin with water. Because of the higher water content, they are paste-like and able to carry higher amounts of aqueous solutions, compared to oleaginous bases. One example is hydrophilic ointment, USP.

Water-soluble bases

Unlike the previous types of ointment bases described, water soluble-bases do not contain oleaginous components. They are easily washed from the skin and are considered "greaseless" bases. Water-soluble bases are typically used for the incorporation of solid substances into a base. One example is polyethylene glycol ointment, NF.

Interpreting the prescription order

The Latin abbreviation "ung" denotes ointment prescriptions. The pharmacist must note the amount to be dispensed and the relative amounts of each ingredient, usually given on a w/w basis or in parts. The stability (physical and chemical) of the ingredients should be confirmed.

Calculating the prescription

When calculating for ointment prescriptions or other topical solid/semi-solid dosage forms, the pharmacist typically converts from percent w/w to the actual amount of a substance in grams.

Compounding the product

Two methods are available for manufacture of compounded ointments. For most pharmacies, the method of spatulation is the most useful method for dispersing solid materials and other ingredients into an ointment base. A pill tile or ointment slab is used to geometrically dilute and disperse the ingredients into the ointment base. The ingredients are placed in the center of the ointment slab and pre-weighed ointment base is slowly added and mixed with the ingredients, geometrically, until the entire ointment base is added to the mixture. The second method involves heating of the ointment base and addition of the other ingredients into the molten base. This method works well as long as the drug, base and other ingredients are not heat labile. If any of the ingredients are heat sensitive, the first method must be used to disperse the ingredients into the ointment base.

Compounding and Calculations Review

Pastes

Description of delivery system

Pastes contain higher solids content than ointments but are made in a similar manner. They contain the same bases, only in smaller amounts, which make a stiff semisolid base for the delivery of pharmaceutical products. Examples of pastes include oral pastes and topical pastes for the delivery of drugs or other therapeutic agents.

Specialty excipients for compounding

(Refer to Ointments.)

Interpreting the prescription order

(Refer to Ointments.)

Creams

Description of delivery system

Creams are semisolid oil-in-water emulsions containing medicinal substances used for topical administration. They are easily applied and spread effectively over the affected area. Unlike ointments, they are readily washed from the skin with water. Creams may also be used for rectal or vaginal administration because of their high water content.

Lotions

Description of delivery system

Lotions are emulsion systems designed to hydrate the skin, act as an emollient in order to protect the skin, and act as a carrier for drugs. Lotions spread well on the skin and are useful to cover large surface areas of the skin. Emulsions are composed of a water phase and an oil phase that are dispersed, one within the other, either as an oil-in-water or water-in-oil emulsion, where the first term refers to the internal phase and the second term refers to the external phase. The surfactants and the relative amounts of each component determine the type of emulsion formed. Surfactants with a low hydrophilic/lipophilic balance (HLB) will make water-in-oil emulsions whereas surfactants with high HLB values tend to make oil-in-water emulsions. The type of emulsion formed will determine the washability of the lotion from the skin. Oil-in-water emulsions tend to be washed from the skin more easily than water-in-oil emulsions. If a drug is incorporated into the lotion, it should be added to the phase in which it is most soluble, prior to emulsification of the two phases.

Interpreting the prescription order

A prescription for a lotion typically contains the oil and water phases that should be mixed and, if one is needed, the drug substance. The relative amounts of each component are included but must be calculated (reduced or enlarged) for the given amount to be dispensed. The pharmacist must be aware of the properties of emulsions in order to prevent "breaking" of the emulsion, which is an irreversible phase separation of the emulsion.

Compounding the product

To make a lotion, the procedure involves heating the two phases separately to melt the components and mixing them to form the emulsion. The order of addition is important to ensure proper emulsion preparation. To make an emulsion, the oil-soluble components are added together and melted and, in a separate beaker, the water-soluble components are mixed and heated a few degrees above the temperature of the oil phase. The internal phase is added to the external phase with mixing. The mixture must be stirred vigorously until the mixture cools and the emulsion is formed and set. If the stirring is not sufficient, the emulsion may break.

Gels

Description of delivery system

Gels are water-based semisolid materials that may contain medicinal substances for topical, vaginal, rectal, and ophthalmologic administration. With the addition of a gelling agent, the viscosity of the aqueous solution increases due to cross-linking of the polymeric molecules. Gels can contain cosolvents such as alcohol or propylene glycol. Because of the high water content, they require the addition of a preservative such as a paraben or chlorhexidine gluconate.

Compounding and Calculations Review

Specialty excipients for compounding

Pluronic™ (poloxamer) makes a thermoplastic gel that when dissolved in water has a low viscosity at low temperatures (e.g., 5° C), but the viscosity increases with increasing temperature (e.g., 25° C). It can be purchased in various grades that differ in molecular weight and gelling properties.

Carbopol™ (carbomer) is a solid polymer of acrylic acid that is a weak acid. When dispersed in a suitable solvent and neutralized with a base (e.g., sodium hydroxide or triethanolamine [TEA]), cross-linking between the polymeric chains causes gelation. Carbopol is available in various molecular weight distributions that have different properties.

Interpreting the prescription order

Prescriptions involving gels typically list the active ingredient and some type of gelling material. Because not all gels are the same, and because the intended use can affect the choice of gelling agent, the pharmacist must ensure that the proper gelling agent be used for the specific application. Occasionally the gelling agent is not listed and the pharmacist must decide on the appropriate type and level. The ingredients may be listed on a percentage w/w or parts basis that must be converted to the amount needed for the prescription.

Calculating the prescription

The prescription order for gels is calculated similarly to ointments and creams, since the final product is a semi-solid. However, during the compounding, some of the components are liquid, so proper volumes (based on density) are used for the weights given.

Compounding the product

Following the calculations, the appropriate weights and/or volumes of the ingredients should be mixed in order to ensure homogeneity. Depending on the gelling agent used, the mode of gelation will determine the final step. For Pluronic gels, the final solution need only be allowed to warm to room temperature to increase the viscosity of the gel. The pharmacist should ensure that the preparation has fully gelled prior to dispensing. Since other ingredients were added to the preparation, the dilution effect can prevent the gel from solidifying at room temperature and may require additional amounts of the gelling agent Pluronic. When Carbopol is used as the gelling agent, the final step involves neutralization with a base to cause the cross-linking and gelation. The pharmacist should use caution when adding the neutralizing agent such that the gel formed is homogenous in nature and lacks clumps from poor mixing. Adding an overage of neutralizing agent, effectively alkalinizing the mixture, will cause the gel to break, resulting in a watery mass. Therefore, the neutralizing agent should be added just to the point of gelation.

Aqueous Nasal Sprays

Description of delivery system

Development and testing of aqueous nasal sprays must comply with specific guidelines as described by the Food and Drug Administration. Nasal spray solutions or suspensions are used for administration of topical or systemic medications via the nasal route. Because of their route of administration, it is important that the drug be sterile and be applied in a suitable fashion by a calibrated nasal spray pump. For the most part, the guidelines regarding nasal sprays regulate performance of the pump and will not be discussed here. The contents of the nasal spray solution are typically filtered through a sterilizing membrane prior to dispensing, to prevent microbial contamination. Preservatives can also be added for prevention of microbial growth.

Interpreting the prescription order

The prescription order lists the ingredients, the mode of administration, and the dose of each administration. The pump used will determine the exact volume expelled during each spray that will be used in the calculations. Similar to solutions, the relative amounts of each ingredient will typically be listed as parts or percentages.

Calculating the prescription

Aqueous nasal sprays should be calculated on a per-spray basis or per-actuation basis. Many of the commercially available pumps dispense or spray 100 mL per dose, but the overall dose delivered through-the-valve must be calculated prior to dispensing. For potent or low dose drugs, the dose delivered through-the-valve should be calculated for a given pump lot prior to compounding, to ensure the most precise dosing. The dose delivered through-the-valve is calculated by taking an initial weight measurement of the filled and primed nasal spray (using water), spraying it 10 times followed by a second weight measurement. By subtracting the final weight from the initial weight and dividing by ten, the dose in "µg per actuation" is calculated. If the density of the solution is known, then the volumetric dose can also be calculated. For most aqueous preparations, the density is assumed to be 1 and the µg per actuation is assumed to be µL sprayed.

Compounding the product

The product is compounded similarly to sterile preparations. The final compounded product should be filtered through a 0.22-µm sterile filter.

Compounding and Calculations Review

Suppositories

Rectal suppositories

Description of delivery system

Rectal suppositories are cylindrical or cone shaped solid dosage forms that are intended to be inserted into the rectum for topical or systemic delivery of medications. Patients who are vomiting or are unable to take oral medications may benefit from this type of delivery route. Rectal suppositories are designed to either melt or dissolve in the rectal vault and release the medication to either be absorbed across the rectal membrane or exhibit a local effect on the membrane. The suppository base used will determine the release mechanism.

Specialty excipients for compounding

The excipients used for the manufacture of suppositories are the suppository bases along with a lubricant for the suppository mold. The lubricant is typically of an opposite hydrophilicity as the suppository base. Some common bases and lubricants are listed below.

Oleaginous bases

Cocoa Butter, NF is a triglyceride that melts between 30-36°C, so therefore, melts at body temperature, but is a solid at room temperature. However, cocoa butter exhibits several polymorphs or different crystalline forms that will display different melting behavior and rate. If cocoa butter is quickly heated well above the minimum melting temperature, the resulting crystal will be the metastable crystal, also known as the α crystal, which has a lower melting point than the original crystal (β form) and may not solidify at room temperature. Therefore, it is important to slowly melt the cocoa butter. Also, the addition of other substances, such as drugs, may cause a melting point depression of the base. This can be alleviated by the addition of substances like cetyl esters wax or beeswax to increase the temperature of solidification of the cocoa butter. Witepsol is an oleaginous suppository base consisting of triglyceride esters, saturated fatty acids and mono- and diglycerides that has a melting point in the range of 40-45°C. Witepsol will not melt as fast during the insertion of the suppository, which is beneficial to the patient.

Water-soluble bases

Polyethylene glycol is designed to dissolve in the fluids of the rectum or vagina rather than melt. Because of this, the melting point of the suppository is well above body temperature. Furthermore, the suppository does not melt during handling and insertion.

Lubricants

Propylene glycol is useful for the lubrication of molds when using oleaginous bases. Mineral oil is useful for the lubrication of suppository molds when using water-soluble bases.

Interpreting the prescription order

The prescription will call for a certain amount of drug to be contained in each suppository. The calculations must take into account the size of the suppository mold and the amount of drug contained in each suppository. The size of the mold or the amount of base needed for each suppository may vary between pharmacies and even within pharmacies that have several molds. The mold should be calibrated to ensure that the pharmacist knows the amount of material needed for each type of suppository base. When dispensing to a patient, the directions should include the method for insertion as well as a statement to unwrap the suppository or remove it from its primary packaging.

Calculating the prescription

The number of suppositories multiplied by the amount needed for each suppository is calculated. An overage amount of two suppositories is recommended in case there is some waste and to ensure enough material during manufacture. A typical mold can make 10-12 suppositories, so if a prescription called for 8 suppositories containing 10 mg of sumatriptan, the total amount of drug needed is 100 mg (assuming an overage of 2 suppositories). If the suppository mold holds 2 g of cocoa butter per suppository, the total amount of cocoa butter would be 10 x 2 g = 20 g - 100 mg (sumatriptan) = 19.9 g of cocoa butter.

Compounding the product

Using the previous example, the cocoa butter and drug are weighed. The cocoa butter is slowly heated to near 40°C with stirring. Once the base is melted, the drug is added slowly with mixing to disperse. After the mold has been lubricated with propylene glycol, the cocoa butter/drug dispersion is slowly poured into the mold, making sure each mold is filled completely, and allowed to cool. Once cooled to room temperature, the excess cocoa butter is scraped from the mold and the mold taken apart to release the suppositories. The finished suppositories are wrapped in a suitable primary wrap (aluminum foil) and dispensed. Plastic molds are also available for preparation and dispensing. Patients must be advised to unwrap the suppositories prior to insertion.

Compounding and Calculations Review

Vaginal suppositories

Description of delivery system

Vaginal suppositories are similar to rectal suppositories in shape and function. However, they are typically designed to dissolve in the vagina where the drug is released to exhibit a local effect, rather than a systemic effect. They are made in a similar fashion to rectal suppositories but the suppository bases may differ because of the physiologic differences between the rectum and the vagina. Diseases, such as yeast infections, bacterial infections, and many others are commonly treated with vaginal suppositories. Also, contraceptive vaginal suppositories are used that contain spermicidal agents, such as nonoxynol-9.

Parenteral Dosage Forms

Important Terms

Subcutaneous injection (SC) – administration below the skin in the subcutaneous region.

Intramuscular Injection (IM) – administration into the muscular tissue. Typically to the arm, thigh, or buttocks.

Intraarterial Injections (IA) – administration directly into arterial blood vessels.

Intrathecal Injections (IT) – administration into the space surrounding the spinal cord.

Intracardiac Injections (IC) – administration directly into the heart.

Intravenous Injection (IV) – injection into venous blood vessels which is the most common form of parenteral administration.

Aseptic – lacking organisms or biological materials which may cause local infection or sepsis when injected directly into the blood stream.

Aseptic Technique – a technique utilized by pharmacists to compound sterile parenteral medications that minimizes the introduction of biological materials such as bacteria.

Compounding and Calculations Review

Questions

Powders

1. Example prescription order:

   Tolnaftate 1% foot powder
   Tolnaftate 1% w/w
   Zinc oxide 5% w/w
   Talc 20% w/w
   Fragrance 3 gtt
   Corn starch qs
   Mft pulv DTD 20 g
   Sig: Apply pulv to feet AD bid for rash

   How often should this prescription be administered?
   A. Twice daily
   B. Three times daily
   C. Four times daily
   D. Every other day
   E. Every 2 hours

2. How many grams of corn starch are needed to complete the prescription?
   A. 20 grams
   B. 10 grams
   C. 14.8 grams
   D. 7.4 grams
   E. 1.48 grams

3. How many grams of corn starch are needed if the prescription called for 30 grams to be dispensed?
   A. 22.2 grams
   B. 2.22 grams
   C. 4.44 grams
   D. 30 grams
   E. 7.88 grams

4. How many grams of tolnaftate are needed if the prescription called for 30 grams to be dispensed?
   A. 3 grams
   B. 0.3 grams
   C. 0.03 grams
   D. 30 grams
   E. 20 grams

5. How many parts tolnaftate are there contained in the total mixture?
   A. 1 part tolnaftate per 200 parts mixture
   B. 1 part tolnaftate per 100 parts mixture
   C. 1 part tolnaftate per 300 parts mixture
   D. 1 part tolnaftate per 50 parts mixture
   E. 1 part tolnaftate per 99 parts mixture

6. Which of the following auxiliary labels should be included with the prescription?
   A. Shake well
   B. Not to be taken by mouth
   C. For the ear
   D. For rectal use only
   E. For the eye

7. Example prescription order:

   Atropine sulfate   1.4 mg
   Blue tracer dye   1.4 mg
   Sodium bicarbonate qs 10 g
   Mft: pulv   DTD 300 g
   Sig: 2 tsp po for procedure

   What quantity of atropine is required for this prescription?
   A. 1.4 mg
   B. 1400 mg
   C. 42 g
   D. 0.42 g
   E. 0.042 g

8. How many grams of atropine are administered with each dose?
   A. 1.4 g
   B. 0.0014 g
   C. 4.2×10^{-6} g
   D. 4.2 g
   E. 0.0042 g

9. What is the % w/w of atropine in the prescription?
   A. 1.4%
   B. 2.5%
   C. 3.6%
   D. 0.014%
   E. 0.0014%

10. What is the intended site of administration of this powder?
    A. The right eye
    B. The left eye
    C. Both ears
    D. The left ear
    E. The right ear

11. How often should the prescription be administered?
    A. Three times daily
    B. Twice daily
    C. Four times daily
    D. Every other day
    E. Every 3 hours

12. How many grams of miconazole are needed to prepare the prescription?
    A. 5 grams
    B. 4 grams
    C. 6 grams

Compounding and Calculations Review

D. 3 grams

E. 2 grams

13. How many grams of boric acid powder will be needed to prepare the prescription?

A. 90 grams

B. 95 grams

C. 5 grams

D. 98 grams

E. 15 grams

14. Which of the following auxiliary labels should be included on the prescription label?

A. For external use only

B. Keep in refrigerator

C. Shake well

D. For the ear

E. A and D only

15. How many milligrams of misoprostol are needed to complete this prescription?

Misoprostol 0.0027% mucoadhesive powder

misoprostol   400 μg

Polyethylene oxide   200 mg

HPMC   qs   15 g

Mft: pulv   DTD 30 g

Sig: as directed

A. 800 mg

B. 400 mg

C. 1 mg

D. 0.4 mg

E. 0.8 mg

16. How many grams of misoprostol are required if the prescription calls for 60 g to be dispensed?

A. 0.0016 g

B. 0.016 g

C. 0.08 g

D. 0.8 g

E. 8 g

17. How many grains are to be dispensed for this prescription?

A. 4.6296 gr

B. 46.296 gr

C. 462.96 gr

D. 4629.6 gr

E. 231.48 gr

18. If the specific gravity of this powder was 1.3, how many milliliters would the final preparation occupy?

A. 30 mL

B. 40 mL

C. 39 mL

D. 23.1 mL

E. 231 mL

19. What does the term "pulv" mean on the prescription order?

A. Powder

B. Ointment

C. Tablet

D. Capsule

E. Gel

20. How many parts of misoprostol are there per part of polyethylene oxide?

A. 1 part misoprostol per 250 parts polyethylene oxide

B. 1 part misoprostol per 500 parts polyethylene oxide

C. 1 part misoprostol per 100 parts polyethylene oxide

D. 1 part misoprostol per 750 parts polyethylene oxide

E. 1 part misoprostol per 375 parts polyethylene oxide

21. What is the weight percent of misoprostol in the preparation?

A. 2.7%

B. 0.27%

C. 27%

D. 0.0027%

E. 0.027%

Capsules

1. Example prescription order:

Acetaminophen 160 mg

Chlorpheniramine maleate 2 mg

Pseudoephedrine HCl 10 mg

Lactose qs

Mft caps (#2) DTD: 6

Sig: 1-2 caps po tid prn allergies

If the smallest amount weighable for the balance used to measure the ingredients is 70 mg, which of the following ingredients require the use of an aliquot?

A. Acetaminophen

B. Chlorpheniramine maleate

C. Pseudoephedrine HCl

D. Lactose

E. Pseudoephedrine HCl and chlorpheniramine maleate

2. What weight of acetaminophen is required to fill eight capsules, in grains?

A. 1.98 gr

B. 19.8 gr

C. 198 gr

D. 1980 gr

E. 0.198 gr

3. What weight of pseudoephedrine HCL is required to fill 10 capsules, in grains?

A. 1.54 gr

B. 15.4 gr

C. 0.154 gr

D. 154 gr

E. 1540 gr

4. How many ounces of powder are required for the final preparation, if #2 capsules hold 350 mg lactose?

   A. 0.07 ounces
   B. 0.7 ounces
   C. 7 ounces
   D. 70 ounces
   E. 700 ounces

5. If a #2 capsule holds 350 mg lactose, how many milligrams of lactose are needed for each capsule?

   A. 200 mg
   B. 350 mg
   C. 178 mg
   D. 250 mg
   E. 300 mg

6. What is the percentage w/w of acetaminophen in the preparation?

   A. 45.7%
   B. 22.85%
   C. 30%
   D. 60%
   E. 42.5%

7. How often should this preparation be administered?

   A. Twice daily as needed
   B. Once daily as needed
   C. Three times daily as needed
   D. Four times daily as needed
   E. Every 3 hours

8. Which of the following auxiliary labels should be included on the prescription?

   A. Shake well
   B. Not to be taken by mouth
   C. For external use only
   D. For the ear
   E. None of the above

9. How often should this preparation be administered?

   Dehydroepiandrosterone   50 mg
   Lactose   qs
   Mft: caps (size #2)   DTD: 10
   Sig: 1 capsule po qid

   A. Once daily
   B. Twice daily
   C. Four times daily
   D. Three times daily
   E. Every four hours

10. If a #2 size capsule holds 350 mg of lactose, what is the percentage w/w of dehydroepiandrosterone in each capsule (assuming no overage)?

A. 28%

B. 14.3%

C. 24.6%

D. 30%

E. 22.5%

11. How many grams of lactose will be required to fill this prescription?

   A. 3 grams
   B. 6 grams
   C. 3.5 grams
   D. 7 grams
   E. 1.75 grams

12. How many grams of dehydroepiandrosterone are required to fill 12 capsules?

   A. 600 g
   B. 60 g
   C. 0.6 g
   D. 6 g
   E. 0.06 g

13. How many grains of lactose are required to complete the prescription, if a #2 capsule will hold 350 mg lactose?

   A. 5.4 gr
   B. 5.4×10^4 gr
   C. 46.296 gr
   D. 0.54 gr
   E. 0.054 gr

14. How many parts of dehydroepiandrosterone are there per part of lactose?

   A. 1 part dehydroepiandrosterone per 7 parts lactose
   B. 1 part dehydroepiandrosterone per 6 parts lactose
   C. 1 part dehydroepiandrosterone per 10 parts lactose
   D. 1 part dehydroepiandrosterone per 5 parts lactose
   E. 1 part dehydroepiandrosterone per 4 parts lactose

15. What quantity of lactose is required to complete this prescription?

   Estradiol   1 mg
   Estriol   8 mg
   Estrone   1 mg
   Progesterone   150 mg
   Lactose   qs   280 mg
   Mft: 100 capsules
   Note: 1 capsule shell will hold 280 mg of lactose
   Sig: 1 capsule po bid

   A. 1.2g
   B. 120mg
   C. 12g
   D. 0.012g
   E. 24g

16. What is the concentration (%w/w) of estriol in the capsule formulation?

Compounding and Calculations Review

A. 5.67%
B. 2.23%
C. 2.86%
D. 1.25%
E. 0.029%

17. How many grams of progesterone will be dosed to the patient after 30 days?

A. 8 g
B. 0.9 g
C. 9 g
D. 0.8 g
E. 2.5 g

Tablets

1. Example prescription order:

    Loratadine 10 mg
    Pseudoephedrine HCl 15 mg
    Lactose 100 mg
    Microcrystalline cellulose 24 mg
    Magnesium stearate 1 mg
    Mft: 150 mg tablets DTD: 200
    Sig: 1 tab po tid prn allergies/congestion

    What is the total amount of powder needed, including a 10% overage of powder?

    A. 33 grams
    B. 30.3 grams
    C. 15 grams
    D. 60 grams
    E. 45 grams

2. How often should the product be administered?

    A. Once daily
    B. Twice daily as needed
    C. Three times daily as needed
    D. Every other day as needed
    E. Every 3 hours

3. What percentage strength (w/w) is the pseudoephedrine in each tablet?

    A. 5%
    B. 10%
    C. 1%
    D. 1.5%
    E. 0.1%

4. What weight of pseudoephedrine HCl, in grains, is required to fill the prescription, including a 10% overage?

    A. 46.75 gr
    B. 4.675 gr
    C. 467.5 gr
    D. 46750 gr
    E. 4675 gr

5. What weight of loratadine, in grams, is required to complete the prescription, including a 10% overage?

    A. 2.02 g
    B. 202 g
    C. 2020 g
    D. 0.202 g
    E. 20.2 g

6. What is the ratio strength for loratadine?

    A. 1:2
    B. 1:1.5
    C. 2:1.5
    D. 1:5
    E. 1:0.75

Troches and Lozenges

1. Example prescription order:

    Sodium fluoride 50 mg
    Sorbitol qs
    Mft 10 lozenges (each lozenge mold will hold 2 grams of material)
    Sig: 1 loz bid

    How often should the preparation be administered?

    A. Once daily
    B. Twice daily
    C. Four times daily
    D. Three times daily
    E. Every 2 hours

2. How many grams of sodium fluoride are required to complete the preparation including a 20% overage?

    A. 600 g
    B. 0.60 g
    C. 6.0 g
    D. 60 g
    E. 0.51 g

3. If the specific gravity of the molten material is 0.98, how many milliliters will each mold hold?

    A. 2.04 mL
    B. 20.4 mL
    C. 1.96 mL
    D. 19.6 mL
    E. 0.98 mL

4. How many total grams of sorbitol are needed to complete the preparation?

    A. 20 grams
    B. 19.5 grams
    C. 30 grams
    D. 10 grams
    E. 15 grams

Compounding and Calculations Review

5. What is the amount of sodium fluoride in ___% w/w?

   A. 2.5%
   B. 5%
   C. 10%
   D. 0.25%
   E. 0.025%

Solutions

1. Example prescription order:

   Phenobarbital 20 mg
   Syrup NF 10% v/v
   Glycerin 5% v/v
   Alcohol 5% v/v
   Methylparaben 0.1% w/v
   Propylparaben 0.01% w/v
   Flavor 0.5 gtt
   Water qs 5 mL
   Mft syrup DTD ii oz
   Sig: ii tsp po tid for seizures

   How many milliliters of the preparation will be dispensed?

   A. 30 mL
   B. 15 mL
   C. 60 mL
   D. 120 mL
   E. 45 mL

2. If phenobarbital is available in a 25-mg/mL stock solution, how many milliliters are required to complete the preparation?

   A. 96 mL
   B. 9.6 mL
   C. 0.96 mL
   D. 960 mL
   E. 0.096 mL

3. If the specific gravity of Syrup NF is 1.3, how many grams would be required to complete the preparation?

   A. 4.6 g
   B. 0.46 g
   C. 7.8 g
   D. 0.78 g
   E. 2.3 g

4. How many milliliters should be administered for each dose?

   A. 15 mL
   B. 30 mL
   C. 10 mL
   D. 5 mL
   E. 60 mL

5. How often should the preparation be administered?

   A. Once daily
   B. Twice daily
   C. Three times daily
   D. Four times daily
   E. Every 3 hours

6. How many milligrams of phenobarbital are required to complete the preparation?

   A. 120 mg
   B. 240 mg
   C. 20 mg
   D. 40 mg
   E. 60 mg

7. How many milliliters of Syrup NF are needed to complete the preparation?

   A. 6 mL
   B. 12 mL
   C. 24 mL
   D. 48 ml
   E. 10 mL

8. How many parts of methylparaben are there per part of phenobarbital?

   A. 1 part methylparaben to 4 parts phenobarbital
   B. 1 part methylparaben to 8 parts phenobarbital
   C. 1 part methylparaben to 1 part phenobarbital
   D. 1 part methylparaben to 16 parts phenobarbital
   E. 1 part methylparaben to 10 parts phenobarbital

9. Example prescription order for questions 8, 9, and 10:

   Meperidine HCl 2.5 g
   Phenol 200 mg
   Sterile water for injection qs 100 mL
   Mft nasal solution DTD 15 mL
   Sig: 2 gtt each nostril qid prn

   What is the percentage w/v of meperidine in the preparation?

   A. 0.25%
   B. 2.5%
   C. 5%
   D. 10%
   E. 15%

10. If meperidine is available in a 10% stock solution, how many milliliters are required to complete the preparation?

    A. 3.75 mL
    B. 375 mL
    C. 37.5 mL
    D. 0.375 mL
    E. 0.0376 mL

11. How many milligrams of phenol are needed to compound the preparation?

    A. 15 mg
    B. 200 mg

C. 100 mg

D. 30 mg

E. 5 mg

12. How often should the preparation be administered?

A. Three times daily as needed

B. Four times daily as needed

C. Twice daily as needed

D. Every other day as needed

E. Every 4 hours

13. Which of the following auxiliary labels should be included on the label of the preparation?

A. For the nose

B. Not to be taken by mouth

C. Shake well

D. A and B only

E. None of the above

Suspensions

1. Example prescription order:

Metronidazole 0.24 g

Xanthan gum 0.9% w/v

Water qs 250 mL

Mft susp DTD 100 mL

Sig: Give 0.5 mg/kg body weight bid for intestinal parasite (cat weighs 10.5 lb)

How many grams of xanthan gum are needed for this preparation?

A. 0.9 g

B. 9 g

C. 0.09 g

D. 18 g

E. 2.7 g

2. What is the percentage strength of metronidazole in this preparation?

A. 0.096%

B. 9.6%

C. 4.3%

D. 0.043%

E. 0.43%

3. How many grains of metronidazole are required if the prescription calls for 150 mL to be dispensed?

A. 2.2 gr

B. 0.22 gr

C. 0.0093 gr

D. 9.3 gr

E. 93 gr

4. How often should this preparation be administered?

A. Once daily

B. Twice daily

C. Three times daily

D. Every other day

E. Four times daily

5. How many milligrams of metronidazole are needed for the preparation?

A. 0.96 mg

B. 0.0096 mg

C. 96 mg

D. 0.096 mg

E. 240 mg

6. How many milliliters of the preparation should be administered per dose?

A. 5.37 mL

B. 2.48 mL

C. 4.8 mL

D. 6.2 mL

E. 10 mL

7. Which of the following auxiliary labels should be included with this preparation?

A. Shake well

B. For external use only

C. Not to be taken by mouth

D. A and B only

E. All of the above

8. Example prescription order:

Sulfamerazine 10.0 g

Carbopol 934P 0.5 g

Sodium lauryl sulfate 0.02 g

Sodium saccharin 0.125 g

Methylparaben 0.2% w/v

Propylparaben 0.02% w/v

Citric acid 0.2 g

2 N Sodium hydroxide solution 5.0 mL

Flavor 5 gtt

40% w/v sucrose qs 100 mL

Mft susp DTD 2 oz

Sig: 3/4 tsp po qd for infection prophylaxis for 1 month

How many milliliters of the final suspension will be dispensed?

A. 20 mL

B. 30 mL

C. 60 mL

D. 120 mL

E. 240 mL

9. If the specific gravity of 2 N sodium hydroxide is 1.2, how many grams of 2 N sodium hydroxide are required to complete the preparation?

A. 3.6 g

B. 36 g

C. 2.5 g

Compounding and Calculations Review

D. 25 g
E. 0.25 g

10. If the only sucrose solution available is Syrup NF (85% sucrose), how many parts Syrup NF and water are required to make the 40% sucrose solution?

   A. 4 parts Syrup NF and 4.5 parts water
   B. 6 parts Syrup NF and 6.5 parts water
   C. 1 part Syrup NF and 5 parts water
   D. 3 parts Syrup NF and 2 parts water
   E. 5 parts Syrup NF and 1 part water

11. How many milliliters of drug product are given for each dose?

   A. 2.5 mL
   B. 3.75 mL
   C. 11.25 mL
   D. 15 mL
   E. 5 mL

12. How often is the sulfamerazine suspension intended to be administered?

   A. Once daily
   B. Twice daily
   C. Four times daily
   D. Every other day
   E. Information not given

13. How many milliliters of sodium hydroxide are needed to compound the preparation?

   A. 5 mL
   B. 3 mL
   C. 6 mL
   D. 1.5 mL
   E. 10 mL

14. If the sodium lauryl sulfate is available as a 1% stock solution, how many milliliters are needed to prepare the preparation?

   A. 1.2 mL
   B. 2.4 mL
   C. 4.8 mL
   D. 0.2 mL
   E. 5 mL

Sterile Solutions

1. Example prescription orders:

   Albuterol sulfate 1 mg/mL
   Benzalkonium chloride 0.01% w/v
   Normal saline qs 1.0 mL
   Mft nebulizer solution DTD 20 mL
   Sig: Use 2 milliliters in nebulizer tqid prn wheezing

   How many mg of albuterol sulfate is delivered in each dose?

   A. 1 mg
   B. 2 mg
   C. 4 mg
   D. 8 mg
   E. 15 mg

2. How often should this preparation be administered?

   A. Once daily as needed
   B. Three times daily as needed
   C. Three to four times daily as needed
   D. Four times daily as needed
   E. Every 3-4 hours

3. How many milligrams of benzalkonium chloride are needed for the preparation?

   A. 2 mg
   B. 4 mg
   C. 20 mg
   D. 40 mg
   E. 200 mg

4. If benzalkonium chloride is available as a 0.1% stock solution, how many milliliters of the stock solution are needed to make the prescription?

   A. 5 mL
   B. 2 mL
   C. 4 mL
   D. 6 mL
   E. 10 mL

Ointments

1. Example prescription order:

   Hydrocortisone 0.5% w/w
   Methylparaben 0.1% w/w
   Propylparaben 0.01% w/w
   White petrolatum qs
   Mft ung DTD 10 g
   Sig: Apply to affected area qod for 1 month

   How many grams of hydrocortisone are required in the preparation?

   A. 0.05 g
   B. 0.5 g
   C. 5 g
   D. 15 g
   E. 25 g

2. If the specific gravity of the final ointment preparation is 1.1, how many milliliters would it occupy?

   A. 9.09 mL
   B. 90.9 mL
   C. 11 mL
   D. 1.1 mL
   E. 110 mL

Compounding and Calculations Review

3. How many grams of white petrolatum are required to dilute to the desired weight of 10 grams?

   A. 9.94 g
   B. 99.4 g
   C. 4.97 g
   D. 0.497 g
   E. 14.9 g

4. How many grams of methylparaben are specified in the prescription drug order?

   A. 0.1 g
   B. 0.01 g
   C. 0.2 g
   D. 0.25 g
   E. 0.5 g

5. How often must the preparation be administered?

   A. Four times daily
   B. Three times daily
   C. Once daily
   D. Every other day
   E. Every 12 hours

6. What does the term "ung" mean in the prescription order?

   A. Powder
   B. Cream
   C. Gel
   D. Ointment
   E. Capsule

7. Which of the following auxiliary labels should be included on the prescription label?

   A. Shake well
   B. For external use only
   C. Not to be taken by mouth
   D. All of the above
   E. B and C only

8. Example prescription order:

   Anhydrous lanolin 10% w/w
   Cetyl esters wax 18% w/w
   Yellow wax 30% w/w
   Liquid petrolatum 42% w/w
   Mft ung DTD 15 g
   Sig: Apply to lips q 2-3 h prn chapping

   How often should this preparation be administered?

   A. Once daily
   B. Four times daily as needed
   C. Every 2 to 3 hours as needed
   D. 2 to 3 times per day as needed
   E. Every 8 hours

9. How many grams of anhydrous lanolin are needed for this preparation?

   A. 3 g
   B. 5 g
   C. 1.5 g
   D. 15 g
   E. 30 g

10. How many grams of cetyl esters wax are needed for this preparation?

    A. 27 g
    B. 2.7 g
    C. 18 g
    D. 36 g
    E. 0.27 g

11. How many grams of yellow wax are needed for this preparation?

    A. 18g
    B. 36g
    C. 30g
    D. 9g
    E. 4.5g

12. How many grams of liquid petrolatum are needed for this preparation?

    A. 25.2 g
    B. 12.6 g
    C. 6.3 g
    D. 42 g
    E. 21 g

13. If the specific gravity of liquid petrolatum is 0.89, how many milliliters are used in the preparation?

    A. 14.2 mL
    B. 7.08 mL
    C. 21 mL
    D. 12.6 mL
    E. 0.07 mL

14. How many parts of cetyl esters wax are required in the preparation, compared to liquid petrolatum?

    A. 1 part cetyl esters wax per 10 parts liquid petrolatum
    B. 1 part cetyl esters wax per 4.66 parts liquid petrolatum
    C. 1 part cetyl esters wax per 2.33 parts liquid petrolatum
    D. 1 part cetyl esters wax per 5.6 parts liquid petrolatum
    E. 1 part cetyl esters wax per 2.5 parts liquid petrolatum

15. Which of the following auxiliary labels should be included on the prescription label?

    A. Shake well
    B. For external use only
    C. Not to be taken by mouth
    D. All of the above
    E. B and C only

Compounding and Calculations Review

Pastes

1. Example prescription order:

    Zinc oxide ointment 53 g
    White petrolatum 17 g
    Mineral oil 25 g
    White Wax 5 g
    Mft dtd 30 g
    Sig: apply to affected area qid prn

    What is the amount of zinc oxide ointment needed for the preparation?

    A.   53 g
    B.   15.9 g
    C.   31.8 g
    D.   60 g
    E.   30 g

2. If zinc oxide ointment contains 20% zinc oxide and 15% mineral oil in white petrolatum, how many total grams of white petrolatum are contained in the preparation?

    A.   15.44 g
    B.   1.544 g
    C.   154.4 g
    D.   27.34 g
    E.   2.734 g

3. What is the amount of white petrolatum needed for the preparation?

    A.   10 g
    B.   17 g
    C.   34 g
    D.   5.1 g
    E.   10.2 g

4. If the specific gravity of mineral oil is 0.89, how many milliliters are needed for the preparation?

    A.   10 mL
    B.   25 mL
    C.   8.4 mL
    D.   28.1 mL
    E.   15 mL

5. How many grams of white wax are needed for the preparation?

    A.   3 g
    B.   5 g
    C.   1.5 g
    D.   10 g
    E.   15 g

6. How many parts white wax is there, compared to zinc oxide ointment?

    A.   1 part white wax per 5 parts zinc oxide ointment
    B.   1 part white wax per 10.6 parts zinc oxide ointment
    C.   1 part white wax per 20.4 parts zinc oxide ointment
    D.   1 part white wax per 15 parts zinc oxide ointment
    E.   1 part white wax per 1 part zinc oxide ointment

Creams

1. Example prescription order:

    Cetyl esters wax 125 g
    Yellow wax 100 g
    Mineral oil 560 g
    Sodium borate 5 g
    Water qs 1000 g
    Mft: cream DTD 15 g
    Sig: apply to hands q 2-3 h prn dryness

    If the density of the cream is 1.1 g/mL, how many milliliters will be dispensed to the patient?

    A.   0.22 mL
    B.   909 mL
    C.   13.6 mL
    D.   20 mL
    E.   30 mL

2. If a 5% sodium borate stock solution in water is available, how many milliliters are required?

    A.   2 mL
    B.   1.5 mL
    C.   3 mL
    D.   15 mL
    E.   2.5 mL

3. How often should this prescription be administered?

    A.   Every 4 hours
    B.   Twice daily as needed
    C.   Five times daily as needed
    D.   Two to three times daily as needed
    E.   Every 2-3 hours as needed

4. How many grams of cetyl esters wax are required to make the product?

    A.   1.875 g
    B.   2 g
    C.   5 g
    D.   5.245 g
    E.   125 g

5. What is the amount of cetyl esters wax required, in % w/w?

    A.   5%
    B.   10%
    C.   12.5%
    D.   15%
    E.   20%

6. If the density of mineral oil is 0.89 g/mL, how many milliliters will be added to make this preparation?

A. 8 mL
B. 10 mL
C. 9.4 mL
D. 15 mL
E. 630 mL

7. How many parts of cetyl esters wax are in the preparation?

A. 1 part cetyl esters wax per 100 parts cream
B. 1 part cetyl esters wax per 8 parts cream
C. 1 part cetyl esters wax per 10 parts cream
D. 1 part cetyl esters wax per 1 part cream
E. 1 part cetyl esters wax per 20 parts cream

Lotions

1. Example prescription order:

Dimethicone 0.75 g
Cetyl alcohol 1.00 g
Petrolatum 3.00 g
Stearic acid 4.50 g
Mineral oil 6.00 g
Propylparaben 0.05 g
Glycerin 5.00 g
TEA 1.25 g
MgAL silicate 0.50 g
Methylparaben 0.10 g
Lactic acid 0.50 g
Water qs 100 g
Mft lotion DTD 15 g
Sig: Apply to face bid ud. Discontinue if redness occurs.

If the specific gravity of the final preparation is 1.2, how many milliliters will the lotion occupy?

A. 12.5 mL
B. 18 mL
C. 1.25 mL
D. 125 mL
E. 180 mL

2. If lactic acid is available in a 25-mg/mL stock solution in water, how many milliliters of the stock solution are required?

A. 3 mL
B. 4 mL
C. 3.5 mL
D. 5 mL
E. 10 mL

3. What percent lactic acid is included in this preparation, in w/w?

A. 0.25%
B. 0.5%
C. 0.75%
D. 1%
E. 2%

4. How many parts of methylparaben are required compared to lactic acid?

A. 1 part methylparaben per 2 parts lactic acid
B. 1 part methylparaben per 4 parts lactic acid
C. 1 part methylparaben per 10 parts lactic acid
D. 1 part methylparaben per 5 parts lactic acid
E. 1 part methylparaben per 20 parts lactic acid

5. If the specific gravity of mineral oil is 0.89, how many milliliters are needed for compounding this prescription drug order?

A. 3 mL
B. 5 mL
C. 1.01 mL
D. 2.37 mL
E. 10 mL

Gels

1. Example prescription order:

Capsaicin 20 mg
Methylparaben 50 mg
Carbomer 934P 1.0 g
Ethanol (95%) 40 mL
Triethanolamine 4-5 gtts
Water 60 mL
Mft gel DTD 15 g
Sig: Apply to hands qod prn arthritis pain

What is the concentration of capsaicin in % w/w?

A. 0.4%
B. 0.133%
C. 0.02%
D. 0.05%
E. 0.5%

2. If methylparaben is available as a 1.25% stock solution, in ethanol, how many milliliters are required?

A. 5 mL
B. 3 mL
C. 4 mL
D. 6 mL
E. 8 mL

3. If the SAW on the balance used is 70 mg and a 10-mL graduated cylinder is available, which of the following procedures could be used to measure the capsaicin?

A: Dissolve 80 mg capsaicin in 4 mL ethanol and take 2 mL of that solution to add to the preparation.
B: Dissolve 60 mg capsaicin in 8 mL ethanol and take 3 mL of that solution to add to the preparation.
C: Dissolve 100 mg capsaicin in 5 mL ethanol and take 3 mL of that solution to add to the preparation.
D: Dissolve 100 mg capsaicin in 10 mL ethanol and take 2 mL of that solution to add to the preparation.

Compounding and Calculations Review

E. Dissolve 50 mg capsaicin in 4 mL ethanol and take 0.5 mL of that solution to add to the preparation.

4. If the dropper used to add the TEA is calibrated to 20 drops/mL, how many milliliters are added if 5 drops are used?
    A. 2.5 mL
    B. 0.25 mL
    C. 4 mL
    D. 0.4 mL
    E. 25 mL

5. How often should this prescription be administered?
    A. Four times daily as needed
    B. Every other day as needed
    C. Twice daily as needed
    D. Three times daily
    E. Once daily

6. Example prescription order:

    Scopolamine HBr 0.3% w/v
    Methylparaben 0.1% w/v
    Poloxamer (20% w/w) qs 10 mL
    Mft gel DTD 3 x 0.1 mL/syringe
    Sig: Apply contents of one syringe behind ear 1 h before travel ud.

    How many milligrams of scopolamine HBr are included in this preparation?
    A. 0.2 mg
    B. 1 mg
    C. 0.9 mg
    D. 0.25 mg
    E. 0.5 mg

7. If the specific gravity of the final preparation is 1.2, how many grams are applied behind the ear?
    A. 0.12 g
    B. 0.24 g
    C. 0.083 g
    D. 0.83 g
    E. 1.2 g

8. If poloxamer is available as a 30% solution, how many parts of poloxamer 30% and water are required to make the 20% poloxamer?
    A. 1 part water and 2 parts 30% poloxamer
    B. 1 part water and 3 parts 30% poloxamer
    C. 2 parts water and 5 parts 30% poloxamer
    D. 4 parts water and 2 parts 30% poloxamer
    E. 1 part water and 6 parts 30% poloxamer

9. How many milligrams of methylparaben are included in this preparation?
    A. 0.2 mg
    B. 0.4 mg

C. 0.5 mg
D. 0.3 mg
E. 0.1 mg

10. What does "ud" mean, as stated in the patient directions?
    A. Both ears
    B. The left ear
    C. As directed
    D. Before lunch
    E. After dinner

Aqueous Nasal Sprays

1. Example prescription order:

    Dihydroergotamine mesylate 0.25 g
    Ethanol, 95% 2.00 mL
    Glycerin 5.00 mL
    Methylparaben 0.20 g
    Sterile water for injection qs 100 mL
    Mft metered nasal spray DTD 30 mL
    Sig: sprays 2 each nostril qd

    If ethanol is available in 100% and 50% solutions, how many milliliters of 50% ethanol solution must be mixed with 100% ethanol to make 1 L of the 95% ethanol?
    A. 100 mL
    B. 900 mL
    C. 300 mL
    D. 250 mL
    E. 500 mL

2. Methylparaben is available as a 3% stock solution in ethanol, how many milliliters are needed to complete the preparation?
    A. 2 mL
    B. 5 mL
    C. 2.4 mL
    D. 1 mL
    E. 8 mL

3. What is the percentage of dihydroergotamine, in w/v?
    A. 0.3%
    B. 0.2%
    C. 0.25%
    D. 0.15%
    E. 0.10%

4. If the density of glycerin is 0.92, how many grams of glycerin will be needed for this preparation?
    A. 1.38 g
    B. 1.4 g
    C. 3 g
    D. 2.5 g
    E. 2 g

Compounding and Calculations Review

5. If after 10 sprays using the nasal pump there is a loss in weight of 2.5 mg, what is the dose delivered through the valve (DDV), in mL (assuming a specific gravity of 1)?

   A. 25 mL
   B. 2.5 mL
   C. 0.25 mL
   D. 250 mL
   E. 0.025 mL

6. Using the DDV calculated in the question above (#5), how many mg of Dihydroergotamine mesylate are delivered with each dose?

   A. 0.01875 mg
   B. 1.875 mg
   C. 0.1875 mg
   D. 62.5 mg
   E. 0.0625 mg

7. Morphine sulfate 200 mg

   Naltrexone 2 mg

   0.9% sodium chloride injection qs 100 mL

   Nft: Nasal spray 20 mL

   Sig: 1 actuation each nostril q4h prn pain

   Before compounding the above prescription, 20 mL of water was added to the aqueous pump and primed. The weight of the primed nasal spray was 30 g. After 10 actuations of the nasal spray, the weight was 28.4 g. Based on this information, what is the dose of morphine delivered through the valve (density of water is 1)?

   A. 3.2 mg/actuation
   B. 320 mcg/actuation
   C. 640 mcg/actuation
   D. 32 mg/actuation
   E. 460 mcg/actuation

8. Before compounding of the above prescription, 20 mL of ethanol (density is 0.8 g/mL) was added to the aqueous pump and primed. The weight of the primed nasal spray was 30 g. After 10 actuations of the nasal spray, the weight was 29.1 g. Based on this information, what is the dose of naltrexone delivered through the valve?

   A. 2.25 mcg/actuation
   B. 2.25 mg/actuation
   C. 1.8 mcg/actuation
   D. 1.8 mg/actuation
   E. 225 mcg/actuation

9. Assuming that the volume of water delivered through the valve is 115 μL, what is the maximum dose of morphine that is delivered per day?

   A. 27.6 mg
   B. 2.76 mg
   C. 276 mcg
   D. 27.6 mcg
   E. 2.76 mcg

Rectal Suppositories

1. Example prescription order:

   Benzocaine 50 mg

   Menthol 20 mg

   Resorcin 10 mg

   Zinc oxide 300 mg

   Witepsol H35 qs 100%

   Mft: sup DTD VI

   Sig: 1 sup pr q 8 h prn hemorrhoid pain

   How often should the suppositories be administered?

   A. Every 4-6 hours as needed
   B. Every 8 hours as needed
   C. Four times per day
   D. As needed
   E. Every 6 hours as needed

2. If the SAW on the balance used is 100 mg, which of the following procedures could be used to measure the resorcin, assuming a two-suppository overage?

   A. Measure 100 mg resorcin and geometrically dilute to 200 mg with zinc oxide. Remove 120 mg of the mixture that contains 80 mg resorcin.
   B. Measure 90 mg resorcin and geometrically dilute to 180 mg zinc oxide. Remove 160 mg of the mixture that contains 80 mg resorcin.
   C. Measure 500 mg resorcin and geometrically dilute to 1000 mg with zinc oxide. Remove 250 mg of the mixture that contains 80 mg resorcin.
   D. Measure 50 mg resorcin and geometrically dilute to 200 mg with zinc oxide. Remove 10 mg of the mixture that contains 80 mg resorcin.
   E. Measure 60 mg resorcin and geometrically dilute to 300 mg with zinc oxide. Remove 150 mg of the mixture that contains 80 mg resorcin.

3. If the suppository mold used held 3 mL and the specific gravity of the molten mixture is 1.1, how many grams of Witepsol are required, assuming a two-suppository overage?

   A. 17.52 g
   B. 1.752 g
   C. 23.36 g
   D. 0.2336 g
   E. 2336 g

4. How many milligrams of benzocaine are required to fill this preparation assuming a two-suppository overage?

   A. 100 mg
   B. 200 mg
   C. 300 mg
   D. 400 mg
   E. 500 mg

5. How many grams of Witepsol are required to fill this prescription if each suppository weighs 2 grams and assuming no suppository overage?

    A. 6.48 grams
    B. 5.236 grams
    C. 2.35 grams
    D. 4.5 grams
    E. 8 grams

Vaginal Suppositories

1. Example prescription order:

    Metronidazole 40 mg
    Water 5%
    PEG base qs 100%
    Mft: sup DTD #4
    Sig: sup 1 pv qhs for infection

    What will be the total quantity of material needed if the mold makes suppositories that weigh 2 grams each (assume no overage)?

    A. 10 grams
    B. 7 grams
    C. 8 grams
    D. 6 grams
    E. 4 grams

2. When should the patient administer this medication?

    A. In the morning before breakfast
    B. Twice daily
    C. After dinner
    D. At bedtime
    E. Before lunchtime

3. What will be the total amount of PEG base needed for this prescription, if each suppository weighs 2 grams (assume no overage)?

    A. 7.44 grams
    B. 5.36 grams
    C. 6.34 grams
    D. 10.25 grams
    E. 11.34 grams

4. How many mL of water are needed for each suppository?

    A. 3 mL
    B. 5 mL
    C. 0.1 mL
    D. 3.2 mL
    E. 4.5 mL

Compounding and Calculations Review

Basic Principles of Pharmaceutical Calculations

The Metric System

The most widely used units of measure comprise the metric system. It is fundamental in all aspects of pharmacy, from production to dispensing. By convention, the metric system allows for interconversion between units by a factor of 10 (see Table 1). For example, 1 meter is 1/10 as large as 1 dekameter. The basic units of length, weight and volume are meters, grams, and liters, respectively. The multiples of these basic units are denoted by the addition of a prefix and are outlined in Table 1.

Table 1. The Metric System Convention

Prefix Factor × basic unit

pico- 10^{-12}	nano- 10^{-9}	micro- 10^{-6}
milli- 10^{-3}	centi- 10^{-2}	deci- 10^{-1}
deka- 10^{1}	hecto- 10^{2}	kilo- 10^{3}

To convert grams to picograms, one would divide the value in grams by 10^{-12} grams. For example:

Example: Convert 3.65 grams to picograms.

Answer: 3.65 grams x 1 picogram/10^{-12} grams = 3.65 x 10^{12} picograms

Apothecaries

Common Systems

Although the metric system is the official system for weights and measures as stated in the United States Pharmacopoeia and National Formulary (USP/NF), the common systems of measurement are still used in pharmacy, and therefore should be recognized. Typically, suppliers and manufacturers of substances that are sold to individual pharmacies or pharmaceutical manufacturers use the avoirdupois system of measurement. Pharmacists when dispensing medications use the apothecaries' system.

Table 2: Apothecaries Fluid Measure

	Gallons (gal)	Quart (qt)	Pint (pt)	Fluidounce	Fluid dram	Minim
Gallon	1	4	8	128	1024	61440
Quart		1	2	32	256	15360
Pint			1	16	128	7680
Fluidounce				1	8	480
Fluiddram					1	60
Minim						1

Table 3: Apothecaries Weight Measure

	Pound (lb)	Ounce	Dram	Scruple	Grain (gr)
Pound (lb)	1	12	96	288	5760
Ounce		1	8	24	480
Dram			1	3	60
Scruple				1	20
Grain (gr)					1

Avoirdupois

Table 4: Avoirdupois System

	Pound (lb)	Ounce (oz)	Grain (gr)
Pound (lb)	1	16	7000
Ounce (oz)		1	437.5
Grain (gr)			1

Compounding and Calculations Review

Conversion Between Systems

Table 5. Conversion Between Systems

Volume

1 mL = 16.23 minums
1 minum = 0.06 mL
1 fluid dram = 3.69 mL
1 fluid ounce = 29.57 mL
1 pt = 473 mL
1 gallon = 3785 mL

Weight

1 g = 15.432 grains
1 kg = 2.20 lbs (avoir.)
1 grain = 0.065 g or 65 mg
1 oz (avoir) = 28.35 g
1 ounce (apothecary) = 31.1 g
1 lb (avoir.) = 454 g
1 lb (apoth.) = 373.2 g

Other

1 oz (avoir.) = 437.5 gr
1 ounce (apoth.) = 480 gr
1 gallon = 128 fluid ounces

Density, Specific Gravity, and Specific Volume

Density

The density of a substance is its mass per unit volume, or the weight of a material required to fill a specific volume at a specific temperature. At 4°C the density of water is one, meaning there is 1 g for every milliliter of water. All other densities are based on this convention, using water as a reference point. To find the density of other substances, one would need to find what volume is taken up by a known mass of that substance and divide that mass by its volume. For example:

Example: Find the density of ethanol if 100 mL weighs 78.9 g.
Answer: Density = 78.9 g/100 mL = 0.789 g/mL

Specific gravity

The specific gravity of a substance is the ratio of its weight to the weight of a standard at a specific temperature, which is water for liquid and solid substances. The specific gravity may be calculated by dividing the weight of a substance by the weight of an equal amount of water. When given a specific gravity, it is assumed that it is in relation to water. For example:

Example: What is the specific gravity of 10 mL of ethanol that weighs 7.89 g and if 10 mL of water weighs 10 g?
Answer: Specific gravity = 7.89/10 g = 0.789

Specific volume

Unlike specific gravity, which is a ratio of weights of equal volume, specific volume is a ratio of volumes of equal weight at a specific temperature. Similar to specific gravity, water is used as the standard for liquids and solids. The specific volume is found by dividing the volume of a substance by the volume of water of an equal weight. For example:

Example: What is the specific volume of 10 g ethanol that has a volume of 12.67 mL?
Answer: Specific volume = 12.67 mL/10 mL = 1.267

Compounding and Calculations Review

Basic Pharmaceutical Calculations

Ratios

A ratio is the relation of two quantities expressed as the quotient of one divided by the other. Therefore, the ratio of 4 capsules to 5 capsules is 4/5, which is typically written as 4:5 to show the relationship as a ratio rather than a fraction. The ratio of 4 capsules to 2 capsules or 4/2 does not equal 2. Solvable fractions are left in the ratio form to show that it is a relationship, or operation, rather than a true fraction. However, ratios can be reduced, such that 4/2 equals 2/1 or 2:1.

Proportions

A proportion is a statement of equality between two ratios, typically written in one of the following ways:

$a/b = c/d$
$a:b = c:d$
$a:b :: c:d$

The proportions are read a is to b as c is to d, where a and d are known as the extremes and b and c are the means. The product of the means equals the product of the extremes, which allows one to find a missing term by algebraic means. The following example illustrates this point.

Example: If 6 liters of a sodium chloride solution contain 5 grams of sodium chloride, how many liters will contain 2 grams of sodium chloride?
Answer: 5 grams/6 liters = 2 grams/X liters, therefore, (2 grams)(6 liters)/5 grams = X liters = 2.4 liters

Aliquots

When the amount required for a prescription or compound exceeds the limit of precision for a measuring instrument or is below the smallest amount measurable, the method of aliquoting can be used to precisely weigh out and dispense the correct dose. The aliquot method involves weighing or measuring an amount above the smallest amount measurable and then diluting it down so as to achieve a measurable dilution containing the correct amount of drug.

Aliquots involving solid dispersions

The following procedure can be used to satisfy the aliquot method:

1. First calculate the desired dilution by setting up a ratio as follows:

    $a/c = b/d$
    where:
    a = the amount of substance needed
    b = the smallest amount weighable (SAW)
    c = a × some multiple in order to get above the smallest amount weighable
    d = b × the same multiple in c

2. From this you will know that a is the amount needed and b is the amount weighed out. Then dilute b down to d and measure out c. The amount measured in c will contain the desired amount (a).

Example: How would you measure 30 mg of chlorpheniramine maleate (SAW for the balance you are using is 70 mg), and then dilute to 20 g with lactose?
Answer: 30 mg (amount needed)/90 mg (30 mg x 3) = 70 mg (SAW)/210 mg (70 mg x 3)

Weigh out 70 mg of chlorpheniramine maleate, then dilute with lactose to 210 mg by geometrically mixing with 140 mg of lactose (210 mg–70 mg). From this dilution, measure out 90 mg of the powder, which contains 30 mg of chlorpheniramine maleate (the amount desired). To complete the question, dilute that to 20 g by adding 19.910 g lactose (20,000 mg–90 mg).

Compounding and Calculations Review

Aliquots involving solid-in-liquid dispersions

Aliquoting a solid using a liquid as the diluent requires that the solubility of the solid in that liquid be known. Because we must measure an amount greater than the SAW for the balance or measuring device used, the quantity of liquid used to dilute the solid must be sufficient to completely solubilize the drug. Furthermore, when using a graduated cylinder, there is also a limit of sensitivity for that measuring device. As a general rule, graduated cylinders can accurately measure volumes equal to 20% or greater than the total volume of the container. For example, a 50-mL graduated cylinder can accurately measure 10 mL or greater in volume. The following example shows one method for achieving a proper aliquot of a solid diluted with a liquid.

Example: Prepare the following prescription if the solubility of theophylline is 25 mg/mL and the SAW of the balance is 70 mg.
> Theophylline 50 mg
> Water qs 100 mL

Answer: First, measure enough theophylline to be above the SAW for the balance. This is achieved by measuring 100 mg. Since the solubility of theophylline is 25 mg/mL, use enough water to dilute the 100 mg of theophylline to be below this solubility limit, which could be 4 mL or more of water. So, the procedure is:

1. Weigh out 100 mg of theophylline
2. Dissolve in 4 mL of water
3. Take from this dispersion 2 mL, which will contain the desired 50 mg of theophylline. Note: use a 10-mL graduated cylinder to measure this volume.
4. Qs to 100 mL with water to complete the prescription.

The procedure for liquid-in-liquid dispersions is similar and requires knowing the miscibility of the two liquids used.

Dimensional Analysis

For most conversions or calculations involving units, the method of dimensional analysis is a useful tool for keeping track of the units involved in order to ensure proper calculations. This method involves setting up a calculation such that all of the units cancel except for the desired unit for the given calculation.

Example: Convert 50 µg/mL to g/L using dimensional analysis.
Answer: (50 µg/1 mL) x (1000 mL/1 L) x (1 mg/1000 µg) x (1 g/1000 mg) = 0.05 g/L

In this example, all of the units are canceled except for the grams and liters, which proves that the answer calculated is the correct conversion, assuming the ratios used are correct.

Dosage Calculations

When calculating doses for a patient, it is important to take into account the age, weight, sex, and surface area of the individual, as well as the delivery device. Various equations have been designed for calculating dosages based on age, weight, and body surface area.

Dosage Adjustment for Pediatric Patients

Because the pharmacokinetics and pharmacodynamics of medications delivered to pediatric patients differs from that of adults, the dose must be adjusted. Several equations have been developed to take into account the patient's age and/or weight in determining dosage adjustments.

Young's Rule:
> (Age/(age + 12)) x adult dose = dose for child

Cowling's Rule:
> (Age at next birthday (in years) x adult dose) /24 = dose for child

Fried's Rule for Infants:
> (Age (in months)/150) x adult dose = dose for child

Clark's Rule:
> (Weight (in lb)/150 (average weight of adults in lb)) x adult dose = dose for child

Compounding and Calculations Review

Dosage Adjustment Based on Body Weight

For drugs in which weight influences efficacy or toxicity, the dose must be adjusted for patients who do not meet the average adult weight of 70 kg. Typically, doses involving these drugs are on a per kg basis, such as 150 µg/kg. If the patient's weight is given in lb, it must be converted to kilograms and the amount calculated from the given dose per kg. This convention is commonly used, especially for potent or toxic drugs that have a narrow therapeutic index, and is the most common dosing method.

Dosage Adjustment Based on Body Surface Area

Determination of body surface area (BSA) is more precise for dosage adjustments compared to adjustments based on age and body weight. Because several factors can effect the weight of a patient, it is more desirable to calculate a dose based on surface area rather than weight alone. For example, a 300-lb, 6-foot-tall male body builder would have significantly different drug distribution and pharmacokinetics when compared to a 300-lb, 5-foot-tall obese patient, which would be reflected in the surface area calculations. The most widely used nomogram for the calculation of surface area is shown in Figures 1 and 2, which take into account both weight and height.

Body Surface of Adults

Nomogram for determination of body surface from height and mass[1]

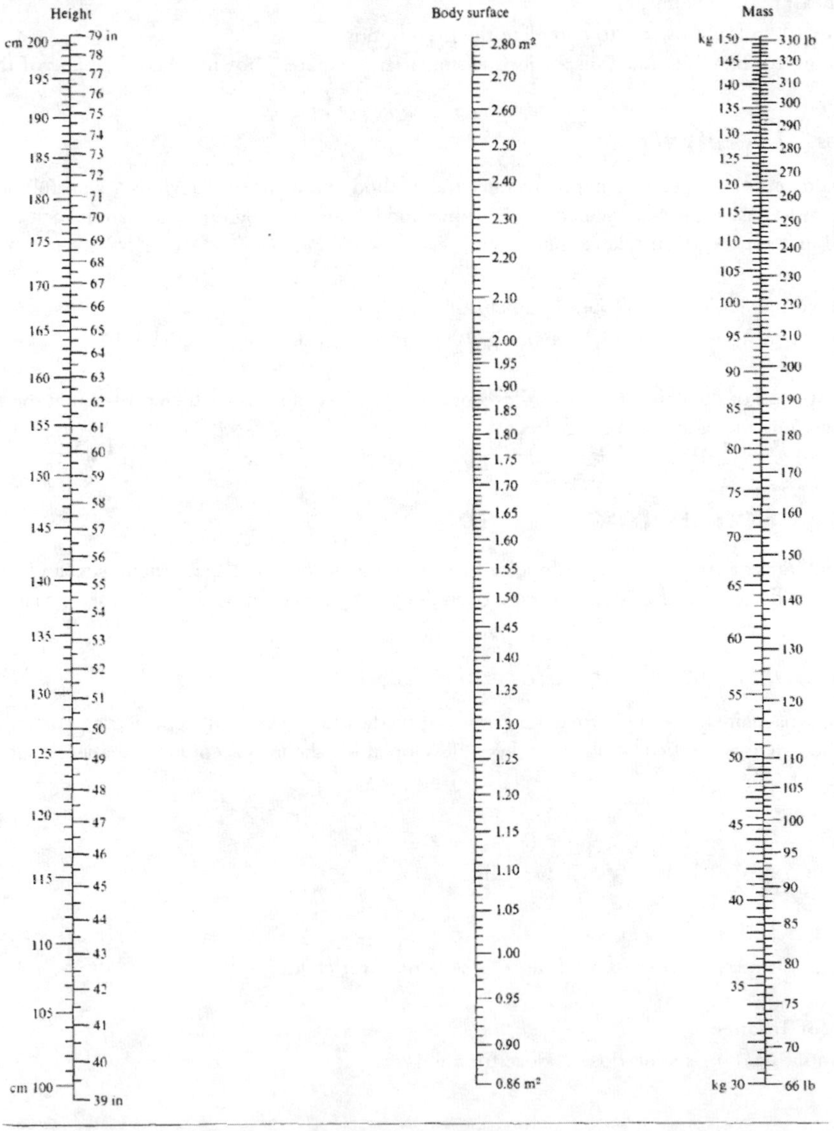

[1] From the formula of Du Bois and Du Bois, *Arch. intern. Med.*, 17, 863 (1916): $S = M^{0.425} \times H^{0.725} \times 71.84$,
or $\log S = \log M \times 0.425 + \log H \times 0.725 + 1.8564$ (S: body surface in cm², M: mass in kg, H: height in cm).

Figure 1. Body surface area nomogram for adults, from Geigy Scientific Tables, Eighth Edition, Vol. 1, C. Lentener (1981).

Compounding and Calculations Review

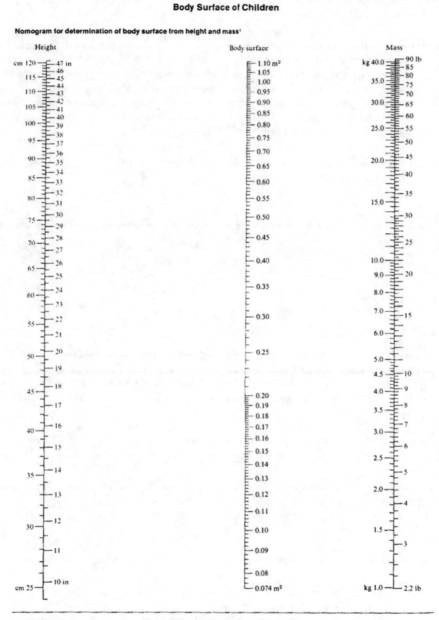

Body Surface of Children

Nomogram for determination of body surface from height and mass[1]

Height	Body surface	Mass

' From the formula of DuBois and DuBois, *Arch. intern. Med.*, 17, 863 (1916): $S = M^{0.425} \times H^{0.725} \times 71.84$, or $\log S = \log M \times 0.425 + \log H \times 0.725 + 1.8564$ (*S*: body surface in cm²; *M*: mass in kg; *H*: height in cm).

Figure 2. Body surface area nomogram for children, from Geigy Scientific Tables, Eighth Edition, Vol. 1, C. Lentener (1981).

Drawing a straight line from the known height to the known weight intersects the surface area column at the estimated surface area for that patient. Once the surface area is known, the following equation can be used to adjust the dose of a potent medication, based on the average adult surface area:

(BSA of patient (m²)/1.73 m² (average adult BSA)) x adult dose = approximate dose for the patient

Dosage Calculations Involving Various Delivery Devices

For the most part, directions for administration of medications to patients are given in a manner relative to the ability of the patient to understand. This is typically achieved by using tablespoons (tbs) or teaspoons (tsp) for liquid preparations. One tablespoon corresponds to 15 mL, whereas one teaspoon corresponds to 5 mL. The accepted general cractice is that the direction should be written in either tablespoons or teaspoons for ease of administration unless a measuring device is supplied to the patient for milliliter doses.

Compounding and Calculations Review

Example: How many teaspoons would the patient take if the prescription calls for 10 mL?
Answer: 10 mL x (1 tsp/5 mL) = 2 tsp

So, the directions are written so that the patient administers 2 teaspoonfuls per dose, rather than 10 mL.

Many times, pediatric patients receive prescriptions involving a certain number of drops per dose. For these prescriptions, a calibrated dropper is supplied and the number of drops/mL is known or determined such that the desired dose can be accurately administered. Although there are variations between droppers, most commercially available droppers are calibrated to deliver 20 drops of water per milliliter. Because water is not always used as the diluent and if the number of drops per milliliter is unknown, the pharmacist should determine the actual number of drops per milliliter for that given liquid prior to dispensing. A dropper can be calibrated by counting the number of drops needed to fill a given volume.

Example: If a pharmacist counted 30 drops of a medication while filling a 10-mL graduated cylinder to the 3-mL mark, how many drops per milliliter does this dropper dispense?
Answer: (30 drops/3 mL) = (x drops/1 mL) = 10 drops/mL

Example: If the prescription called for 0.8 mL of the drug product to be dispensed per dose, how many drops should be specified on the prescription label?
Answer: 0.8 mL x (10 drops/1 mL) = 8 drops

Concentration

Percentage of Strength

Many of the pharmaceutical preparations that are encountered during compounding or dispensing involve the use of percentages. The percentage sign (%) represents a ratio of 1 part of a substance to 100 parts of another substance or of the mixture. For example, in a 1% liquid preparation, this corresponds to 1 g of solute in 100 grams of total mixture, which in most cases is 1 gram per 100 mL of total mixture. There are three ways to express percentage strength, depending on the components.

Percent weight-in-volume (% w/v):

This corresponds to 1 gram of solute in 100 mL of total solution (solute and solvent) or the total volume regardless of the solvent type. In some instances, the term mg% is used to denote the number of milligrams of solute in 100 mL of total solution.

Example: What is the percentage strength w/v of 2.5 grams of a substance contained in 400 mL of an aqueous solution?
Answer: (2.5 g/400 mL) = (X g/100 mL) = 0.625% w/v

Percent volume-in-volume (% v/v)

This corresponds to the number of milliliters of liquid solute in 100 mL of the total volume (solute and solvent) of the preparation.

Example: What is the percentage strength v/v of 10 milliliters of a substance contained in 1000 mL of an aqueous solution?
Answer: (10 mL/1000 mL) = (X mL/100 mL) = 1% v/v

Percent weight-in-weight (% w/w)

This corresponds to the number of grams of solute or drug in 100 grams of the total weight (solute and diluent) of the preparation.

Example: What is the percentage strength w/w of 15 grams of a substance contained in 500 mg of a solid dispersion?
Answer: (15 g/500 g) = (X g/100 g) = 3% w/w

Ratio Strength

Ratio strength is a method of expressing concentration in the form of a ratio and is typically used to express concentration of dilute solutions or liquid preparations. Much like the percentage strength designations, the ratio strength is the ratio of parts of solute contained in some parts of a solvent or total mixture. For example, 2 parts of chlorpheniramine maleate contained in 100 parts of total solution is ratio strength and is written as 2:100. The first term is reduced to 1 such that the ratio in the previous example is 1:50 or 1 part chlorpheniramine maleate to 50 parts total solution. If the parts are liquid then one would use milliliters. Likewise, one would use grams for solid materials. So, in the previous example, the ratio 1:50 would be 1 gram of chlorpheniramine maleate contained in 50 mL of the total solution.

Compounding and Calculations Review

Dilutions

Dilutions involve taking a liquid or solid solution or dispersion of a known concentration and reducing the strength or concentration by adding a diluent of a known volume or weight. When making dilutions, it is easiest to convert ratio strength to percentage strength in order to perform the calculations. Dilutions of liquids, solids, alcoholic solutions, and the method of alligation will be discussed.

Dilution of liquids and solids

There are two methods to calculate the percentage strength of a diluted solution for both liquids and solids. The following examples illustrate dilution of liquids and solids.

Example: What is the percentage strength if 250 mL of a 5% (w/v) ciprofloxacin IV solution is diluted to 1 liter?
Answer:

Method 1: Set up the proportion:

(Initial quantity) x (initial concentration) = (final quantity) x (final concentration)
(250 mL) x (5%) = (1000 mL) x (X %)
X = 1.25% (w/v)

Method 2: Knowing the quantity of dissolved solute, calculate the new concentration:

From the question, 5 g are dissolved per 100 mL of solution. So, for 250 mL, there are 12.5 g of ciprofloxacin. Set up the following ratio:
12.5 g/1000 mL = X/100 mL
X = 1.25 or 1.25% (w/v)

Example: What is the volume needed to dilute 300 mL of a 10% (w/v) lidocaine HCl solution in order to make a 2% solution?
Answer: (300 mL) x (10%) = (X mL) x (2%)
X = 1500 mL

Dilution of alcohol

When water is used as a diluent for alcoholic solutions, there is an appreciable contraction in the volume. This complicates the methods previously described for the dilution of liquids. The same proportion method can be used. However, after calculating the final volume needed or the amount of water to add, one must qs to that amount rather than add the calculated volume of water. The following example illustrates this point.

Example: How many milliliters of water are needed to dilute 200 mL of 95% (v/v) ethanol to make a final concentration of 38%?
Answer: (200 mL) x (95%) = (X mL) x (38%)
X = 500 mL total solution
Therefore, use 200 mL of 95% (v/v) ethanol and enough water to make 500 mL.

Alligations

The method of alligation is used when solutions of different concentrations are mixed. The calculations allow one to make a solution of a given concentration or to find the concentration of the final mixture, each of which is calculated somewhat differently.

Finding the concentration of a mixture

This method is used when mixing two or more solutions of varying concentrations and known volumes, in order to determine the final concentration.

Example: What is the concentration of sodium chloride in percent strength of a mixture of 200 mL of 20% (w/v) sodium chloride, 300 mL of 15% (w/v) sodium chloride, and 400 mL of 30% sodium chloride?
Answer:

20 x 200	4000
15 x 300	4500
30 x 400	12000 +

Total: 900
20500 ÷ 900 mL = 22.8%

Compounding and Calculations Review

Making a solution of a known dilution with two or more solutions of known concentrations

This type of alligation is termed alligation alternate and it allows one to calculate the relative number of parts of two or more components of known concentrations that can be mixed to form the desired dilution. The concentration of the desired solution must lie between the concentrations of the available solutions, meaning that it must be stronger than its weakest component and weaker than its strongest component. The following example illustrates this method.

Example: How much 15% dextrose and 2% dextrose solutions are needed to make a 5% dextrose solution?
Answer: To solve this problem, a ratio is set up between the known components and the difference between the known components and the desired mixture is calculated to form the final ratio to be mixed, as follows:

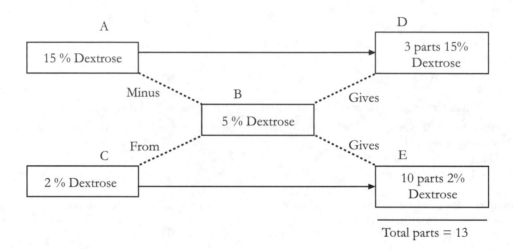

Figure 3.

In other words, % solution A minus % solution B (desired concentration) equals number of parts of solution C, which is given in E; and % solution B (desired concentration) minus % solution C equals number of parts of solution A, which is given in D. So, in this example, mixing 3 parts of the 15% dextrose solution and 10 parts of the 2% dextrose solution will make 13 parts of 5% dextrose solution.

Milliequivalents and Normality

Earlier in this chapter the units for concentration of solute dissolved in an aqueous solution were discussed. For the most part, the units of concentration are grams per liter or % (w/v). However, in the United States, solutions of electrolytes are almost exclusively discussed as milliequivalents (mEq). This unit of measure takes into account the chemical potential of the electrolyte solution and is related to the total number of ionic charges in solution. The normality of a solution is the number of equivalents per liter of solution. In order to convert from the unit of weight to the unit of mEq, the valence and molecular weight of the ionic substance must be known. The equation used for conversion is as follows:

$$mEq = (mg \times valence)/MW$$
and
$$mg = (mEq \times MW)/valence$$

Example: How many mEq of potassium are in 1 liter of a 1% (w/v) KCl solution?
Answer: Molecular weight of KCl = 74.5
mg of KCl = 1000 mL x (1 g/100 mL) x (1000 mg/1 g) = 10,000 mg
mEq = (10,000 mg x 1)/74.5 = 134.23 mEq KCl

Milliosmoles

For intravenous preparations, the osmotic pressure exerted by the solution is important for determining what effect it will have on biological membranes. The osmotic pressure is proportional to the total number of particles in solution. This is termed the osmolarity of the solution and has the unit of milliosmoles (mOsm). For non-electrolytes, 1 mmol of the substance corresponds to 1 mOsm.

Compounding and Calculations Review

However, for electrolyte solutions, the degree of dissociation becomes important in calculating the total number of species in solution. Because of this, the calculated values of osmolarity may differ slightly from experimentally determined values. The osmolarity can be calculated using the following equation:

mOsm/L = (weight of substance (g/L)/MW(g)) x number of species x 1000

Example: If a 2-liter solution contains 3 grams of KCl, what does this correspond to in mOsm/L?
Answer: ((3 g/2 L)/74.5 g) x 2 (K and Cl) x 1000 = 40.3 mOsm/L

The term osmolality is occasionally used to describe the concentration of species in solution. Osmolality represents the number of mOsm per kilogram of solvent, versus per liter of solvent in the case of osmolarity. When using osmolality, the solvent must be weighed unless it is water, which has a specific gravity of 1. The equation used for osmolarity is applicable to osmolality, but rather than using g/L, that term is replaced by g/kg.

Tonicity

The tonicity of a solution is related to the osmotic pressure of the solution and how that pressure relates to the bodily fluids to which the solution is being compared. Solutions with equal osmolarities are termed isosmotic, while solutions that have the same osmolarities as body fluids to which they are being compared are termed isotonic. The tonicity or degree of difference between the osmolarities is a significant factor in the distribution of water between physiological membranes. When cells are exposed to hypertonic solutions, water will diffuse out of the cell according to the principle of osmosis and likewise, hypotonic solutions will cause the cell to swell as water diffuses into the cell. For most applications, 0.9% (w/v) sodium chloride is considered isotonic. For calculations involving other species, a sodium chloride equivalent is used to relate the tonicity of the other species to the tonicity of sodium chloride. For example, lidocaine HCl has a sodium chloride equivalent equal to 0.22, so 1 gram of lidocaine HCl exhibits the same tonicity as 0.22 g of sodium chloride in solution. This relationship allows for the calculation of isotonic solutions comprising various species. If a drug is added to the solution, the sodium chloride equivalent can be calculated and subtracted from the amount of tonicity adjusting agent (typically sodium chloride or dextrose) required to make an isotonic solution.

Example: How many grams of sodium chloride are required to make the following prescription?
    Lidocaine HCl 100 mg
    Purified water qs 100 mL
    Sodium chloride qs to make an isotonic solution
Answer:
    1. Calculate the sodium chloride equivalent for the lidocaine HCl (Table 2 gives the sodium chloride equivalent for lidocaine HCl):

Table 2. Sodium Chloride Equivalents

Substance	Molecular Weight	Ions	i	Sodium Chloride Equivalent
Atropine sulfate	695	3	2.6	0.12
Benzalkonium chloride	360	2	1.8	0.16
Boric Acid	61.8	1	1.0	0.52
Cocaine hydrochloride	340	2	1.8	0.16
Dextrose	180	1	1.0	0.18
Ephedrine hydrochloride	202	2	1.8	0.29
Glycerin	92	1	1.0	0.34
Lidocaine hydrochloride	289	2	1.8	0.22
Mannitol	182	1	1.0	0.18
Phenobarbital sodium	254	2	1.8	0.24
Phenylephrine hydrochloride	204	2	1.8	0.32
Pilocarpine hydrochloride	245	2	1.8	0.24
Potassium chloride	74.5	2	1.8	0.76
Potassium penicillin G	372	2	1.8	0.18
Sodium chloride	58	2	1.8	1.00
Sodium iodide	150	2	1.8	0.39
Tetracaine hydrochloride	301	2	1.8	0.18
Tobramycin	468	1	1.0	0.07
Urea	60	1	1.0	0.59
Zinc chloride	136	3	2.6	0.62

Compounding and Calculations Review

Sodium chloride equivalent = 0.22 × 100 mg = 22 mg NaCl

2. Calculate the total amount of sodium chloride needed to make the solution isotonic:
   0.9% = (0.9 g/100 mL) x 100 mL = 0.9 g or 900 mg

3. Subtract the lidocaine HCl sodium chloride equivalent from the total amount of sodium chloride needed to make the solution isotonic:
   900 mg - 22 mg = 878 mg NaCl that must be added to the prescription to make it isotonic

Calculations For Sterile Products

Reconstitution of Dry Powders

Most suspensions and many parenteral medications are prepackaged as powders that must be reconstituted to form the suspension or solution. This is typically due to limited stability of the medication when in the reconstituted form. Pharmacists who receive prescriptions for powders for reconstitution should observe the packaging and follow the directions whenever possible. Occasionally, a physician may write a prescription which requires a concentration that is not outlined in the packaging and it must be calculated to ensure that the proper amount of water or diluent is added to achieve the desired concentration. It is important to note that in some cases the powder which is reconstituted adds to the volume of the final solution or dispersion. For this reason, it is imperative that the pharmacist read the label directions to see if the prescription in question displays this type of behavior. Below are some examples of these types of calculations:

POWDER DOES NOT CONTRIBUTE TO FINAL VOLUME:

Example: A pharmacist receives a prescription for Vancomycin 150 mg/mL in a syringe for injection. The pharmacist is supplied with Vancomycin 1 g in a 20 mL vial. The label directions instruct that to form a 100 mg/mL solution, add 10 mL of diluent. How would the pharmacist compound the desired concentration?

Answer: In this case, the powder does not significantly affect the final volume of the solution. This can be seen from the directions on the label, since it is known that the vial contains 1 g of vancomycin and it takes exactly 10 mL to form a 100 mg/mL solution. To make the desired concentration, the pharmacist would calculate the following:

100 mg/mL x 10 mL = 150 mg/mL x (X) mL

(X) = 6.67 mL

POWDER DOES CONTRIBUTE TO FINAL VOLUME:

Example: A pharmacist receives a prescription for Penicillin G Potassium 200,000 units/mL for injection. The pharmacist is supplied with Penicillin G Potassium 5,000,000 units. The label directions instruct that to form a 500,000 units/mL solution, the pharmacist should add 8 mL of diluent. How would the pharmacist compound the desired concentration?

Answer: In this case, the powder does significantly affect the final volume of the solution. This can be seen from the directions on the label, since it is known that the vial contains 5,000,000 units of penicillin G potassium and it takes 8 mL to form a 500,000 unit/mL solution. To make the desired concentration, the pharmacist must first determine the volume occupied by the powder:

From the problem it can be seen that the final volume is:

5,000,000 units x (1 mL / 500,000 units) = 10 mL

Since 8 mL of diluent is required to make the 10 mL solution, the volume occupied by the dry powder is 10 mL - 8 mL = 2 mL.

Next, the pharmacist will need to determine the final volume of the solution at the desired concentration:

5,000,000 units x (1 mL / 200,000 units) = 25 mL

Because 2 mL of that is occupied by the dry powder, the amount of diluent needed to reconstitute is 25 mL - 2 mL = 23 mL of diluent.

Compounding and Calculations Review

Parenteral Nutrition

Parenteral nutrition, also known as hyperalimentation, refers to the feeding of patients through an intravenous or central line. Calculations for parenteral nutrition involve electrolyte and caloric intake calculations.

Caloric intake requirements

The level of caloric intake (kcal) which is required for a patient can be calculated using the Harris-Benedict equation for the resting metabolic energy requirements (RME)

MALES
$$RME = 66 + (13.7 \times W) + (5 \times H) - (6.8 \times A)$$

FEMALES
$$RME = 655 + (9.6 \times W) + (1.8 \times H) - (4.7 \times A)$$

where W is weight in kilograms, H is height in centimeters, and A is age in years. The caloric intake is achieved through administration of lipids, amino acids and dextrose sterile solutions. For the purpose of calculations, amino acids provide 4 kcal/g, dextrose provides 3.4 kcal/g, whereas lipids provide 1 kcal/mL for a 10% solution or 10 kcal/g lipid. Other components which will be added will be calculated similarly to mEq calculations or concentration as described previously.

Example: A 170 cm, 70 year old female patient weighing 60 kg was admitted to the hospital and a prescription for parenteral nutrition was provided to the pharmacy. Using the Harris-Benedict equation, what is the caloric intake which is required for this patient?

$$RME = 655 + (9.6 \times 60) + (1.8 \times 170) - (4.7 \times 70)$$
$$RME = 655 + 576 + 306 - 329$$
$$RME = 1208 \text{ kcal}$$

If the prescription called for a protein level of 0.75 g/kg, what level of amino acids should be added to the parenteral nutrition and how many milliliters of a 50% dextrose solution should be added to fulfill the remaining caloric intake requirement?

Part 1:
    60 kg x 0.75 g/kg = 45 g Amino Acid
    45 g x 4 kcal/g = 180 kcal provided by the amino acids

Part 2:
    Total kcal required = 1208
    Kcal of protein = 180
    Kcal required by dextrose = 1208 - 180 = 1128

For a 50% solution of dextrose, there are 50 g of dextrose per 100 mL of the solution or 0.5 g/mL. We know that there is 3.4 kcal/g, so:

$$(3.4 \text{ kcal} / 1 \text{ g}) = (1128 \text{ kcal} / X \text{ g})$$
$$X = 331.8 \text{ g dextrose is required}$$

From the 50% solution, the amount of dextrose to be added would be:

$$(0.5 \text{ g} / 1 \text{ mL}) = (331.8 \text{ g} / X \text{ mL})$$
$$X = 663.6 \text{ mL of the dextrose solution is required}$$

Flow Rate Calculations for Parenteral Administration

Most calculations involving parenteral medications are a determination of flow rate to achieve a desired pharmacokinetic profile. For the most part, commercial medications provide literature which explains typical flow rates, depending on the patient age, weight and health status (renal and hepatic status). The calculations described in this section will focus on achieving a desired flow rate with given parameters, such as dose, route of administration and time scale. Parenteral medications can be broken into sub categories such as large volume and small volume. Large volume parenterals are typically for longer periods of time and are generally for maintenance of fluid and electrolytes. Small volume parenterals include piggyback medications, syringe administration and other smaller volume parenteral medications.

Compounding and Calculations Review

The pharmacist will generally be given a desired volume over a desired length of time. In this case, the pharmacist will need to determine the required flow rate to achieve the prescribed dose.

Example: A pharmacist receives a drug order for the administration of 2000 mL of D_5NS over a 12 hour period. If the IV administration instrument is calibrated to deliver 10 drops/mL, how many drops per minute must be administered to the patient to achieve the desired dose of D_5NS?

(2000 mL / 12 hr) x (1 hr / 60 min) x (10 drops / 1 mL) = 27.8 drops/min

Questions

Basic Principles of Pharmaceutical Calculations

1. Convert 1.45 mg to picograms.

   A. 1.45 picograms
   B. 1.45×10^{-4} picograms
   C. 3.45×10^{-7} picograms
   D. 1.45×10^{-9} picograms
   E. 1.45×10^{9} picograms

2. How many fluid ounces are contained in 5 quarts?

   A. 1.6 fluid ounces
   B. 16 fluid ounces
   C. 160 fluid ounces
   D. 1600 fluid ounces
   E. 0.16 fluid ounces

3. If a bulk powder purchased by a pharmacist weighs 3 lb, what is its corresponding weight in grains?

   A. 2.1×10^{4} gr
   B. 2.1×10^{3} gr
   C. 2.1×10^{2} gr
   D. 2.1×10^{-4} gr
   E. 2.1×10^{-3} gr

4. If a prescription calls for 2.5 mg/kg and the patient weighs 110 lb, what is the dose to be delivered for this patient?

   A. 75 mg
   B. 700 mg
   C. 125 mg
   D. 2.5 mg
   E. 25.2 mg

5. Substance A is poured into a graduated cylinder to the 100-mL mark and then weighed. What will the density be if the weight was 94 g for the 100 mL?

   A. 0.25 g/mL
   B. 0.5 g/mL
   C. 1.06 g/mL
   D. 0.94 g/mL
   E. 9.4 g/mL

Compounding and Calculations Review

6. A prescription calls for 2 g of a pharmaceutical liquid. If the density of the pharmaceutical liquid is 0.976 g/mL, what will be the corresponding amount in mL?

   A. 3.73 mL
   B. 5.2 mL
   C. 1.987 mL
   D. 1.952 mL
   E. 2.05 mL

7. A new pharmaceutical active substance has a specific gravity of 1.02. How many milliliters does 2 grams of this substance occupy?

   A. 2.78 mL
   B. 3.56 mL
   C. 1.96 mL
   D. 3.92 mL
   E. 3.05 mL

8. If the specific gravity of a substance is 0.956, what is the specific volume?

   A. 1.05
   B. 0.956
   C. 2.10
   D. 1.46
   E. 0.87

9. How many grains are contained in 1.5 kg of a raw material?

   A. 23149 gr
   B. 35648 gr
   C. 25785 gr
   D. 25468 gr
   E. 49845 gr

10. What is the specific gravity of 30 mL of mineral oil that weighs 6.5 g and if 10 mL of water weighs 10 g?

    A. 0.22
    B. 3.5
    C. 7.8
    D. 10.8
    E. 20.5

11. If the specific gravity of a liquid substance is 6.5, what is the volume occupied by 9 grams of the material?

    A. 5.2 mL
    B. 1.38 mL
    C. 230 mL
    D. 25.4 mL
    E. 45.2 mL

Basic Pharmaceutical Calculations

1. If a prescription calls for 5 g of sodium chloride, how many milliliters of a stock solution are needed if every 1000 mL contains 20 g?

   A. 300 mL
   B. 400 mL
   C. 250 mL
   D. 25 mL
   E. 40 mL

2. Using the aliquot method, how would a pharmacist measure 30 mg of pseudoephedrine HCl if the SAW for the balance he or she is using is 70 mg and the diluent is lactose?

   A. Weigh 80 mg pseudoephedrine HCl and dilute to 300 mg with lactose. From this mixture, remove 90 mg that will contain the necessary 30 mg pseudoephedrine HCl.
   B. Weigh 60 mg pseudoephedrine HCl and dilute to 240 mg with lactose. From this mixture, remove 120 mg that will contain the necessary 30 mg pseudoephedrine HCl.
   C. Weigh 70 mg pseudoephedrine HCl and dilute to 210 mg with lactose. From this dilution, remove 90 mg that will contain the necessary 30 mg pseudoephedrine HCl.
   D. Both b and c are correct.
   E. None of the above.

3. How would a pharmacist measure 15 mg of methylparaben using ethanol as a diluent, if the SAW for the balance is 80 mg and a 20 mL graduated cylinder is available?

   A. Dissolve 60 mg methylparaben in 10 mL ethanol and take 2 mL from the solution, which will contain 15 mg methylparaben.
   B. Dissolve 90 mg methylparaben in 12 mL ethanol and take 2 mL from the solution, which will contain 15 mg methylparaben.
   C. Dissolve 120 mg methylparaben in 5 mL ethanol and take 3 mL from the solution which will contain 15 mg methylparaben.
   D. Dissolve 0.5 g methylparaben in 100 mL ethanol and take 10 mL from the solution which will contain 15 mg methylparaben.
   E. Dissolve 0.3 g methylparaben in 50 mL ethanol and take 20 mL from the solution, which will contain 15 mg methylparaben.

4. Convert 50 mg/mL to µg/L using dimensional analysis.

   A. 5×10^{7} µg/L
   B. 5×10^{5} µg/L
   C. 5×10^{2} µg/L
   D. 5×10^{-7} µg/L
   E. 5×10^{-2} µg/L

5. 750 mL of D_5W runs for 5 hours. Calculate the flow rate in mL/hr and mL/min.

   A. 130 mL/hr, 3 mL/min
   B. 160 mL/hr, 5 mL/min
   C. 150 mL/hr, 2.5 mL/min
   D. 155 mL/hr, 2.8 mL/min
   E. 130 mL/hr, 2.5 mL/min

Compounding and Calculations Review

6. One liter of NS runs for 8 hours at 700 drops/hour. What is the drop factor?

    A. 7.5 drops/mL
    B. 2.5 drops/mL
    C. 3 drops/mL
    D. 5.6 drops/mL
    E. 7 drops/mL

Dosage Calculations

1. Calculate the dose needed for a 3-month-old infant if the adult dose is 500 mg ciprofloxacin per dose.

    A. 10 mg
    B. 300 mg
    C. 150 mg
    D. 800 mg
    E. 100 mg

2. What is the dose for a 15-kg child if the adult dose is 65 mg?

    A. 25.2 mg
    B. 30.4 mg
    C. 65 mg
    D. 58 mg
    E. 14.3 mg

3. If the dose of a given drug is 2 mg/kg, what is the dose for a 200-lb adult male?

    A. 182 mg
    B. 204 mg
    C. 15 mg
    D. 84 mg
    E. 18.2 mg

4. If a patient weighs 300 lb and is 5'11" tall, what is the dose, based on body surface area, if the normal dose for an adult is 300 mg?

    A. 300 mg
    B. 200 mg
    C. 434 mg
    D. 450 mg
    E. 150 mg

5. A prescription is brought into the pharmacy directing that 30 mL is to be administered for each dose. What is the dose in teaspoons?

    A. 6 tsp
    B. 4 tsp
    C. 2 tsp
    D. 8 tsp
    E. 5 tsp

6. If a prescription calls for 2 tablespoons per day, how many milliliters are required for a 30-day prescription?

    A. 90 mL
    B. 900 mL

C. 500 mL
D. 850 mL
E. 50 mL

7. If a pharmacist determines while calibrating a dropper bottle that 30 drops filled a 10-mL graduated cylinder to the 5-mL mark, what is the calibration in drops/mL?

    A. 8 drops/mL
    B. 6 drops/mL
    C. 8.5 drops/mL
    D. 4 drops/mL
    E. 6.5 drops/mL

8. A prescription calls for 1.2 mL to be administered for each dose. If a dropper is calibrated to deliver 5 drops/mL, what is the required dose in drops?

    A. 6 drops
    B. 5 drops
    C. 10 drops
    D. 20 drops
    E. 3 drops

9. If a dropper bottle holds 30 mL and the dropper is calibrated to deliver 5 drops/mL, how many 15-drop doses can be administered?

    A. 15
    B. 10
    C. 4
    D. 20
    E. 8

10. You have an order for 1.5 mg of epinephrine. If your stock solution is 1:1000, how many mL should you dispense?

    A. 1.5 mL
    B. 2.5 mL
    C. 5 mL
    D. 0.5 mL
    E. 6 mL

11. You have an order for Lanoxin 0.8 mg IV. Your stock is available in 500 mcg/2 mL. How many mL should you dispense?

    A. 2.3 mL
    B. 3.2 mL
    C. 5 mL
    D. 1.6 mL
    E. 9 mL

Concentration

1. What is the percentage strength (w/v) of 50 mg of cefuroxime dissolved in water to make a 500 mL D_5W solution?

    A. 0.2%
    B. 0.1%
    C. 0.01%

Compounding and Calculations Review

D.   2.5%
E.   0.025%

2. What is the percentage strength (w/w) for zinc oxide if 20 grams are mixed with 80 grams petrolatum?

    A.   25%
    B.   20%
    C.   15%
    D.   30%
    E.   22.5%

3. Convert 50% w/v to ratio strength.

    A.   1:2
    B.   1:4
    C.   2:5
    D.   2:1
    E.   1:1

4. What is the percentage strength of the final solution if 250 mL of 1% lidocaine HCl is diluted to 500 mL?

    A.   2%
    B.   1%
    C.   0.5%
    D.   1.5%
    E.   10%

5. How many milliliters of water are needed to dilute 500 mL of 90% ethanol to a 50% concentration?

    A.   500 mL
    B.   800 mL
    C.   400 mL
    D.   900 mL
    E.   600 mL

6. What is the concentration of KCl in percentage strength of a mixture of 300 mL 5% KCl, 400 mL 2% KCl, 250 mL 8 % KCl, and 400 mL 7.5% KCl?

    A.   2.5%
    B.   5.4%
    C.   3.2%
    D.   8.5%
    E.   4.5%

7. How many mEq of KCl are in 200 mL of a 5% KCl solution?

    A.   100 mEq
    B.   200 mEq
    C.   1.34 mEq
    D.   13.4 mEq
    E.   134.23 mEq

8. How many mOsm/L of KCl are present in 1000 mL of a 5% solution?

    A.   1342 mOsm/L
    B.   342 mOsm/L
    C.   2345 mOsm/L
    D.   13.42 mOsm/L
    E.   134.2 mOsm/L

9. Which of the following is considered to be isotonic?

    A.   0.9% NaCl
    B.   0.45% NaCl
    C.   0.225% NaCl
    D.   1.8% NaCl
    E.   0.75% NaCl

10. How many grams of sodium chloride are required to make the following prescription?

    Cocaine HCl 10 mg
    Purified water qs 100 mL
    Sodium chloride qs to make an isotonic solution

    A.   898.4 mg
    B.   89.84 mg
    C.   98.65 mg
    D.   8.98 mg
    E.   8.98 Kg

11. You have a vial of potassium solution that contains 20 mEq of potassium per 5 mL. You add 2.5 mL to a one liter IV bag. What is the final concentration of potassium in the bag?

    A.   0.41 mEq/mL
    B.   0.15 mEq/mL
    C.   0.30 mEq/mL
    D.   0.01 mEq/mL
    E.   0.09 mEq/mL

12. A one liter bag of ½ NS contains 22.5 mEq of sodium. The flow rate is 25 drops/min, with a drop factor of 15 drops/ mL. What is the hourly dose of sodium?

    A.   2.45 mEq/hr
    B.   2.25 mEq/hr
    C.   2.33 mEq/hr
    D.   2.56 mEq/hr
    E.   2.16 mEq/hr

13. A 0.8% solution of lidocaine is flowing at 50 mL/hr. What is the hourly dose?

    A.   500 mg/hr
    B.   400 mg/hr
    C.   360 mg/hr
    D.   460 mg/hr
    E.   510 mg/hr

Calculations for Sterile Products

1. A physician orders atropine sulfate 0.8 mg. Using a stock atropine sulfate of 0.4 mg/mL, calculate the volume of atropine that is needed to complete the physician's order.

Compounding and Calculations Review

A. 2.6 mL
B. 3 mL
C. 2 mL
D. 1.8 mL
E. 10 mL

2. An emergency room doctor orders 50 units of U100 insulin stat. Using a 1-cc syringe, how much insulin would you dispense?

A. 0.5 mL
B. 0.6 mL
C. 0.25 mL
D. 1 mL
E. 0.3 mL

3. A hospital physician orders 100,000 Units of penicillin to be added to a 1 L bag of saline and infused over 4 hours. Your infusion is set at 8 drops/mL. What is the flow rate in drops/minute?

A. 33.3 drops/minute
B. 50 drops/minute
C. 20 drops/minute
D. 55 drops/minute
E. 65 drops/minute

4. 500 mL of NS is infused at 55 mL/hr. How long will the infusion go?

A. 3 hours
B. 7.5 hours
C. 10 hours
D. 15 hours
E. 9 hours

5. 450 mL of D_5W ½ NS is delivered in 100 minutes. Your drop factor is 10 drops/mL. Calculate the flow rate in drops/min.

A. 49 drops/min
B. 30 drops/min
C. 25 drops/min
D. 45 drops/min
E. 52 drops/min

6. 250 mL of saline is infusing at 25 mL/hr. How much saline does the patient receive in 30 minutes?

A. 13.6 mL
B. 12.5 mL
C. 10 mL
D. 9.8 mL
E. 15 mL

7. The label on a drug vial says to reconstitute with 8 mL of water to get 10 mL of a 400,000 Units/mL solution. You add 10 mL by mistake. What would the resulting concentration of the drug be?

A. 333,333 Units/mL
B. 450,300 Units/mL

C. 500,100 Units/mL
D. 300,000 Units/mL
E. 555,555 Units/mL

8. An order for heparin is 1000 Units/hr in 1 L D_5W, to be infused for 4 hours. Calculate the amount of heparin to add to the IV.

A. 4000 Units
B. 5500 Units
C. 3300 Units
D. 4500 Units
E. 3000 Units

9. You reconstitute a vial of drug with 4 mL of saline. The vial contains 500 mg of drug. What is the final concentration of drug in the vial?

A. 132 mg/mL
B. 160 mg/mL
C. 125 mg/mL
D. 100 mg/mL
E. 400 mg/mL

10. How much dextrose is contained in 450 mL of D_5W?

A. 22.5 g
B. 32.9 g
C. 43.6 g
D. 52.9 g
E. 20.3 g

11. You add 4 g of drug to 1 liter of NS. The hourly dose is to be 240 mg. Calculate the flow rate. How long will the IV run?

A. 18 hr
B. 15 hr
C. 17 hr
D. 13 hr
E. 12 hr

12. An IV solution of heparin contains 2500 Units in 250 mL and takes 2 hours to infuse. How much drug is infused in 30 minutes?

A. 625 Units
B. 700 Units
C. 550 Units
D. 330 Units
E. 600 Units

13. There is an order for lidocaine 15 mg subcutaneously. Stock is a 1% solution. How many mL of lidocaine are required?

A. 3.2 mL
B. 2.6 mL
C. 1.5 mL
D. 1.9 mL
E. 3.5 mL

Compounding and Calculations Review

14. You have an order for Depo-Provera 0.45 g. Stock is available in 500 mg/10 mL vial. How much volume should you dispense?

    A. 5 mL
    B. 8 mL
    C. 6 mL
    D. 9 mL
    E. 3 mL

15. How many mEq of sodium are in 100 mL of saline? (MW = 23 (sodium) and 35 (chlorine))

    A. 16.5 mEq
    B. 15.5 mEq
    C. 13.9 mEq
    D. 23 mEq
    E. 58 mEq

16. You add 1 g of aminophylline to 500 mL of NS. The patient is to receive 60 mg/hr. What is the flow rate?

    A. 10 mL/hr
    B. 15 mL/hr
    C. 22 mL/hr
    D. 39 mL/hr
    E. 30 mL/hr

17. 30 mL of a 10% solution contains _____ g of drug.

    A. 0.3
    B. 30
    C. 13
    D. 300
    E. 3

18. You have an order for 500 mL of NS to run for 3 hours. Your infusion rate is set at 8 drops/mL. The flow rate in drops/min would be:

    A. 22 drops/min
    B. 24 drops/min
    C. 33 drops/min
    D. 16 drops/min
    E. 30 drops/min

19. A 6% solution would be:

    A. 6 g/100 mL
    B. 60 g/L
    C. 60 g/100 mL
    D. A and B
    E. None

20. You add 4 mL of a 350 mg/mL solution of methotrexate to 500 mL saline. What is the final concentration in the bag?

    A. 2.2 mg/mL
    B. 3.3 mg/mL
    C. 2.8 mg/mL
    D. 2.0 mg/mL
    E. 3.0 mg/mL

21. How many milligrams of drug are in 30 mL of a 1:10,000 solution?

    A. 30 mg
    B. 3 mg
    C. 300 mg
    D. 30 g
    E. 0.3 mg

Appendixes

Appendix A

NAPLEX® Competency Statements

NAPLEX® Blueprint

The NAPLEX® Competency Statements

The NAPLEX® Competency Statements provide a blueprint of the topics covered on the examination. They offer important information about the knowledge, judgment, and skills you are expected to demonstrate as an entry-level pharmacist. A strong understanding of the Competency Statements will aid in your preparation to take the examination.

Area 1

Assure Safe and Effective Pharmacotherapy and Optimize Therapeutic Outcomes
(Approximately 54% of Test)

1.1.0 Obtain, interpret and evaluate patient information to determine the presence of a disease or medical condition, assess the need for treatment and/or referral, and identify patient-specific factors that affect health, pharmacotherapy, and/or disease management.

1.1.1 Identify and assess patient information including medication, laboratory and disease state histories.

1.1.2 Identify and/or use instruments and techniques related to patient assessment and diagnosis.

1.1.3 Identify and define the terminology, signs, and symptoms associated with diseases and medical conditions.

1.1.4 Identify and evaluate patient factors, genetic factors, biosocial factors, and concurrent drug therapy that are relevant to the maintenance of wellness and the prevention or treatment of a disease or medical condition.

1.2.0 Identify, evaluate, and communicate to the patient or health-care provider, the appropriateness of the patient's specific pharmacotherapeutic agents, dosing regimens, dosage forms, routes of administration, and delivery systems.

1.2.1 Identify specific uses and indications for drug products.

1.2.2 Identify the known or postulated sites and mechanisms of action of pharmacotherapeutic agents.

1.2.3 Evaluate drug therapy for the presence of pharmacotherapeutic duplications and interactions with other drugs, food, diagnostic tests, and monitoring procedures.

1.2.4 Identify contraindications, warnings and precautions associated with a drug product's active and inactive ingredients.

1.2.5 Identify physicochemical properties of drug substances that affect their solubility, pharmacodynamic and pharmacokinetic properties, pharmacologic actions, and stability.

1.2.6 Interpret and apply pharmacodynamic and pharmacokinetic principles to calculate and determine appropriate drug dosing regimens.

1.2.7 Interpret and apply biopharmaceutic principles and the pharmaceutical characteristics of drug dosage forms and delivery systems, to assure bioavailability and enhance patient compliance.

1.3.0 Manage the drug regimen by monitoring and assessing the patient and/or patient information, collaborating with other health care professionals, and providing patient education.

1.3.1 Identify pharmacotherapeutic outcomes and endpoints.

1.3.2 Evaluate patient signs and symptoms, and the results of monitoring tests and procedures to determine the safety and effectiveness of pharmacotherapy.

1.3.3 Identify, describe the mechanism of, and remedy adverse reactions, allergies, side effects and iatrogenic or drug-induced illness.

1.3.4 Prevent, recognize, and remedy medication non-adherence, misuse or abuse.

1.3.5 Recommend pharmacotherapeutic alternatives.

Area 2

Assure Safe and Accurate Preparation and Dispensing of Medications
(Approximately 35% of Test)

2.1.0 Perform calculations required to compound, dispense, and administer medication.

2.1.1 Calculate the quantity of medication to be compounded or dispensed; reduce and enlarge formulation quantities and calculate the quantity of ingredients needed to compound the proper amount of the preparation.

2.1.2 Calculate nutritional needs and the caloric content of nutrient sources.

2.1.3 Calculate the rate of drug administration.

2.1.4 Calculate or convert drug concentrations, ratio strengths, and/or extent of ionization.

2.2.0 Select and dispense medications in a manner that promotes safe and effective use.

2.2.1 Identify drug products by their generic, brand, and/or common names.

2.2.2 Determine whether a particular drug dosage strength or dosage form is commercially available, and whether it is available on a nonprescription basis.

2.2.3 Identify commercially available drug products by their characteristic physical attributes.

2.2.4 Interpret and apply pharmacokinetic parameters and

Appendix A

NAPLEX® Competency Statements

quality assurance data to determine equivalence among manufactured drug products, and identify products for which documented evidence of inequivalence exists.

2.2.5   Identify and communicate appropriate information regarding packaging, storage, handling, administration, and disposal of medications.

2.2.6   Identify and describe the use of equipment and apparatus required to administer medications.

2.3.0   Prepare and compound extemporaneous preparations and sterile products.

2.3.1   Identify and describe techniques and procedures related to drug preparation, compounding, and quality assurance.

2.3.2   Identify and use equipment necessary to prepare and extemporaneously compound medications.

2.3.3   Identify the important physicochemical properties of a preparation's active and inactive ingredients; describe the mechanism of, and the characteristic evidence of incompatibility or degradation; and identify methods for achieving stabilization of the preparation.

National Association of Boards of Pharmacy® and the NAPLEX/MPJE Bulletin. © 2006, National Association Boards of Pharmacy, Mount Prospect, Illinois.

Area 3

Provide Health Care Information and Promote Public Health
(Approximately 11% of Test)

3.1.0   Access, evaluate, and apply information to promote optimal health care.

3.1.1   Identify the typical content and organization of specific sources of drug and health information for both health-care providers and consumers.

3.1.2   Evaluate the suitability, accuracy, and reliability of information from reference sources by explaining and evaluating the adequacy of experimental design and by applying and evaluating statistical tests and parameters.

3.2.0   Educate the public and health-care professionals regarding medical conditions, wellness, dietary supplements, and medical devices.

3.2.1   Provide health care information regarding the prevention and treatment of diseases and medical conditions, including emergency patient care.

3.2.2   Provide health care information regarding nutrition, lifestyle, and other non-drug measures that are effective in promoting health or preventing or minimizing the progression of a disease or medical condition.

3.2.3   Provide information regarding the documented uses, adverse effects and toxicities of dietary supplements.

3.2.4   Provide information regarding the selection, use and care of medical/surgical appliances and devices, self-care products, and durable medical equipment, as well as products and techniques for self-monitoring of health status and medical conditions.

A & O
Alert and oriented

A&P
Auscultation and percussion

A1
Abortus-1

AA
Alcoholics Anonymous

AAFP
American Academy of Family Physicians

AAP
American Academy of Pediatrics

ABD
Abdomen

ABG
Arterial blood gases

AC
Before meals

AC and HS
Before meals and at bedtime

AC & HS
Before meals and at bedtime

ACE
Angiotensin converting enzyme

ACIP
Advisory Committee on Immunization Practices (CDC)

Adj BW
Adjusted body weight

AHFS
American Hospital Formulary Service

AIDS
Acquired immunodeficiency syndrome

Alk Phos
Alkaline Phosphatase

ALL
Acute lymphocytic leukemia

ALP
Alkaline phosphatase

ALT
Alanine aminotransferase

AM
Morning

AMA
Against medical advice

ANA
Antinuclear antibody

Anti-ds DNA
Anti-double-stranded deoxyribonucleic acid

Anti-HAV
Antibody to hepatitis A virus

Anti-HBc
Antibody to the hepatitis B core antigen

Anti-Hbe
Antibody to the hepatitis 'e' antigen

Anti-HBs
Antibody to the hepatitis B surface antigen

Anti-HCV
Antibody to the hepatitis C virus

AP
Anterior-posterior

APAP
Acetaminophen

ARF
Acute renal failure

ASA
Aspirin

ASCVD
Atherosclerotic cardiovascular disease

AST
Aspartate aminotransferase

ATC
Around the clock

Appendix B

Abbreviations

AUC
Area under the concentration time curve

AV
Arteriovenous

Baso
Basophils

BCG
Bacille Calmette-Guérin

bid
Twice a day

BKA
Below knee amputation

BM
Total cells counted in bone marrow

BM
Bowel movement

BM-Bx
Bone marrow-biopsy

BP
Blood pressure

BPH
Benign prostatic hypertrophy

bpm
Beats per minute

BRBPR
Bright red blood per rectum

BS
Bowel sounds

BSA
Body surface area

BUN
Blood urea nitrogen

c/c/e
Clubbing/cyanosis/edema

C3
Complement component 3

C4
Complement component 4

Ca
Calcium

CA-125
Cancer antigen 125

CABG
Coronary artery bypass graft

CAD
Coronary artery disease

CAP
Community acquired pneumonia

CAPD
Continuous ambulatory peritoneal dialysis

CBC
Complete blood count

CC
Chief Complaint

CCE
Clubbing, cyanosis, edema

CDC
Centers for Disease Control and Prevention

CEA
Carcinoembryonic antigen

CHF
Congestive heart failure

CINV
Chemotherapy-induced nausea & vomiting

CK
Creatine kinase

CKMB
Creatine kinase myocardial band

Cl
Chloride

Cl_{cr}
Creatinine clearance

CML
Chronic myelogenous leukemia

CMV
Cytomegalovirus

CN
Cranial nerves

CNS
Central nervous system

CO$_2$
Carbon dioxide (pCO$_2$ = peripheral or arterial carbon dioxide)

COMT
Catechol-O-methyltransferase

COPD
Chronic obstructive pulmonary disease

COX
Cyclooxygenase

COX-2
Cyclooxygenase-2

CrCl
Creatinine clearance

CSF
Cerebral spinal fluid

CT
Computed tomography

CTA
Clear to auscultation

CTX
Chemotherapy

CV
Cardiovascular

CVA
Cerebrovascular accident

CVA
Costovertebral angle

CVAT
Costovertebral angle tenderness

CVD
Cisplatin, vinblastine, dacarbazine

CXR
Chest x-ray

D. bili
Direct bilirubin

D$_5$W
Dextrose 5% in water

DBP
Diastolic blood pressure

DEXA
Dual energy x-ray absorptiometry

DIP
Distal interphalangeal

DM
Diabetes mellitus

DMARD
Disease-modifying antirheumatic drug

DNA
Deoxyribonucleic acid

DOE
Dyspnea on exertion

DTR
Deep tendon reflex

E.C.
Enteric coated

ECASA
Enteric coated aspirin

ECG
Electrocardiogram

ED
Emergency department

EGD
Esophagogastroduodenoscopy

EKG
Electrocardiogram

Appendix B

Abbreviations

ELISA
Enzyme linked immunosorbent assay

EMS
Emergency medical services

ENDO
Endocrine

EOMI
Extra-ocular movements (or muscles) intact

EOS
Eosinophils

ESR
Erythrocyte sedimentation rate

ESRD
End-stage renal disease

EtOH
Ethanol

EXT
Extremities

FAC
Fluorouracil, doxorubicin (Adriamycin), cyclophosphamide

FBG
Fasting blood glucose

FDA
Food and Drug Administration

FEV1
Forced expiratory volume in 1 second

FSH
Follicle stimulating hormone

FT_3
Free triiodothyronine

FT_4
Free thyroxine

FT_4I
Free thyroxine index

FTA-ABS
Fluorescent treponemal antibody absorption

FVC
Forced vital capacity

G-1
Gravida-1

G-4
Gravida-4

GAD
Generalized anxiety disorder

GBS
Guillain-Barré Syndrome

GC
Gonococci or gonococcal infection

GEN
General appearance or presentation

GERD
Gastroesophageal reflux disease

GI
Gastrointestinal

GPC
Gram-positive cocci

gtt
Drop

GU
Genitourinary

H/O
History of

H_2RA
Histamine-2 receptor antagonist

HA
Headache

HAART
Highly active antiretroviral therapy

HAV
Hepatitis A virus

HbA_{1c}
Hemoglobin A_{1c}

Appendix B

Abbreviations

HBc
Antigen hepatitis B core antigen

HbcAg
Hepatitis B core antigen

HBe
Antigen hepatitis B 'e' antigen

HBIG
Hepatitis B immune globulin

HBs
Antigen hepatitis B surface antigen

HbsAg
Hepatitis B surface antigen

HCG
Human chorionic gonadotropin

HCO$_3$
Bicarbonate

Hct
Hematocrit

HCTZ
Hydrochlorothiazide

HD
Hemodialysis

HEENT
Head, ear, eyes, nose, and throat

HER2
Human epidermal growth factor receptor-2

Hgb
Hemoglobin

HiB
Haemophilus Influenzae, type B

HIV
Human immunodeficiency virus

HJR
Hepatojugular reflux

HLA
Human leukocyte antigen

HPI
History of present illness

HR
Heart rate

HS
At bedtime

HSM
Hepatosplenomegaly

HSV
Herpes simplex virus

HTN
Hypertension

IBW
Ideal Body Weight

IgG
Immunoglobulin G

IgM
Immunoglobulin M

IL-2
Interleukin-2

IM
Intramuscular

INH
Isoniazid

Inorganic Phos
Inorganic phosphorus

INR
International normalized ratio

IP
Intraperitoneal

IU
International Units

IV
Intravenous

IVDA
Intravenous drug abuse

Appendix B

Abbreviations

IVP
Intravenous push

IVPB
Intravenous piggy back

JNC VI
Sixth report of the Joint National Committee on Prevention, Detection, Evaluation, and Treatment of High Blood Pressure

JVD
Jugular venous distention

K
Potassium

kcal
Kilocalorie

LDH
Lactate dehydrogenase

LDL
Low-density lipoprotein

LE
Lower extremity

LES
Lower esophageal sphincter

LFTs
Liver function tests

LH
Luteinizing hormone

LHRH
Luteinizing hormone releasing hormone

LLL
Left lower lobe

LLQ
Left lower quadrant

LMP
Last menstrual period

LPF
Low power field

LTC
Long-term care

Lymph
Lymphocytes

m/r/g
Murmurs/rubs/gallops

MAO-A
Monoamine oxidase type A

MAO-B
Monoamine oxidase type B

MCH
Mean corpuscular hemoglobin

MCHC
Mean corpuscular hemoglobin concentration

MCP
Metacarpophalangeal

MCV
Mean corpuscular volume

MDI
Metered dose inhaler

Mg
Magnesium

MI
Myocardial infarction

MIC
Minimum inhibitory concentration

MIU
Million international units

MMR
Mumps, Measles, and Rubella

MMSE
Mini-mental status exam

Monos
Monocytes

MRI
Magnetic resonance imaging

MRSA
Methicillin resistant Staph aureus

MTP
Metatarsophalangeal

MU
Million units

MUGA
Multiple-gated acquisitions of data

MVA
Motor vehicle accident

MVI
Multivitamin

MWF
Monday, Wednesday, Friday

N/V
Nausea and vomiting

NA
Narcotics Anonymous

NA
Not applicable

Na
Sodium

NAD
No apparent (acute) distress

NC/AT
Normocephalic, atraumatic

NCAT
Normal cephalic, atraumatic

NEURO
Neurological

Neut
Neutrophils

NG
Nasogastric

NIH
National Institutes of Health

NKA
No known allergies

NKDA
No known drug allergies

NL
Normal

NPO
Nothing by mouth

NS
Nasal spray

NSAID
Nonsteroidal anti-inflammatory drug

NSR
Normal sinus rhythm

NT/ND
Nontender, nondistended

o/p
Ova or parasites

O_2
Oxygen (pO_2 = peripheral or arterial oxygen)

OA
Osteoarthritis

OB/GYN
Obstetrician/Gynecologist

OC
Oral contraceptive

OHSS
Ovarian hyperstimulation syndrome

OSHA
Occupational Safety and Health Administration

OTC
Over the counter

OU
Both eyes

P
Puffs

Appendix B

Abbreviations

P-1
Para-1

P-4
Para-4

PC
After meals

PCA
Patient controlled analgesia

PCN
Penicillin

PCP
Pneumocystis carinii *pneumonia*

PCP
Primary care physician

PD
Parkinson's disease

PERRLA
Pupils equal, round, and reactive to light and accommodation

Ph-
Philadelphia chromosome negative

Ph+
Philadelphia chromosome positive

Phos
Inorganic phosphorus

PIP
Proximal interphalangeal

Plt
Platelets

PMN
Polymorphonuclear leukocyte

po
By mouth (oral)

PO_4
Phosphate

ppd
Pack(s) (of cigarettes) per day

PPD
Purified protein derivative

prn
As needed

PSA
Prostate specific antigen

PT
Prothrombin time

PTT
Partial thromboplastin time

PUD
Peptic ulcer disease

PVD
Peripheral vascular disease

q
Every

q am
Every morning

qd
Once a day

q hs
At bedtime

qid
Four times a day

qod
Every other day

q wk
Every week

RA
Rheumatoid arthritis

RBC
Red blood cells

RDA
Recommended daily allowance

RDW
Red (cell) distribution width

REM
Rapid eye movement

RF
Rheumatoid factor

ROM
Range of motion

RPR
Rapid plasma reagin

RR
Respiratory rate

RRR
Regular rate and rhythm

RSV
Respiratory syncytial virus

RUE
Right upper extremity

RUQ
Right upper quadrant

Rx
Prescription

S/P
Status post

S_1
First heart sound

S_2
Second heart sound

S_3
Third heart sound (abnormal)

S_4
Fourth heart sound (abnormal)

SBP
Systolic blood pressure

SCr
Serum creatinine

SE
Status epilepticus

Segs
Neutrophils

SEM
Systolic ejection murmur

Serum Cr
Serum creatinine

SGPT
Serum glutamic pyruvic transaminase

SHBG
Sex-hormone binding globulin

Sig
Directions

SL
Sublingual

SLE
Systemic lupus erythematosus

Sp
Species

SQ
Subcutaneous

SR
Sustained release

SSRI
Selective serotonin reuptake inhibitor

STD
Sexually transmitted disease

Subq
Subcutaneous

SULFAS
Sulfonylureas

Sx
Symptoms

T. bili
Total bilirubin

T_4
Levothyroxine

Appendix B

Tart
Tartrate

TB
Tuberculosis

TDT
Terminal transferase

TG
Triglycerides

TIA
Transient ischemic attack

TIBC
Total iron binding capacity

tid
Three times a day

TM
Tympanic membrane

TMP/SMX
Trimethoprim/sulfamethoxazole

TNF
Tumor necrosis factor

TPHA
T. pallidum hemagglutination assay

TSH
Thyroid Stimulating Hormone

TT$_3$
Total triiodothyronine

TT$_4$
Total thyroxine

TTS
Transdermal therapeutic system

UC
Ulcerative colitis

ud
As directed

UE
Upper extremity

URI
Upper respiratory infection

USP DI
United States Pharmacopeia Drug Information

USP NF
United States Pharmacopeia National Formulary

UTI
Urinary tract infection

UV
Ultraviolet

UVA
Ultraviolet-A

UVB
Ultraviolet-B

UVC
Ultraviolet-C

VA
Veterans Affairs

Vd
Volume of distribution

VLDL
Very low-density lipoprotein

VS
Vital signs

WBC
White Blood Cells

WD
Well-developed

WD,WN
Well-developed, well-nourished

WNL
Within normal limits

yo
Years old

Appendix C

Laboratory Values

Nondrug Reference Ranges for Common Laboratory Tests in Traditional and SI Units[a]

Laboratory Test	Reference Range Traditional Units	Conversion Factor	Reference Range SI Units	Comment
Alanine aminotransferase (ALT)	0–30 IU/L	0.01667	0–0.50 μkat/L	SGPT
Albumin	3.5–5 g/dL	0.00	35–50 g/L	
Ammonia	30–70 μg/dL	0.587	17–41 μmol/L	
Aspartate aminotransferase (AST)	8–42 IU/L	0.01667	0.133–0.700 μkat/L	SGOT
Bilirubin (direct)	0.1–0.3 mg/dL	17.10	1.7–5 μmol/L	
Bilirubin (total)	0.3–1.0 mg/dL	117.10	5–17 μmol/L	
Calcium	8.5–10.8 mg/dL	0.25	2.1–2.7 mmol/L	
Carbon dioxide (CO_2)	24–30 mEq/L	1.000	24–30 mmol/L	Serum bicarbonate
Chloride	96–106 mEq/L	1.000	96–106 mmol/L	desirable
Cholesterol (HDL)	>10 mg/dL	0.026	>1.55 mmol/L	desirable
Cholesterol (LDL)	100 <130 mg/dL	0.026	<3.36 mmol/L	males
Creatine kinase (CK)	25–90 IU/L (males)	0.01667	0.42–1.50 μkat/L	females
	10–70 IU/L (females)		0.17–1.17 μkat/L	adults
Serum creatinine (SCr)	0.7–1.5 mg/dL	88.40	62–133 μmol/L	
Creatinine clearance (CrCl)	90–140 mL/min/1.73 m²	0.017	1.53–2.38 mL/sec/1.73 m²	
Folic acid	150–540 ng/mL	2.266	340–1020 nmol/L	GGTP
g-Glutamyl transpeptidase	0–30 U/L (but varies)	0.01667	0–0.50 μkat/L (but varies)	
Globulin	2–3 g/dL	10.00	20–30 g/L	fasting
Glucose (fasting)	<110 mg/dL	0.056	6.1 mmol/L	males
Hemoglobin (Hgb)	14–18 g/dL	0.622	8.7–11.2 mmol/L	females
	12–16 g/dL		7.4–9.9 mmol/L	
Iron	50–150 μg/dL	0.179	9–26.9 μmol/L	TIBC
Iron-binding capacity	250–410 μg/dL	0.179	45–73 μmol/L	LDH
Lactate dehydrogenase	100–210 IU/L	0.01667	1667–350 nmol/L, 1.7–3.2 μkat/L	Lactic acid
Serum lactate (venous)	0.5–1.5 mEq/L	1.000	0.5–1.5 mmol/L	
Serum lactate (arterial)	0.5–2.0 mEq/L	1.000	0.5–2.0 mmol/L	
Magnesium	1.5–2.2 mEq/L	0.500	0.75–1.1 mmol/L	
5′ Nucleotidase	1–11 U/L (but varies)		0.01667 0.02–0.18 μkat/L (but varies)	
Phosphate	2.6–4.5 mg/dL		0.85–1.48 mmol/L	
Potassium	3.5–5.0 mEq/L	1.000	3.5–5.0 mmol/L	
Sodium	136–145 mEq/L	1.000	136–145 mmol/L	
Total serum thyroxine (T_4)	4–12 μg/dL	12.86	51–154 nmol/L	Total T_4
Triglycerides	<150 mg/dL	0.0113	<1.26 mmol/L	Adults >20 yo
Total serum triiodothyronine (T_3)	78–195 ng/dL	0.0154	1.2–3.0 nmol/L	Total T_3
Urea nitrogen, blood	8–20 mg/dL	0.357	2.9–7.1 mmol/L	BUN
Uric acid (serum)	3.4–7 mg/dL	59.48	202–416 μmol/L	

[a]Some laboratories are maintaining traditional units for enzyme tests.

Appendix D

State Boards of Pharmacy

Alabama State Board of Pharmacy

Herbert "Herb" Bobo, Executive Secretary
10 Inverness Center, Suite 110
Birmingham, AL 35242
205/981-2280
fax 205/981-2330 hbobo@albop.com
www.albop.com

Alaska Board of Pharmacy

Sher Zinn, Licensing Examiner
P.O. Box 110806, Juneau, AK 99811-0806
907/465-2589
fax 907/465-2974
sher_zinn@commerce.state.ak.us
www.commerce.state.ak.us/occ/ppha.htm

Arizona State Board of Pharmacy

Harlan "Hal" Wand
Executive Director
4425 W. Olive Avenue, Suite 140
Glendale, AZ 85302
623/463-3844
623/934-0583 fax
www.pharmacy.state.az.us
hwand@azsbp.com

Arkansas State Board of Pharmacy

Charles S. Campbell, Executive Director
101 E Capitol, Suite 218
Little Rock, AR 72201
501/682-0190
501/682-0195 fax
charlie.campbell@arkansas.gov
www.arkansas.gov/asbp

California State Board of Pharmacy

Patricia F. Harris
Executive Officer
400 R Street, Suite 4070
Sacramento, CA 95814
916/445-5014
916/327-6308 fax
www.pharmacy.ca.gov
patricia_harris@dca.ca.gov

Colorado State Board of Pharmacy

Wendy Anderson, Program Director
1560 Broadway, Suite 1310
Denver, CO 80202-5143
303/894-7754
303/894-7764 fax
wendy.anderson@dora.state.co.us
www.dora.state.co.us/pharmacy

Connecticut Commission of Pharmacy

Anne-Christine Vrakas, Board Administrator
165 Capitol Ave, State Office Bldg, Room 147
Hartford, CT 06106
860/713-6070
860/713-7242 fax
Anne-christine.vrakas@ct.gov
www.ct.gov/dcp/si te/default .asp

Delaware State Board of Pharmacy

David W. Dryden, R.Ph., JD
Executive Secretary
P.O. Box 637
Dover, DE 19903
302/739-4798
302/739-3071 fax
ddryden@state.de.us
www.professionallicensing.state.dc.us

District of Columbia Board of Pharmacy

Bonnie Rampersaud, Executive Director
717 14th St NW, Suite 600
Washington, DC 20005
202/724-4900
202/727-8471 fax
graphelia.ramseur@dc.gov
www.dchealth.dc.gov

Florida Board of Pharmacy

Rebecca Poston, Executive Director
4052 Bald Cypress Way, Bin# C04
Tallahassee, FL 32399-3254
850/245-4292
850/413-6982 fax
Pharmacy@doh.state.fl.us
www.doh.state.fl.us/mqa

Georgia State Board of Pharmacy

Lisa Durden, Executive Director
Professional Licensing Boards
237 Coliseum Dr, Macon, GA 31217-3858
478/207-1610
478/207-1633 fax
ldurden@sos.state.ga.us
www.sos.state.ga.us/plb/pharmacy

Guam Board of Examiners for Pharmacy

Teresita L. G. Villagomez
Acting Administrator
P.O. Box 2816
Hagatna, GU 96932
671/735-7406
671/735-7413 fax
tlgvillagomez@dphss.govguam.net

Hawaii State Board of Pharmacy

Lee Ann Teshima
Executive Officer
P.O. Box 3469
Honolulu, HI 96801
808/586-2694
808/586-2689 fax
pharmacy@dcca.state.hi.us

Idaho Board of Pharmacy

Richard K. Mick Markuson, R.Ph.
Executive Director
3380 American Terrace, Suite 320
Boise, ID 83706
208/334-2356
208/334-3536 fax
www.accessidaho.org/bop
rmarkuson@bop.state.id.us

Illinois Department of Professional Regulation

Kim Scott, Pharmacy Board Liaison
320 W Washington, 3rd Floor
Springfield, IL 62786
217/782-8556
217/782-7645 fax
PRFGROUP10@idfpr.com
www.idfpr.com

Indiana Board of Pharmacy

Marty Allain, Director
402 W Washington St, Room W072
Indianapolis, IN 46204-2739
317/234-2067
317/233-4236 fax
pla4@pla.in.gov
www.in.gov/pla/bandc/isbp/

Iowa Board of Pharmacy Examiners

Lloyd K. Jessen, B.S., R.Ph., JD
Executive Director/Secretary
400 S.W. 8th Street, Suite E
Des Moines, IA 50309-4688
515/281-5944
515/281-4609 fax
www.state.ia.us/ibpe
lloyd.jessen@ibpe.state.ia.us

Kansas State Board of Pharmacy

Debra L. Billingsley, Executive Secretary/Director
Landon State Office Bldg.
900 Jackson Street, Room 560
Topeka, KS 66612-1231
785/296-4056
785/296-8420 fax
pharmacy@pharmacy.state.ks.us
www.kansas.gov/pharmacy

Kentucky Board of Pharmacy

Michael A. Burleson, Executive Director
Spindletop Administration Bldg, Suite 302
2624 Research Park Drive
Lexington, KY 40511
859/246-2820
859/246-2823 fax
mike.burleson@ky.gov
http://pharmacy.ky.gov

Louisiana Board of Pharmacy

Malcolm J. Broussard, R.Ph.
Executive Director
5615 Corporate Boulevard, Suite 8E
Baton Rouge, LA 70808-2537
225/925-6496
225/925-6499 fax
www.labp.com
mbroussard@labp.com

Maine Board of Pharmacy

Geraldine L. "Jeri" Betts
Board Administrator
Department of Professional/Financial Regulation
35 State House Station
Augusta, ME 04333
207/624-8625
207/624-8637 fax
207/624-8563 TTY
www.maineprofessionalreg.org
geraldine.l.betts@dhmh.state.me.us

Maryland Board of Pharmacy

LaVerne George Naesea, MSW
Executive Director
4201 Patterson Avenue
Baltimore, MD 21215-2299
410/764-4755
410/358-9512 fax
lnaesea@dhmh.state.md.us

Massachusetts Board of Registration in Pharmacy

James D. Coffey, Interim Director
239 Causeway St, 2nd Floor
Boston, MA 02114
617/973-0950
617/973-0983 fax
james.d.coffey@state.ma.us
www.mass.gov/dpl/boards/ph/index.htm

Appendix D

State Boards of Pharmacy

Michigan Board of Pharmacy

Rae Ramsdell, Director
Licensing Division
611 W. Ottawa, 1st Floor, P.O. Box 30670
Lansing, MI 48909-8170
517/335-0918
517/373-2179 fax
rhramsd@michigan.gov
www.michigan.gov/healthlicense

Minnesota Board of Pharmacy

Cody C. Wiberg, Executive Director
2829 University Ave SE, Suite 530
Minneapolis, MN 55414-3251
651/201-2825
651/201-2837 fax
Cody.Wiberg@state.mn.us
www.phcybrd.state.mn.us

Mississippi State Board of Pharmacy

Leland "Ma" McDivitt
Executive Director
P.O. Box 24507
Jackson, MS 39225-4507
601/354-6750, ext. 106
601/354-6071 fax
lmcdivitt@mbp.state.ms.us
www.mbp.state.ms.us

Missouri Board of Pharmacy

Kevin E. Kinkade, R.Ph.
Executive Director
P.O. Box 625
Jefferson City, MO 65102
573/751-0091
573/526-3464 fax
www.ecodev.state.mo.us/pr/pharmacy
kkinkade@mail.state.mo.us

Montana Board of Pharmacy

Starla Blank, Executive Director
P.O. Box 200513, 301 S Park Ave., 4th Floor
Helena, MT 59620-0513
406/841-2371
406/841-2305 fax
dlibsdpha@mt.gov
http://mt.gov/dli/bsd/license/bsd_boards/pha_board/
board_page.asp

Nebraska Board of Examiners in Pharmacy

Becky Wisell, B.S.
Executive Secretary
P.O. Box 94986
Lincoln, NE 68509-4986

402/471-2118
402/471-3577 fax
www.hhs.state.ne.us
becky.wisell@hhss.state.ne.us

Nevada State Board of Pharmacy

Larry L. "Larry" Pinson, Executive Secretary
555 Double Eagle Ct., Suite 1100
Reno, NV 89521
775/850-1440
775/850-1444 fax
pharmacy@govmail.state.nv.us
http://bop.nv.gov

New Hampshire Board of Pharmacy

Paul G. Boisseau, R.Ph., Sc.D. (Hon)
Executive Secretary
57 Regional Drive
Concord, NH 03301-8518
603/271-2350
603/271-2856 fax
www.state.nh.us/pharmacy
nhpharmacy@nhsa.state.nh.us

New Jersey State Board of Pharmacy

Joanne Boyer, Executive Director
124 Halsey Street
Newark, NJ 07101
973/504-6450
973/648-3355 fax
boyerj@dca.lps.state.nj.us
www.state.nj.us/lps/ca/boards.htm

New Mexico Board of Pharmacy

William Harvey, Executive Director/Chief Drug Inspector
5200 Oakland NE, Suite A
Albuquerque, NM 87113
505/222-9830
505/222-9845 fax
william.harvey@state.nm.us
www.state.nm.us/pharmacy

New York Board of Pharmacy

Lawrence H. Mokhiber, R.Ph.
Executive Secretary
89 Washington Ave., 2nd Floor W.
Albany, NY 12234-1000
518/474-3817, ext. 130
518/473-6995 fax
www.op.nysed.gov
pharmbd@mail.nysed.gov

North Carolina Board of Pharmacy

Jack William "Jay" Campbell IV, Executive Director
P.O. Box 4560
Chapel Hill, NC 27515-4560
919/246-1050
919/246-1056 fax
jcampbell@ncbop.org

North Dakota State Board of Pharmacy

Howard C. Anderson, Jr., R.Ph.
Executive Director
P.O. Box 1354
Bismarck, ND 58502-1354
701/328-9535
701/258-9312 fax
ndboph@btinet.com
www.nodakpharmacy.com/NDBP/ndbp.html

Ohio State Board of Pharmacy

William T. Winsley, M.S., R.Ph.
Executive Director
77 S. High Street, Room 1702
Columbus, OH 43215-6216
614/466-4143
614/752-4836 fax
www.state.oh.us/pharmacy
exec@bop.state.oh.us

Oklahoma State Board of Pharmacy

Bryan H. Potter, B.S. Pharm, R.Ph.
Executive Director
4545 Lincoln Boulevard, Suite 112
Oklahoma City, OK 73105-3488
405/521-3815
405/521-3758 fax
www.state.ok.us/~pharmacy
pharmacy@oklaosf.state.ok.us

Oregon State Board of Pharmacy

Gary A. Schnabel, R.Ph., RN
Executive Director
State Office Building, Suite 425
800 N.E. Oregon Street, #9
Portland, OR 97232
503/731-4032
503/731-4067 fax
www.pharmacy.state.or.us
pharmacy.board@state.or.us

Pennsylvania State Board of Pharmacy

Melanie A. Zimmerman, R.Ph.
Executive Secretary
P.O. Box 2649
Harrisburg, PA 17105-2649

717/783-7156
717/787-7769 fax
www.dos.state.pa.us/bpoa/phabd/mainpage.htm
st-pharmacy@state.pa.us

Puerto Rico Board of Pharmacy

Magda Bouet, Executive Director
Department of Health, Board of Pharmacy
Call Box 10200
Santurce, PR 00908
787/724-7282
787/725-7903 fax
mbouet@salud.gov.pr

Rhode Island Board of Pharmacy

Catherine A. Lordy, Chief of the Board
3 Capitol Hill, Room 205
Providence, RI 02908-5097
401/222-2837
401/222-2158 fax
www.health.state.ri.us/hsr/pharmacy/htm
cathyc@doh.state.ri.us

South Carolina Board of Pharmacy

Lee Ann Bundrick, Administrator
110 Centerview Drive, Suite 306, Kingstree Building
Columbia, SC 29210
803/896-4700
803/896-4596 fax
www.llr.state.sc.us/pol/pharmacy
bundricl@mail.llr.state.sc.us

South Dakota State Board of Pharmacy

Dennis M. Jones, B.S., R.Ph.
Executive Secretary
4305 S. Louise Avenue, Suite 104
Sioux Falls, SD 57106
605/362-2737
605/362-2738 fax
www.state.sd.us/dcr/pharmacy
dennis.jones@state.sd.us

Tennessee Board of Pharmacy

Terry Webb Grinder, Interim Executive Director
Tennessee Department of Commerce and Insurance
Board of Pharmacy
500 James Robertson Parkway, 2nd Floor, Davy Crockett Tower
Nashville, TN 37243-1149
615/741-2718
615/741-2722 fax
terry.grinder@state.tn.us
www.state.tn.us/commerce/boards/pharmacy

Appendix D

State Boards of Pharmacy

Texas State Board of Pharmacy

Gay Dodson, R.Ph.
Executive Director
William P. Hobby Building
333 Guadalupe, Tower 3, Suite 600, Box 21
Austin, TX 78701-3942
512/305-8000
512/305-8082 fax
www.tsbp.state.tx.us
gay.dobson@tsbp.state.tx.us

Utah Board of Pharmacy

Division of Occupational and Professional Licensing
Diana L. Baker, Manager
P.O. Box 146741
Salt Lake City, UT 84114-6701
801/530-6179
801/530-6511 fax
www.dopl.utah.gov
dbaker@utah.gov

Vermont Board of Pharmacy

Peggy Atkins, Board Administrator
Office of Professional Regulation
26 Terrace Street, Drawer 09
Montpelier, VT 05609-1106
802/828-2875
802/828-2465 fax
www.vtprofessionals.org/pharmacists
cpreston@sec.state.vt.us

Virgin Islands Board of Pharmacy

Lydia T. Scott, Executive Assistant
Department of Health
Roy L. Schneider Hospital, 48 Sugar Estate
St. Thomas, VI 00802
340/774-0117, ext. 5078/5074
340/777-4001 fax
lydia.scott@usvi-doh.org

Virginia Board of Pharmacy

Elizabeth Scott Russell, Executive Director
6603 W Broad Street, 5th Floor
Richmond, VA 23230-1712
804/662-9911
804/662-9313 fax
scotti.russell@dhp.virginia.gov
www.dhp.state.va.us/pharmacy/default.htm

Washington State Board of Pharmacy

Lisa Salmi, Acting Executive Director
P.O. Box 47863
Olympia, WA 98504-7863
360/236-4825

360/586-4359 fax
Lisa.Salmi@doh.wa.gov
https://fortress.wa.gov/doh/hpqa1/HPS4/Pharmacy/default.htm

West Virginia Board of Pharmacy

William T. Douglass, Jr., JD
Executive Director
232 Capitol Street
Charleston, WV 25301
304/558-0558
304/558-0572 fax
www.wvbop.com
wdouglass@wvbop.com

Wisconsin Pharmacy Examining Board

Tom Ryan, Bureau Director
1400 E. Washington Avenue
P.O. Box 8935
Madison, WI 53708-8935
608/266-8098
608/267-3816 fax
www.drl.state.wi.us
tom.ryan@drl.state.wi.us

Wyoming State Board of Pharmacy

James T. Carder, R.Ph.
Executive Director
1720 S. Poplar Street, Suite 4
Casper, WY 82601
307/234-0294
307/234-7226 fax
http://pharmacyboard.state.wy.us
wypharmbd@wercs.com

Answers

Answers

Case 1 Angina Pectoris

1. The answer is C (1.3.4)

Cocaine users may develop ischemic chest discomfort that is indistinguishable from the unstable angina secondary to coronary atherosclerosis. The widespread use of cocaine makes it mandatory to consider this cause, because its recognition mandates special management, according to guidelines by the American College of Cardiology (ACC) and the American Heart Association (AHA). Beta-blockers are thought by many to be contraindicated in cocaine-induced coronary spasm, because there is evidence that beta-adrenergic blockade augments cocaine-induced coronary artery vasoconstriction. Others believe that if the patient has a high sympathetic state with sinus tachycardia and hypertension, then beta-blockers should be used. According to treatment guidelines, beta-blockers are indicated for cocaine-positive patients that are hypertensive (systolic blood pressure greater than 150 mmHg) or present with sinus tachycardia (pulse greater than 100 min^{-1}). WP does not fit either of these criteria.

2. The answer is C (1.1.0)

Any patient with two fasting plasma glucose levels of 126 mg/dL (7.0 mmol/L) or greater is considered to have diabetes mellitus. If WP is currently fasting and a subsequent fasting blood glucose test demonstrates levels of 126 mg/dL (7.0 mmol/L) or greater, he could be diagnosed with diabetes. Atypical presentations of angina do occur in patients with autonomic dysfunction as a result of diabetes. Diabetes occurs in about one fifth of patients with unstable angina and is an independent predictor of adverse outcomes. It is associated with more extensive coronary artery disease, unstable lesions, frequent comorbidities, and less favorable long-term outcomes with coronary revascularization, especially with percutaneous transluminal coronary angioplasty. Diabetes is an independent risk factor in patients with unstable angina. Although beta-blockers may mask the symptoms of hypoglycemia or lead to it by blunting the hyperglycemic response, they should nevertheless be used with appropriate caution in diabetics with acute coronary syndrome.

3. The answer is A (2.2.0)

The rationale for nitroglycerin use in unstable angina is extrapolated from pathophysiological principles and extensive, although uncontrolled, clinical observations. Most studies of nitrate treatment in unstable angina have been small and uncontrolled, and there are no randomized, placebo-controlled trials that address reduction in cardiac events. Nitroglycerin reduces myocardial oxygen demand while enhancing myocardial oxygen delivery through effects on both the coronary and peripheral vasculature. Nitrate use within 24 hours after sildenafil or the administration of sildenafil in a patient who has received a nitrate within 24 hours has been associated with profound hypotension, myocardial infarction, and even death as a result of exaggerated nitroglycerin-mediated vasodilatation.

Tolerance to the hemodynamic effects of nitrates is dose and duration dependent and typically becomes important after 24 hours of continuous therapy with any formulation. An effort must be made to use non-tolerance-producing nitrate regimens, such as lower dose and intermittent dosing.

4. The answer is E (2.2.4)

The steady-state serum digoxin level in patients receiving the average digoxin dose in the DIG trial averaged between 0.8 ng/mL and 0.9 ng/mL (therapeutic range 0.5–2.0 ng/mL). Higher maintenance doses of digoxin (0.375 mg per day) were used in the PROVED and RADIANCE trials, but there was no evidence that increasing the dose in the range 0.2–0.39 mg per day resulted in any symptomatic improvement. There are several lines of evidence showing that the risk of digoxin toxicity rises rapidly when trough serum digoxin levels are above 1.0 ng/mL. A drug-drug interaction exists between verapamil and digoxin that can double digoxin levels if doses are not adjusted. Adverse reactions to digoxin are usually dose-dependent and occur at dosages higher than those needed to achieve a therapeutic effect. The principal manifestations of digoxin toxicity include cardiac arrhythmias (ectopic and reentrant cardiac rhythms and heart block), gastrointestinal tract symptoms (anorexia, nausea, vomiting, and diarrhea) and neurologic symptoms (visual disturbances, headache, weakness, dizziness, and confusion).

5. The answer is B (1.2.0)

In unstable angina, the primary benefits of beta-blockers are due to effects on beta1-adrenergic receptors that decrease cardiac work and myocardial oxygen demand. Some beta-blockers have partial agonist activity, also called intrinsic sympathomimetic activity, and may not decrease heart rate and blood pressure at rest. The initial choice of agents includes metoprolol, propranolol, or atenolol. Esmolol can be used if an ultrashort-acting agent is required. The usual dose of metoprolol for angina is 50 to 200 mg twice daily. Patients with significant COPD who may have a component of reactive airway disease should be administered beta-blockers very cautiously; initially, low doses of a beta1-selective agent should be used. If there are concerns about possible intolerance to beta-blockers, initial selection should favor a short-acting beta1-specific drug such as metoprolol. Mild wheezing or a history of COPD mandates a short-acting cardioselective agent at a reduced dose rather than the complete avoidance of a beta-blocker. Patients with significant sinus bradycardia (heart rate less than 50 bpm) or hypotension (systolic blood pressure less than 90 mmHg) generally should not receive beta-blockers until these conditions have resolved.

6. The answer is B (1.2.1)

No trial has directly compared the efficacy of different doses of aspirin in patients who present with unstable angina. However, trials in secondary prevention of stroke, myocardial infarction, death, and graft occlusion have not shown an added benefit for aspirin doses of greater than 80 and 160 mg per day

Answers

but have shown a higher risk of bleeding. The prompt action of aspirin and its ability to reduce mortality rates in patients with suspected acute myocardial infarction enrolled in the ISIS-2 trial led to the recommendation that aspirin be initiated in the ED as soon as the diagnosis of acute coronary syndrome is made or suspected. In patients who are already receiving aspirin, it should be continued. Contraindications to aspirin include intolerance and allergy (primarily manifested as asthma), active bleeding, hemophilia, active retinal bleeding, severe untreated hypertension, an active peptic ulcer, or another serious source of gastrointestinal or genitourinary bleeding. By irreversibly inhibiting cyclooxygenase-1 within platelets, aspirin prevents the formation of thromboxane A2, thereby diminishing platelet aggregation promoted by this pathway but not by others. Trials in secondary prevention of stroke, myocardial infarction, death, and graft occlusion have not shown an added benefit for aspirin doses of greater than 80 and 160 mg per day but have shown a higher risk of bleeding. An overview of trials with different doses of aspirin in long-term treatment of patients with coronary artery disease suggests similar efficacy for daily doses ranging from 75 to 324 mg.

7. The answer is D (3.1.2)

The weights of evidence used by the ACC, AHA, and many other associations to rank recommendations are: (A) if the data were derived from multiple randomized clinical trials that involved large numbers of patients and intermediate, (B) if the data were derived from a limited number of randomized trials that involved small numbers of patients or from careful analyses of nonrandomized studies or observational registries, and (C) when expert consensus was the primary basis for the recommendation. The customary classifications I, II, and III are used when describing final recommendations for both patient evaluation and therapy. Class I is assigned when conditions for which there is evidence and/or general agreement that a given procedure or treatment is useful and effective. Class II recommendations are conditions for which there is conflicting evidence and/or a divergence of opinion about the usefulness/efficacy of a procedure or treatment. Class III is information for which there is evidence and/or general agreement that the procedure/treatment is not useful/effective and in some cases may be harmful.

8. The answer is A (1.2.1)

Morphine sulfate has potent analgesic and anxiolytic effects, as well as hemodynamic effects that are potentially beneficial in unstable angina. Morphine causes venodilation and may produce modest reductions in heart rate and systolic blood pressure to further reduce myocardial oxygen demand. Morphine has not been shown to reduce mortality rates in patients with unstable angina. Unless contraindicated by hypotension or intolerance, morphine may be administered along with intravenous nitroglycerin, with careful blood pressure monitoring, and may be repeated every 5 to 30 minutes as needed to relieve symptoms and maintain patient comfort. The major adverse reaction to morphine is an exaggeration of its therapeutic ef-

fect, causing hypotension, especially in the presence of volume depletion and/or vasodilator therapy.

9. The answer is E (3.2.2)

All statements are correct and should be included in counseling WP on smoking and heart disease. Referral to a smoking cessation program and the use of nicotine patches or gum are recommended. Bupropion, an anxiolytic agent and weak inhibitor of neuronal uptake of neurotransmitters, has been effective when added to brief regular counseling sessions in helping patients to quit smoking.

10. The answer is D (2.2.0)

To avoid the loss of drug when using the 30- and 40-mg prefilled syringes, do not expel the air bubble from the syringe before the injection. Administration should be alternated between the left and right anterolateral and left and right posterolateral abdominal wall. Mild local irritation, pain, hematoma, ecchymosis, and erythema may follow injection and can be worsened by rubbing the injection site.

Case 2 Heart Failure

1. The answer is B (1.1.2)

An assessment of ejection fraction (EF) is necessary to definitively diagnose heart failure. BNP testing is gaining popularity, but should not be used alone to make or confirm a diagnosis. Elevated BNP levels are seen in other settings such as COPD, renal failure, and pulmonary embolus. A chest x-ray might show cardiomegaly or infiltrates, but neither of these would be diagnostic of heart failure.

2. The answer is B (3.2.1)

Though there are many good drugs for heart failure, some of which are proven to decrease mortality, the disease is not curable without cardiac transplantation. Most patients with heart failure will require three or four medications for this disease (angiotensin converting enzyme inhibitor, beta blocker, diuretic, and possibly digoxin or spironolactone) in order to comply with evidence-based treatment guidelines. Even if a patient can be symptomatically managed with one or two drugs, this is not recommended.

3. The answer is E (2.1.3)

5 mcg/kg/min (96.4 kg) = 482 mcg/min

482 mcg/min (1mg / 1000 mcg) (250 mL / 500 mg) (60 min / hr) = 14.5 mL/hr

250 mL (1 / 14.5 mL/hr) = 17 hr

4. The answer is C (1.2.2)

Dopamine and dobutamine work predominantly via stimulation of β_1-adrenergic receptors in the heart. Nesiritide (Natrecor) is intravenous B-type natriuretic peptide. Nesiritide mimics the actions of endogenous natriuretic peptide. Nitroglycerin acts to decrease preload in heart failure.

5. The answer is E (3.1.1)

Hawthorn and coenzyme Q10 are herbal products that have been used for heart failure with limited success. Controlled clinical trial data on these two herbals in heart failure are very limited and often conflicting.

6. The answer is D (1.2.1)

The RALES trial assessed the effect of adding spironolactone (25 mg) to standard heart failure regimens of patients with recent or current NYHA Class IV disease. Mortality decreased significantly in the group receiving spironolactone.

7. The answer is C (1.2.4)

Beta blockers are generally contraindicated in patients with heart block or severe bradycardia/hypotension. Though beta blockers may mask the signs and symptoms of hypoglycemia in a diabetic patient, this is not a contraindication to their use.

8. The answer is B (1.3.3)

Digibind is an antidote for digoxin toxicity. It works by binding with digoxin molecules so they can be excreted by the kidneys. Digibind should be used for patients who are experiencing signs and symptoms of digoxin toxicity (i.e., life-threatening ventricular arrhythmias, severe or progressive bradycardia, second- or third-degree heart block) or adult patients with an acute ingestion of greater than 10 mg of digoxin. Digibind should not generally be administered to asymptomatic patients with mild elevations in serum levels. In these cases, digoxin can be held until levels return to therapeutic range.

9. The answer is A (1.2.4)

Amiodarone, a Class III antiarrhythmic, has beneficial effects in heart failure. Class Ia agents (quinidine and procainamide) should be used with great caution in heart failure due to their negative inotropic effect. Class Ic agents (flecainide and propafenone) should not be used in patients with cardiac disease because of increased mortality in this population.

10. The answer is E (1.3.5)

Eplerenone (Inspra) is a new selective aldosterone receptor antagonist. Because of its selectivity, there are fewer adverse effects associated with it than with spironolactone (especially gynecomastia).

Case 3 Hypertension

1. The answer is E (1.1.2)

All three choices are natural consequences of hypertension. Their development is hastened when the patient received no, or incomplete, treatment.

Answers

2. The answer is C (1.1.1)

The following is the classification scheme for systolic blood pressure:

Optimal <120 mmHg
Normal <130 mmHg
High-normal 130–139 mmHg
Stage 1 HTN 140–159 mmHg
Stage 2 HTN 160–179 mmHg
Stage 3 HTN >180 mmHg

3. The answer is C (3.3.2)

Weight loss can effectively reduce blood pressure and lower AJ's cholesterol. African American and elderly patients with high blood pressure are typically more sodium-sensitive and can ordinarily benefit from sodium restriction. AJ's current alcohol intake of three servings of beer per week does not increase his blood pressure from baseline. Only patients with an excessive intake of alcohol will benefit from reducing alcohol use.

4. The answer is B (1.1.4)

Unlike diastolic hypertension, the incidence of systolic hypertension is not dependent on sex or race. There is a clear correlation between advancing age and systolic hypertension.

5. The answer is A (1.3.2)

Thiazide diuretics are the drug of choice because of their superior efficacy in treating systolic hypertension and low ADR profile. Beta-blockers and dihydropyridine calcium channel blockers are also effective.

6. The answer is E (1.2.4)

Alpha blockers, adrenergic blockers, and high-dose diuretics can exaggerate postural changes in blood pressure. Central alpha-2 agonists, like clonidine, can cause cognitive dysfunction in the elderly.

7. The answer is D (1.2.4)

As they can increase serum uric acid levels, thiazide diuretics should be used with caution in patients with hyperuricemia or a history of gout.

8. The answer is C (1.2.4)

Alpha blockers can cause slight decreases in LDL levels. Beta blockers can increase triglycerides and decrease HDL levels. Calcium channel blockers have no effect on serum lipids.

9. The answer is B (3.2.2)

NSAIDs do not generally raise blood pressure, but they can often offset the blood pressure reductions caused by antihypertensive medications.

10. The answer is A (1.2.1)

Procardia XL is the brand name for extended-release nifedipine. Calan SR is the brand name for extended-release verapamil.

Answers

DynaCirc CR is the brand name for controlled-release isradipine. Cardizem SR is the brand name for sustained-release diltiazem. Toprol XL is the brand name for extended-release metoprolol.

Case 4 Myocardial Infarction

1. The answer is B (1.2.0)

Thrombolytic therapy is not a realistic option in patients who present more than 24 hours after the onset of chest pain. By this time the clot is more stable and less likely to respond to the chemical thrombolysis. Neither past history (more than 2–4 weeks out) of peptic ulcer disease nor advanced age are appropriate contraindications to the use of a thrombolytic.

2. The answer is D (1.2.4)

Moderate chronic hypertension is not a contraindication to the use of a thrombolytic. History of any hemorrhagic stroke, a nonhemorrhagic stroke within the past year, and known intracranial bleeding are all absolute contraindications. Recent internal bleeding and current anticoagulant use are relative contraindications.

3. The answer is A (1.3.0)

After the onset of symptoms, there is a decline in efficacy associated with thrombolytic therapy the later a drug is started. The problem occurs in identifying when a patient has progressed from unstable angina to MI.

4. The answer is E (1.3.3)

Aspirin 325 mg either swallowed, chewed, or sucked will give an immediate antiplatelet effect and reduce mortality. Enoxaparin or heparin is useful in the prevention of ischemia, and morphine, usually given in 2-mg IV doses, relieves pain, reduces anxiety, and reduces sympathetic tone, preload, and myocardial oxygen demand.

5. The answer is C (1.2.0)

Clopidogrel is a potent oral antiplatelet agent with a once daily dosing and a low degree of hematological toxicity, which has the best risk versus benefit ratio. Ticlopidine is also a potent oral antiplatelet agent and has demonstrated benefits in patients with stroke who experience aspirin failures; however, the high degree of life-threatening neutropenia and thrombocytopenia makes ticlopidine a less correct answer. Tirofiban and abciximab are both injectable antiplatelet agents not intended for long-term use. Amiodarone has no antiplatelet activity.

6. The answer is D (1.3.0)

Under current NCEP guidelines, any patient with CAD should strive to lower LDL cholesterol levels to <100 mg/dL.

7. The answer is E (1.3.0)

All statements are true and directly affect the management of KP.

8. The answer is C (1.1.4)

The following factors have been shown to place a post-MI patient at risk of death within 30 days post-MI: age >70 years, decreased left ventricular function, hypertension, atrial fibrillation, tachycardia, large infarct size, anterior wall infarct location, previous AMI, and female sex.

9. The answer is E (1.1.2)

All of the data listed are indicative of MI.

10. The answer is B (1.2.1)

Lovastatin is the generic of Mevacor. Atorvastatin is the generic of Lipitor. Simvastatin is the generic of Zocor. Pravastatin is the generic of Pravachol. Cerivastatin is the generic of Baycol, which was removed from the market due to increased risk of serious liver damage.

Case 5 Shock

1. The answer is E (1.3.1)

Untreated cardiogenic shock is associated with an 82%–97% mortality rate.

2. The answer is B (1.3.1)

The most likely causes of cardiogenic shock in this situation is acute myocardial infarction with extensive ventricular damage. Hypertension with coronary artery disease and hyperlipidemia with caffeine and/or tobacco use will not cause cardiogenic shock.

3. The answer is E (1.3.5)

Sodium bicarbonate is not indicated for treatment of cardiogenic shock. In the management of cardiogenic shock, it is critical to optimize initial fluid resuscitation. If cardiogenic shock, decreased cardiac output with persistent systemic hypotension despite adequate intravascular volume, persists, then vasopressor or inotropic agents should be initiated. Initiating vasopressor agents and inotropic agents before aggressive fluid management will worsen cardiac output and perfusion to vital organs.

4. The answer is A (1.2.1)

Aggressive fluid resuscitation with NaCl 0.9% infusion is the cornerstone of initial treatment of cardiogenic shock. Administration of nesiritide would worsen hypotension. The manufacturer's recommended starting dose is $0.01 \mu g/kg/min$ not $0.1 \mu g/kg/min$. Dopamine would be a reasonable second step once fluid resuscitation has been optimized, but dopamine may make the patient more tachycardic. Drotrecogin alpha is used in the treatment of septic shock and is not recommended in treatment of cardiogenic shock. Administration of a furosemide infusion would worsen hypotension.

5. The answer is B (1.3.5)

The hemodynamic parameters suggest the patient is now fluid resuscitated since the Pulmonary Artery Wedge Pressure (PAWP) is slightly greater than the top of the range (8–12 mmHg). But this patient is still hypotensive (both BP and MAP are low) and tachycardic resulting in a low cardiac output. In addition, the Systemic Vascular Resistance Index (SVRI) is increased. The combination of decreased cardiac output and increased systemic vascular resistance is strongly suggestive of cardiogenic shock. Since further fluid resuscitation will worsen pulmonary congestion and increase PCWP, an inotropic agent would provide the most benefit for improving cardiac output of the heart.

6. The answer is A (1.3.5)

Nesiritide, nitroglycerin, and norepinephrine are not inotropes. Nitroglycerin would not increase cardiac index and may further aggravate hypotension. Nesiritide would worsen hypotension. Norepinephrine is a vasopressor that is indicated for severe hypotension (systolic <70 mmHg). Dopamine is generally reserved for hypotension associated with bradycardia or immediately post-resuscitation. Dobutamine is a ß-adrenergic agent that has a dose-dependent increase in myocardial contractility, therefore cardiac output increases.

7. The answer is B (1.3.5)

As discussed above, dobutamine increases myocardial contractility but it has little effect on systemic vascular resistance. Phenylephrine works as a pure β_1-agonist and therefore has no effect on cardiac output. Vasopressin has emerged as a useful therapy in septic shock and possibly in shock secondary to trauma, its usefulness in cardiogenic shock is not established. Both dopamine and norepinephrine have both inotropic and vasopressor effects; however, norepinephrine is generally reserved for therapeutic failures using dopamine or when the systolic BP is less than 70 mmHg. This is due to its more potent peripheral vasoconstrictive effects.

8. The answer is A (1.2.4)

The ß-adrenergic effects of the catecholamines can cause tachydysrhythmias which may cause an increase in myocardial oxygen demand sufficient to cause ischemia. The α-adrenergic effects may cause severe capillary vasoconstriction if extravasation occurs (this can be treated with phentolamine injected intradermally). Lactic acidosis can occur due to increases glycogenolysis, peripheral vasoconstriction resulting in peripheral anaerobic metabolism (early) or even after improvement in peripheral circulation allows for mobilization of peripherally produced lactate (late). Bradycardia is not associated with catecholamine use.

9. The answer is D (1.2.6)

Dopamine has a very short elimination half life ~2 minutes, as does its active metabolite norepinephrine. So plasma levels will reach steady state in a very short time period; however, it is wise to allow the patient to stabilize hemodynamically between each dosing change; 30–60 minutes is a conservative approach. Maintaining the hemodynamic parameters (MAP, HR and CI) in the normal ranges indicates the patient is no longer dependent on the drug. Normal adult renal perfusion usually results in urine output greater than 0.5 mL/kg/min.

10. The answer is E (1.3.3)

All three statements are correct.

Case 6 Thromboembolic Disorders

1. The answer is C (1.1.0)

The American College of Chest Physicians (ACCP) recommends anticoagulation in patients with atrial fibrillation greater than 48 hours to minimize the risk of atrial thrombi formation. Patients with atrial fibrillation and other risk factors for stroke, including hypertension, mitral stenosis, increasing age, and previous transient ischemic event or stroke, should receive anticoagulation with warfarin, unless other contraindications exist. Warfarin should not be used in pregnancy as it is pregnancy Category X.

2. The answer is B (3.1.0)

Vitamin K is a cofactor necessary for the formation of clotting factors II, VII, IX, and X, as well as proteins C and S. Warfarin acts by inhibiting the enzymes responsible for the conversion of vitamin K in the liver. By decreasing the supply of vitamin K available to serve as a cofactor, warfarin slows the rate of synthesis of these clotting factors. Increasing levels of dietary vitamin K will promote clotting factor formation, thereby decreasing the effect of warfarin and the patient's INR. It is important for patients to maintain a consistent and moderate consumption of foods containing vitamin K, avoiding sudden changes in amounts of high vitamin K foods. Green tea beverages and spinach contain very high levels of vitamin K (classified as >200 mcg per 100-g serving). Broccoli contains high levels of vitamin K (classified as 100–200 mcg per 100-g serving). Corn contains low levels of vitamin K (<50 mcg per 100-g serving). Garlic nutritional supplements can cause an increased anticoagulation effect. These categories are stated as found in Chapter 19 of DiPiro's *Pharmacotherapy*, 6th ed.

3. The answer is B (1.1.1)

Warfarin is metabolized by the cytochrome P450 hepatic system. It is a substrate of CYP450 2C8/9 and 2C19. Gemfibrozil is an inhibitor of CYP450 2C8/9 and 2C19. By inhibiting warfarin's metabolism through this hepatic system, concomitant use of gemfibrozil with warfarin may result in increased INR and increased anticoagulant effect. Hydrochlorothiazide is not metabolized by the CYP450 system and has no known interactions with warfarin. Metoprolol is a substrate of 2D6

Answers

and 2C19. It has no known effect on the metabolism of warfarin, and therefore has no known interactions.

4. The answer is D (1.2.6)

The time required for warfarin's full effect to be achieved is based on the half-lives of the coagulation proteins that are inhibited. Because prothrombin has a long half-live of 60–100 hours, it can take 8 to 15 days for maximum therapeutic effect of warfarin to be achieved.

5. The answer is B (1.1.0)

Epistaxis can be an adverse effect when INR levels are too high; however, it is not usually reason for complete discontinuation of warfarin. Patients should be instructed to call their health care provider in the event of bleeding signs for INR determination and possible dosage adjustment or held doses. Easy bruising may also occur with warfarin, especially in the elderly or in patients whose INR level is too high. It can be minimized by attaining the appropriate dosage, but is generally not an indication for discontinuation. Warfarin-induced skin necrosis is a rare but serious adverse event which can progress to necrotic gangrene. If this diagnosis is suspected, warfarin should be immediately discontinued. Often, warfarin is never initiated again; if it is decided to restart, extreme caution should be used.

6. The answer is D (1.2.0)

The ACCP guidelines recommend an INR range of 2.0–3.0 as ideally therapeutic in atrial fibrillation.

7. The answer is A (1.3.0)

Addition of amiodarone to the regimen can increase the effects of warfarin, resulting in a supratherapeutic INR.

8. The answer is D (1.2.2)

ACCP recommends that patients who undergo cardioversion to normal sinus rhythm receive warfarin treatment for at least 4 weeks following effective cardioversion. Full atrial contraction following cardioversion may not be achieved for 3 to 4 weeks and patients still require anticoagulation to continue to prevent the formation of a thrombus.

9. The answer is C (3.2.2)

Warfarin dose, based on INR, can be adjusted to compensate for dietary vitamin K consumption. Changes in consumption pattern will result in a nontherapeutic INR if the dose of warfarin remains unchanged.

10. The answer is D (1.2.3)

Coenzyme Q10 and St. John's Wort can potentially cause a decrease in INR. Cranberry juice and Vitamin E may cause an increase in INR. Saw palmetto is not commonly thought to interfere with warfarin and INR.

Case 7 Asthma

1. The answer is B (3.2.4)

Peak flow meters are helpful in monitoring patients with asthma. Blood pressure and blood glucose fluctuations (A and D) are not associated with asthma. Aero Chamber and InspirEase (C and E) are delivery devices.

2. The answer is C (1.1.1)

Based on MT's past medical history he should be diagnosed with mild persistent asthma. He is experiencing more than two asthmatic episodes per week and has significantly increased his albuterol use. In this case a medication for long-term control should be prescribed. Fluticasone is an inhaled corticosteroid which is a potent anti-inflammatory agent. Use of inhaled corticosteroids to "control" asthma has been shown to improve asthma control and normalize lung function to prevent irreversible airway damage. Salmeterol (B) is the generic name of Serevent. Theophylline and glycopyrrolate (D and E) may be used in the treatment of asthma, but neither agent is preferred because of documented modest clinical effectiveness.

3. The answer is C (3.2.2)

Inhaled albuterol is the drug of choice for acute asthma exacerbation (I). It is not necessary for MT to discontinue sports at this time (III), but he should be cautious of triggers such as viral illness, changes in weather, and tobacco smoke (II).

4. The answer is A (1.2.1)

From the PMH, it appears that MT has seasonal allergies that result in an asthma exacerbation. Zyrtec is an antihistamine and does not treat bronchospasm (B), inadequate oxygen exchange (C), contact dermatitis (D), or rapid heart rate (E).

5. The answer is B (1.2.4)

Salmeterol is a long-acting beta-agonist indicated for use in asthma (A) and does not have an immediate onset of action. Thus, it should only be used in a regimen that also includes a short-acting beta-agonist (E). It has an FDA-labeled indication for children (C) greater than or equal to 12 years of age with the oral inhaler. The inhaled powder (diskus) is indicated in children greater than or equal to 4 years of age. Although a spacer device (D) may be useful in some patients, it is not required for use of the medication.

6. The answer is C (1.2.0)

For exercise-induced asthma, dosing 30–60 minutes prior to exercise is appropriate. It is not indicated for acute relief of bronchospasm (D). The long duration of action (A, E) of salmeterol allows for twice-daily dosing for most patients.

7. The answer is E (2.2.5)

The switch to HFA inhalers is a major public health venture to protect the earth's ozone layer. The HFA inhalers have different physical properties than the CFCs (I). Because of the different properties, different suspending agents are used in the HFA inhalers. This may cause them to feel and taste different than the CFC inhalers (II). Although cleaning is important for all inhalers, HFA inhalers become blocked by residue, which forms around the exit hole. Therefore, it is particularly important to clean them so the spray is not blocked (III). HFA inhalers come packaged in moisture-resistant pouches. Canisters should be discarded after 200 sprays or 3 months after removal from the foil pouch, whichever comes first.

8. The answer is D (1.2.4)

For the short-term, the potential changes in behavior and appetite will be most significant for MT and his mother (D). With short-term therapy (A), (B), (C), and (E) are not a primary concern. If MT's mother raises questions about these effects, they should be addressed. Likewise, if MT should require multiple short courses of corticosteroids over a 12-month period, these long-term issues become more important.

9. The answer is B (1.1.2)

Patients with severe respiratory distress may not exchange air well at all and may, therefore, not wheeze (A) because of poor airflow. Patients frequently respond only in short sentences (C) to conserve energy. Cyanosis may be seen but is not always present (E). Beta-agonists (D) are the treatment of choice.

10. The answer is E (3.2.1)

Use of a spacer or holding chamber may increase lung delivery over MDI alone in patients with poor MDI technique (I). Use of a spacer or holding chamber device improves lung deposition and reduces systemic absorption by decreasing oral bioavailability (II). When spacers or holding devices are used with inhaled corticosteroids, decreased systemic absorption results in decreased systemic adverse reactions (III). Children often have difficulty actuating an inhaler device properly; the use of a spacer helps them administer the dose appropriately.

Case 8 Chronic Obstructive Pulmonary Disease

1. The answer is B (1.1.3)

Asthma is generally considered a reversible disease whereas COPD is generally progressive and irreversible. Although many of the medications used to treat the two conditions are similar, they are different disease processes. Family history, although it may be important in patients with asthma, does not appear to contribute to the development of COPD.

2. The answer is C (1.1.1)

Spiriva (tiotropium) is an anticholinergic agent and may cause dry mouth. The drug is administered via a dry powder inhaler and patients should be instructed not to swallow the capsules,

but to use them in the inhaler. Tiotropium does not affect depression.

3. The answer is A (1.2.2)

Tiotropium is an anticholinergic agent. Epinephrine and isoproterenol (C and E) are sympathomimetic agents. Theophylline (B) does not possess anticholinergic activity. Fluticasone (D) is a corticosteroid.

4. The answer is E (1.2.1)

Adding albuterol might be beneficial for BG as its mechanism of bronchodilation is different from tiotropium. The daily maximum recommended dose of tiotropium is 18 mcg (A). Combivent (a combination of ipratropium and albuterol [D]) might also be an option for BG but adding it to his regimen without stopping his tiotropium would result in too much anticholinergic effect and is considered a duplication of therapy. His Flomax (B) is for BPH and his Norvasc (C) is for HTN. Increases in either of these agents would not benefit BG's emphysema.

Other alternatives for BG include adding theophylline or an inhaled ß₂ agonist.

5. The answer is E (3.2.1)

Patients with COPD should receive a pneumococcal vaccine and a yearly influenza vaccine. Pulmonary function tests do not need to be followed at each office visit. While spirometry can be used to monitor disease progression, an interval of at least 12 months is suggested to improve the reliability of the measurements.

6. The answer is C (1.2.4)

Cough is an important protective mechanism in patients with COPD, and cough suppressants, such as Robitussin DM (C), should not be used. Acetaminophen (A), multivitamins (B), and Tums (D) do not present any contraindications in patients with COPD. While the use of saw palmetto (E) is not problematic in patients with COPD, its use might be problematic in this patient who is on therapy for BPH and he should talk with his doctor about its use.

7. The answer is A (1.2.2)

Tiotropium acts through inhibition of c-GMP. Beta-agonists stimulate beta receptors (E) and increase c-AMP (C).

8. The answer is A (1.2.4)

The anticholinergic activity of tiotropium can aggravate symptoms of narrow-angle glaucoma. A related product, ipratropium, is used as symptomatic treatment of perennial rhinitis (FDA-labeled indication) and asthma (off-label use).

9. The answer is A (1.1.4)

Smoking history is a primary risk factor for the development of COPD. Other significant risk factors include age and occupation. Although traditionally viewed as a male-dominated

Answers

disease, the incidence in women is increasing with increased rates of smoking in this gender group.

10. The answer is B (3.1.1)

While there is a lot of good information on the Internet, there is also a good chance of finding information that is of questionable origin or bias when searching is done randomly on a health-related topic through a search engine. A safer alternative would be to start with a reliable site and use the links provided by that site to obtain additional information.

Case 9 Rhinitis (Perennial)

1. The answer is D (1.2.2)

By directly stimulating alpha receptors in the vasculature, pseudoephedrine shrinks swollen nasal mucous membranes, which helps improve nasal patency. It also indirectly releases norepinephrine from storage sites, which further stimulates alpha receptors causing vasoconstriction.

2. The answer is E (3.2.4)

All of these methods have been demonstrated to be effective in decreasing the concentration of dust mites in the home.

3. The answer is E (1.3.5)

All are viable options with this patient. Although the use of an intranasal corticosteroid may not be the most favored option for this patient due to previous experience, it has been shown to be very effective for allergic rhinitis symptoms. Not all second-generation antihistamines are alike, however, they all have more favorable side effect profiles than the first generation. Singulair has been approved for use in allergic rhinitis and may be effective for this patient.

4. The answer is C (1.2.4)

Cromolyn is considered one of the safest medications for the treatment of allergic rhinitis. It is well tolerated with only minimal nasal irritation. Side effects with fluticasone are generally minimal but may include nasal irritation, burning, or bleeding (A). Pseudoephedrine may cause central nervous system side effects such as insomnia, dizziness, nervousness, and agitation (D). Oxymetazoline may cause rhinitis medicamentosa if used for more than 3 or 5 days (E).

5. The answer is C (1.3.5)

Fluticasone is one of the more potent corticosteroids available, so switching to a different intranasal corticosteroid spray would not likely lead to improved symptom control. Data are not available that would support increasing the dose above standard to obtain improved symptom control. Adding two antihistamines is not effective, and adding cromolyn to fluticasone would not likely improve symptoms. Patients who remain symptomatic despite optimal avoidance measures and pharmacotherapy are generally candidates for immunotherapy.

6. The answer is E (1.1.4)

Immunotherapy is a mainstay of therapy for those patients who have failed pharmacotherapy and avoidance measures. The patient needs to adhere to a schedule of weekly allergy injections for several months. Eventually, patients will be maintained on injections every 2 or 4 weeks for a duration of approximately 3 to 5 years.

7. The answer is A (1.3.3)

Injections are administered subcutaneously. If standard injection practices are followed, there should be essentially no risk for the development of infection or hematoma. Because immunotherapy is administering an allergen in which patients have demonstrated a positive IgE reaction (Type I hypersensitivity), there is a small risk for the development of an anaphylactic reaction.

8. The answer is D (1.3.3)

The first line of treatment for anaphylaxis is epinephrine. Data are mixed concerning the best route of administration. Either IM or SQ have been effective. Diphenhydramine can also be administered shortly after the epinephrine (B). The key to effectively treating anaphylaxis is to act quickly. Delaying treatment can lead to detrimental consequences for the patient (C). Oxygen and nebulized albuterol are not part of the standard first line of treatment. (A, E)

9. The answer is C (1.2.2)

Intranasal corticosteroids have been demonstrated to have broad anti-inflammatory activity. These actions include the ability to decrease microvascular permeability, which leads to a reduction in nasal edema (i.e., congestion). They have also been demonstrated to decrease mucus production.

10. The answer is C (3.2.1)

Allergic rhinitis is a chronic inflammatory condition. After a genetically susceptible individual is exposed to an allergen, the development of IgE antibodies occurs. These antibodies then attach to mast cells and basophils. If the patient is re-exposed to the offending allergen, the allergen cross-links the IgE antibodies, causing the release of inflammatory mediators from the mast cell or basophil. This process also leads to increased, not decreased, production of eosinophils.

Case 10 Smoking Cessation

1. The answer is C (1.1.2)

JB states he thinks about quitting but does not think this is a good time. He has not formally set a quit date or thought about a plan for quitting, therefore, offering him nicotine replacement products is premature.

At each visit patients should be assessed for tobacco use. If they use tobacco, assess whether they are willing to quit. If so, provide appropriate counseling on options (pharmacologic and non-pharmacologic) available. If patients aren't yet willing to quit, providing motivation can get them thinking about quitting.

If the pharmacist discusses JB's medical problems and relates them to smoking this may help JB become more motivated to quit. For example, smoking can worsen GERD, erectile dysfunction, and increase blood pressure. JB's COPD and lung function also may improve with tobacco cessation. Relapse prevention techniques should be addressed once a patient has quit using tobacco. Examples include: encourage abstinence, reward successes, and offering tips to minimize weight gain associated with cessation.

2. The answer is D (1.2.3)

Smoking can increase the metabolism of caffeine. If JB quits smoking the metabolism may normalize causing stimulating effects of caffeine to be more pronounced. Increased levels of caffeine may increase JB's risk of tachycardia.
Smoking has no effect on Combivent, sildenafil, famotidine, or saw palmetto levels or metabolism.

3. The answer is A (1.1.3)

Common symptoms of nicotine withdrawal include craving for tobacco, irritability, anxiety, difficulty concentrating, restlessness, headache, and drowsiness. Gastrointestinal disturbances are also common, but gastrointestinal reflux symptoms/heartburn might improve with smoking cessation. Lower clearances of caffeine may cause his heart rate to increase, but palpitations/dizziness would be unlikely. These symptoms are not usually seen as part of the nicotine withdrawal syndrome.

JB should be counseled regarding the symptoms of nicotine withdrawal. Smokers with higher nicotine intake may be more likely to experience nicotine withdrawal symptoms. As a general rule, those who use more than 16 cigarettes per day and a "regular" (vs. "light") cigarette may have a greater daily intake of nicotine. Nicotine content, however, varies significantly by brand. Actual nicotine intake also varies with a person's individual smoking technique (frequency and depth of inhalation).

4. The answer is D (1.3.2)

Smokers develop tolerance to the effects of nicotine over time. When nicotine is stopped abruptly, withdrawal symptoms may occur. Withdrawal symptoms reach maximal intensity 24–48 hours after cessation and diminish in intensity over 2 weeks. The desire to smoke (cravings) can persist for months to years after cessation.

5. The answer is C (1.2.1)

The nicotine spray can cause nasal irritation and congestion and should be avoided in patients with severe reactive airway disease. The nicotine replacement products can be used in patients with coronary artery disease as long as the patient has not experienced a myocardial infarction in the past 14 days or has an arrhythmia or angina.

6. The answer is C (3.2.4)

The best initial strength of the patch is unknown. The usual starting dose is either 21 mg (24-hour patch) or 15 mg (16-hour patch). Those who are very nicotine dependent may require higher starting doses, which may be achieved with multiple patches. Lower doses may be beneficial in those who smoker fewer cigarettes, weigh less than 45 kg, or have cardiovascular disease.

Because JB is smoking 1/2 pack per day, he may be initiated on a lower than usual starting dose of nicotine.

7. The answer is D (3.2.4)

JB is experiencing strong cravings in the morning on awakening most likely due to low levels of nicotine. The 16-hour patch is applied in the morning, but levels of nicotine drop off around bedtime. Switching to a 24-hour patch will provide JB with a steady level of nicotine throughout the day and night. Levels of nicotine should remain high enough in the morning that strong urges to smoke and cravings are minimized.
Increasing the dose of the 16-hour patch will not improve the urge to smoke in the morning. Switching to bupropion may improve urges to smoke, but this is not due to low levels of nicotine.

Utilizing the combination of nicotine patch and gum is a common way for patients that are heavy smokers (who typically smoke more than 20 cigarettes per day) to have both a steady level of nicotine throughout the day and handle strong cravings by using a short acting nicotine replacement product. This strategy won't help decrease early morning cravings for JB because he would still be receiving only 16 hours of nicotine replacement. Switching to nicotine spray will not provide a continual level of nicotine or help with early morning cravings. Because the spray closely mimics the nicotine delivery of smoking, more (up to 46%) individuals are likely to continue the use of this product 12 months after cessation.

8. The answer is A (2.2.5)

It is important to counsel patients not to smoke while using the patch, especially those with cardiovascular disease. (JB has had coronary artery disease for 10 months, but no chest pain for 6 months). Concurrent use of the patch and smoking may result in high levels of nicotine and increase the risk of serious cardiovascular complications. Use of the patch (without smoking) has less cardiovascular risk than smoking.
It should also be stressed to JB to rotate the placement of the patch on a daily basis. Rotation of the patch is essential for prevention of skin irritation. Skin reactions are the most common adverse effect seen with nicotine patches but are usually not serious.

Use of the nicotine patch is unlikely to increase the risk of seizures or worsen erectile dysfunction.
It would also be important to explain to JB how to properly dispose of the nicotine patches. Used patches should be folded, replaced in the original "aluminum" pouch, and placed in a secure trash can. The nicotine remaining in used patches is significant enough to cause serious harm to small pets or children if touched or ingested.

Answers

9. The answer is C (1.2.4)

Patients with a history of anorexia, bulimia, or other eating disorders have a lower threshold for seizures. Zyban, or bupropion, can also lower the seizure threshold, making a history of eating disorders, or seizure disorders, relative contraindications to bupropion. Other relative contraindications include allergy/sensitivity to bupropion. None of his other conditions should be affected by bupropion. The symptoms of his acid reflux, COPD, and erectile dysfunction may improve or stabilize with smoking cessation.

10. The answer is B (2.2.5)

The nicotine lozenge comes in two strengths; 2 mg and 4 mg. The 2-mg strength is recommended for those who wait 30 minutes after awakening to smoke. The 4-mg strength is recommended for those who smoke within 30 minutes of awakening.

The bite and park (or chew and park) method is useful for nicotine gum. If the lozenge is chewed and swallowed, the amount of nicotine that enters the bloodstream is greatly reduced.

While utilizing any form of nicotine replacement therapy, it is advised to not smoke cigarettes.

Each lozenge contains: 4 calories, 1 g carbohydrates, and no sugar. Therefore, it should not increase blood glucose levels in those with diabetes.

Only one lozenge should be used at a time, and the manufacturer recommends not to exceed 20 lozenges a day with either the 2- or 4-mg dose. If this amount is exceeded, the risk of nicotine overdose increases. Symptoms of overdose include nausea, vomiting, dizziness, diarrhea, weakness, and rapid heartbeat. Patients should be educated to call their physician should any of these symptoms occur.

Case 11 PUD—H. pylori-related

1. The answer is D (1.1.3)

Patients with PUD typically present with epigastric pain, which often occurs during the night. However, symptoms associated with other acid-related disorders, e.g., gastroesophageal reflux disease, dyspepsia, as well as other diseases, e.g., gall bladder disease, and gastric cancer often overlap. Therefore, the diagnosis of PUD cannot be based solely on the patient's symptoms.

2. The answer is B (1.1.0)

Most individuals infected with Helicobacter pylori are asymptomatic. Most peptic ulcers are Helicobacter pylori-positive. However, nonsteroidal anti-inflammatory drug-related ulcers may occur in the absence of Helicobacter pylori. Eradication of Helicobacter pylori heals peptic ulcers and reduces ulcer recurrence. Helicobacter pylori has been linked to gastritis, peptic ulcers, and gastric cancer, but only a small percent will develop gastric cancer in the long term.

3. The answer is C (1.2.0)

Three-drug regimens containing two antibiotics (e.g., clarithromycin and amoxicillin) and a proton pump inhibitor (PPI) are the preferred first-line regimens used to eradicate Helicobacter pylori, heal peptic ulcers, and relieve ulcer symptoms. The PPI-based three-drug regimen containing ciprofloxacin has not been widely studied and therefore cannot be recommended as first line. Regimens that contain only one antibiotic are no longer recommended because of variable eradication rates and the increased possibility for antibiotic resistance. The four-drug bismuth-based regimen, although effective, is less likely to foster adherence as it requires four medications and more frequent daily dosing than the PPI-based three-drug regimen.

4. The answer is D (1.3.5)

Regimens that contain amoxicillin (or any other penicillin such as dicloxacillin) must be avoided in patients with a documented allergy to penicillin. The PPI-based three-drug regimen containing clarithromycin and metronidazole avoids the use of amoxicillin in penicillin allergic individuals, and there is evidence to support similar eradication rates as a PPI, clarithromycin and amoxicillin. The PPI-based three-drug regimen containing tetracycline has not been widely studied and, therefore, cannot be recommended at this time. Regimens that contain only one antibiotic are not recommended because of variable eradication rates and the increased possibility for antibiotic resistance. Single agents, e.g., PPI daily, are no longer recommended for use in Helicobacter pylori-positive ulcer patients because they do not eradicate the infection and they are associated with high rates of ulcer recurrence and the need for long-term maintenance therapy.

5. The answer is A (1.3.5)

You may substitute any PPI for another when used in recommended dosages as all available PPIs are considered to be interchangeable. You should not substitute any of the H_2-receptor antagonists or bismuth subsalicylate for a PPI, ampicillin for amoxicillin, or azithromycin for clarithromycin as there is insufficient evidence to support the efficacy of these substitutions in the three-drug eradication regimen.

6. The answer is C (1.3.1)

Recurrence of epigastric pain is the most cost-effective parameter to monitor in a patient with uncomplicated PUD as it serves as a surrogate marker for incomplete ulcer healing or failure to eradicate the infection. Serology should not be used post eradication because it takes 6 months to 1 year for the antibodies to Helicobacter pylori to return to baseline after successful eradication. The urea breath test, when given at least 4 weeks post completion of the eradication regimen, confirms eradication, but it is costly and is not routinely used to monitor eradication. Abdominal x-ray may confirm ulcer healing, but not eradication. Although endoscopy will confirm ulcer healing and a biopsy can be taken to determine eradication, it is invasive and much to costly for a patient with an uncomplicated ulcer.

7. The answer is E (3.2.0)

Advise patients taking metronidazole about the disulfiram-like reaction and the need to avoid alcohol-containing foods, beverages, and medications. There are no clinically important interactions between metronidazole and milk products, citrus foods or beverages, caffeinated or carbonated beverages.

8. The answer is B (1.3.3)

Sodium bicarbonate should be avoided as sodium is readily absorbed resulting in fluid retention, which may increase blood pressure. Antacids that contain calcium, magnesium, magaldrate (complex of magnesium and aluminum) or aluminum salts are acceptable for use as they do not result in fluid retention.

9. The answer is C (1.3.3)

Magnesium-containing salts are associated with a dose-dependent diarrhea, whereas aluminum-containing salts are associated with constipation. When magnesium hydroxide is combined with aluminum hydroxide in the same antacid, diarrhea will predominate. Calcium salts, sodium bicarbonate, and bismuth subsalicylate are usually not associated with diarrhea.

10. The answer is A (1.2.3)

Atenolol is primarily renally eliminated and does not interact with cimetidine. Cimetidine inhibits the hepatic CYP-450 metabolism of theophylline, warfarin, phenytoin, and diazepam in a dose-dependent manner and may cause clinically important drug interactions. The lower nonprescription doses of Tagamet HB are less likely to interact, but patients should be advised to avoid concomitant use of cimetidine and drugs metabolized by the CYP-450 enzyme system.

Case 12 GERD-esophagitis

1. The answer is A (1.1.3)

Heartburn occurs most often in the absence of esophageal mucosal injury. In fact, most patients who experience heartburn do not have endoscopically proven esophagitis. Alternatively, most patients with endoscopically proven esophagitis do complain of heartburn. However, neither the frequency nor the severity of the heartburn directly correlates with the severity of the underlying esophageal mucosal injury.

2. The answer is D (1.1.3)

Heartburn and regurgitation are the most common typical symptoms of GERD. However, GERD is also associated with atypical (extraesophageal) manifestations that are also related to the long-term (chronic) abnormal reflux of gastric contents into the esophagus. Dental erosions, chronic laryngitis, coughing, choking, hoarseness, asthma, bronchitis, and noncardiac chest pain are all atypical manifestations of GERD.

3. The answer is D (1.2.1)

PPIs are the drugs of choice for healing esophagitis because they provide the most rapid rate of esophageal healing when compared to the other drug regimens. When used in standard recommended PPI dosages (e.g., pantoprazole 40 mg daily) the PPIs are superior to standard (e.g., ranitidine 150 mg bid) and high-dose (e.g., famotidine 40 mg bid) H$_2$RAs. High-dose esomeprazole (40 mg tid) exceeds the usually recommended daily dosage for esophageal healing and is not indicated as the patient has "moderate" erosive esophagitis. If a higher esomeprazole dosage is required, it should be increased to 40 mg twice daily. There is insufficient evidence to support the use of sucralfate for esophageal healing.

4. The answer is E (1.2.0)

When used in recommended esophageal-healing daily dosages (omeprazole 20 mg, lansoprazole 30 mg, rabeprazole 20 mg, pantoprazole 40 mg, or esomeprazole 20–40 mg qd), the PPIs provide similar rates of esophageal healing. In patients with severe erosive esophagitis, esomeprazole 40 mg qd may provide superior esophageal healing to 20 mg qd.

5. The answer is B (1.2.0)

The antisecretory effect of a PPI is maximized if given when the parietal cells are actively secreting gastric acid. This is best accomplished by taking the PPI about 30 minutes before breakfast as this permits adequate absorption of the PPI prior to ingestion of the meal. Eating a meal stimulates the parietal cells to actively secrete acid. PPIs should not be taken on an empty stomach because most parietal cells are not actively secreting acid at that time. Taking a PPI after a meal will delay absorption of the PPI and its effect on acid. Although a single daily dose of a PPI is recommended to be taken in the morning prior to breakfast, it may be taken 30 minutes prior to lunch or dinner. Taking the PPI at bedtime is problematic in GERD because patients should refrain from eating at least 2–3 hours prior to bedtime. When a second dose is needed, the PPI is given 30 minutes before breakfast and 30 minutes before dinner.

6. The answer is A (1.3.0)

GERD is a chronic disease. Symptomatic relapse after treatment has been withdrawn occurs in up to 90% of patients within 6 months. Most patients will require long-term maintenance therapy. Although the duration of maintenance therapy for this patient is unknown at this time, the preferred long-term management is to continue Protonix 40 mg qd for an additional 2–3 months and then re-evaluate. Since this patient was asymptomatic on Protonix 40 mg qd there is no need to add Zantac to the regimen. The most effective maintenance therapy is often the same drug regimen that was used to heal the esophagitis. Standard (and even higher) H$_2$RA dosages are

Answers

not as effective as a PPI when used to maintain remission. In addition, the potential for tolerance to develop to the H$_2$RA exists. There is insufficient evidence to support the prn use of PPIs (e.g., Prilosec OTC) as maintenance therapy in patients with GERD.

7. The answer is D (3.2.0)

PPIs are FDA-approved for long-term maintenance therapy in patients with GERD. The approval for the maintenance therapy indication was based on substantial evidence that supported the long-term safety of PPIs for at least 1 year. However, there is no limit placed on the duration of long-term use as long as the PPI is indicated as safety data beyond 1 year has now been published. Long-term PPI use does not cause irreversible acid inhibition when the drug is discontinued. There is no evidence to date to indicate that long-term PPI use is linked to esophageal cancer or cardiotoxicity in humans. Although a theoretical concern exists (based on animal data), there is no evidence to indicate that long-term PPI use is associated with gastric cancer in humans.

8. The answer is C (1.2.5)

H$_2$RAs inhibit histamine at the H$_2$-receptor and, therefore, are susceptible to the development of tolerance. Evidence suggests that tolerance to the antisecretory effect most likely occurs within several days to several weeks when H$_2$RAs are taken daily on a scheduled basis. Tolerance can be avoided by taking an H$_2$RA prn (occasionally) rather than continuously. Tolerance has not been associated with low dosages or with duration of treatment. Tolerance to the antisecretory effect of an H$_2$RA may explain why a patient who initially obtained symptom relief no longer responds to treatment. Because PPIs do not act at a receptor, they do not appear to be susceptible to the development of tolerance.

9. The answer is C (2.2.5)

The most important reason why PPI tablets and granules should not be chewed or crushed before swallowing is that the PPI is acid-labile and will be degraded by the low intragastric pH. In addition, the PPI is likely to become prematurely protonated (activated) in the acidity of the stomach. The enteric-coating on the tablet and the granules protect the PPI from the acidic contents of the stomach. Once the enteric-coated tablet/granules pass into the duodenum, the enteric coating dissolves, the PPI is released, and then absorbed. It is unlikely that the uncoated PPI causes pharyngitis or esophageal injury. Salivary bicarbonate does not degrade the active drug. Although the taste is most likely bad, this is not the most important reason why PPI tablets/granules should not be chewed or crushed.

10. The answer is E (2.2.1)

The antacids (aluminum hydroxide and magnesium carbonate) are the "active" ingredients in this product. The alginic acid is listed as an "inactive" ingredient. When chewed or swallowed, the alginic acid reacts with bicarbonate to create a foam

barrier or "raft" which floats on the stomach acid. When reflux occurs, this foam barrier theoretically is first to contact the esophageal mucosa providing protection against the acid-pepsin content of the stomach.

Case 13 Constipation—Chronic (Rx)

1. The answer is D (1.1.3)

Although there is no universally accepted clinical definition of chronic constipation, the FDA defines chronic constipation as lasting longer than 6 months. Most clinicians differentiate acute (temporary or occasional) from chronic constipation by the duration of "persistent" constipation. Patients with persistent constipation that lasts for longer than 3 months and do not respond to nonprescription therapy are likely to have chronic constipation.

2. The answer is B (1.1.0)

Endocrine disorders such as diabetes mellitus or hypothyroidism; neurologic disorders such as Parkinson's disease, spinal cord injury, or multiple sclerosis; and psychological disorders including depression, anxiety, or eating disorders are all associated with an increased risk of constipation. Ulcerative colitis is associated with diarrhea, abdominal pain, and gastrointestinal bleeding.

3. The answer is C (1.1.1)

The sigmoidoscopy or colonoscopy, barium enema, stool guaiac, and an abdominal examination are all important in the evaluation of a patient with suspected chronic constipation. Sigmoidoscopy, colonoscopy, and the barium enema help to determine whether an underlying cause of constipation exists, e.g., obstruction. The stool guaiac determines the presence of occult blood in the stool. The fecal fat test is used to evaluate patients with steatorrhea, which is most often associated with diarrhea.

4. The answer is E (1.3.2)

Saline laxatives such as magnesium citrate draw water into the small intestines until it reaches the colon, where it is eliminated. These agents produce watery diarrhea and in some cases a complete catharsis with one or two doses. Precautions associated with the use of saline laxatives include patients with signs/symptoms of dehydration and fluid/electrolyte disturbances. Patients, such as JB, who require prolonged laxative use should also avoid frequent or continuous use of saline laxatives, as they may lead to fluid/electrolyte disturbances. Magnesium-containing saline laxatives should be avoided in renal failure because magnesium accumulates secondary to decreased renal elimination. There is no reason why a patient with drug-induced constipation should avoid the intermittent use of a saline laxative unless one of the above precautions exists.

5. The answer is D (2.2.1)

The primary active ingredient in Miralax is polyethylene glycol 3350. This agent is FDA-approved for temporary constipation, but it is also used by physicians for the treatment of chronic constipation.

6. The answer is A (1.3.3)

The continuous long-term use of stimulant laxatives such as senna has been linked to cathartic colon, tolerance, and colonic cancer. Although self-treating patients are instructed to seek medical attention if symptoms persist beyond 7 days of treatment with these agents, many people continue to use stimulants long-term without further medical evaluation. Alternatively, physicians will use stimulants intermittently to treat chronic constipation. Although controversial, there are those who believe that the evidence to support cathartic colon, tolerance, and colon cancer is insufficient and not of good quality. Until more definitive information is available, it is prudent for the pharmacist to advise patients to limit treatment with stimulants to 7 days unless under the care of a physician. Saline laxatives, emollients, lubricants, and polyethylene glycol 3350 have not been associated with these conditions.

7. The answer is A (1.2.0)

Tegaserod, lactulose, or lubiprostone are preferred for the treatment of chronic idiopathic constipation because there is sufficient evidence to support their efficacy and safety. The most recent drug FDA-approved for this indication is lubiprostone, which is a locally acting chloride channel activator that enhances intestinal secretion, thereby increasing intestinal motility and passage of stool. Although polyethylene glycol 3350 is often used to treat chronic constipation, it is only FDA-approved for short-term use (2 weeks). Mineral oil and castor oil should not be used to treat chronic constipation because of the potential adverse effects associated with their use. Alosetron is not indicated for the treatment of chronic constipation. It is used to treat severe diarrhea associated with IBS.

8. The answer is C (1.3.1)

The most important parameters to monitor to assess the effectiveness of lactulose is stool frequency and consistency. Although it is not necessary to strive for daily bowel movements in this patient, the dose of lactulose should be adjusted to produce more frequent and softer stools. More than two stools/day and/or watery stools suggest the need for a dose reduction. Relief of abdominal pain and bloating may not be readily achieved as these are side effects associated with lactulose. Although hydration status (fluid and electrolytes), stool color and stool guaiac should be monitored, they are not indicative of drug efficacy.

9. The answer is B (1.2.2)

Tegaserod is a 5-HT$_4$ serotonin receptor agonist, which stimulates peristaltic reflex and intestinal secretions. It also inhibits visceral sensitivity.

10. The answer is E (1.2.0)

Constipation often returns when tegaserod is discontinued. The FDA does not limit the duration of treatment with tegaserod when used to treat chronic constipation. Although patients may experience diarrhea when treatment with tegaserod is initiated, the diarrhea usually resolves with continued dosing and is seldom severe or warrants discontinuation. There is evidence to support the efficacy of tegaserod in relieving abdominal pain and bloating as well as straining associated with constipation. Because food decreases its oral bioavailability, tegaserod should be taken prior to and not with a meal.

Case 14 Diarrhea (Self-treat with OTC)

1. The answer is A (1.1.1)

The most likely cause of MD's acute diarrhea is infectious. Viruses, e.g., rotavirus and Norwalk virus are common especially in young children and this individual works in a child day care center. Bacteria that cause diarrhea are often associated with ingestion of contaminated food, drink or travel. Protozoa, e.g., Giardia lamblia, is also associated with acute diarrhea. Food intolerance, dietary deficiencies, and medication do not appear to be related to her acute onset of diarrhea. MD does not reveal any medical conditions, such as IBD or IBS, that are typically associated with chronic (present for more than 1 month) diarrhea.

2. The answer is D (1.1.4)

All of the above individuals are considered to be at high risk for developing infectious diarrhea except those who are lactase deficient and unable to digest dairy, e.g., milk, cheese, ice cream, etc. Recall that MD works at a child day care center. Staff and children in day care centers are at increased risk because infectious organisms spread so easily by person-to-person contact via fecal contamination of hands, toys, diaper changing areas, flush handles on toilets, etc. Patients in acute and long-term care facilities are at increased risk of infectious diarrhea because of multiple causes including nosocomial infections. Recent travelers to "high-risk" countries, e.g., Mexico, and campers are at increased risk of acute infectious diarrhea secondary to ingestion of fecally contaminated food or water (including ground water). Men who have anal sex and prostitutes are at risk of developing infectious diarrhea through the oral-fecal route. Homosexual men are also at risk of developing infectious diarrhea related to gay bowel syndrome and AIDS.

3. The answer is C (1.3.3)

Numerous medications may initiate diarrhea in a specific patient. However, certain medications are more likely to cause diarrhea than others. Antibiotic-associated (e.g., clindamycin) diarrhea is a common manifestation of antibiotic therapy.

Answers

Magnesium-containing antacids and misoprostol are both associated with a dose-dependent increase in diarrhea. Cardiac drugs (e.g., quinidine, digoxin), gout medication (e.g., colchicine), prokinetic drugs (e.g., metoclopramide), and antidepressants (e.g., SSRIs), may cause diarrhea. Laxatives (in addition to those containing magnesium) may also be a source of diarrhea. Sucralfate is an aluminum-containing salt which is associated with constipation.

4. The answer is B (1.1.3)

Responses to the pharmacist's questions indicate that MD is most likely mildly dehydrated. This assessment is based on the number of stools/day (3), duration of diarrhea (24 hours), presence of dry mouth, increased thirst, slight decrease in urination, and absence of fever. Moderate to severe abdominal cramping, a longer duration of diarrhea, increased stool frequency, fever, lethargy, orthostasis, tachycardia, and decreased blood pressure are all signs and symptoms of moderate to severe dehydration.

5. The answer is A (1.1.0)

Individuals, such as MD, who have mild diarrhea and abdominal cramping of less than 3 days duration are acceptable candidates for self-treatment if there are no other exclusions to self-treatment. However, individuals with exclusions to self-treatment, such as diarrhea of 3 days or longer, severe abdominal cramping or diarrhea, protracted vomiting, fever and chills, blood or mucus in the stool, and women who are pregnant or breast-feeding, should be referred for further medical evaluation. Fluid and electrolyte disturbances are more likely to be associated with prolonged diarrhea and protracted vomiting. In addition, prolonged diarrhea and vomiting, severe abdominal cramping and diarrhea, fever and chills, and blood or mucus in the stool may be associated with a more serious condition or disorder.

6. The answer is D (1.2.1)

The treatment of diarrhea is aimed at fluid replacement when dehydration exists. Alert patients should be given ORS for rehydration and maintenance until the diarrhea ceases. These agents are intended to provide rapid restoration of fluid, electrolytes (sodium, potassium, chloride, citrate) and carbohydrates. There is no evidence to indicate that an ORS shortens the duration of diarrhea or reduces stool frequency. Commercial ORS's are superior to Gatorade, cola beverages, and fruit juices because they contain sufficient amounts of appropriate electrolytes and glucose. Although many pharmacists prefer that ORS be used under the supervision of a physician (especially pediatric patients), these agents are available without prescription and do not require physician oversight.

7. The answer is E (1.2.0)

The recommended self-treatment dose for loperamide is 4 mg initially; 2 mg after each bowel movement; up to 8 mg/24 hours. The dosage if supervised or prescribed by a physician is 4 mg initially, 4 mg after each bowel movement; up to 16 mg/24 hours. The total daily dosage is limited to 8 mg/24 when self-treating versus 16 mg/24 hours when under the direction of a physician.

8. The answer is D (1.3.3)

Patients should be advised that loperamide may cause drowsiness or dizziness and that they should observe caution while driving or performing other tasks requiring alertness, coordination, or physical dexterity. Nausea, flatulence, and skin rash are uncommon. Increased appetite has not been reported.

9. The answer is B (1.2.1)

Each Lomotil tablet contains 2.5 mg of diphenoxylate and 0.025 mg of atropine, a chemical that prevents the use of diphenoxylate for illicit drug purposes. When used in recommended dosages, the amount of atropine in this product does not contribute to the antidiarrheal effect of diphenoxylate, does not reduce abdominal cramping, and does not reduce the side effects profile. Neither the diphenoxylate nor the atropine has an anti-inflammatory effect on the bowel.

10. The answer is C (2.2.1)

Kaopectate antidiarrheal products now contain bismuth subsalicylate as the active ingredient. Originally, Kaopectate contained kaolin and pectin but was reformulated to contain attapulgite when there was insufficient evidence to support the efficacy of the combination product. During the time the product contained attapulgite, the manufacturer promoted it as a "salicylate-free" antidiarrheal. In January, 2003, the manufacturer, reformulated the product again to contain bismuth subsalicylate and dropped the attapulgite from the formulation. The labeling at that time stated "new and improved" formulation indicating in small letters that the product now contained a salicylate. If MD decides to purchase Kaopectate, she should be informed that it now contains a salicylate. To add to the confusion, the manufacturer also includes in its Kaopectate product line Kaopectate Stool Softener, which contains docusate calcium. Docusate calcium is a stool softer and, therefore, should not be used to treat diarrhea. Loperamide is not included in any of the Kaopectate antidiarrheal products.

Case 15 Inflammatory Bowel Disease—Ulcerative Colitis

1. The answer is A (1.1.0)

Unlike Crohn's disease, which may affect any part of the GI tract from mouth to anus, UC affects primarily the mucosa and submucosa of the rectum and the left or descending colon, with the rectum involved in >90% of the cases. In some patients, the entire colon (ascending, transverse, and descending) may be involved. Lesions develop in the rectum and spread proximally; however, initial disease may involve the entire colon. Distal UC may be described as proctitis or proctosigmoiditis depending on the location of mucosal inflammation. In UC, surgery is curative. The risk of colon cancer is greater in patients with UC than in the general population and in patients with Crohn's disease. The predominant signs and symptoms of UC are related to the underlying intestinal disease and include diarrhea, GI bleeding, and abdominal pain. Patients with UC may also present with extraintestinal manifestations.

2. The answer is B (1.1.3)

CF presents with signs/symptoms of moderate UC characterized by disease location (rectum and part of colon), frequency of stools/day (5 to 6/day), the presence of abdominal pain and GI bleeding, weight loss, and tachycardia (HR 90). Mild UC usually involves the rectum and possibly the sigmoid colon, with stool frequency of less than 4/day; abdominal pain, GI bleeding, weight loss, tachycardia and fever are usually absent. Severe and/or life-threatening UC is consistent with involvement of the rectum and entire colon, increased stool frequency (greater than 6/day), severe abdominal pain and bleeding, persistent fever, absence of bowel sounds, anemia and other markers of disease severity. UC may be complicated by GI problems such as perianal fissures, fistula, abscesses, pseudopolyps, obstruction, and toxic megacolon.

3. The answer is D (1.1.4)

The most likely cause of exacerbation of CF's ulcerative colitis at this time was the discontinuation of Asacol. She had discontinued sulfasalazine and hydrocortisone enema previously. Although there is data to suggest that diet and stress may have contributed, they were not the most likely cause of this patient's worsening UC.

4. The answer is C (1.1.3)

Many extraintestinal manifestations are associated with UC or CD and may precede or accompany the underlying intestinal disorder. These manifestations may be related to the clinical activity of the inflammatory process or to its anatomic location. The arthritis and arthralgias (including joint pain), skin, eye (iritis), and mouth (aphthous ulcers) manifestations occur more often in patients with UC and Crohn's colitis than in patients with CD of the small intestine. The arthritis is usually asymmetric and affects the joints of the knees, hips, ankles, wrists, and elbows. In most patients, it parallels the activity and severity of the bowel disease, often subsiding with therapy, colectomy, or spontaneous remission. Poor appetite and weight loss are related to the intestinal manifestations of UC. Malaise and headache are not considered extraintestinal manifestations of UC, but may be associated with certain medications used to treat UC.

5. The answer is E (1.3.3)

Dyspepsia, headache, nausea, vomiting, and malaise are all considered dose-dependent side effects of sulfasalazine. In most cases, these effects subside when the sulfasalazine dose is re-

duced. Alternatively, therapy can be initiated at a low dose and then titrated upward. Skin rash, fever, and hemolytic anemia are important examples of side effects that occur independent of the sulfasalazine dose.

6. The answer is D (1.2.5)

Asacol is a 5-ASA enteric-coated tablet with dissolution characteristics that permit release of the active drug (5-ASA) in the terminal ileum and colon. Eudragit-S, the pH-sensitive Asacol tablet coating, is designed to deliver effective concentrations of 5-ASA to the colon with low systemic absorption. Studies with Eudragit-S-coated preparations have shown that the coating begins to dissolve at the level of the terminal ileum and/or the proximal colon in both normal volunteers and patients with active ulcerative colitis Pentasa is a time-dependent dosage form in which granules continuously release 5-ASA in the small intestine and colon.

7. The answer is D (1.2.0)

When Asacol is used to treat mild to moderate active UC, the recommended adult dosage is 800 mg tid (2.4 g/d). Lower dosages (1.6 g/day) are effective for maintenance of remission.

8. The answer is C (1.3.1)

The most important endpoint of treatment in this patient is to treat the acute attack in order to induce remission. Once remission is induced, the most important goal of therapy is to maintain remission. There is no medical "cure" for either UC or CD. Maintaining weight and proper nutrition, avoiding anemia and nutritional deficiencies, and reducing psychological stress as well as increasing a sense of well-being should all be goals of treatment over time. However, the most important therapeutic endpoints for this patient at this time are to induce and maintain remission.

9. The answer is A (1.2.1)

A small number of UC patients are unable to discontinue corticosteroids (steroid-dependent) or do not respond to corticosteroids (refractory). If the patient is taking more than 15 mg/day of prednisone for 6 months or longer, treatment with an immunomodulator (azathioprine or 6-MP) or surgery should be considered because of the adverse effects associated with chronic corticosteroid use at these dosages. The immunomodulator should be discontinued if the corticosteroid dose cannot be tapered. In those patients who do respond, an attempt to taper the immunomodulator should be considered after several years because of the risk of malignancy associated with long-term use. Some clinicians, however, will continue the immunomodulator indefinitely as recurrence occurs within a few months of withdrawal. Azathioprine and 6-MP are not used to reduce the dose of 5-ASA in patients requiring 5-ASA maintenance therapy. Because their effect takes 2 to 3 months, azathioprine and 6-MP are not used to treat acute IBD or serve as bridge to cyclosporine therapy. Azathioprine and 6-MP are not used to decrease the side effects associated with cyclosporine therapy.

Answers

10. The answer is B (2.2.1)

Olsalazine, sulfasalazine, and balsalazide are all broken down in the colon by colonic bacteria to 5-ASA. Mesalamine is another name for 5-aminosalicylic acid. Infliximab is a monoclonal antibody.

Case 16 Adverse Effects of Drugs on the Liver

1. The answer is C (1.3.3)

Nicotinic acid preparations, such as Niacor (I), have been associated with hepatocellular necrosis with moderate elevation of hepatic transaminases. ACE-inhibitors, including Capoten (captopril), Vasotec (enalapril) (II), and Zestril (lisinopril), have been associated with cholestatic and mixed hepatocellular/cholestatic injury. Starlix (nateglinide) (III) is generally not regarded as a hepatotoxic agent.

2. The answer is B (1.3.3)

LW's dark urine, light-colored stools, pruritus, jaundice, hyperbilirubinemia, and high alkaline phosphatase concentration suggest cholestatic liver injury. In addition, high serum concentrations of AST and ALT suggest hepatocellular damage, as well. Thus, LW's presentation is consistent with mixed hepatocellular-cholestatic liver injury. Hepatic cholestasis and jaundice have been reported with the use of estrogen-containing oral contraceptives, such as Triphasil-28 (I). Jaundice is usually noted during the first 6 months of therapy, and often during the first cycle of use. The hepatotoxic effects of Lamisil (II) are also usually cholestatic in nature. Augmentin (amoxicillin-clavulanic acid) (III) has been associated with a mixed hepatocellular-cholestatic liver injury pattern or delayed cholestatic jaundice that usually has a benign course. Adults over the age of 30 appear to be at greatest risk.

3. The answer is D (2.2.1)

Triphasil-28 is a triphasic oral contraceptive containing 30 μg of ethinyl estradiol with 0.05 mg of levonorgestrel (six tablets), 40 μg of ethinyl estradiol with 0.075 mg of levonorgestrel (five tablets), and 30 μg of ethinyl estradiol with 0.125 mg of levonorgestrel (ten tablets).

4. The answer is A (1.3.3)

Although current clinical studies have yielded no evidence of hepatotoxicity with Avandia, liver function testing is recommended prior to initiating therapy and periodically thereafter due to the structural similarity with the known hepatotoxin troglitazone. Glucophage and HCTZ (hydrochlorothiazide) are generally not regarded as hepatotoxic agents.

5. The answer is A (3.1.1)

The drug monographs in AHFS Drug Information (I) contain information regarding the adverse effects, precautions, and contraindications of drug products. American Drug Index (II) monographs detail the manufacturer, composition, available forms, dosage, and use of drug products. The Merck Index (III) contains monographs of chemicals, drugs, and biological substances that detail the chemical abstract registry numbers and names, molecular formula, structure, physical data, use, and therapeutic category of the included entities.

6. The answer is D (1.3.2)

Baseline liver function tests are recommended in patients receiving isoniazid therapy, however follow-up testing is not routinely indicated for all patients receiving treatment. Routine measurements of hepatic function are not necessary during treatment unless patients have baseline abnormalities or are at increased risk of hepatotoxicity (e.g., hepatitis B or C virus infection, alcohol abuse). Peripheral neurotoxicity is a dose-related adverse effect of isoniazid therapy, and is uncommon at conventional doses. The risk is increased in persons with other conditions that may be associated with neuropathy such as nutritional deficiency, diabetes, HIV infection, renal failure, and alcoholism, as well as for pregnant and breastfeeding women. Pyridoxine supplementation would be recommended for LW due to her history of diabetes. Patients taking ethambutol (but not isoniazid) should be questioned regarding possible visual disturbances at each monthly visit due to the potential risk of retrobulbar neuritis. This effect is dose-related, with minimal risk at a daily dose of 15 mg/kg.

7. The answer is E (1.3.2)

Hepatitis is the most severe toxic effect of isoniazid. The drug is associated with hepatocellular necrosis accompanied by marked elevation of hepatic transaminases such as ALT (E).

8. The answer is C (1.2.2)

In vitro studies have demonstrated that Lamisil is an inhibitor of CYP2D6-mediated metabolism (C).

9. The answer is E (3.2.2)

Daily monitoring of feet, wearing shoes both indoors and outdoors, and keeping feet clean and dry should help to decrease the risk of subsequent foot ulcers in LW. These practices may decrease the risk of bacterial and fungal infections, or lead to early identification of a potential foot care issue.

10. The answer is B (1.3.1)

The LDL cholesterol goal for patients with coronary heart disease (CHD) and CHD risk equivalents (i.e., diabetes, other forms of atherosclerotic disease, and multiple risk factors that confer a 10-year risk for CHD >20%) is <100 mg/dL. A recent update to the Adult Treatment Panel III guidelines suggests an optional LDL goal of <70 mg/dL in patients who are at very high risk. Factors that favor a decision to reduce LDL levels to <70 mg/dL include: (1) the presence of established CVD plus multiple major risk factors (especially diabetes), (2)severe and poorly controlled risk factors (especially continued cigarette smoking), (3) Multiple risk factors of the metabolic syndrome (especially high triglycerides >= 200 mg/dL plus non-HDL >= 130mg/dL with low HDL (<40mg/dL), and (4) patients with acute coronary syndromes.

Case 17 Hepatitis

1. The answer is A (3.2.1)

Rebetol is extremely teratogenic. It is contraindicated in pregnant females or in males whose female partners are pregnant. Extreme care must be taken to avoid pregnancy of female patients and female partners of male patients. The manufacturer recommends two adequate methods of birth control and monthly pregnancy testing up to 6 months after cessation of therapy. Ribavirin may cause nonserious nasal itching and stuffiness in as many as 20% due to a histamine like effect. However, BT should be monitored for worsening asthma symptoms possibly due to ribavirin. Unlike interferons, ribavirin does not commonly adversely affect immune or white blood cell function. Most hematological side effects involve RBCs, which may lead to anemia. Hence, fatigue, shortness of breath, and palpitations may represent a significant drop in hemoglobin, anemia, and need for prompt medical evaluation.

2. The answer is B (3.1.0)

The hepatitis C virus exists as many different genotypes and constantly mutates, thus escaping the host's immune response (very similar to HIV). This results in a higher incidence of chronic disease and thwarts vaccine development. Hence, there is no vaccine against hepatitis C. According to the CDC, chronic HCV infection develops in up to 75%–85% of persons. Of these, 60%–70% will have persistent or fluctuating ALT elevations indicating active liver disease, while the remaining 30%–40% of chronically infected persons will have normal ALT levels. Non-A, non-B hepatitis was first recognized because of its association with blood transfusion. Discovery of HCV by molecular cloning in 1988 showed that non-A, non-B hepatitis was primarily caused by HCV infection. In 1989, most non-A, non-B hepatitis became referred to as hepatitis C.

3. The answer is D (1.3.3)

Common side effects associated with interferons, including peginterferons, are worse during the first few weeks of treatment, especially after the first injection. Most self-limiting side effects diminish with continued therapy. Injections of the IFN-alpha component should be administered subcutaneously, not IM. In relapses after IFN-alpha monotherapy, 24–48 weeks of combination therapy is indicated, depending on the viral genotype, viral response at 24 weeks, and the patient's ability to tolerate therapy. Either ibuprofen or acetaminophen may be used to attenuate fever and myalgia associated with interferon therapy.

4. The answer is C (1.3.3)

Peginterferon (pegylated interferon) is produced by adding an inert polyethylene glycol molecule to alpha interferon. Currently, there are two available peginterferons: peginterferon alpha 2a (Pegasys) and peginterferon 2b (PEG-Intron). Pegylation modifies some of the drug's pharmacokinetic properties, thus prolonging half-life. Peginterferons can be given once per week, compared to standard interferon, which must be given several times per week, making peginterferons more convenient to the patient. Peginterferons are more active than standard interferon in inhibiting HCV, which results in higher sustained response rates. However, the side effects profile is similar to the standard interferons. Because of the improved administration convenience and superior efficacy, peginterferons are replacing standard interferons in the management of HCV.

5. The answer is E (1.1.4)

Patients with anti-HCV, HCV RNA, elevated serum ALT, and evidence of chronic hepatitis on liver biopsy, who have no contraindications, should be offered combination therapy with peginterferon and ribavirin. Generally, lower viral loads (<2 million copies/mL) correlate with response to therapy. According to the CDC, patients with chronic hepatitis C generally circulate virus at levels of 10^5 to 10^7 genome copies per milliliter. Persons with advanced liver disease with cirrhosis typically do not respond well and are not considered good candidates for combination therapy. Genotyping should only be used as a guide to predict likelihood of response and treatment duration. Most people in the United States have genotype 1a or 1b, which are less responsive to therapy than genotypes 2 and 3. However, having genotype 1 alone should not preclude offering combination therapy to an otherwise suitable candidate because some patients with this genotype will benefit.

6. The answer is B (3.3.2)

Body piercing and tattooing are only potential sources of transmission if contaminated equipment or supplies are used. Blood and blood products appears to be the primary reservoir responsible for hepatitis C transmission. IV drug use is the most common mode of transmission.

7. The answer is E (1.3.2)

Interferons are well known to potentially cause anxiety, depression, irritability, personality changes, and possibly suicide. All patients should be screened for active psychiatric illness prior to IFN/Rib therapy and monitored and treated during therapy. SSRIs are reportedly helpful in the management. Interferons can cause mild to severe myelosuppression, while ribavirin can cause hemolytic anemia. Furthermore, ribavirin should not be used in patients with pre-existing anemia or with significant CAD or angina. Ribavirin has been associated with stroke, angina, and acute myocardial infarction in patients at risk for these.

8. The answer is B (1.2.4)

ACE inhibitors are contraindicated in patients who have renal

Answers

artery stenosis, a history of angioedema, or who are pregnant. Beta-blockers may be inappropriate for patients with asthma, and loop diuretics may be inappropriate for patients with gout.

9. The answer is A (1.3.1)

Advair is a combination of a steroid and a long-acting β_2-agonist. It does not require the same coordination as a metered-dose inhaler does. The β_2-agonist in Advair is not indicated for reversal of acute bronchoconstriction.

10. The answer is B (1.2.1)

Serevent is salmeterol. Atrovent is ipratropium bromide. Ventolin is one of the trade names for albuterol.

Case 18 Osteoarthritis

1. The answer is A (1.2.1)

The American College of Rheumatology recommends acetaminophen up to 1 gram QID as initial therapy for osteoarthritis (A). Acetaminophen is effective and safe. Recent studies have indicated that acetaminophen is not as effective as NSAIDs but remains the initial drug of choice due to superior safety. If the response is inadequate, then NSAIDs, tramadol, or opioids should be considered (B, C, D). Of these, NSAIDs are preferred unless a contraindication is present. Opioids are helpful for acute pain exacerbations but are not recommended for long-term use due to the potential for tolerance and dependence. Hyaluronic acid is indicated only for OA of the knee when other treatments have failed (E).

2. The answer is E (1.3.2)

Hepatic enzymes (AST and ALT) should be checked at baseline then periodically (annually) (I). For diclofenac it is recommended to also check AST and ALT within 4 weeks after initiating therapy. Increased liver enzymes and drug-induced hepatitis are rare adverse effects associated with NSAID therapy. A CBC should be checked periodically to detect hematologic adverse effects (II). NSAIDs can cause nephrotoxicity due to effects on renal prostaglandins. Serum creatinine should be checked within a few days to a week after initiating therapy, then periodically, especially in patients at risk (III).

3. The answer is B (2.1.1)

Small studies have shown that topical NSAIDs are effective for treatment of OA. However, no topical NSAID is commercially available in the U.S. at this time. To compound 50 grams of 5% ibuprofen cream you would need 2500 mg of ibuprofen (B). A 5% cream would contain 5 grams of ibuprofen per 100 grams of cream; therefore, to make 50 grams of cream it would take 2.5 grams, or 2500 mg.

4. The answer is B (2.2.1)

The generic name of Celebrex is celecoxib; the brand name for

piroxicam is Feldene (A). Lodine is the brand name for etodolac; Orudis is the brand name for ketoprofen (C). Relafen is the brand name for nabumetone; Naprosyn is the brand name for naproxen (D). Voltaren is the brand name for diclofenac (E).

5. The answer is E (1.2.3)

NSAIDs inhibit platelet aggregation and can increase the effects of warfarin (A). The INR should be monitored closely and patients should watch for signs/symptoms of bleeding. NSAIDs can increase the serum levels of lithium and phenytoin; use caution and monitor drug levels closely (B, C). NSAIDs reduce the renal clearance of lithium. Ibuprofen, and possibly other NSAIDs, may inhibit the hepatic microsomal enzymes responsible for phenytoin metabolism, leading to increased phenytoin levels. NSAIDs can decrease the effects of antihypertensives, especially ACE inhibitors (lisinopril) and diuretics; monitor blood pressure closely (D). Various mechanisms are involved in this interaction. NSAIDs do not interact with ranitidine or other H_2-receptor antagonists (E).

6. The answer is A (1.1.3)

Crepitus is a crackling noise heard when the joint is moved (A). It results from the rubbing of bone fragments. Swelling and joint enlargement may also be noted on physical exam and are findings consistent with OA (B, E).

7. The answer is C (1.3.3)

NSAIDs can cause photosensitivity. Patients should be instructed to avoid the sun or wear sunscreen (I). The most common adverse effect of NSAIDs is GI upset. Patients should be counseled to take the medication with food to decrease GI upset (II). Other adverse effects of NSAIDs include inhibition of platelet aggregation, fluid retention and peripheral edema, increased liver enzymes (rare; most frequent with diclofenac), rarely CNS effects (drowsiness, dizziness, headache, depression, confusion, tinnitus) and hypersensitivity reactions (bronchospasm, urticaria). Nephrotoxicity and NSAID-induced ulcers may also occur. Cough is not an adverse effect of NSAIDs (III).

8. The answer is A (1.2.2)

At the time of this writing celecoxib was the only COX-2 selective NSAID available (I). Rofecoxib and valdecoxib have been removed from the market. Other COX-2 selective NSAIDs are in the pipeline. Meloxicam, nabumetone, and etodolac have some COX-2 specificity but still have a potent effect on COX-1 (I, II).

9. The answer is C (3.2.3)

The main adverse effect with glucosamine is GI discomfort (C). Other adverse effects include drowsiness and headache. In clinical trials, adverse effects were not significantly different from placebo. Various studies, including a 3-year, randomized, placebo-controlled study in adults with OA of the knee have found glucosamine to be effective for the symptoms of OA

(B). One study has suggested that it may have disease-modifying properties. Research suggests that glucosamine must be taken for at least 1 month before improvement in symptoms can be expected (A). Conflicting reports exist regarding glucosamine's effects on blood glucose levels, with recent evidence suggesting that glucosamine does not increase glucose levels in patients with diabetes. Patients with diabetes can use glucosamine for OA but should closely monitor their blood glucose levels (D). Glucosamine is a dietary supplement and, therefore, not regulated by the FDA (E). A reputable manufacturer should be recommended to help ensure product reliability.

10. The answer is D (3.2.2)

The American College of Rheumatology recommends a number of non-drug measures, including education, self-management programs, support groups, physical therapy, occupational therapy, exercise programs (aerobic, stretching, strengthening, and range of motion exercises), assistive devices (wedge insoles, cane, brace, orthotic shoes), heat or cold treatment, and weight loss. Weight loss decreases symptoms and disability and is important in reducing the biomechanical force on weight-bearing joints. Even a 5-lb weight loss can be beneficial (II). Exercise is important to improve or maintain joint mobility (III). Exercises should be taught and then observed before the patient exercises at home, to ensure safety and effectiveness. Inactivity or rest can worsen symptoms and disability by leading to further deconditioning and weight gain (I).

Case 19 Rheumatoid Arthritis

1. The answer is B (1.1.3)

Migraine headaches are not included in the classification criteria for the diagnosis of RA. According to the American College of Rheumatology criteria, patients must have four of the following seven findings: 1) morning stiffness lasting at least 1 hour (A), 2) arthritis of three or more joints simultaneously, 3) arthritis of hand joints (C), 4) symmetric arthritis (D), 5) rheumatoid nodules, 6) positive serum rheumatoid factor (E), and 7) radiographic changes (erosions and bony decalcification). The first four criteria must be present for at least 6 weeks. This patient has five of the seven criteria and, therefore, may be classified as having RA. This patient also has an elevated erythrocyte sedimentation rate (ESR) and C-reactive protein, which are nonspecific indicators of inflammation that are usually elevated in RA. She also complains of afternoon fatigue, which may be seen as part of the prodromal symptoms associated with early onset RA.

2. The answer is E (1.2.1)

NSAIDs provide symptomatic relief of RA by virtue of their analgesic and anti-inflammatory properties (I). They will not prevent joint erosions or otherwise slow the progression of the underlying disease. Therefore, they should not be used as sole treatment but as adjunctive therapy for symptom relief. Corticosteroids (e.g., prednisone) have anti-inflammatory and immunosuppressive properties that make them useful for RA treatment (II). They improve symptoms and functional status. Corticosteroids are not recommended as monotherapy because they do not appear to alter the disease course and are associated with significant adverse effects. They are beneficial as bridge therapy to control pain and synovitis while DMARDs are taking effect; in short-term high-dose bursts for acute flares; or as adjunctive, continuous, low-dose therapy when DMARDs do not provide adequate disease control. Disease-modifying antirheumatic drugs (DMARDs) are the cornerstone of therapy for RA (III). They have the potential to reduce or prevent joint damage, preserve joint function, reduce total health care costs, and maintain patient productivity. The American College of Rheumatology recommends that DMARDs be initiated within 3 months of establishing the diagnosis of RA in all patients except those with only minimal disease controlled by NSAIDs. Methotrexate is the DMARD of choice for initial therapy, especially for patients whose RA is more active.

3. The answer is C (3.2.2)

Nonpharmacologic treatments for RA include instruction in joint protection, conservation of energy, and a home program of joint range of motion (I) and strengthening (II) exercises. Patients should also regularly participate in exercise programs, including aerobic exercises. These can help maintain joint function and psychological well being. Patients and their families also need education about the disease. Physical therapy and occupational therapy may be needed to improve the patient's ability to engage in activities of daily living. Surgery should be considered in patients who have unacceptable levels of pain, loss of range of motion, or limitation of function because of structural joint damage. This patient does not meet these criteria for surgery at this time (III).

4. The answer is D (3.2.4)

Signs and symptoms of myelosuppression include extreme fatigue, easy bruising and bleeding, and frequent infections (II, III). Patients should be instructed to report these symptoms to their physician as soon as possible. The American College of Rheumatology recommends monitoring CBC with differential and platelets at baseline, monthly for the first 6 months, then every 1 to 2 months thereafter. Dark urine is not associated with myelosuppression (I). It can be a sign of liver dysfunction and should certainly be reported to the physician.

5. The answer is C (1.3.2)

Methotrexate therapy is associated with the following toxicities, which require monitoring: myelosuppression, hepatic fibrosis, cirrhosis, and pulmonary infiltrates or fibrosis. The American College of Rheumatology recommends baseline evaluation of CBC with differential and platelets, creatinine, LFTs (AST, ALT, albumin) (I), alkaline phosphatase, chest radiograph within previous year (II), and hepatitis B and C serol-

Answers

ogy in high-risk patients. Subsequent monitoring should include CBC, creatinine, and LFTs monthly for the first 6 months then every 1–2 months thereafter. Annual chest x-rays are also recommended. Methotrexate does not affect thyroid function. Monitoring of TSH (thyroid-stimulating hormone) is not needed (III).

6. The answer is D (1.2.1)

Methotrexate is a folic acid antagonist and can cause folic acid deficiency when given chronically for the treatment of rheumatoid arthritis. Folate deficiency may be associated in part with methotrexate toxicity, and folic acid supplementation has been shown to mitigate some of methotrexate's adverse effects (e.g., GI disturbances, mouth or gastrointestinal ulcerations, and perhaps alopecia). Importantly, concomitant folic acid does not reduce the efficacy of methotrexate. The addition of folic acid does not permit methotrexate dosage reduction (A), enhance methotrexate efficacy (B), shorten methotrexate's onset time (C), or prevent teratogenicity from methotrexate (E).

7. The answer is A (1.2.1)

NSAIDs are generally continued at the previous effective dose when DMARD therapy is initiated (A). There is a lag time before the onset of effect of the DMARD, and analgesic and anti-inflammatory activity is needed during that period (B, C, E). With methotrexate, the time to benefit is typically 1–2 months with maximum response taking 6–12 months. There is no need to increase the NSAID dose beyond the previous effective dose (D). The lowest effective dose should always be used as higher doses of NSAIDs are associated with more adverse effects. If disease remission is achieved with the DMARD, a slow taper of the NSAID may be attempted while continuing the DMARD at the effective dose as long as the patient tolerates the drug and continues to benefit from it. In these patients, as needed use of NSAIDs may be adequate. Continuous treatment with an NSAID may not be necessary if the patient is adequately treated with a DMARD.

8. The answer is B (1.3.5)

Hydroxychloroquine is effective for early, milder disease and is the best tolerated DMARD. It is an appropriate initial agent (B). Sulfasalazine is also effective for early, milder disease but is contraindicated in this patient with a sulfa allergy (C). Prednisone should not be used without DMARDs (A). Corticosteroids can be used as a bridge to effective DMARD therapy (i.e., while waiting for DMARD to take effect). Adalimumab is indicated for moderate to severe RA in patients with inadequate response to other DMARDs (D). This is mainly due to a lack of long-term safety data and expense. Infliximab is indicated for RA patients with an incomplete response or flare-up of disease activity while receiving low-dose methotrexate therapy. It is only approved for use in combination with methotrexate (E). The combination results in synergy and enhanced duration of response.

9. The answer is A (1.3.0)

Gastrointestinal side effects can be minimized by initiating sulfasalazine at a low dose and titrating gradually (D), dividing the dose evenly throughout the day, and using the enteric-coated tablet (A). Products that are enteric-coated should not be taken with milk or antacids as this may cause the coating to dissolve in the stomach instead of the intestines (B). Sulfasalazine may cause myelosuppression (C). The American College of Rheumatology recommends that a CBC with differential be monitored at baseline, every 2–4 weeks for the first 3 months, then every 3 months thereafter. Headache is the dose-limiting side effect, not diarrhea (E). If headache develops during the titration period, the dose should be decreased and titrated more slowly.

10. The answer is C (2.2.1)

The generic of Arava is leflunomide; Enbrel is the brand name of etanercept (A). The generic of Humira is adalimumab; Kineret is the brand name of anakinra (B). The brand name of infliximab is Remicade (D). The generic of Imuran is azathioprine; Azulfidine is the brand name of sulfasalazine (E).

Case 20 Acid/Base Disorders

1. The answer is A (1.1.1)

The arterial pH is the determinant of acidemia versus alkalemia. A pH <7.35 is defined as acidemia and pH >7.45 is alkalemia.

2. The answer is B (1.1.1)

The pCO_2 determines respiratory acidosis versus alkalosis. A high pCO_2 concentration is respiratory acidosis, and a low pCO_2 concentration is respiratory alkalosis.

3. The answer is B (1.1.1)

Venous HCO_3 determines metabolic acidosis versus alkalosis. High venous HCO_3 is metabolic alkalosis, and low HCO_3 is metabolic acidosis.

4. The answer is C (1.1.2)

Anion gap is defined as the serum sodium minus the sum of the serum chloride and bicarbonate concentrations and is useful in determining the cause of metabolic acidosis, such as ketoacidosis, lactic acidosis, renal failure, or methanol and ethylene glycol intoxication. For this patient it is calculated as 120 - (83 + 13) = 24.

5. The answer is D (1.1.2)

Low arterial pH and venous HCO_3 concentrations along with high arterial pCO_2 are indicative of a mixed respiratory and metabolic acidosis. The metabolic acidosis was secondary to pancreatitis and diabetes. The respiratory acidosis is secondary to respiratory arrest.

6. The answer is D (1.1.2)

Diabetes, increased lactate levels, and pancreatitis are etiologies of this patient's acidemia. Hypertension is not a major contributor to the development of the acidosis.

7. The answer is D (1.2.6)

Intravenous sodium bicarbonate is the drug of choice for the correction of an acute severe acidotic state. Shohl's and oral sodium bicarbonate are used in chronic conditions and when the GI tract is functional. Hydrochloric acid is never used to treat acidotic states.

8. The answer is A (3.2.3)

Chronic use of sodium bicarbonate tablets can lead to milk-alkali syndrome. Sodium bicarbonate tablets should not be taken if patient is hypocalcemic. Sodium bicarbonate is a treatment option for hyperkalemia.

9. The answer is C (3.2.2)

Angiotensin converting enzyme inhibitors are known to cause cough, rash, and loss of taste in some patients. Hypovolemia and diuretics could contribute to hypotension. These agents are associated with hyperkalemia.

10. The answer is C (1.1.1)

Serum osmolarity can be estimated with the formula (2 x sodium concentration) + glucose concentration/18) + (BUN/2.8). Based on a sodium concentration of 120 mEq/L, a glucose concentration of 1358 mg/dL, and a BUN of 63 mg/dL, the calculated osmolarity is 339 mOsm/L, with a normal range of 280–300 mOsm/L.

Case 21 Dietary Supplements

1. The answer is D (1.3.3)

Glucosamine is an aminosugar (proteoglycan). Glucosamine is thought to act intracellularly and, therefore, does not appear to contribute to blood glucose levels. In animal studies, however, glucosamine sulfate was shown to cause insulin resistance. A few small studies in humans have assessed the effects of intravenous glucosamine sulfate on insulin levels and glucose. The majority of studies suggest glucosamine does not have clinically significant effects on insulin resistance or glucose metabolism. It is unknown if glucosamine sulfate worsens diabetes or contributes to insulin resistance in patients with diabetes. Patients with diabetes wishing to use glucosamine sulfate products may do so; however, adequate blood glucose monitoring is required. Hyperglycemia is not a recognized clinical side effect of glucosamine. Glucosamine sulfate and chondroitin sulfate are generally well tolerated. Gastrointestinal disturbances like nausea have been observed in clinical trials (A). Heartburn has been reported in patients taking glucosamine sulfate or chondroitin sulfate. Often, these symptoms are mild.

A patient suffering from GERD may experience a worsening of reflux symptoms (B). Abdominal pain has been reported by patients taking glucosamine sulfate in clinical trials (C). Flatulence has been reported with glucosamine sulfate (E).

2. The answer is E (1.2.2)

Glucosamine has been well studied for preventing pain and symptoms associated with osteoarthritis. Currently, there is no clinical evidence to support the use of glucosamine in rheumatoid arthritis. Glucosamine-containing products have a very slow onset of action. Since glucosamine sulfate needs to be incorporated into the cartilage structures and is used to prevent the cartilage breakdown, it may take a while to see a benefit. In clinical trials, symptoms of pain and joint function mobility improved over a 1–3 week period. In some patients, improvements were noted after 1–2 months. MS should know that Glu-droitin should not be used "as needed" to alleviate his acute osteoarthritis pain. He should take Glu-droitin on a regular basis either one capsule three times daily or three capsules once daily. Both of these regimens appear to be effective, and the once-daily regimen may help with compliance (A). Animal studies show that NSAIDs, when used chronically, can cause cartilage breakdown. NSAIDs, however, are very effective analgesics, especially in patients with acute osteoarthritis-related pain. Since NSAIDs function to inhibit inflammation and associated pain, there is no reason why glucosamine-containing products would be contraindicated. MS may use the ibuprofen, short term, to control the acute pain. Glu-droitin may be used concurrently to prevent further cartilage breakdown, minimize joint space narrowing, and prevent further episodes of joint pain (B). The duration of analgesia afforded by glucosamine-containing products is not clearly established. However, in clinical trials, patients experienced a return of osteoarthritis-related pain within 1 month of glucosamine discontinuation. MS should know that Glu-droitin should be continued indefinitely and that his osteoarthritis pain symptoms may reappear within 1 month if he discontinues the product (C). Glucosamine sulfate has an estimated molecular weight of 179. Radiolabeled studies suggest that glucosamine sulfate is absorbed through the gastrointestinal tract. There is evidence that glucosamine is taken up by cartilage cells as well as by other organs (liver, pancreas) (D).

3. The answer is B (2.2.1)

Glucosamine sulfate has been studied the most in clinical trials for osteoarthritis. Studies suggest improvements in joint pain and mobility. The sulfate component of glucosamine serves to impart polarity within the structure of cartilage. This polarity is necessary in maintaining cartilage strength. MS may want to select a product that contains glucosamine sulfate as the single ingredient; this would be an inexpensive alternative to Glu-droitin. Glucosamine chlorhydrate is the same as glucosamine hydrochloride and has not been studied as well as glucosamine sulfate in knee osteoarthritis. Products that contain glucosamine chlorhydrate may cost more than products containing other glucosamine products, may not be as effec-

Answers

tive, and may lead to consumer confusion when selecting a product (A). Glucosamine hydrochloride has been studied to a lesser degree than glucosamine sulfate. The most recent evidence suggests that patients treated with glucosamine hydrochloride do not display significant improvements in pain and stiffness but may experience some improvement in joint mobility. Until more information is available, the value of glucosamine hydrochloride remains unknown (C). Glucosamine hydroiodide should be avoided as there are no clinical studies assessing efficacy in osteoarthritis. Furthermore, glucosamine hydroiodide may contribute to undiagnosed thyroid disease and can interfere with thionamide therapy in those patients with Grave's disease (D). N-acetyl glucosamine (NAG) has not been studied in clinical trials in adults with knee osteoarthritis. Some experts believe NAG to be a poor substrate for cartilage synthesis in humans. A recent in vitro NAG study suggests that it has anti-inflammatory properties. More research is needed before NAG can be recommended for knee osteoarthritis. The addition of ingredients like NAG contribute to the high cost of combination glucosamine products (E).

4. The answer is C (1.3.3)

Manganese is added to combination glucosamine products, often in large amounts. Manganese deficiencies have lead to abnormal bone and joint development. While these deficiencies can occur, it is unlikely that the typical Western diet is manganese deficient to the extent that would lead to abnormal bone and joint formation. The U.S. RDA for manganese in adults is 1.8–2.3 mg daily. Some combination glucosamine products may provide approximately 288 mg daily, which is unnecessary and far exceeds the RDA. Small amounts of potassium are added to glucosamine products for stability. The amount added is typically very small (1–2 mEq potassium per capsule) and is unlikely to be of concern to MS (A). Zinc is often added to a variety of combination glucosamine products; however, the amount of elemental zinc provided is very small (1.6 mg) and is well below the RDI for adults (15 mg/day) (B). Sodium is often added during the manufacturing process to stabilize the glucosamine formulation. The amount of sodium added is small but varies widely by manufacturer. Some glucosamine products can provide up to 160 mg of sodium daily. While this is certainly not enough to cause hypernatremia, it may contribute to this patient's total dietary sodium intake. This is especially important in MS, who appears to have some component of sodium-dependent hypertension and is maintaining a low-sodium diet (3 g/day) (D). Copper is not commonly added to combination glucosamine products (E).

5. The answer is E (2.2.1)

The manufacturer does not have to prove that any dietary supplement is safe. In fact, after a product is on the market, the FDA must prove that a dietary supplement is unsafe before any restrictions can be imposed on the manufacturer. Any dietary supplement that carries a structure-function claim on the label must also carry this disclaimer (A). Dietary supplement manufacturers must base the structure-function claims on their interpretation of scientific evidence. This evidence, however, does not have to be presented to the FDA nor does it have to be made publicly available (B). Manufacturers that wish to use the structure-function claim must notify the FDA within 30 days after the product is made available to consumers. If the structure-function claim is judged misleading or if the claim appears to promote the product as a drug, the FDA may have the manufacturer revise the label (C). The FTC is responsible for regulating dietary supplement advertising. Dietary supplement labeling claims are regulated by the FDA (D).

6. The answer is D (3.2.1)

Manufacturers claim that chondroitin sulfate inhibits cartilage-destroying enzymes on the basis of animal and in vitro studies. Currently, there are no studies in humans with knee osteoarthritis to support this effect. Glucosamine sulfate has been studied for up to 3 years in one clinical trial without serious side effects; however, long-term safety data are still needed (A). Historical evidence and anecdotal evidence suggests glucosamine sulfate and chondroitin sulfate appear safe; however, serious side effects may not have been reported and are currently unknown. MS should know that side effects may not appear until later into therapy and that continuous monitoring by his physician is important (B). Experts do not agree on the exact mechanism of action, but most research suggests glucosamine sulfate/chondroitin sulfate helps strengthen existing cartilage and prevents further cartilage erosion (C). End-stage degenerative osteoarthritis does not appear to respond well to glucosamine sulfate. Many experts believe that the cartilage cells have been destroyed by a lack of nutrients and resulting ischemia and that glucosamine uptake is minimal and, therefore, ineffective. Mild to moderate osteoarthritis tends to respond better to glucosamine supplementation. MS should respond to glucosamine sulfate therapy since he has mild joint space narrowing (E).

7. The answer is D (2.2.1)

A 200-mg chondroitin sulfate dose has not been studied. Clinical trials have used 400 mg three times daily. Other dosing has included 1200 mg once daily with similar results. Chondroitin sulfate is a repeating sequence of glucosamine sulfate and aminosugars (A). The molecular weights of glucosamine sulfate and chondroitin sulfate vary depending on the manufacturing process; however, chondroitin sulfate maintains a much larger molecular weight compared to glucosamine sulfate (B). Clinical trials involving chondroitin sulfate as a single agent have reported improvements in joint mobility and a decrease in subjective pain compared to placebo (C). The effectiveness of chondroitin sulfate appears equal to glucosamine sulfate, and it is likely to function in a similar way to prevent cartilage breakdown (E).

8. The answer is E (1.2.2)

Coenzyme Q 10 appears to have a role in angina since it has significant antioxidant properties. Two well-designed clinical trials have assessed the value of coenzyme Q 10 in patients with angina and myocardial infarction. Improvements in lipoprotein (a) concentration (a marker for atherosclerosis) and increases in high-density lipoprotein cholesterol (HDL-C) levels were observed. While this evidence appears promising, coenzyme Q 10 should not be used in place of conventional treatment options. Coenzyme Q 10 may have a role when used in combination with conventional treatment options. Coenzyme Q 10 has not been studied for lowering cholesterol (A). Coenzyme Q 10 has been studied as an adjunct for its effects in reducing high blood pressure. Many uncontrolled studies have shown reductions in blood pressure. Only one well-designed trial has shown an average systolic blood pressure reduction of 10 mmHg and a reduction on diastolic blood pressure of 7 mmHg. The reductions in blood pressure appeared 3–4 weeks into therapy. MS should know that while studies show coenzyme Q 10 may reduce blood pressure, it is not an antihypertensive agent. It is unknown if MS will be able to decrease the dose or discontinue his prescription antihypertensives (B). Coenzyme Q 10 has also been studied for heart failure. The best designed clinical trial that used Swan-Ganz measurements of cardiac output and echocardiography did not show any significant difference between coenzyme Q 10 and placebo. It is unknown if coenzyme Q 10 has any affect on heart muscle function (C). Coenzyme Q 10 has been studied for cardiomyopathy. The evidence for cardiomyopathy is conflicting. Some research suggests no improvements in heart muscle function, exercise tolerance, or electrocardiogram evidence. One study suggests that benefits are seen when replacing low endogenous levels of coenzyme Q 10 levels (<1.2 μg/mL). The value of replacing coenzyme Q 10 based on blood levels requires further study (D).

9. The answer is A (3.2.1)

Patients who begin HMG-CoA reductase inhibitors have lower than normal coenzyme Q 10 levels. Clinical trials have found a 25%–32% decrease in serum coenzyme Q 10 levels after initiating HMG-CoA reductase inhibitors. The metabolic consequences of low coenzyme Q 10 levels are unknown. HMG-CoA is a precursor for coenzyme Q 10. Coenzyme Q 10 is composed of a benzoquinone with 10 isoprene units. The 10 isoprene units are unique to humans (B). Coenzyme Q 10 has been studied for its antioxidant effects and functions as a natural antioxidant in the blood by blocking free radical scavengers. For this reason, some clinicians use coenzyme Q 10 with HMG-CoA reductase inhibitors to ultimately prevent rhabdomyolysis. There are no clinical studies, however, to support this theory (C). Supplementing coenzyme Q 10 to achieve blood levels between 2 and 3 μg/mL is commonly used in clinical trials. The value of replacing low coenzyme Q 10 levels is not known (D). Although the exact amount of antioxidant activity between coenzyme Q 10 and HMG-CoA reductase inhibitors has not been compared, the HMG-CoA reductase inhibitors are considered more potent antioxidants. HMG-CoA reductase inhibitors have been shown to reverse the atherosclerotic process in blood vessels, and some are used to prevent myocardial infarction. This same level of evidence has not been

shown with coenzyme Q 10 (E).

10. The answer is E (1.3.2)

Agranulocytosis is not a recognized side effect of coenzyme Q 10. Gastrointestinal distress is the most common side effect reported with coenzyme Q 10. Symptoms reported include nausea, diarrhea, and heartburn (A). Although rare, maculopapular rash has been reported in patients receiving coenzyme Q 10 (B). Thrombocytopenia has been reported rarely in patients receiving coenzyme Q 10 (C). In clinical trials, CNS side effects such as irritability, headache, and dizziness have been reported. Typically, these side effects have occurred in <1% of patients (D).

Case 22 Fluids and Electrolytes

1. The answer is D (1.1.2)

The patient is acidemic with an elevated PCO_2, a lowered bicarbonate, and an increased anion gap. Because the pH is low with the increased PCO_2, there is a respiratory acidosis, and with decreased bicarbonate, there is a metabolic acidosis. There is also a metabolic alkalosis because the sum of the excess anion gap and measured bicarbonate is greater than the normal bicarbonate concentration.

2. The answer is B (1.1.1)

The anion gap = sodium – (chloride + bicarbonate) = 144 - (101 + 19) = 144 - 120 = 24

3. The answer is E (1.1.2)

The history of vomiting can cause metabolic alkalosis. Metabolic acidosis can be caused by sepsis, NSAIDs overdose, and renal failure. Metabolic acidosis may also be caused by toxic ingestion of methanol, ethylene glycol, and starvation.

4. The answer is B (1.1.2)

Hypomagnesemia can be caused by both pancreatic insufficiency and drug inducement but not in this specific case. The possible etiology for the hypomagnesemia in this case is the patient's alcoholism. Other possible causes for SM's hypomagnesemia are vomiting, protein-calorie malnutrition, and renal impairment. Other causes of hypomagnesemia include short-bowel syndrome, malabsorption syndromes, excessive laxative use, prolonged diarrhea, diabetic ketoacidosis, excessive sweating, and lactation.

5. The answer is C (1.3.3)

Some common causes of drug-induced hypomagnesemia include aminoglycosides, amphotericin B, diuretic medications, pentamidine, cisplatin, and cyclosporine.

6. The answer is B (1.2.6)

When serum magnesium levels are less than 1.2 mg/dL or

Answers

symptomatic, patients should be given parenteral magnesium therapy. If patients are asymptomatic with a magnesium level between 1.2 mg/dL and 1.8 mg/dL, patients can be started with parenteral magnesium at lower doses or supplemented with oral magnesium products.

7. The answer is E (1.3.1)

The main organ systems that are affected involve the cardiovascular and neuromuscular systems. Symptoms of hypomagnesemia include neuromuscular hyperactivity, psychiatric effects, and cardiac effects. Chvostek's and Trousseau's signs and convulsions are reported as symptoms of hypomagnesemia.

8. The answer is C (1.1.2)

Ketoacidosis causes increased anion gap metabolic acidosis (>13 mEq). Nonanion gap metabolic acidosis can be caused by GI bicarbonate loss, renal bicarbonate loss, hydrochloric acid administration, and posthypocapnia.

9. The answer is A (1.1.1)

SM has renal failure and sepsis. Both of these conditions may lead to increased anion gap. Ketoacidosis and methanol poisoning can also cause increased anion gap, but neither condition is present in this case.

10. The answer is C (2.3.3)

A 50% solution of $MgSO_4$ is available for injection in 10-mL or 2-mL vials or ampules. The 50% solution should be diluted to 20% before injection to prevent venous sclerosis and pain. 2 g $MgSO_4$ in 6 mL of 0.9% NaCl should only be administered by IV bolus in extreme life-threatening situations. IV bolus is associated with flushing, sweating, and pain.

Case 23 Herbal Therapy

1. The answer is E (1.2.3)

For the herbs listed, both garlic and ginkgo have antiplatelet effects and have been associated with actual case reports of bleeding. The evidence for ginseng's effect is based on in vitro studies showing platelet inhibition. All of these herbs should be discontinued for 7–10 days preoperatively and postoperatively to avoid potential bleeding complications. In cases where general anesthesia is used, botanicals with sedative-hypnotic properties, like kava and valerian, should also be avoided. At recommended dosing, tapering of kava and valerian would not be necessary. One case report of withdrawal symptoms, however, was reported in a patient using 4–10 times the recommended dose of valerian.

2. The answer is D (1.3.3)

Both Panax ginseng and American ginseng (Panax quinquefolius) may lower blood glucose, which could adversely affect JL's diabetes. Panax ginseng has also been linked to stimulatory side effects, such as agitation, hypertension, and insomnia, which could complicate his history of hypertension, anxiety, and insomnia. These stimulatory side effects may be related to methylxanthines in the plant. Decreases in blood pressure have also been reported with Panax ginseng use, so blood pressure should be monitored the first few weeks after starting this herb, especially in persons taking anti-hypertensive medications.

3. The answer is A (1.3.1)

JL's LDL is high and his HDL is low. In addition to lowering LDL, simvastatin also has the indication of raising HDL. A 20-mg dose is likely to increase HDL by about 8%. His current medication should be given an adequate therapeutic trial before changes in therapy are made. Niacin should not be added at this time, as it could adversely affect this patient's blood glucose and is more of a second- to third-line agent in patients with type 2 diabetes. Garlic's effect on reducing total cholesterol is mild, 4%–6%, and is not significant in persons who are already on a heart-healthy diet. Garlic does not appear to affect HDL, and its effect on reducing LDL has not been individually studied. Ginkgo and evening primrose oil are unlikely to affect cholesterol. Evening primrose oil is primarily used for premenstrual symptoms and breast pain.

4. The answer is B (1.2.1)

Ginkgo is the only botanical that may actually improve cognitive function in patients with dementia. It also has been shown to increase pain-free walking distance in persons with peripheral vascular disease. Ginkgo does not have a significant affect on any of the other conditions listed.

5. The answer is C (2.3.3)

Ginseng is derived from the root of the ginseng plant. Botanical names for ginseng include Panax ginseng (Chinese or Korean variety), Panax quinquefolius (American variety), Panax notoginseng (Sanchi variety), and Panax japonicus (Japanese variety). Other plants referred to as ginseng that are not in the Panax family include Eleutherococcus senticosus (Siberian ginseng) and Pfaffia paniculata (Brazilian ginseng). The latter two are not standardized by ginseng content. Botanical names for garlic, gingko, and kava are Allium sativum, Ginkgo biloba, and Piper methysticum, respectively. There are many species of valerian, the most common of which is Valeriana officinalis.

6. The answer is E (1.3.1)

Diphenhydramine has both sedative and hypnotic properties, which could add to memory impairment and anticholinergic properties. This could cause urinary retention and exacerbate benign prostatic hypertrophy (BPH). The other products listed (kava, valerian, and alprazolam) could worsen memory impairment through sedative hypnotic affects but will not affect BPH. Ginseng could exacerbate this patient's insomnia and agitation, a symptom that can accompany Alzheimer's disease.

7. The answer is A (2.3.3)

Saw palmetto is standardized by its content of fatty acids and sterols. The other standardizations are those for garlic (alliin or allicin), ginseng (ginsenosides), St. John's wort (hyericin or hyperforin), and milk thistle (silymarin).

8. The answer is D (3.2.1)

It is good advice for JL to stop smoking and initiate a heart healthy diet to reduce his weight. Although light alcohol intake (1–2 glasses) may actually be beneficial in reducing cardiovascular risk, it is probably not a good idea for JL, due to the risk of memory impairment from the sedative hypnotic effects.

9. The answer is E (1.3.2)

Within the last year, German authorities have reported up to 24 cases of liver damage (1 person died and 3 had liver transplants) that may have been caused by the patients' use of kava. Kava use should be limited to 3 months, and periodic liver function tests should be performed to avoid possible toxicity. Kava does not affect any of the other lab tests listed in A–D.

10. The answer is C (3.2.3)

Gingko products should be standardized to 24% flavonoids and 6% terpenes. Although there is evidence that ginkgo is effective at improving cognition in persons with mild forms of dementia, it has not been shown to have any benefit for improving memory or cognition in healthy seniors or in younger individuals who have used it as a "smart" supplement.

Case 24 Anemias (General)

1. The answer is E (1.1.3)

Irritability, pallor and anorexia are symptoms of vitamin B_{12} deficiency. Neurologic symptoms of vitamin B_{12} deficiency are often nonspecific, such as tinnitus or vertigo. Mr. Hanes has not had his "dizzy spells" worked up to know if they are related to vitamin B_{12} deficiency or another etiology. There is no correlation between the extent of neurologic symptoms and anemia severity.

2. The answer is D (1.1.1)

A complete blood count lab evaluation is needed for diagnosis. MCV would be increased. MCV nls (80–100 fL). Concurrent iron deficiency may mask megaloblastic changes in red blood cells. In that case, the MCV may be normal. One must be alert for iron deficiency anemia in patients using nonsteroidal anti-inflammatory drugs. This patient had a negative stool guaiac. Although this patient has normal thyroid function, pernicious anemia occurs commonly in patients with Hashimoto's thyroiditis. This was part of his past medical history. The Schilling test assesses absorption of vitamin B_{12}. Low urinary excretion of radioactive vitamin B_{12} is found in pernicious anemia.

3. The answer is E (1.3.2)

Drugs should always be considered as a cause of macrocytic anemia. Drugs can cause vitamin B_{12} malabsorption (colchicine, neomycin, para-aminosalicylic acid) or inactivate vitamin B_{12} (nitrous oxide).

4. The answer is E (1.3.1)

Hematologic parameters improve quickly. That is why it is important to have an accurate diagnosis prior to treatment. Neurologic symptoms should also improve quickly, but other symptoms may take longer or never improve. Neurologic signs and symptoms may more likely be reversible if they have been present less than 6 months. Tongue burning or soreness should resolve with adequate therapy.

5. The answer is C (1.1.4)

Inadequate intake, decreased absorption, inadequate transport or inadequate utilization can result in vitamin B_{12} deficiency. Pernicious anemia results from lack of ability to absorb vitamin B_{12}. Deficiency of intrinsic factor may cause decreased absorption of vitamin B_{12}. Inadequate intake may occur in strict vegetarians. Increased serum homocysteine levels may be seen.

6. The answer is A (3.2.3)

Hemoglobin is needed for oxygen carrying capacity. One of the definitions of anemia is a decrease in hemoglobin concentration in blood to a level below the normal physiologic requirement needed for tissue oxygenation. Inflammatory cytokines such as interleukin-1 are involved in the pathogenesis of anemia of chronic disease.

7. The answer is C (2.3.3)

Cyanocobalamin and hydroxocobalamin are very hygroscopic. No reconstitution of the product is necessary.

8. The answer is D (3.2.2)

A diagnosis is essential prior to implementing anemia treatment. Incorrect treatment may obscure the correct diagnosis. Routine lab evaluation can determine the most common anemias. Signs and symptoms are not specific for anemias. If a patient suspects they are anemic, the pharmacist should refer the patient to a physician for a history and physical exam. Iron, folic acid and vitamin B_{12} are available orally over-the-counter. Pharmacists need to be aware that patients with a vitamin B_{12} deficiency, inappropriately treated with folate can have worsening neurologic defects but improvement of macrocytic anemia.

9. The answer is A (1.3.3)

Formulations of intrinsic factor and vitamin B_{12} can cause therapy failure if antibodies form against hog mucosa-derived intrinsic factor. Oral therapy is not routinely recommended for initial therapy but may be used for maintenance therapy in high doses of 1000–2000 µg if patients are compliant.

10. The answer is B (3.2.1)

Answers

As patients monitor their therapy they need to understand that symptom improvement does not mean vitamin B_{12} therapy can be discontinued. Most patients learn to self-administer the drug parenterally at home. Oral therapy can be used as an alternative to parenteral therapy in patients with good compliance and no neurological impairment. Most causes of vitamin B_{12} deficiency require lifetime therapy. A Schilling test may be expensive and not practical to administer to all patients.

Case 25 Coagulation Disorders

1. The answer is D (1.2.1)

Enoxaparin and tinzaparin have been FDA approved for the use of DVT treatment. Dalteparin has been approved for DVT prophylaxis but not for treatment.

2. The answer is D (1.2.1)

1 mg/kg q 12 h or 1.5 mg/kg q24 h for patients with acute DVT without PE. Warfarin therapy is initiated when appropriate (usually within 72 hours of enoxaparin). Enoxaparin should be continued for 5 days and until a therapeutic anticoagulant effort has been achieved (INR 2 to 3).

3. The answer is D (3.2.1)

COPD is not a risk factor for the development of deep venous thrombi.

4. The answer is C (3.2.4)

Instruct patient and family to dispose directly into puncture resistant container, place bleach into container, seal bag, and place in trash. Patients and family should not be instructed to recap syringes.

5. The answer is E (1.1.4)

Patients are more at risk for bleeding with advanced age. All others are risk factors for bleeding. (AFFIRM Trial. *American Heart Journal.* 2005.)

6. The answer is E (1.3.3)

Enoxaparin anticoagulant response is predictable and does not required increased laboratory monitoring. One still needs to monitor for signs and symptoms of bleeding. Unfractionated heparin is not an acceptable alternative in patients that suffer from heparin-induced thrombocytopenia.

7. The answer is D (2.2.1)

Lovenox is enoxaparin, Plavix is clopidogrel, Penetrex is enoxacin, Fragmin is dalteparin, and Arixtra is fondaparinux.

8. The answer is D (1.3.2)

Hypophonia is a weak voice. All others are signs and symptoms of bleeding.

9. The answer is C (1.3.2)

The goal INR for the treatment of deep vein thrombosis (DVT) without complication is in the range of 2.0 to 3.0 with a target of 2.5.

10. The answer is D (1.3.2)

Patient is currently being loaded with 10 mg of warfarin daily. Loading doses of warfarin frequently lead to over-anticoagulation. INR levels should be repeated every 1–2 days until therapeutic.

Case 26 Diabetes Mellitus

1. The answer is B (1.2.4)

Metformin is contraindicated in renal disease or dysfunction (e.g., serum creatinine greater than or equal to 1.4 mg/dL in women and 1.5 mg/dL in men). Metformin is also contraindicated in patients with heart failure requiring pharmacologic therapy. Caution should be used in elderly patients >80 years of age and patients with hepatic disease or acute or chronic alcohol ingestion.

2. The answer is D (3.2.2)

The development of lactic acidosis is often subtle and accompanied by nonspecific symptoms. Patients may experience malaise, myalgia, unusual somnolence, hyperventilation, and/or gastrointestinal symptoms. Nausea and diarrhea are not uncommon with the initiation of metformin, however, these symptoms often subside. If GI symptoms occur later in therapy, they may be caused by excessive build-up of lactate. SW's renal function should be monitored closely to ensure stability.

3. The answer is E (1.2.4)

A meglitinide or an alpha-glucosidase inhibitor have minimal effect on the fasting blood glucose (A, D, E). The meglitinide acts at the same receptor as the sulfonylurea, therefore, this would not provide any additional benefit in combination with a sulfonylurea (A, B, C, E). Since this patient has significant elevations in her fasting blood glucose, the addition of an alpha-glucosidase inhibitor to her current regimen would have minimal benefit. She requires additional therapy that addresses both the fasting and postprandial blood glucose (E).

4. The answer is E (1.3.3)

Weight gain with the thiazolidinediones can be significant (I). Peripheral edema is also a common side effect of monotherapy (4.8%–9.1% of patients) and in combination with insulin (approximately 15% of patients) (II). Mild anemia may occur in 2%–3% of patients (III). The mild anemia would only require baseline CBC and follow-up if the patient develops symptoms (i.e., fatigue).

Answers

5. The answer is E (1.2.6)

Lispro (a rapid-acting insulin example, similar to other rapid-acting insulins such as insulin aspart and insulin glulisine) and regular (a short-acting) insulin, primarily affect the post-prandial BG levels. Their duration of action is too short to effect her fasting BG (A and B). The regular insulin component in the 70/30 mixture should not be given at bedtime, since most patients do not eat their evening meal at bedtime and this would likely result in nocturnal hypoglycemia (C). The single dose of NPH alone or NPH in the 70/30 mixture at bedtime will control the fasting BG levels but will not last for 24 hours (C and D). The insulin glargine has a duration of 24 hours. This will provide control of her fasting BG and continue to work with her daytime oral agents (E).

6. The answer is C (3.2.1)

Hypoglycemia can be a serious complication of insulin and oral hypoglycemic therapy (sulfonylurea). Each patient should know the signs/symptoms and appropriate treatment. The liquids will provide approximately 15 g of carbohydrate that can be readily absorbed (I). Rechecking the BG can ensure that the hypoglycemia has resolved. If the BG has not improved (BG > 80 mg/dL), then 15 g of carbohydrates should again be ingested and the BG checked again after 15 minutes. This is referred to as the "rule of fifteen" (II). A light snack such as a sandwich and milk should also be consumed to prevent additional hypoglycemia. Glucagon is given to the unconscious patient with type 1 diabetes by another individual (III).

7. The answer is E (1.3.2)

Estrogen does increase the HDL-C, but this increase does not translate into a decrease in cardiovascular risk for patients such as SW who are without any history of cardiovascular disease (I, III). In the Women's Health Initiative (WHI), postmenopausal patients using unopposed conjugated equine estrogen (women who have had a hysterectomy) demonstrated no beneficial effect on coronary artery disease. Stroke risk was increased in the study. The U.S. Preventative Task Force recommends against the routine use of unopposed estrogen for the prevention of chronic conditions (III). If estrogen therapy is needed (i.e., to control menopausal symptoms), close monitoring for increases in triglycerides is warranted. This is especially true in diabetic patients, since they often have elevated triglycerides (II).

8. The answer is E (1.1.3)

Keeping the feet clean and dry helps to decrease the risk for the development of bacterial and fungal infections (A). Protective footwear should be worn at all times (B). This is especially important for patients such as SW who have lost some of the feeling in their feet. Diabetic foot care includes daily inspection for sores, cuts, redness, or swelling. Calluses can crack open and provide a site for infection to develop. Patients should know what to look for when examining their feet each day and the significance of the sign or symptom. For example, redness and swelling may indicate an infection.

9. The answer is B (2.1.4)

70/30 insulin is composed of 70% NPH insulin and 30% regular insulin. For example, 0.7 x 30 units = 21 units of NPH and 0.3 x 30 units = 9 units of regular insulin.

10. The answer is E (1.3.1)

Diabetic neuropathy (DN) is a microvascular complication. In the DCCT trial those patients with improved glycemic control reported improvements in their pain related to their diabetic neuropathy (E). SW is at risk for developing diabetic nephropathy from her poorly controlled BG and elevated blood pressure. Ibuprofen, an NSAID, can be nephrotoxic and, therefore, any increase in her dose may adversely effect her renal function. The clearance of her metformin is also dependent on her maintaining adequate renal function. Finally, the ibuprofen may also cause fluid retention and worsen her blood pressure(A). Gabapentin in doses of 1200 mg tid (3.6 g) has been tolerated and increasing by 1200 mg per day (4.8 g) may cause excessive drowsiness (B). The desipramine 75 mg at bedtime is being used for both her depression and DN. SSRIs have not been shown to be as effective for diabetic neuropathy(C). Hot water should not be suggested to those individuals who have lost feeling in their legs or feet (D).

Case 27 Dyslipidemia

1. The answer is C (1.1.1)

CHD risk equivalents carry a risk for major coronary events equal to that of established CHD (>20% per 10 years). They include: diabetes, other clinical forms of atherosclerotic disease (peripheral arterial disease, abdominal aortic aneurysm, and symptomatic carotid artery disease) and multiple risk factors that confer a 10-year risk for CHD >20% (I and II). Hypertension is not a CHD risk equivalent but is a major risk factor for CHD that modifies the LDL goal (III).

2. The answer is E (1.3.1)

The patient has a CHD risk equivalent; therefore, his LDL cholesterol goal is the same as if he had CHD (i.e., a previous heart attack). With ATP III, the classification for normal triglycerides has been reduced to less than 150 mg/dL. The goal for non-HDL-C is 30 mg/dL above the LDL-C goal.

3. The answer is E (3.2.2)

Plant stanols/sterols have been shown to lower LDL cholesterol as much as 17% (I). Cigarette smoking and physical inactivity can contribute to low HDL cholesterol (II and III).

4. The answer is B (1.3.5)

Initial ATP III recommendations indicated that initiating LDL-C lowering drug therapy concurrently with TLC was optional for patients with LDL-C of 100 mg/dL to 129 mg/dL (A). However, based on more recent clinical trial results, updated

Answers

ATP III guidelines now recommend initiation of an LDL-C lowering drug simultaneously with TLC if LDL-C is 100 mg/dL or greater. Before initiating lipid drug therapy, potential secondary causes of dyslipidemia must first be addressed. Improved glucose control can improve lipid levels. In addition, clinical studies have shown that metformin can lower mean fasting serum TG, TC and LDL-C levels with no adverse effects on other lipid levels in patients with type 2 diabetes. Because this patient's diabetes is suboptimally controlled, initiation of metformin is indicated concurrently with TLC given that he has no contraindications (B). After his diabetes control is optimized, additional lipid drug therapy may be considered (C, D, E).

5. The answer is B (1.1.1)

To get to 90 mg/dL, the patient requires a 20% reduction in his current LDL-C level: subtract 90 mg/dL (goal) from 113 mg/dL (current LDL-C level) and divide the result by 113 mg/dL (current LDL-C level). Then, multiply by 100 to change from fraction to percent. Alternatively, divide 90 mg/dL by 113 mg/dL and multiply by 100 to change to percent, then subtract the result from 100.

6. The answer is D (1.2.4)

The patient has no contraindications to pravastatin (I). Because niacin can increase blood glucose levels, especially in patients with diabetes, it should be avoided if possible (II). Because the patient's triglycerides are over 200 mg/dL, the use of colestipol is also a relative contraindication (III). Bile acid sequestrants, such as colestipol, can increase TG, especially if baseline levels are above 200 mg/dL.

7. The answer is C (1.1.1)

The patient's AST level remained within normal limits and exhibited a small increase within the range of normal fluctuations; therefore, he may continue the atorvastatin (A). The patient is not at goal for HDL-C (>40 mg/dL) or TG (<150 mg/dL) (B). For high TG (200–499 mg/dL), non-HDL-C becomes a secondary target of therapy and so should be calculated in this patient to guide further treatment decisions (C). Drug therapy should not be added until after the non-HDL-C level has been determined (D). Therefore, determining percent reduction in TG needed to reach goal is also not yet necessary (E).

8. The answer is B (1.1.1)

VLDL cholesterol is the most readily available measure of atherogenic remnant lipoproteins. The sum of LDL + VLDL cholesterol is termed the non-HDL cholesterol. It is calculated as follows: total cholesterol minus HDL cholesterol. In this patient: 149 mg/dL minus 32 mg/dL equals 117 mg/dL. The goal for non-HDL cholesterol in persons with high serum triglycerides can be set at 30 mg/dL higher than the LDL cholesterol goal on the premise that a VLDL cholesterol level of 30 mg/dL or less is normal. In this patient, the goal for non-HDL-C is 130 mg/dL. He is currently at his goal.

9. The answer is D (1.1.1)

TG-lowering effectiveness: adding fenofibrate > adding Niaspan > adding ezetimibe > increasing to atorvastatin 20 mg daily > changing to simvastatin 10 mg daily

Based on estimated decreases in TG reported in the prescribing information for each agent, the medication change with the greatest potential to decrease TG without compromising LDL-C control would be adding fenofibrate 145 mg daily (D). The medication change with the least potential to lower TG would be changing to the less potent simvastatin (B). Combination therapy provides synergistic effects that have a greater impact on improving lipids as compared to increased doses of monotherapy, which results in relatively small changes in lipids with each doubling of the dose (A). Adding Niaspan would provide less TG reduction than adding fenofibrate but would likely raise HDL-C more than fenofibrate. And while a study of persons with diabetes showed that lower doses (< 1000 mg) had less of an effect on blood glucose, avoidance of this potential drug/disease-state interaction is prudent (C). Adding ezetimibe would provide even less TG reduction and less improvement in HDL-C than adding Niaspan (E). An important consideration is the potential for side effects. Adding fenofibrate increases risk of myopathy and rhabdomyolysis (although likely to a lesser degree given the low, starting dose of atorvastatin in this patient), and adding Niaspan may worsen diabetes. Therefore, the potential benefits must be weighed against the potential risks in each patient.

10. The answer is D (3.2.1)

The diagnosis of the metabolic syndrome is made when at least three of five risk determinants are present. This patient exhibits all five of the risk determinants, which are: abdominal obesity (waist circumference >40 inches in men and >35 inches in women), elevated triglycerides (150 mg/dL or greater), low HDL cholesterol (<40 mg/dL for men and <50 mg/dL for women), elevated blood pressure (130/85 mmHg or greater), and elevated fasting glucose (110 mg/dL or greater) (I). This syndrome is closely linked to a generalized metabolic disorder called insulin resistance, in which the normal actions of insulin are impaired. Excess body fat (particularly abdominal obesity) and physical inactivity promote the development of insulin resistance. Because weight reduction and physical activity target these underlying causes of the metabolic syndrome, they are first-line for treatment of the resulting lipid and nonlipid risk factors (II). Because the lipid and nonlipid risk factors of the metabolic syndrome increase the risk of CHD, treating them will reduce CHD risk. These include treatment of hypertension, use of aspirin in patients with CHD to reduce the prothrombotic state, and treatment of high triglycerides and low HDL cholesterol (III).

Case 28 Obesity

1. The answer is B (1.1.1)

The National Heart, Lung and Blood Institute (NHLBI) has produced The Clinical Guidelines on the Identification, Evaluation, and Treatment of Overweight and Obesity in Adults: The Evidence Report. In this report, overweight is defined as a BMI of 25.0 to 29.9 kg/m² and obesity as a BMI of 30 kg/m². (B, C, E) The cutoff points are based on epidemiological data that show increases in mortality with BMIs above 25 kg/m². A normal BMI is between 18.5 and 24.9 kg/m². The presence of excessive abdominal fat is an independent predictor of cardiovascular morbidity. Waist circumference is a surrogate marker for abdominal fat. Waist circumference provides an easy way to estimate a patient's abdominal fat content before and during weight loss treatment. The waist circumference at which there is an increased relative risk is 40 inches for men and 35 inches for women. (A)

More than half of type 2 diabetes is obesity induced. It is estimated that for every kilogram increase in weight, diabetes risk increases by approximately 9% (D). Obesity is a risk factor for not only type 2 diabetes but also dyslipidemia, hypertension, stroke, gallbladder disease, sleep apnea, and several types of cancer.

2. The answer is E (1.2.4)

Sibutramine has the potential for clinically significant interactions with several classes of drugs. In patients receiving combinations of MAOIs and serotoninergic agents, reports have been made of a potentially fatal "serotonin syndrome." For the same reason, sibutramine should not be given concomitantly with other drugs that either release or block reuptake of serotonin. These drugs include sumatriptan, dihydroergotamine, dextromethorphan, meperidine, pentazocine, fentanyl, lithium, and tryptophan. In the pivotal trials with sibutramine, subjects experienced a slight increase in heart rate and diastolic blood pressure. Therefore, patients with already uncontrolled blood pressure should not be started on sibutramine. However, sibutramine is not contraindicated in patients with well-controlled blood pressure.

3. The answer is D (1.3.1)

The initial weight loss goal recommended by NHLBI is to reduce body weight by approximately 10% from baseline (A, B, C, E). A reasonable timeline for a 10% reduction in body weight is 6 months of therapy. Weight loss as little as 5% to 10% from baseline has been shown to improve cardiovascular risk factors such as blood pressure, dyslipidemia, insulin resistance and other obesity induced disorders such as sleep apnea and osteoarthritis.

4. The answer is C (1.2.4)

While a hypocaloric health diet, increased physical activity, and other life style changes are essential components of any weight management program, drug therapy may be an appropriate option. Pharmacotherapy is considered appropriate in patients with a BMI >29.9 or >27 with additional risk factors such as coronary artery disease. (A, B, C) Pharmacotherapy is never

used alone but rather added to dietary modification, exercise and behavioral strategies. Because of the unpredictable amounts of active ingredients and the potential for harmful effects, APhA and NHLBI do not recommend the use of herbal preparations for weight loss. Furthermore, most herbal formulas have not be studied carefully in randomized trials.

5. The answer is B (1.3.1)

The most common adverse events encountered during sibutramine treatment include headache (reported in approximately 30% of patients receiving sibutramine), dry mouth in 17% of patients, anorexia in 13%, and constipation and insomnia in 11%. (C, D, E) Despite greater weight loss compared to placebo (A), most sibutramine randomized controlled trials show no effect on lowering blood pressure (B).

6. The answer is D (1.3.2)

Clinical experience with sibutramine has shown that patients who will respond to sibutramine will generally exhibit at least 4-lb weight loss during the first 4 weeks of treatment (A, E). Eighty percent of patients who fail to lose 4 lb during the first 4 weeks will not achieve a 5% weight loss after 6–12 months of therapy. Because of the side effect profile of sibutramine, close monitoring of blood pressure and heart rate are necessary especially if the dose is titrated upward (B). Phentermine would not be a good alternative for JH if blood pressure is a problem. Because of the noradrenergic activity of phentermine, it may worsen blood pressure (C).

7. The answer is B (1.2.4)

Sibutramine has the potential for clinically significant interactions with several classes of drugs. In patients receiving combinations of MAOIs and serotoninergic agents, reports have been made of a potentially fatal "serotonin syndrome." For the same reason, sibutramine should not be given concomitantly with other drugs that either release or block reuptake of serotonin. These drugs include sumatriptan, dihydroergotamine, dextromethorphan, meperidine, pentazocine, fentanyl, lithium, and tryptophan.

8. The answer is E (1.1.4)

Topiramate is FDA approved for epilepsy, however one of the most common side effects includes weight loss (B). It has been studied as a weight loss agent and resulted in significant weight loss compared to placebo. However, topiramate was associated with central nervous system side effects including paresthesia, memory and concentration difficulties. Bupropion is an FDA-approved antidepressant and has been shown in clinical trials to produce weight loss comparable to other obesity drugs (D). Pravastatin and metformin are mostly weight neutral (A, C). In contrast, thiazolidinediones (pioglitazone, rosiglitazone) are antidiabetic agents which lead to 3-kg weight gain in average over 6 months (E).

9. The answer is C (3.2.1)

Answers

Chromium picolinate has not been studied in rigorous long term clinical trials alone or in combination with sibutramine (A). Substantial evidence of harm emerged in 2003, when a major study reported more than 16,000 adverse events associated with the use of ephedra-containing dietary supplements, including heart palpitations, tremors and insomnia. The study also found little evidence that ephedra is effective in reducing weight. FDA subsequently determined that ephedra presents an unreasonable risk of illness or injury. In 2004, FDA prohibited the sales of dietary supplements containing ephedra (B). Sibutramine has the potential for clinically significant interactions with several classes of drugs. In patients receiving combinations of MAOIs and serotoninergic agents, reports have been made of a potentially fatal "serotonin syndrome." For the same reason, sibutramine should not be given concomitantly with other drugs that either release or block reuptake of serotonin. These drugs include sumatriptan, dihydroergotamine, dextromethorphan (antitussive agent included in Robitussin DM), meperidine, pentazocine, fentanyl, lithium, and tryptophan (C). The recommended starting dose of sibutramine is 10mg once a day, generally given in the morning. Sibutramine can be taken without regard to the timing of meals (D). Obesity is a chronic condition. Therefore, it is inappropriate to consider the use of pharmacotherapy as a short-term approach alone (E). Effective pharmacotherapy for obesity is likely to require long-term, if not lifelong, treatment.

10. The answer is B (3.2.1)

Sibutramine is a centrally acting weight-loss agent that acts in the CNS, where it inhibits the reuptake of both norepinephrine and serotonin, and that also weakly inhibits dopamine reuptake (B). Unlike phentermine or fenfluramine, sibutramine does not release norepinephrine or serotonin (A).

Case 29 Thyroid Disorders

1. The answer is C (1.2.1)

Synthroid is one brand name for levothyroxine (T_4) (C). Cytomel is T_3, while Thyrolar (liotrix) and Armour Thyroid contain both T_4 and T_3 (A, B, D). Thyrogen is thyrotropin alfa, a recombinant TSH preparation (E).

2. The answer is A (1.2.3)

Estrogens tend to increase serum thyroxine binding globulin (TBG). In a patient with a functioning thyroid gland, a compensatory increase in thyroxine will occur following the administration of estrogen. However, in a patient receiving thyroid supplementation, free levothyroxine may be decreased when estrogens are initiated, thereby increasing thyroid requirements (A). Aluminum-containing antacids, calcium carbonate, and iron-containing products can impair the absorption of levothyroxine but do not affect the dose of levothyroxine (B, D, E). Atorvastatin does not interact with levothyroxine (C).

Administration of levothyroxine should be separated from other medications by at least 4 hours to allow for necessary absorption.

3. The answer is B (1.2.4)

Angina can be worsened by levothyroxine because levothyroxine increases cardiac oxygen consumption even before euthyroidism is achieved (III). Minute doses of levothyroxine, insufficient to reverse hypothyroidism, are often started in elderly patients, patients with underlying cardiac disease, and in patients with long-standing hypothyroidism to avoid precipitating cardiac ischemia. Levothyroxine can be increased on a weekly basis, if tolerated, until empiric replacement doses are reached. Hypercholesterolemia is improved by correction of the hypothyroidism (II). Depression is currently stabilized and treating the hypothyroidism can result in better control of depressive symptoms (I).

4. The answer is E (1.1.2)

All the aforementioned signs and symptoms can be expected to improve once KJ is euthyroid if hypothyroidism is the only causative factor. The classic symptoms of hypothyroidism (fatigue, cold intolerance, constipation, and weight gain) tend to respond within 4–6 weeks of starting T_4 therapy. However, hair loss and changes in skin and nails may take several months to reverse once euthyroidism occurs (I). Levothyroxine is necessary for normal function of multiple-organ systems, including the heart and lungs. Bradycardia and respiratory depression with carbon dioxide retention occurs in severe and long-standing hypothyroidism and may reverse with T_4 replacement (II). Hypercholesterolemia is common in hypothyroidism. Although the rate of cholesterol synthesis is normal in hypothyroidism, the rate of cholesterol clearance is decreased (III).

5. The answer is D (1.3.1)

TSH is the most sensitive index for detecting euthyroidism (D). TSH can be abnormal even if the free thyroxine and the index are within normal limits (A, C). In this patient, the TSH is elevated, indicating hypothyroidism, despite the normal total T_4 and total T_3. Estrogens can increase the thyroxine binding globulin, thereby increasing the amount of total triiodothyronine and total thyroxine measured. The free thyroxine index, free thyroxine, free T_3, and TSH are not affected by changes in thyroid-binding globulin. Measurement of the free or total T_3 level is not helpful in hypothyroidism because many factors, including hypothyroidism, can impair the peripheral conversion of T_4 to T_3 (B, E). Nonthyroidal illnesses and drugs (e.g., conjugated estrogens) can also alter the total T_3.

6. The answer is E (3.2.3)

Levothyroxine is optimally absorbed in the fasting state. Patients should take thyroid medications in the morning about 30 minutes before food or other medications. Food, including dairy products and fiber, can decrease its absorption by about 20% (III). Iron products and antacids can also decrease absorption (I and II).

7. The answer is E (3.2.1)

The onset of levothyroxine is dependent on achieving a steady state of the drug, which takes several weeks (A, B, C, D). Based on its half-life of 7 days, the onset of efficacy is usually after 3 half-lives, or 21 days. Therefore, once the estimated replacement dose of 1.6–1.7 µg/kg/day is taken for at least 21 days, reversal of some of her hypothyroid symptoms, such as fatigue and cold intolerance, can be expected. However, response to therapy will vary from person to person, and it may take longer than 21 days to see improvement in symptoms, depending on individual response to therapy and need for dose adjustment (E). If patients do not see improvement in 4–6 weeks of therapy, they should inform their physician to determine if dose adjustment is needed.

8. The answer is C (1.2.4)

TSH concentration is considered to be the most sensitive and specific monitoring parameter for adjustment of levothyroxine dose (A). Loss of bone density is associated with supraphysiologic doses of levothyroxine as evidenced by the suppressed TSH level (C). Atrial fibrillation has also been reported. Hypercholesterolemia and bradycardia would improve with levothyroxine therapy (B, D). Anemia, if caused by the hypothyroidism, would also improve (E).

9. The answer is B (1.1.4)

The dosage of levothyroxine is correlated with weight; therefore, excessive weight gain could alter her thyroid requirements (III). As KJ ages, the dosage of levothyroxine might also need to be reduced due to an age-related reduction in T_4 elimination. Other factors affecting T_4 dosing include pregnancy, drugs that impair T_4 absorption, and hepatic enzyme inducers (e.g., phenobarbital, phenytoin, and carbamazepine). Renal disease and alcohol intake have no impact on its elimination (I, II).

10. The answer is D (1.2.0)

Because of its shorter half-life (e.g., 1.5 days compared to 7 days for levothyroxine), T_3 (Cytomel) requires multiple daily dosing for efficacy (A, D). Although T_3 is more completely absorbed than T_4 (levothyroxine), it is not recommended for routine replacement because supraphysiologic T_3 levels after ingestion can produce symptoms of mild toxicity in susceptible individuals (B, E). The onset of T_3 is 1–3 days compared to 21 days for T_4 (C).

Case 30 Dialysis Therapy

1. The answer is B (2.2.1)

PhosLo is the brand name for calcium acetate. Calcium carbonate is available generically or under brand names such as Tums and Oscal. The brand name for calcitriol is Calcijex or Rocaltrol. The brand name for sevelamer is Renagel. There are several generic formulations of aluminum hydroxide, although the brand name for this product is Amphogel. All of these products are used as phosphate binders.

2. The answer is E (1.1.1)

The PO_4 level is the primary target in managing phosphate and calcium imbalance leading to renal osteodystrophy and other complications in patients with end stage renal disease. However, calcium and PTH levels must also be kept under control. The calcium X phosphate product is calculated by multiplying the corrected calcium level times the phosphate level. Values greater than 70 are associated with major complications, including vascular and soft tissue calcifications and cardiovascular disease. The corrected calcium level can be estimated with the following equation: corrected calcium = (4-albumin) x 0.8 + reported calcium level. For TT, the corrected calcium level is (4 - 2.4) x 0.8 + 10.3 = 11.6.

Kidney Disease Outcomes Quality Initiative guidelines suggest the following target goals for a dialysis patient such as TT:

PO_4 level: 3.5–5.5 mg/dL

Corrected calcium level: 8.4–9.5 mg/dL

Ca x PO_4: <55 mg^2/dL^2

Intact PTH: 150–300 pg/mL

3. The answer is B (1.2.5)

TT's PO_4 level is > 5.5 mg/dl and must be further reduced. His corrected calcium level is > 9.5 mg/dl and Ca X PO_4 product is > 55 mg^2/dl^2. Changing calcium acetate to calcium carbonate would not be indicated since the calcium carbonate is likely to increase his calcium level even further. Aluminum hydroxide is usually reserved for situations where the PO_4 level is > 7 mg/dl. Sevelamer (Renagel) is a non-calcium containing PO_4 binder and is not associated with hypercalcemia. It can be used in place of calcium containing PO_4 binders or added to these, thus allowing a reduction in dose in calcium containing PO_4 binders. It is currently recommended that the daily dose of calcium containing PO_4 binders not exceed 1500 mg of elemental calcium per day.

4. The answer is B (1.2.1)

Sevelamer is a nonabsorbable hydrogel PO_4 binding agent. It has been shown to reduce LDL cholesterol on average by 30% and elevate HDL cholesterol on average by 18%. Since TT's LDL is elevated (140 mg/dl), the use of sevelamer may have positive effects. Sevelamer has no direct effects on acidosis, anemia, hyperkalemia, or hypertension.

5. The answer is A (1.1.3)

Paricalcitol and doxercalciferol are active vitamin D analogues. Calcitriol is also a vitamin D analogue. Both paricalcitol and doxercalciferol are as effective as calcitriol in reducing PTH secretion but may have a lower incidence of hypercalcemia compared to calcitriol. If hypercalcemia remains an issue, TT can be switched from calcitriol to either paricalcitol or doxercalciferol, but these agents may not be any more effective than calcitriol at suppressing PTH.

Answers

Cinacalcet, an oral calcimetic agent, is approved for use for the treatment of secondary hyperparathyroidism in patients on hemodialysis either as add-on or first-line therapy, although most studies used as add-on therapy. Cinacalcet not only decreases PTH levels, it has also been shown to lower calcium and phosphate levels. Thus if TT's PTH becomes > 300 and his calcium and phosphorous remain high, cinacalcet is the best choice for TT.

6. The answer is E (1.3.3)

More than likely vancomycin was infused too rapidly. Rapid IV administration of vancomycin must be avoided to help prevent infusion-related reactions, such as red man syndrome. Red man syndrome can cause hypotension, flushing, and a rash on the face, neck, chest, and upper extremities. Allergic reactions are also possible, but rare. Doses of 500 mg or 1 g can be given over 1 hour. However, if a patient develops an infusion-related reaction, slowing the rate to 10 mg/min is recommended.

7. The answer is E (1.2.6)

Vancomycin, with its relatively high molecular weight (1500 daltons), is not removed by low-flux (low-permeability) membranes. Because of this ineffective removal of vancomycin, vancomycin can be dosed once every 5–7 days in this type of patient. By contrast, the use of high-flux membranes reduces the vancomycin concentration by approximately 25%. Therefore a typical dosing regimen using a high-flux membrane would be to administer vancomycin at a dose of approximately 7 mg/kg at the end of each dialysis session. This regimen keeps the vancomycin levels within the therapeutic range between dialysis sessions. Vancomycin 500 mg IV q 24 h is not appropriate for HD (hemodialysis) patients unless they happen to be dialyzed daily with a high-flux filter. Vancomycin 1 g IV q 12 h is a standard dose for most patients with normal renal function. Since oral vancomycin is only negligibly absorbed from the GI tract, oral vancomycin therapy is used primarily in the treatment of C. difficile colitis.

8. The answer is C (1.1.4)

Metabolic acidosis is another common problem in dialysis patients. Metabolic acidosis can often be managed by adjusting the dialysate. However, some patients require chronic oral bicarbonate supplementation. Either Bicitra (modified Shohl's solution) or sodium bicarbonate can be given. Bicitra is preferred over sodium bicarbonate because many of these patients have hypertension. Sodium bicarbonate administration in this patient population can exacerbate sodium and water retention. If sodium bicarbonate is used, close monitoring for blood pressure elevations, weight gain, and presence of edema is important. Polycitra is not an appropriate choice for this patient. Although Polycitra is an alkalinizing agent, it contains potassium which can result in hyperkalemia, another common problem in these patients.

9. The answer is D (3.2.3)

Hemodialysis removes water soluble vitamins and folic acid. This removal could lead to vitamin deficiencies and contribute to anemia in this patient population. Nephrovite is a multivitamin specifically made for these patients. Nephrovite contains vitamin C, niacin, pantothenic acid, vitamin B_6, vitamin B_{12}, vitamin B_1, folic acid, and biotin. Hemodialysis has no effect on fat soluble vitamins A, E, or K, and these tend to be elevated in patients on dialysis; therefore, supplementation is not required. Centrum as well as other multivitamins may not have enough of the necessary components and too much in the way of other components such as fat soluble vitamins.

10. The answer is B (1.1.3)

Although all these conditions listed as selections do occur in this patient population and sometimes lead to death in patients with chronic renal failure, cardiovascular disease is the leading cause of death. High cholesterol, high blood pressure, and diabetes are known cardiovascular risk factors in the general population. The same is true in patients with end stage renal disease. As a matter of fact, the mortality due to cardiovascular disease in this population is 10 to 30 times higher then the general population.

Case 31 Dosing of Drugs in Renal Failure

1. The answer is A (1.1.2)

Using the Cockcroft-Gault equation for female patients, the estimated creatinine clearance is 24 mL/min.

$$Cl_{cr} (male) = \frac{body\ wt\ (kg) \times (140 - age\ in\ years)}{serum\ creatine \times 72}$$

$$Cl_{cr} (female) = 0.85 \times Cl_{cr} (male)$$

$$\frac{(52\ kg)(140-73)}{1.7\ mg/dL \times 72} = \frac{3484}{122.4} = 28.46 \times 0.85$$

$$= 24.19\ mL/min.$$

2. The answer is D (1.2.6)

Guaifenesin/hydrocodone syrup is metabolized by the liver and does not require dose adjustment with diminished renal function. Metformin is not recommended for a SCr >1.4 mg/dL in females. Dosing of meperidine, piperacillin/tazobactam, and gentamicin requires adjustment in patients with renal dysfunction.

3. The answer is B (1.2.4)

Meperidine is metabolized by the liver. Normeperidine, one

metabolite, is eliminated primarily by the kidneys and accumulates in renal insufficiency. Normeperidine is a very potent CNS stimulant that can cause seizures in renal patients receiving multiple doses.

4. The answer is D (1.2.4)

Products containing phosphate (such as Fleet's Phospho-Soda [sodium phosphates]), products containing magnesium (such as MOM [magnesium hydroxide]), or products containing sodium salts should be used with caution in renal patients to avoid electrolyte disturbances. A stool softener such as Surfak (docusate calcium) alone is unlikely to be sufficient in a patient taking opiate narcotics. A stimulant laxative must generally be added to help prevent/treat constipation.

5. The answer is D (1.2.6)

For clinical purposes, the clearance of gentamicin (Cl_{Gent}) is usually considered equal to creatinine clearance (Cl_{Cr}). The volume of distribution of gentamicin (Vd_{Gent}) is 0.3 L/kg of adjusted BW in this patient. In normal patients the Vd is estimated based on IBW, but in obese patients the Vd is slightly increased and is better estimated when based on an adjusted BW that adds back about 40% of the mass in excess of the ideal weight.

Adjusted Body Weight (BW) = [(Actual BW- IBW) 0.4] + IBW

$$Vd = (0.3 \text{ L/kg})(\text{adj BW})$$

$$= (0.3 \text{ L/kg})(62.4 \text{ kg})$$

$$= 18.72 \text{ L}$$

For treatment of infections from Pseudomonas, a peak level of 8–10 mcg/mL is desired.

$$Ld = (Vd_{Gent})(\text{desired } Cp_{peak})$$

$$= (18.72 \text{ L})(8 \text{ mcg/mL})$$

$$= 149.76 \text{ mg (rounded to 150 mg)}$$

6. The answer is C (3.1.2)

Facts and Comparisons: Drug Interactions Facts focuses on interactions between medications. Goodman and Gillman's, while having an excellent discussion of aminoglycoside dosing and renal function, does not list methodologies for estimating creatinine clearance. Pharmacotherapy would be expected to list methodologies and discuss clinical applications in various situations. A medical dictionary would define clearance but does not discuss methodologies for estimation in the clinical environment. Griffith's is disease based and would be unlikely to discuss specific calculations.

7. The answer is E (3.2.3)

A large number of herbal products have little or no scientifically valid data available relating to their use. In general, is it best to avoid such herbal agents unless there is reliable scientific information supporting their use.

8. The answer is E (1.2.3)

Metformin is contraindicated in renal dysfunction. The package insert defines renal dysfunction as serum creatinine >1.5 mg/dL in males and >1.4 mg/dL in females. Glynase is glyburide, which the patient is currently taking. Glucotrol (glipizide) is in the same class of drugs as glyburide, a sulfonylurea. The most appropriate choice listed is Actos (pioglitazone), which is indicated for combination therapy with glyburide.

9. The answer is A (2.2.1)

The trade name of losartan is Cozaar. Hyzaar is a combination of losartan and hydrochlorothiazide. The generic name of Diovan is valsartan. The generic name of Atacand is candesartan. The generic name for Avapro is irbesartan.

10. The answer is B (1.2.0)

An appropriate antibiotic might be either piperacillin or ciprofloxacin because Pseudomonas was cultured. However, piperacillin does not come in an oral dosage form. Thus, ciprofloxacin would be the best choice. Since the patient's estimated Cl_{Cr} <30 mL/min, the recommended dosing interval is once daily.

Daptomycin is an intravenous antibiotic that covers gram positive organisms. Azithromycin is an oral macrolide antibiotic that does not cover pseudomonas. Cefazolin is an IV cephalosporin that does not cover pseudomonas.

Case 32 Renal Failure (Acute)

1. The answer is A (1.1.1)

There are three broad categories of acute renal failure (ARF). Prerenal ARF results from a combination of hypotension, hypovolemia, and decreased renal perfusion. The most common causes of prerenal ARF are characterized by circulatory volume depletion, decreased cardiac output, and/or vascular obstruction of the kidneys. Intrinsic ARF indicates damage to the kidney itself. The main causes of intrinsic ARF include acute tubular necrosis, glomerular lesions, accelerated HTN, and hepatorenal syndrome. Postrenal ARF is caused by bladder outlet obstruction (of both kidneys). Postrenal ARF can be attributed to BPH, cervical cancer, crystal formation in the renal pelvis, or tubules, etc.

This patient's renal impairment is likely due to the combination of an ACEI and an NSAID leading to decreased renal perfusion and, thus, pre-renal ARF.

2. The answer is C (2.2.1)

The generic name for Glucotrol XL is glipizide. The generic name for Glucophage is metformin. The generic name for Glycet is miglitol. The generic name for Prandin is repaglinide.

Answers

3. The answer is D (1.3.3)

The afferent arterioles that supply the glomerulus and the efferent arterioles that drain the glomerulus are responsible for maintaining an intraglomerular pressure that is sufficient for ultrafiltration and is dependent on renal perfusion. The patient was hypovolemic with resultant decreased renal perfusion. Naproxen sodium contributed to XNO's acute renal failure (ARF) by causing vasoconstriction of the afferent arterioles, thereby further decreasing renal perfusion. Enalapril also contributed to decreased renal perfusion by causing vasodilation of the efferent arterioles in the glomerulus, effectively removing the beneficial compensatory mechanism for the pre-existing compromised renal blood flow. Metformin is contraindicated in patients with compromised renal function (males with SCr >1.5 mg/dL, females with SCr >1.4 mg/dL) because of the risk of drug accumulation and possible lactic acidosis. Metformin generally does not contribute to decreasing renal function.

4. The answer is C (2.2.0)

Potassium chloride as a sustained release preparation (K-Dur) could reasonably be given at 40 mEq bid with careful monitoring of the serum potassium. Single doses in excess of 80 mEq or daily doses in excess of 100 mEq daily would be of concern in a patient with renal impairment.

5. The answer is D (1.1.2)

The equation to calculate CrCl is as follows: ((140 - Age)(Weight in kg))/ ((72)(SCr)). The result is multiplied by 0.85 for females. XNO's CrCl is ((140 - 38)(100))/((72)(3.0)) = 47.22. (47.22)(0.85) = 40 mL/min.

6. The answer is C (2.2.1)

Levothyroxine is the generic name of Synthroid.

7. The answer is C (2.1.3)

A 50% solution of magnesium sulfate is equivalent to 50 g/100 mL. A dose of 2 g is equal to 4 mL (check: 4 mL x 50 g/100 mL = 2 g), which, when added to 50 mL solution, results in a final volume of 54 mL (50 mL + 4 mL = 54 mL). The final volume is then divided by the 30-minute infusion rate (54 mL/30 min = 1.8 mL/min), then multiplied by 60 to get the final rate of infusion = 108 mL/h (1.8 mL/hr x 60 min/hr = 108 mL/hr).

8. The answer is A (3.1.2)

Trissel's *The Handbook on Injectable Drugs* focuses on IV compatibility and stability information. Neither of the other two references provide in-depth compatibility information.

9. The answer is E (1.2.3)

If alcohol is ingested during Flagyl therapy, then a disulfiram-like reaction—characterized by flushing, headache, nausea, vomiting, sweating, or tachycardia—may occur. Alcohol should be avoided during and for 72 hours after Flagyl therapy. Levaquin can be taken without regard to food; however, administration with antacids decreases the amount of drug available for absorption. Antibiotic therapy should continue until the full course has been taken because of the possibility of resistance and to ensure that the infection has been completely resolved.

10. The answer is D (3.2.2)

Nutrition and exercise programs are important and cost-effective interventions in the treatment of diabetes. Type 2 DM is usually the result of increased insulin resistance and eventual decrease of insulin secretion because of beta cell failure. Physical activity improves blood glucose levels, results in decreased insulin resistance, and helps with weight loss. The increased sensitivity to insulin that results during physical activity can last up to 48 hours after exercise. Therefore, at least 30 minutes of exercise q 48 h is recommended. Every exercise program should be tailored to the individual patient's capacity and coexisting conditions, such as HTN. XNO should also understand the correlation between blood pressure control and glucose control. Recent studies have shown that intensive control of blood pressure in patients with HTN can reduce diabetic complications (such as diabetic nephropathy) by 24%. Cigarette smoking and alcohol use should be avoided, even in social situations. Diabetics already have an increased risk of cardiovascular disease and smoking cigarettes adds an additional risk factor. The effect of alcohol on blood glucose is unpredictable and depends upon the amount of alcohol ingested in relationship to the amount and type of food consumed.

Case 33 Anxiety

1. The answer is E (1.3.3)

Acetaminophen, NSAIDs, opiates, and caffeine can cause rebound headache when overused. Overuse is demonstrated in KT's profile by early refill of her opiate, purchase of multiple bottles of OTC analgesic, and note about tapering medications used for headache. Additionally, 3–5 16-oz Diet Pepsi's per day can cause caffeinism.

2. The answer is A (1.1.2)

Excessive worry is the primary symptom that a patient must have for more days that not for at least 6 months in order to be diagnosed with GAD.

3. The answer is E (3.3.2)

Anxiety is a disease state that is often unrecognized or misunderstood by members of the community. It is most often thought of as a condition that can be controlled by the patient if they try hard enough. Medication can quickly treat the most annoying of the symptoms, but patients must learn coping mechanisms to deal with this disease and to prevent exacerbation. Also, support groups can help the patient learn these techniques and can aid the patient in understanding and accepting the illness. Finally, family education is important so that the disease becomes a reality for those who live with the patient. With this education they will understand what the patient is experiencing and can empathize rather than ostracize.

4. The answer is D (3.3.1)

Regular exercise and good sleep hygiene aid in reducing symptoms of anxiety. Also, exercise may provide an outlet for stress. Changing jobs may or may not help with symptoms of anxiety. There is stress related with any job. The goal is to learn coping strategies to reduce stress and avoid symptoms of anxiety.

5. The answer is C (1.3.3)

Both alcohol and Darvocet-N-100 are CNS depressants which cause somnolence, sluggish thinking and incoordination. These are the symptoms that can occur with Ambien when given in high doses or when interacting with other agents.

6. The answer is C (1.2.0)

Lorazepam and temazepam are the best choice for this patient because of her elevated liver enzymes. Because lorazepam and temazepam will undergo conjugation in the liver, it will not produce active metabolites that are likely to accumulate in a liver that is acutely damaged. The other agent is subject to oxidative metabolism and, therefore, could cause this patient some toxicity and adverse events.

7. The answer is A (1.2.2)

Benzodiazepines facilitate the action of GABA by allowing an influx of chloride ions into the cell.

8. The answer is E (2.2.0)

There is evidence to support the treatment of anxiety disorders with agents that have GABAergic pharmacology.

9. The answer is E (1.3.3)

Rebound insomnia, increased anxiety and seizures are symptoms that can occur with abrupt withdrawal or discontinuation of short half-life benzodiazepine therapy.

10. The answer is D (1.2.5)

The patient is the best judge of what is working and what isn't. The patient did not take the medication as prescribed, but that does not mean she is abusing it. She is upfront with her needs to increase the dose on occasion to treat symptoms. Take the opportunity to talk to the patient and counsel her about the medication and how to monitor therapy.

Case 34 Attention Deficit Hyperactivity Disorder (ADHD) (Child and Adolescent)

1. The answer is D (1.1.2)

Choice I is the Wechsler Intelligence Scale for Children Revised,

which measures intellectual functioning. The Children's Behavior Checklist and Connors Rating Scales can assess degree of symptom severity in ADHD.

2. The answer is D (1.3.5)

Methylphenidate in a form that is effective in once daily dosing eliminates the need to remember later day doses and possible adherence problems as well as the stigma for a school age patient to take medication at school. The same potential side effects exist with either immediate or sustained release preparations but may occur somewhat less frequently with the sustained release forms of methylphenidate. Short-acting forms are absorbed rapidly, reaching peak plasma concentrations in 1–2 hours, with duration of action of 4–5 hours; and as the trough level of the drug is reached, the patient can have discomforting rebound with irritability, low frustration tolerance, increased restlessness, oppositionality, and impaired concentration. The sustained release preparations generally cost more than the immediate release forms. The extended release forms do not produce the immediate euphorigenic effect that substance abusers typically crave; and because extended release forms are given only once in the morning, there is no need to take medication out of the home where it might be diverted more easily for abuse.

3. The answer is E (1.1.1)

A couple decades ago it was common knowledge that children with ADHD grew out of their symptoms at puberty and that psychostimulants would no longer be effective for ADHD symptoms once a patient entered adolescence. These beliefs have been disproven with careful research over recent years; and current statistics show that at least 60%–70% of people diagnosed with ADHD in childhood will continue to have some degree of impairment due to ADHD symptoms in several areas of their daily life into their early adult years. The same stimulant and non-stimulant drug treatments remain as effective in adults with ADHD as in children.

4. The answer is C (1.3.1)

Although hyperactivity usually diminishes into adolescence and young adulthood, both children and adults have most impairment in functioning due to symptoms listed in I and II. With effective treatment children can improve grades and conduct in school, improve self-esteem and peer relationships, and follow parental directives better. Adults are more successful both with work and with social and family relationships and have a lower rate of substance abuse, vehicular violations and accidents, and problems with the law. Stimulant medications and modafinil are used to treat narcolepsy; but impaired wakefulness is not typically a problem associated with ADHD.

5. The answer is D (1.3.1)

Statistics generated from dozens of studies involving thousands of children have shown substantial clinical improvement with the use of a stimulant medication in 70%–90% of patients treated.

Answers

6. The answer is C (1.2.2)

Atomoxetine selectively inhibits the presynaptic norepinephrine transmembrane transporter protein raising the relative concentration of norepinephrine in the synaptic cleft.

7. The answer is C (1.1.3)

Response to stimulant medication is not a diagnostic criterion for ADHD, as 10%–30% of children with ADHD do not show clinical improvement with methylphenidate or amphetamine preparations. Choices I and II are correct along with the requirement that symptoms are not found exclusively during the course of autism or a psychotic disorder; and are not better accounted for by another mental disorder, despite the fact that ADHD is frequently comorbid with several other conditions including depression or bipolar disorder, anxiety disorders, oppositional defiant or conduct disorder, and substance use disorders.

8. The answer is C (2.1.3)

Since 98 pounds equals 44.5 kg, 54 mg/day divided by 44.5 kg equals 1.2 mg/kg/day. The other answers result from failure to convert pounds to kg, or dividing pounds or kg by mg rather than vice versa. The usual dosing of methylphenidate is 1–2 mg/kg/day.

9. The answer is E (1.3.3)

Choices A and B are alpha 2 adrenergic agonists, which by themselves, may be considered third line treatment for ADHD but as an adjunctive to stimulant medication, are useful in ADHD patients with a tic disorder and comorbid aggressive outbursts and for their sedating effect at bedtime. Choices C and D are antidepressant medications that have sedation as a side effect due to blockade of both histamine H_1 receptors and alpha 2 adrenergic receptors. Choice E is correct as it is indicated for anxiety but does not have sedative or hypnotic activity.

10. The answer is D (2.2.1)

Provigil is the brand name of modafinil, Strattera is the brand name of atomoxetine, Concerta is the brand name for methylphenidate HCl in the OROS delivery system, Anafranil is a tricyclic antidepressant in the USA only FDA approved to treat Obsessive Compulsive Disorder and is the brand name for clomipramine, and Dextrostat is a brand name for dextroamphetamine sulfate.

Case 35 Depression

1. The answer is A (1.1.3)

Each is a phase in the process of an individual with co-morbid alcohol dependence and depression. Detoxification and stabilization must be accomplished initially since withdrawal has the potential to be life-threatening and can decrease the likelihood that RB will progress to the other phases. Sobriety and remission of symptoms are longer-term issues. Maintenance of long-term recovery is accomplished with biological and nonbiological techniques that will continue for years following the other two phases.

2. The answer is B (1.2.2)

Although A and B all might minimize the blood pressure elevations of alcohol withdrawal, atenolol or other beta-blockers have been used to decrease some of the autonomic symptoms of withdrawal but must be used with CNS depressants like benzodiazepines to prevent the most serious withdrawal symptoms, i.e., seizures. Simvastatin has minimal autonomic effects. Aspirin might lower temperature as a part of the syndrome but again has minimal autonomic attenuating effects.

3. The answer is A (1.2.4)

I is correct and is included as a warning in the package insert. Duloxetine is a moderately potent inhibitor of CYP 450 2D6 and therefore would not have an effect on the metabolism of simvastatin. Statement III is incorrect since a therapeutic response to any antidepressant medication can result in improvement in sleep and anxiety associated features of depression.

4. The answer is B (1.3.3)

A is incorrect since increasing the dose of an SSRI acutely may worsen symptoms of anxiety. Decreasing the dose is a possibility, but these symptoms are not worsening, just persisting. B is the correct answer. It appears that the anxiety and insomnia may be a part of the alcohol withdrawal syndrome and might be most appropriately managed initially by adjusting the taper with a larger dose of chlordiazepoxide at bedtime. C is incorrect based on the rationale provided for Answer B. Bupropion may also worsen anxiety and sleep and may have some minor effect on decreasing seizure threshold (D). Headaches do not seem to be contributing to the problem, and acetaminophen's effect on the liver must be considered (E).

5. The answer is E (1.1.4)

Alcoholics with depression and depressed patients with alcohol use have been shown to have increased morbidity and mortality compared to patients with major depression without alcohol use. Thus all statements are correct.

6. The answer is D (1.3.3)

Although all antidepressants have the potential to cause weight gain, mirtazapine has been associated with the greatest likelihood of weight gain probably related to its antihistaminergic activity. Other older sedating tricyclic antidepressants such as amitriptyline and doxepin have also been associated with more significant weight gain.

7. The answer is A (1.2.6)

Venlafaxine and sertraline are the serotonergic antidepressants with the least potential for CYP 450-2D6 drug interactions. Bupropion is not a serotonergic antidepressant. Duloxetine does have some serotonergic effects but has a fairly significant effect inhibiting CYP450-2D6. Paroxetine and fluoxetine are potent inhibitors of CYP450-2D6.

8. The answer is C (1.3.3)

A is incorrect since RB denies any alcohol use and continues to improve in many areas associated with his depression. There is no evidence for this as a problem. B is incorrect since delayed orgasm is an uncommon symptom of depression. C is the correct answer as serotonergic antidepressants can negatively affect both sexual desire and performance. E is incorrect. Although beta-blockers may contribute to sexual performance problems, delayed orgasm is unlikely.

9. The answer is B (3.2.2)

A is incorrect in that although St. John's wort does induce CYP-450 enzymes, it is unrelated to this syndrome. B is the correct statement since venlafaxine is a serotonergic and norepinephrine uptake inhibitor with a short half-life and is associated with this discontinuation syndrome. C is incorrect because any alcohol withdrawal syndrome would not exist at this time and has a different characteristic syndrome. E is unlikely since his depression was previously well controlled and somatic symptoms had not been observed previously.

10. The answer is D (3.3.1)

A is incorrect since the reaction is unrelated to need for treatment. B is correct except recurrent episodes need to be treated differently than a single episode. C is incorrect since RB's significant alcohol history, if anything, suggests indefinite treatment. D is correct since three episodes of depression have >90% chance of recurrence. E is incorrect because although weight gain may be a problem associated with antidepressant therapy and could justify a change in the antidepressant or nonantidepressant therapy, it does not justify discontinuing antidepressant therapy given the severity and recurrent nature of RB's depression.

Case 36 Drug Abuse and Alcoholism

1. The answer is D (1.1.2)

Nausea/vomiting and diaphoresis result from opioid withdrawal and alcohol withdrawal. Auditory hallucinations result from alcohol withdrawal.

2. The answer is A (1.1.2)

Alcohol withdrawal is much more likely than the others to result in death. Death due to heroin withdrawal is very rare. The others do not cause life-threatening withdrawal syndromes.

3. The answer is D (1.2.1)

Dolophine® (methadone) and Subutex® (buprenorphine) are approved for the treatment of opiate dependence. Talwin® (pentazocine) is not.

4. The answer is C (1.1.2)

Signs of minor alcohol withdrawal include elevated vital signs (temperature, blood pressure, pulse), GI disturbances (e.g., nausea, vomiting, and/or diarrhea), tremor, diaphoresis, and seizures. Patients in alcohol withdrawal are more likely to have difficulty sleeping than to be sedated. Major alcohol withdrawal includes disorientation, hallucinations, and often agitation.

5. The answer is E (3.2.2)

All three are appropriate ways to dispose of the remainder of the prescription.

6. The answer is A (1.2.4)

Extrapyramidal symptoms are more common with haloperidol. Olanzapine has more sedative and anticholinergic properties.

7. The answer is D (1.2.5)

Lorazepam is metabolized to inactive compounds so it is less likely to accumulate and lead to overdose than the other agents.

8. The answer is E (1.1.3)

Alcohol dependent individuals are often deficient in thiamine, even with normal diets. Impaired glucose utilization associated with thiamine deficiency leads to Wernicke-Korsakoff syndrome. Alcohol dependent patients should receive thiamine, ideally IM or IV, prior to re-feeding or receiving carbohydrate-containing fluids to prevent Wericke-Korsakoff syndrome.

9. The answer is D (1.2.3)

Bupropion and paroxetine are both potent CYP450 2D6 inhibitors. Mirtazapine is not.

10. The answer is E (3.3.2)

Alcoholics Anonymous (AA), cognitive behavioral therapy (CBT), and motivational enhancement therapy (MET) are all examples of nonmedication treatment strategies for substance dependence.

Case 37 Eating Disorders

1. The answer is C (1.1.1)

At the time of admission, the main focus is to stabilize the patient medically. Disruption in menses in women with very low body fat is common. Generally, menses returns with return of the patient's body weight to within normal limits. If menses does not return with weight normalization, an estradiol concentration as well as other hormonal evaluations may be ordered at that time to assist in evaluation of this problem.

Answers

2. The answer is B (1.1.1)

Patient's weight/IBW x 100 = % of IBW. 70 lb = 32 kg. (32 kg/49 kg) x 100 = 65%.

3. The answer is E (1.2.4)

Emetine is the active ingredient in Ipecac Syrup. Ephedra is a main ingredient in many of the herbal weight loss products. Phenolphthalein is the active ingredient in Ex-Lax. All three have been used by anorexia nervosa patients to induce weight loss.

4. The answer is E (1.2.1)

No medications are approved for the treatment of anorexia nervosa. Currently, medication treatment of anorexia nervosa is aimed at the symptomatic relief of the disorder.

5. The answer is E (1.1.4)

Any of the above criteria would signal the need for intervention resulting from the physical effects of anorexia nervosa. At this point, the patient is exhibiting an inability to adequately care for her basic needs. In particular, this includes the need for intake of enough nourishment to sustain body functions and survival.

6. The answer is D (1.2.4)

The tricyclic antidepressants are notorious for causing fatalities resulting from cardiac arrhythmias on overdose or in patients with prior cardiac abnormalities. Patients with anorexia nervosa are especially at risk for cardiac arrhythmias from the possible existence of electrolyte abnormalities and dehydration. Severe constipation can be deadly to a patient who has not eaten for a prolonged period of time. Bowel problems, especially with bowel motility, are common in patients with anorexia nervosa. Bowel obstruction is a risk during the initial refeeding period of treatment. Constipation may aggravate these risks and problems.

7. The answer is B (1.2.2)

Malnutrition results in depletion of tryptophan, the precursor to serotonin. As anorexia nervosa patients are malnourished versus bulimia nervosa patients, they must first regain weight and nutrients before the SSRI will work. Essentially, there is not enough serotonin in the synapse for its reuptake to be blocked.

8. The answer is B (1.2.4)

Fluvoxamine would be the best choice for a patient with anorexia nervosa with a comorbid diagnosis of OCD because of its safety and tolerability profile as well as its FDA approval for OCD. Amitriptyline and clomipramine both have constipation as a common side effect. Severe constipation can be deadly to a patient who has not eaten for a prolonged period of time. Bowel problems, especially with bowel motility, are common in these patients. Bowel obstruction is a risk during the initial refeeding period of treatment. Constipation may aggravate these risks and problems. Nefazodone and bupropion are not indicated for the treatment of OCD.

9. The answer is E (1.3.1)

Depending on the choice of medication, all of the above parameters may be addressed by the use of medications. No medications are approved for the treatment of anorexia nervosa. Thus, medication use is directed toward symptomatic improvement and the symptomatology of the patient.

10. The answer is E (1.3.1)

Preventing relapse, restoring healthy eating habits, and resolving physical complications are all goals for the successful treatment of patients with anorexia nervosa.

Case 38 Obsessive-Compulsive Disorder

1. The answer is D (1.1.2)

The DSM-IV-TR is the main reference source providing the diagnostic criteria for psychiatric disorders. The Covi, BPRS, and HAM-A are rating scales used to assess symptom severity and response to medications and/or psychotherapy. The Simpson-Angus is used to objectively rate extrapyramidal side effects.

2. The answer is B (1.1.2)

Although LF does experience auditory hallucinations and aggression, these symptoms are not core features of OCD. He does have obsessions of organization and compulsions of rearranging furniture and plants.

3. The answer is A (1.2.1)

SSRIs are considered first-line treatment interventions for OCD. Fluvoxamine (Luvox) is an SSRI. Nefazodone is an antidepressant but does not have proven efficacy for the treatment of OCD. Buspirone is used to treat generalized anxiety disorder.

4. The answer is C (1.2.6)

The correct recommended starting dose for paroxetine is 20 mg.

5. The answer is B (3.2.1)

Higher doses, not lower, are generally required to treat OCD. OCD patients usually require longer periods of time (~10–12 weeks) to realize beneficial effects from SSRIs. Paroxetine is comparable to fluoxetine with regard to mechanism of action and side effect profile. Paroxetine has been studied in OCD and has an FDA indication for the treatment of OCD.

6. The answer is A (1.3.3)

Decreased sexual functioning and nausea are common side effects related to paroxetine and other SSRIs. An increase in DBP is not a side effect associated with the SSRIs and it is more likely to be a side effect seen with the SNRI venlafaxine.

7. The answer is C (2.2.3)

To gain FDA approval, generic drug products must be, according to the FDA, "bioequivalent to a brand name drug in dosage form, safety, strength, route of administration, quality, performance characteristics and intended use." The active ingredient has to be the same, but the inactive ingredients do not need to be identical between the two products.

8. The answer is E (3.1.1)

All three resources would provide information regarding fluoxetine-induced hyponatremia.

9. The answer is D (1.2.3)

Risperidone (D) is an atypical antipsychotic that is recognized as first-line for the treatment of psychotic symptoms. It also has some evidence for its use as an augmentation agent in OCD. Haloperidol (A) and thioridazine (B) are typical antipsychotics and are associated with debilitating side effects, such as extrapyramidal symptoms and tardive dyskinesia. Clozapine (C), another atypical antipsychotic, is primarily reserved for treatment-refractory patients owing to side effects and the risk of agranulocytosis. Buspirone (E) is not an antipsychotic.

10. The answer is A (1.2.3)

Risperidone is primarily metabolized by P450 2D6, and fluoxetine is a potent inhibitor of this enzyme. Thus fluoxetine inhibits the metabolism of risperidone. Although fluoxetine (or the active metabolite, norfluoxetine) also inhibit other enzyme systems, those enzyme systems are not thought to be significantly involved in the metabolism of risperidone.

Case 39 Schizophrenia

1. The answer is C (1.3.3)

NMS causes leukocytosis rather than leukopenia; and along with the other listed signs and symptoms, can include dysphagia, incontinence, mutism, and fluctuating level of consciousness from mild confusion to coma. It is thought to be related to dopamine deficiency associated with dopamine antagonists, sudden discontinuation of antiparkinsonian drugs, and on occasion the abrupt withdrawal of an antipsychotic medication. Emergency treatment starts with immediate discontinuation of the causal medication, IV hydration, antipyretic medication, cooling blanket or ice pack, dopamine agonists (e.g., IV levodopa/carbidopa, amantadine, bromocriptine, dantrolene, ropinirole), muscle relaxants (e.g., benzodiazepines), and nasal O_2.

2. The answer is E (2.2.2)

These are the only dosage strengths commercially available at present for Risperdal Consta brand of risperidone long-acting injection; and consists of biodegradable polymer microspheres suspended in a water-based diluent.

3. The answer is B (1.1.2)

Choice A is the Yale-Brown Obsessive-Compulsive Scale and is a measure of obsessive compulsive symptoms. Choices C and D rate medication side effects, so they are incorrect. Choice E is a clinician rating of patient's level of function, not symptoms, so it is also incorrect. Choice B is correct because it measures symptom severity including positive and negative symptoms in schizophrenia.

4. The answer is C (1.2.4)

Risperidone blocks alpha-1 adrenergic receptors, thus inducing orthostatic hypotension, including the possibility of syncope. This risk can be minimized by initiating treatment with BID dosing and using lower doses in geriatric or debilitated patients. Pre- and post-marketing studies of risperidone have not shown any effect on the rate or extent of GI absorption when taken either with or without food or beverages; however, risperidone oral solution has been shown not to be compatible with cola drinks or tea. Risperidone is not associated with bone marrow suppression, which is the reason that weekly or biweekly blood monitoring is required with clozapine therapy.

5. The answer is E (3.2.3)

Rauwolfia serpentine has high affinity for alpha 2 adrenergic and D2 dopamine receptors and is thought to have some antipsychotic properties; although reserpine which is derived from this plant can cause severe depression. Periwinkle (Catharanthus roseum), kava-kava (Piper methysticum), Ma Huang (Mormon tea or Square tea), and mandrake (Mandragora officinarum) can cause psychosis. An illegal herb commonly abused for its hallucinogenic property (Psilocybe semilanceta) has the "street name" magic mushrooms.

6. The answer is C (1.3.4)

By having RMcW report to the clinic on a more frequent and regular basis to receive depot injections (e.g., fluphenazine or haloperidol decanoate, Risperdal Consta), his clinical status can be more closely monitored, recurring problems he has with p.o. medications can be averted, and deterioration prevented. Changing from a typical to an atypical antipsychotic would lower the risk for akathisia, EPS, and dystonia as well as improving negative symptoms and cognitive function, eliminate the need for other medications to alleviate side effects, and possibly reduce the urge to self-medicate with drugs or alcohol thus aiding better adherence. Every other day regimens are not necessarily associated with improved medication adherence; and no currently available antipsychotic medication has a recommended dosing schedule of qod.

7. The answer is D (2.2.1)

Risperdal is the trade name for risperidone. Zyprexa is the proprietary name for olanzapine, Seroquel is quetiapine, Geodon is the trade name of ziprasidone, and Clozaril is clozapine, which is also available generically.

Answers

8. The answer is A (1.1.3)

Positive symptoms of schizophrenia include hallucinations, delusions, and disorganized thought process. Negative symptoms include impaired cognition, flat or constricted affect, poverty of speech, anhedonia, avolition, and social withdrawal. In this list, only choice A is a negative symptom of schizophrenia.

9. The answer is D (3.2.2)

Except for the development of insulin resistance leading to type II diabetes, schizophrenia and use of antipsychotic medications are not particularly associated with gastrointestinal disorders. Patients with schizophrenia have an increased risk of abnormal glucose regulation, lipid abnormalities, increased appetite and weight gain all of which are exacerbated by treatment with antipsychotic medication. Diabetes can present initially with diabetic ketoacidosis; and lead to long-term morbidity and mortality from micro- and macrovascular complications. Weight gain resulting in abdominal obesity, elevated cholesterol and more highly elevated triglycerides with resulting atherosclerosis and hypertension greatly increase the incidence of myocardial infarction and cerebrovascular accidents. In addition there are frequently concomitant medications prescribed with antipsychotics including mood stabilizers, anxiolytics, and anticholinergics with exacerbation of appetite and weight gain, lethargy, and sedating side effects increasing the difficulty of patients being consistent with physical activity and healthful nutrition.

10. The answer is A (1.2.3)

Risperidone is metabolized via the CYP 2D6 isoenzyme. Paroxetine is a strong inhibitor of this enzyme system and can raise the plasma concentration of risperidone nearly four-fold. RMcW's side effects are likely a result of increased concentration of risperidone with increased dopaminergic, histaminic, and alpha-adrenergic blockade resulting from decreased metabolism of risperidone via CYP 2D6.

Case 40 Alzheimer's Disease

1. The answer is A (1.1.1)

Patients with dementia have cognitive deficits, including memory impairment and either aphasia, apraxia, agnosia, or executive dysfunction and related functional impairment. Alzheimer's disease, the most common dementia, is a degenerative disease with a slowly progressive course. There are other degenerative dementias which are less common. Vascular dementia is the second most common form of dementia and is thought to be caused by small infarcts in the brain.

There are a number of "reversible causes" of dementia. Reversal of the problem does not usually bring about marked improvement but can arrest further deterioration. Metabolic disorders such as severe hypothyroidism or hyperthyroidism can cause symptoms of dementia. Patients with a thyroid disorder and dementia do not necessarily have Alzheimer's disease. An elevated erythrocyte sedimentation rate is a marker for inflammation, such as might be seen in patients with cancer or vasculitis. Ferritin is a marker for diseases that cause heme deposits. Untreated syphilis can lead to neurosyphilis which can cause progressive dementia. A comprehensive metabolic profile (CMP) measures liver and renal functions, which can indicate associated encephalopathies, and electrolyte disturbances, such as hyponatremia and hypercalcemia, which can cause mental status changes. Vitamin B_{12} or folic acid deficiencies can cause dementia, depression and neuropathy. These tests are not used to determine risk factors for Alzheimer's disease or vascular dementia, nor are they prognostic indicators or required as baseline laboratory testing prior to starting therapy.

2. The answer is B (3.2.1)

The answer is a social worker. Occupational therapists assess patients' cognitive and physical functioning to determine if patients can live independently. Occupational therapists provide assistive devices and alternative strategies as needed to optimize the patients' ability to perform activities of daily living (self-care, such as feeding oneself or dressing) and instrumental activities of daily living (independent living, such as shopping or writing checks). A social worker provides information on respite care, social services available in a community, and alternative living situations. A physical therapist assesses and treats problems of physical functioning, relieving pain and improving mobility. A neuropsychologist provides cognitive testing that can be mapped to specific areas of brain function. Physicians are frequently asked to provide information on these questions but this is not their area of expertise and they might defer to a social worker if available.

3. The answer is B (1.1.4)

Of the five choices, uncontrolled hypertension is the most likely risk factor for vascular dementia. Atrial fibrillation is a very important risk factor because the fibrillating atria can create emboli that cause strokes. Other probable risk factors include smoking, hyperlipidemia, diabetes mellitus and atherosclerotic cardiovascular disease. Although there are no studies of the treatment of vascular dementia, aspirin is often used to prevent small infarcts that cause vascular dementia. Blood pressure reduction is also important. The blood pressure goal is controversial in the elderly. Her blood pressure should be lowered to around 144 mmHg systolic, which was done in the Systolic Hypertension in the Elderly Program (SHEP) study. Medications with prominent central nervous systems effects such as clonidine, methyldopa and reserpine should be avoided when possible. There are data supporting the use of acetylcholinesterase inhibition in vascular dementia and more limited information supporting the use of memantine.

4. The answer is B (1.1.4)

Statement I is an old hypothesis about Alzheimer's disease but is not consistent with current knowledge. Alzheimer's disease is not an inevitable part of the aging process. Statement II is not true, in fact, high cholesterol may lead to higher concentrations of beta-amyloid. A controlled pilot study indicates that atorvastatin, a drug that lowers cholesterol, may be of some benefit in Alzheimer's disease. Case reports indicate that statins may also cause confusion. Statement III is the major current hypothesis regarding the etiology of this disease. People who have the allele apolipoprotein E epsilon4 have accumulation of beta-amyloid protein in the brain and are at increased risk for Alzheimer's disease.

5. The answer is E (1.2.4)

Statements I, II, and III include diseases where acetylcholinesterase inhibitors should be avoided when possible. Asthma and COPD can be vagally-mediated and further cholinergic stimulation may worsen these conditions. Peptic ulcer disease can theoretically be worsened by enhanced cholinergic stimulation. The acetylcholinesterase inhibitors have been shown to cause bradycardia through increased cholinergic innervation and should not be used in patients with heart block.

6. The answer is B (1.3.5)

Donepezil (Aricept) 5 mg 1 po daily is correct. Donepezil, rivastigmine, tacrine and galantamine are acetylcholinesterase inhibitors and have not been shown to have important differences in efficacy. There are no direct comparisons of these agents in clinical trials. Tacrine is rarely used due to hepatotoxicity and the qid regimen. Rivastigmine is the only acetylcholinesterase inhibitor which inhibits butyrylcholinesterase as well as acetylcholinesterase but the clinical significance is unknown. Donepezil is a once-a-day medication; rivastigmine and galantamine are administered bid. The doses of rivastigmine and galantamine listed above are not starting doses. It is important to slowly titrate acetylcholinesterase inhibitors to avoid side effects. Hydergine, a blend of ergoloid mesylates, has been used to treat Alzheimer's disease but efficacy has never been shown. There are little published data available on the use of memantine in mild-moderate Alzheimer's disease. Gingko biloba has minor positive effects in Alzheimer's disease.

7. The answer is C (1.3.5)

Nonsteroidal anti-inflammatory agents may provide protection against developing Alzheimer's disease, but they cause too many side effects to be used routinely. They may be of use to guide development of new drugs to prevent Alzheimer's disease. Several clinical trials have shown that estrogen use increases the chance of developing dementia. Vitamin E, at 1000 IU bid, was shown in one clinical trial to lengthen the time to enter long-term care, but did not improve cognition. Also, a recent meta-analysis shows increased mortality associated with vitamin E doses over 400 IU daily. High doses of vitamin E can prolong bleeding time and should not be used in RM since she is taking warfarin.

8. The answer is B (3.1.2)

The results are controversial, since the improvement from donepezil is transient and the benefit when measured by cognitive testing is small. Having an epsilon4 allele is a positive risk factor for progression to Alzheimer's disease, and donepezil appears to have the most benefit in this group. A p value = 0.03 means that there is a 3% likelihood that a particular result is due to chance rather than a valid outcome of the study. A hazard ratio of 0.64 means that 64% of patients developed Alzheimer's disease compared to 100% in the placebo group, that is, there is a 34% reduction in risk of developing Alzheimer's disease by using donepezil.

9. The answer is A (1.1.3)

Delirium means that there is acute onset of confusion, associated with waxing and waning and impaired consciousness or concentration. It often occurs in a patient with underlying dementia. It is usually associated with deterioration in a medical condition, such as due to the addition of a new drug, an infection, or worsening of a chronic disease, such as heart failure. A chronically depressed mood can produce a clinical presentation similar to dementia (often called "pseudodementia") in the elderly. This can be treated with antidepressant therapy. Alzheimer's disease is a slowly progressive disease and does not present with an acute onset. RM has several other risk factors for episodic confusion. Her sodium is low; hyponatremia can cause confusion. She is taking a long-acting sulfonylurea that can predispose to hypoglycemia. Since she has a Hb_{A1c} of 7 and an elevated blood glucose, there may be periods of time when she has hypoglycemia.

10. The answer is C (1.3.3)

The usual starting dose of donepezil is 5 mg daily, with an increase at 6 weeks to 10 mg daily to maximize the effect of the drug. Patients generally have fewer side effects with gradual dosage titration of all the acetylcholinesterase inhibitors. However, some patients have significant early side effects, such as nausea and vomiting, and cannot tolerate even a low dose of the acetylcholinesterase inhibitor. Switching to an alternative acetylcholinesterase inhibitor is sometimes a successful strategy. Other side effects include worsening confusion, anorexia, bradycardia and syncope. Not every patient responds to donepezil or the other acetylcholinesterase inhibitors. The beneficial effects are modest rather than dramatic.

Case 41 Pain Management

1. The answer is B (1.1.3)

Patient-controlled analgesia (PCA) would be the most appropriate of the three choices. The patient's INR is elevated, which does not make him a good candidate for IM or epidural administration.

2. The answer is B (1.2.6)

No correlation exists between a patient's body weight and dos-

Answers

age requirements. Likewise, no maximum dose of morphine exists. Choice III is the typical initial dosing regimen for IV PCA morphine.

3. The answer is D (1.2.3)

Because of GS's elevated INR, low HCT, and renal insufficiency, an NSAID would not be a good selection. Given his renal insufficiency, meperidine would not be a good recommendation because of the potential accumulation of its active metabolite. Codeine conversion to morphine may be inhibited by Prozac; also, he has had itching with codeine in the past.

4. The answer is B (1.2.6)

Typical conversion of IV to oral morphine is 1:3. Thus, 60 mg IV morphine approximately equates to 180 mg oral morphine. Oral morphine to oral oxycodone conversion ranges from 1:1 to 2:1. Thus, the amount of oxycodone would be 90–180 mg. The oxycodone dose listed would be too small.

5. The answer is E (2.2.1)

Morphine 15- and 30-mg tablets and oxycodone 5-mg tablets are available in an immediate release tablet formulation in the exact size of the dose being prescribed.

6. The answer is C (3.2.2)

Promethazine has not been shown to enhance analgesia; moreover, it may have an anti-analgesic effect.

7. The answer is C (1.2.2)

Opioid receptors have been located both in the brain and spinal cord. Opioids have no direct effect on serotonin receptors.

8. The answer is A (2.1.1)

Calculation: 0.6 mL x 50 mg/mL = 30 mg
30 mg/30 mL = 1 mg/mL final concentration

9. The answer is E (3.2.2)

When acute pain patients were evaluated for their risk of addiction when using opioid analgesics for treatment of their pain, the risk is very low (<0.1%).

10. The answer is E (1.3.3)

No known difference exists among agents regarding renal effects. NSAIDs may be particularly beneficial in bone pain from its inflammatory component. They are additive to the analgesic activity of opioids because they work via different mechanisms.

Case 42 Parkinson's Disease

1. The answer is E (1.1.2)

The definitive diagnosis of PD requires pathologic confirmation of Lewy bodies and depigmentation of the substantia nigra within the brain. Therefore, diagnosis is dependent on physical examination and patient interview. The cardinal clinical features of PD are T-R-A-P: Tremor at rest, Rigidity, Akinesia/bradykinesia, and Postural instability. Individually, these physical findings are nonspecific, but as a whole, they constitute Parkinsonism.

A rhythmic, "pill rolling," tremor of the hand and upper extremities is the most visible, yet least disabling symptom. This tremor generally occurs at rest (i.e., rest tremor). Patients may also demonstrate postural tremor (occurs when arms are held outstretched in a fixed posture). An action tremor (detectable on finger-to-nose testing) may be also be present but is less common than rest and postural tremor.

Rigidity is commonly encountered upon passive flexion of the elbow or wrist as well as knee and ankle joints. Common problems associated with rigidity include impairment of basic activities of daily living (e.g., buttoning a shirt, putting on earrings), difficulty arising from a chair, and inability to turn over in bed. The presence of facial, truncal, and lower extremity rigidity often manifests as a lack of facial expression ("masked facies"), stooped posture, and difficultly turning, respectively. The masking of facial expression is often an early symptom of PD and may be misinterpreted as apathy, unfriendliness, or depression.

Akinesia and bradykinesia are terms used to describe absence and slowness of movement, respectively. Difficulty with initiating and executing learned movements contributes substantially to the development of functional impairment (e.g., significant interference with employability, ability to manage household/business affairs, performing basic activities of daily living, and worsening of gait). The combination of bradykinesia and rigidity often contributes to a characteristic slow, shuffling gait; micrographia; and reduced arm swing.

Postural instability or poor balance is a disabling symptom of advanced disease. Often a slow, shuffling gait is transformed into a rapid, festinating gait with a tendency to fall forward. Retropulsion with a tendency to fall backwards also occurs. As a result, patients are at greater risk for injuries due to falls.

Although not considered a cardinal feature, "freezing," or sudden, episodic inhibition of motor function, is not uncommon and also contributes to falls. Patients may report that their "feet are stuck to the floor" and that they have difficulty initiating steps (start hesitation) or turns (turn hesitation). Freezing is often exacerbated by anxiety or when perceived obstacles (e.g., doorways, turnstiles) are encountered.

In addition to the primary motor features, nonmotor symptoms are also very common and significantly impair quality of life. Examples include anxiety, bladder incontinence, constipation, dementia, depression, drooling, dysphagia, erectile dysfunction, olfactory deficit, orthostatic hypotension, pain, paresthesias, seborrheic dermatitis, sleep disturbances, sweating, and temperature intolerances.

As motor and nonmotor symptoms can be pharmacologically exacerbated, clinicians should routinely screen for drugs that can exacerbate any of these conditions.

2. The answer is E (1.1.3)

Immediate release carbidopa/levodopa formulations are available in dosage strengths of 10/100 mg, 25/100 mg, and 25/250 mg. The sustained-release formulations are available in dosage strengths of 25/100 mg and 50/200 mg. The dosage of carbidopa is always expressed first, followed by the dosage of levodopa. Therefore, the carbidopa/levodopa 25/100-mg tablet contains 25 mg of carbidopa and 100 mg of levodopa. Dyskinesias are involuntary choreiform movements involving the head, neck, torso, and extremities. Peak-dose dyskinesias occur predictably and are the result of excessive "peak" levels of levodopa. Increasing the levodopa dosage will worsen dyskinesias. Therefore, therapeutic management strategies are aimed at reducing levodopa dosage. Nonselective monoamine oxidase inhibitors (MAOIs), such as phenelzine (Nardil) and tranylcypromine (Parnate), inhibit both types of MAO (Type A and B) and are contraindicated with levodopa-containing products because of the risk of hypertensive crisis. Recall that even with the concurrent administration of carbidopa, a certain amount of levodopa still undergoes peripheral conversion to dopamine, a monoamine. If MAO-A is inhibited, the metabolism of peripheral dopamine is reduced. The excess peripheral dopamine is then available for conversion to norepinephrine and epinephrine, thus increasing the risk of hypertensive crisis.

3. The answer is A (1.3.3)

Immediate release carbidopa/levodopa formulations (conventional and orally disintegrating tablets) are available as 10/100 mg, 25/100 mg, and 25/250 mg tablets. SJ is currently on carbidopa/levodopa 10/100 mg tid. This provides only 30 mg carbidopa per day and is not enough to provide adequate saturation of the enzyme dopa decarboxylase. Approximately 75–100 mg of carbidopa is required to saturate the peripheral stores of dopa decarboxylase (some patients may require up to 200 mg/d). Therefore, it would be appropriate to switch SJ to the 25/100 mg formulation. The primary function of carbidopa is to inhibit peripheral dopa decarboxylase. Recall that levodopa in the peripheral circulation is converted to dopamine by the enzyme dopa decarboxylase and that dopamine cannot cross the blood-brain barrier. The peripheral dopamine can induce nausea and vomiting by stimulating the chemoreceptor trigger zone of the area postrema, which is located outside the blood-brain barrier. Therefore, the combination product carbidopa/levodopa not only allows more levodopa to enter the brain (and to be subsequently converted to dopamine), but it also reduces the prevalence of nausea and vomiting. It may be useful to think of the Latin-derived term "sinemet" as meaning "without emesis" or "without metabolism."

A second alternative would be to coadminister each dose of carbidopa/levodopa with food. Because levodopa is absorbed in the duodenum, the associated reduction in gastric emptying time helps to attenuate levodopa "peaks." However, because diet-derived, large, neutral amino acids (i.e., histidine, isoleucine, leucine, methionine, phenylalanine, tryptophan, tyrosine, valine) may compete with levodopa for passage across the duodenal mucosa or the blood-brain barrier, a low protein snack is preferred. In patients with early Parkinson's disease, such as SJ, this drug-food interaction is of minimal clinical significance. To enhance adherence and minimize nausea, SJ should be advised to take his carbidopa/levodopa with breakfast, lunch, and dinner and to report any signs of reduced drug efficacy. As the Parkinson's disease progresses, some patients become increasingly sensitive to changes in carbidopa/levodopa bioavailability. In such instances, administration of carbidopa/levodopa should occur 30 minutes before or 2 hours after a high-protein meal. However, this may not be practical in all situations and some patients require consultation with a dietitian to redistribute their protein intake. If SJ continued to experience nausea despite receiving 75–100 mg carbidopa per day and coadministration with food, the use of supplemental carbidopa (available as the product Lodosyn) at a starting dose of 12.5–25 mg taken 30 minutes before carbidopa/levodopa may be tried.

Another alternative would be to prescribe an antiemetic agent. Antiemetic agents with central antidopaminergic activity (e.g., droperidol, metoclopramide, prochlorperazine) can worsen Parkinsonism and should be avoided. Antiemetics that do not worsen parkinsonism include trimethobenzamide (Tigan), serotonin (5HT$_3$)-receptor blockers (e.g., dolasetron, granisetron, ondansetron), and the peripheral dopamine receptor blocker, domperidone (not available in the United States).

4. The answer is D (1.1.3)

Centrally acting anticholinergic agents are effective in the management of Parkinson's disease. Examples include benztropine (Cogentin), biperiden (Akineton), diphenhydramine (Benadryl), procyclidine (Kemadrin), and trihexyphenidyl (Artane). In general, symptomatic improvement is modest and favors tremor control. Quaternary anticholinergic agents that do not readily cross the blood-brain barrier are not useful for Parkinson's disease. Examples of quaternary anticholinergics include glycopyrrolate (Robinul) and propantheline (Pro-Banthine). Centrally acting anticholinergics are also useful for treating extrapyramidal side effects (EPS) such as acute dystonic reactions caused by antipsychotic agents. When providing pharmaceutical care to SJ, it would be important to monitor for common anticholinergic-associated side effects. In general, the elderly are more sensitive to anticholinergic side effects and many clinicians use these agents cautiously in older patients especially in patients who have a history of confusion as a side effect from other drugs or who have a history of cognitive impairment. Side effects to monitor for include confusion, dry mouth (xerostomia), drowsiness, urinary retention, and constipation. Additional side effects include hallucinations, elevated intraocular pressure, blurred vision, pupil dilation, decreased sweating, tachycardia, and erectile dysfunction. If unaddressed, clinically significant sequelae may result from several of these side effects. Dry mouth can alter taste sensation and result in decreased appetite and nutritional intake. Additionally, dry mouth may result in poor retention of dentures.

Answers

Drowsiness may cause the patient to feel lethargic and fatigued. Urinary retention can exacerbate benign prostatic hypertrophy in males. Constipation can result in impaction, abdominal discomfort, and ileus. Confusion and hallucinations can reduce the patient's ability to perform activities of daily living and may also cause distress among caregivers. Elevated intraocular pressure can exacerbate glaucoma. Decreased sweating can impair the body's ability to regulate core body temperature and may result in heat stroke during hot weather. Erectile dysfunction can have a negative impact on quality of life for both the patient and his partner.

5. The answer is C (1.3.3)

Common side effects of all dopamine agonists are drowsiness, hallucinations, and nausea. Other side effects include confusion, vivid dreams, peripheral edema, and orthostatic hypotension. Many of these effects can be minimized with slow dose titration and it may require several weeks to months to achieve the therapeutic maintenance dose. Ropinirole and pramipexole are non-ergotamine dopamine agonists. Bromocriptine and pergolide are ergotamine-derived dopamine agonists which have been associated with inducing fibrosis of cardiac valve, pulmonary, and retroperitoneal tissue.

6. The answer is A (3.2.0)

Flumadine is a brand name of rimantadine and the brand name for amantadine is Symmetrel. Amantadine has FDA approved labeling for the management of parkinsonism and also for the prevention and treatment of respiratory tract illness caused by influenza A virus. Amantadine-induced livedo reticularis occurs in up to 5% of patients. This is a vascular cutaneous reaction that is benign and reversible upon drug discontinuation. It is characterized by a reddish-purple, fishnet-patterned mottling of the upper or lower extremities and often accompanied by ankle edema.

7. The answer is C (1.2.7)

Sinemet CR is a sustained release tablet formulation of carbidopa/levodopa (25/100 mg; 50/200 mg) and should not be crushed, chewed, or dissolved. However, the 50/200-mg tablet is scored and may be halved with a tablet splitter. Peripheral bioavailability of Sinemet CR is less than that of standard release Sinemet and a 10%–30% higher total daily levodopa dosage is required for comparable therapeutic effects. Unlike standard release Sinemet, the sustained-release tablet must be taken with food to improve bioavailability. Food increases gastric retention and allows greater tablet erosion. Hence, a greater amount of levodopa is released and is available for subsequent absorption in the duodenum.

8. The answer is D (3.2.0)

Apomorphine is a subcutaneously administered dopamine agonist and will potentiate the activity of levodopa. Therefore, Answer I is false.

Within the striatum, two types of dopamine receptors are involved in motor control: the D_1 and D_2 receptors. Agents that block striatal dopamine receptors will reduce the efficacy of levodopa. Haloperidol (Haldol), a butyrophenone, is used to manage psychotic behavior as well as other conditions associated with agitation. Haloperidol will cross the blood-brain barrier and block striatal dopamine (D_2) receptors. Another butyrophenone, droperidol (Inapsine), an agent used for management of nausea and vomiting, will also block striatal D_2 receptors. Chlorpromazine (Thorazine) is a centrally acting phenothiazine agent used to manage psychotic behavior; it will also block striatal dopamine (D_2) receptors. Other centrally acting phenothiazines that will block striatal D_2 receptors include fluphenazine (Prolixin), mesoridazine (Serentil), perphenazine (Trilafon), prochlorperazine (Compazine), thioridazine (Mellaril), thiothixene (Navane), trifluoperazine (Stelazine), and triflupromazine (Vesprin). The atypical antipsychotics are less specific for striatal D_2 receptors. Clozapine and quetiapine are less likely to interfere with levodopa activity, while olanzapine and risperidone are more likely.

Metoclopramide (Reglan) is commonly used to treat nausea and symptoms associated with gastroparesis. This agent will also block striatal D_2 receptors. Another agent useful in managing gastroparesis, nausea and vomiting is domperidone (Motilium). Although this drug blocks D_2 receptors, it does not cross the blood-brain barrier and, therefore, does not antagonize the central effects of levodopa. At the time of this writing, domperidone is not available in the United States.

9. The answer is A (2.1.1)

SJ is having difficulties remembering to take his afternoon dose of carbidopa/levodopa. The purpose of converting to Sinemet CR is to reduce the dosage frequency with the goal of improving adherence. SJ is currently taking standard release carbidopa/levodopa 25/100 mg po tid. This is equivalent to 75 mg carbidopa and 300 mg levodopa per day. When switching to the sustained-release formulation, the first step is to calculate a new total daily dosage. In this case, the manufacturer recommends an increase of 10%–30% total daily levodopa dose (to compensate for reduced levodopa bioavailability associated with the sustained-release tablet matrix). This calculates to a range of 330–390 mg levodopa per day. Next, the dosing frequency must be reduced by approximately 30%–50% (to compensate for the slower and more continuous release of drug from the tablet matrix). Since a tid regimen is equivalent to three doses/day, a 33% reduction calculates to two doses/day or a bid regimen. Since Sinemet CR is available as 25/100 mg or 50/200 mg tablet formulations, the correct answer is Sinemet CR 50/200 mg: one tablet po bid. The tid and qid regimens are incorrect (answers B, D, and E) because conversion to Sinemet CR requires a reduction in dosing frequency, not an increase. Answer C is incorrect because conversion to Sinemet CR requires an increase in total daily levodopa dose, not a reduction.

10. The answer is A (3.1.1)

Recommending SJ and his wife seek information in a medical textbook is inappropriate for several reasons. Medical textbooks are written to provide information on diagnosing or treating a disease. SJ and his wife are requesting additional information to help them cope and adapt to the disease as patient and caregiver. Additionally, the language in medical textbooks is often very technical and may be difficult for SJ and his wife to interpret. If SJ or his wife had a scientific background, then perhaps a medical textbook may be a useful educational supplement. The other answers are all appropriate. Support groups are an excellent source of educational, emotional, and social support (for both patients and caregivers). Groups specific to the patients' demographic characteristics (e.g., stage of disease, ethnicity, and gender) may offer greater appeal to some patients. Nonprofit Parkinson's disease organizations are also useful sources of information and include the National Parkinson Foundation and the American Parkinson Disease Association.

Case 43 Seizure Disorder

1. The answer is E (2.2.2)

Carbamazepine has a chew tablet, extended-release capsule, extended-release tablet and suspension. The suspension must be shaken well and administered three to four times a day to ensure stable concentrations. The extended-release capsule may be swallowed whole or opened and placed on a small amount of applesauce for the patient to swallow, not chew. The patient should drink fluids after administration to make sure the mixture is completely swallowed. The extended-release tablet should be swallowed whole and not chewed or broken.

2. The answer is D (2.2.1)

Lorazepam is the generic name for Ativan. Valium (diazepam), Klonapin (clonazepam), Xanax (alprazolam) and Versed (midazolam) are other benzodiazepines. Diazepam or midazolam may also be used to stop a seizure. Alprazolam and clonazepam do not have an IV formulation available.

3. The answer is D (2.1.1)

The nurse has the 2 mg/mL vial. Therefore, she should administer 2 mL to the patient to provide a dose of 4 mg. If the nurse had the 4 mg/mL vial, she could administer 1 mL to the patient.

4. The answer is D (1.2.6)

The half-life of carbamazepine during therapy initiation or after single doses is approximately 21–28 days. As carbamazepine is an autoinducer, the half-life decreases dramatically to an average of 15 hours. Carbamazepine levels should be obtained 21–28 days after initiation.

5. The answer is C (1.3.3)

Carbamazepine is not associated with an increase in kidney stone formation. Topiramate and zonisamide are the two anticonvulsants with this adverse effect. Carbamazepine may cause a rash during therapy. A patient should stop the medication and call the physician immediately. Dizziness and drowsiness may occur at drug initiation and dose escalations. This usually resolves after continued therapy. Other adverse effects of carbamazepine include leukopenia, thrombocytopenia and anemia. Hyponatremia may also be seen but this usually occurs more often in the elderly.

6. The answer is B (1.2.6)

The therapeutic concentration range for carbamazepine is 4–12 mcg/mL. Phenytoin's therapeutic range is 10–20 mcg/mL. Phenobarbital's therapeutic range is 10–40 mcg/mL. Therapeutic concentrations have not been well defined for the newer generation anticonvulsants as clinical outcome has not shown to correlate with specific concentration ranges.

7. The answer is D (3.2.1)

If witnessing a person have a seizure, help the person to the floor and cushion their head. Remove any sharp items from their hands and move any close furniture. Take off any eye glasses the patient may be wearing. Loosen any restrictive clothing such as a tie. Turn their head to the side or roll the person to the side to prevent aspiration. Do not place anything in the mouth. Many believe that placing an object in the mouth will prevent the tongue from being bitten or swallowed. A person can not swallow their tongue and during a seizure a person does not bite off their tongue. They may bite it but it is usually not severe. Placing an object in the mouth can increase the risk of aspiration and cause more harm to the patient.

8. The answer is E (1.1.1)

As SB has a sulfa allergy, he should not be prescribed zonisamide. Zonisamide is structurally related to the sulfonamides. Lamotrigine and topiramate may be used as an adjunct therapy. Phenytoin and valproic acid may be used as monotherapy for generalized tonic-clonic seizures.

9. The answer is B (1.3.3)

Vitamin D and calcium should be supplemented in patients on anticonvulsants, especially growing children. Bone mineral density decreases have been seen in patients on carbamazepine, phenobarbital, phenytoin and valproic acid. It is postulated that anticonvulsants may increase the catabolism of vitamin D, impair bone resorption and formation and impair calcium absorption. Vitamin C, B, and E may be supplemented in SB but he is not at risk for these deficiencies because of anticonvulsant therapy.

Answers

10. The answer is D (1.3.1)

The American Academy of Neurology has guidelines for discontinuing anticonvulsants in seizure free patients. They recommend that discontinuation may be considered if the patient has been seizure free for 2–5 years, has a single seizure type, has a normal neurologic exam and IQ and the EEG normalized while on treatment. There is no reference regarding dose of medication for a specified time for discontinuing an anticonvulsant.

Case 44 Bone Marrow Transplantation

1. The answer is C (1.3.3)

Antiemetics are required because this is a highly emetogenic regimen (Hesketh level 5). Busulfan at these doses is well-documented to lower the seizure threshold, so prophylactic anticonvulsants should be started and continued for 48–72 hours after the drug is finished. While diarrhea can occur, it is unlikely, and antidiarrheals would not need to be scheduled at this time.

2. The answer is A (1.2.3)

Itraconazole significantly inhibits the metabolism of cyclosporine at the cytochrome P450 3A4 hepatic enzymes, increasing cyclosporine levels and generally requiring a 50%–60% reduction in dose to prevent toxic cyclosporine levels. Ciprofloxacin and valacyclovir and lansoprazole and prednisone have no significant interactions.

3. The answer is C (1.3.3)

Cyclosporine is the likely cause due to its vasoconstrictive effects on the afferent arteriole. Cyclophosphamide rarely causes hypertension and never this late after infusion. Prednisone can raise blood pressure secondary to fluid retention and electrolyte effects, but it would be unlikely to occur this rapidly or as significantly when she was previously normotensive.

4. The answer is B (1.3.3)

Clonidine (A) and methyldopa (C) are third- or fourth-line agents for hypertension, and nitroglycerin (D) would be for a hypertensive urgency, which this case is not at a diastolic pressure of 96 mmHg. Dihydropyridine calcium channel blockers would be chosen over other types since one of the ways they exert their effect is via relaxation of the afferent arteriole in the kidney, which is where cyclosporine acts to cause hypertension. Verapamil is a nondihydropyridine calcium channel blocking agent.

5. The answer is C (2.2.4)

The only oral form currently available is the 2-mg tablet. Generally, the tablets of each dose are placed in empty 00-size capsules to decrease the number of items swallowed per dose. The IV form is dosed on the same interval but at 0.8 mg per 1 mg oral busulfan. Once daily busulfan is experimental at this time, and the dosing is still being worked out.

6. The answer is C (2.1.1)

The square root of Ht x Wt/3600 = BSA. 158.5 cm x 86 kg/3600 = 3.786. The square root of 3.786 gives a BSA of 1.95 m². 1.95 m² x 15 mg/m² = 29.2 mg. Actual body weight is used over ideal unless otherwise directed.

7. The answer is D (1.2.5)

Low doses such as this do not require sodium bicarbonate to alkalinize the urine and increase the solubility of methotrexate. At doses higher than 1 g/m² this is commonly done and is generally considered the standard of care to protect renal tubules from methotrexate precipitation.

8. The answer is B (3.2.3)

Valerian is a potential CYP 3A4 inhibitor and could make her cyclosporine levels unpredictable, increasing her risk for toxicity. SAMe is not used for insomnia, the FDA doesn't currently review herbal supplements, and trazodone isn't a benzodiazepine, making all of the other choices incorrect.

9. The answer is A (2.2.5)

The oral solution is equally bioavailable to the capsules of the microemulsion (Neoral). It adsorbs onto plastic, so to make each dose palatable it is mixed in glass with a metal spoon and consumed immediately. This is generally done with room temperature liquids, and additional diluent (milk, juice, etc.) is then used to rinse out the glass and ensure that the full dose has been consumed. It would be taken at the same times and intervals as the capsules.

10. The answer is B (2.2.1)

Any A/B rated micro-emulsion that is a Neoral equivalent, whether capsule or liquid form, would be an appropriate substitution. Macro-emulsion products, like Sandimmune or its equivalents, would not give similar blood cyclosporine levels. It is often prudent to verify that levels don't change significantly as you change products but in general they are substitutable.

Case 45 Breast Cancer

1. The answer is C (1.3.3)

All of the following are side effects of doxorubicin except for peripheral neuropathy. Peripheral neuropathy is a common adverse effect of Taxol (paclitaxel) chemotherapy.

2. The answer is E (1.2.1)

MESNA is oxidized to dimesna which in turn is reduced in the kidney back to mesna, supplying a free thiol group which binds to and inactivates acrolein, the urotoxic metabolite of ifosfamide and cyclophosphamide.

Dexrazoxane exhibits cardioprotective effects when infused 15 minutes prior to an anthracycline chemotherapy agent. The mechanism is believed to be iron chelation following intracellular hydrolysis to ultimately inhibit the generation of free radicals that can be damaging to the myocardium following an anthracycline dose. It is not used up front as standard of care. Dexrazoxane is indicated for reducing the incidence and severity of cardiomyopathy associated with doxorubicin in women with metastatic breast cancer who have received a cumulative doxorubicin dose of 300 milligrams/square meter and will continue receiving doxorubicin to maintain tumor control.

Naloxone is an opioid antagonist used to treat reversal of an opioid overdosage.

Flumazenil is used as a benzodiazepine receptor antagonist.

Leucovorin is used to diminish the toxicity and counteract the effect of high doses of folic acid antagonists, such as methotrexate.

3. The answer is B (1.3.3)

Palonosetron (Aloxi) has the longest T1/2 of all the 5-HT$_3$ antagonists with an elimination half-life of 30 to 40 hours. Chemotherapy is classified by emetogenicity into five categories (Hesketh levels) based on the incidence of nausea and vomiting without antiemetic prophylaxis. Chemotherapy-induced nausea and vomiting can be life-threatening if not treated appropriately in a timely manner (e.g., electrolyte disturbances). CINV can last for several days (1–7 days) but is often preventable with appropriate antiemetic therapy.

4. The answer is C (1.3.5)

Emend is a new anti-emetic FDA approved in 2004. It is currently approved for: (1) prophylaxis for chemotherapy-induced nausea and vomiting, due to highly emetogenic chemotherapy, including high-dose cisplatin; and (2) prophylaxis for chemotherapy-induced nausea and vomiting, due to moderately emetogenic chemotherapy.

There is a clinical trial looking at Emend usage with cyclophosphamide/doxorubicin or epirubicin chemotherapy regimen. This would be a viable option for treatment of patients with nausea.

Ativan is an additive anti-emetic option when dexamethasone and Compazine are not providing relief.

Zofran is most effective for chemotherapy nausea/vomiting when it is used within 24 hours of the infusion.

5. The answer is A (1.2.3)

The concurrent administration of anthracyclines and trastuzumab increased the incidence and severity of cardiac dysfunction during clinical trials. Trastuzumab monotherapy has been associated with the development of ventricular dysfunction and congestive heart failure, and these cardiotoxic effects are enhanced by the presence of anthracyclines.

6. The answer is A (2.1.3)

The correct answer would be 279 mL/h.

Since the total Taxol dose is 175 mg and the concentration is 6 mg/mL. The total volume of the Taxol for the dose of 175 mg is 29.2 mL. When added to the 250-mL bag the total volume would be 279 mL. Since the IV is infusing over 1 hour the correct infusion rate would be 279 mL/h.

7. The answer is D (1.2.1)

Antiestrogen therapy is indicated for all breast cancer patients whose tumor is positive for estrogen receptors. A poorly differentiated tumor has no bearing on whether a patient will benefit from tamoxifen therapy. Depending on whether a patient is pre- or post-menopausal depends on whether Tamoxifen or Arimidex (anastrozole) is used in postmenopausal patients for adjuvant treatment.

8. The answer is E (1.3.3)

Tamoxifen is associated with all of the adverse events listed.

9. The answer is D (3.2.3)

Since CF's hemoglobin is <11 and she is having symptoms of anemia, i.e., extreme fatigue, initiation of a erythropoietin stimulator is recommended. The most appropriate dose would be Procrit 40,000 units SC weekly or Aranesp 200 mcg SC every 2 weeks. Aranesp used every 2 weeks would coincide with her chemotherapy schedule. With a serum iron <70 mcg/dL, Ferritin <100 ng/mL, or transferrin saturation <20%, it is also recommended to start iron therapy. Without adequate iron stores the Aranesp or Procrit would not be able to effectively maintain erythpoiesis. Ferrous sulfate 325 mg PO TID would be the best option for iron replacement.

10. The answer is E (3.2.1)

All of the above are true regarding breast cancer screening guidelines. These guidelines can be accessed at:

www.cancer.org/docroot/NWS/content/NWS_1_1x_ Updated_Breast_Cancer_Screening_Guidelines_Released.asp

Case 46 Gastrointestinal Cancer

1. The answer is B (1.2.2)

5-Fluorouracil is a pyrimidine antimetabolite that inhibits the enzyme thymidylate synthase, thereby blocking DNA synthesis.

2. The answer is C (2.2.1)

5-Fluorouracil is commonly referred to as 5-FU. FUDR is floxuridine, an antimetabolite sometimes given through hepatic artery infusion for liver metastases. 5-FC is flucytosine (an antifungal agent). UFT is an investigational combination of tegafur and uracil. Tegafur is a prodrug of 5-FU and uracil inhibits dihydropyrimidine dehydrogenase (DPD), the enzyme that breaks down 5-FU. CPT-11 is the investigational designa-

Answers

tion of irinotecan, a topoisomerase I inhibitor often combined with 5-FU and leucovorin for colon cancer treatment.

3. The answer is B (2.1.0)

Based on the height and weight the patient's BSA is 2.03 m², making the correct daily dose of 5-fluorouracil 860 mg.

4. The answer is C (1.2.0)

When administering 5-fluorouracil and leucovorin for the treatment of colon cancer, leucovorin should be infused prior to 5-FU. Leucovorin is a reduced form of folic acid which can potentiate the effects of 5-FU by stabilizing the ternary complex of thymidylate synthetase. In order to be most effective, the reduced folate needs to be available when 5-FU binds to thymidylate synthetase. 5-Fluorouracil should not be mixed in the same bag as leucovorin because recent evidence has found them to be incompatible.

5. The answer is B (1.2.4)

Mucositis and myelosuppression are the main dose-limiting toxicities of 5-fluorouracil. Myelosuppression is greater when 5-FU is given by bolus, and mucositis predominates when 5-FU is given by continuous infusion. Nausea and vomiting associated with 5-fluorouracil and leucovorin is mild and not dose limiting. Alopecia (loss of hair) is minimal with 5-FU and would not limit dosing of the drug.

6. The answer is C (1.2.1)

Oxiliplatin has been approved as a first- or second-line treatment of metastatic colorectal cancer. It is given in combination with 5-fluorouracil and leucovorin. Therefore, it would be the next line of treatment for MW. Cytarabine, paclitaxel, and doxorubicin do not have significant activity in colorectal cancer. Interferon has some activity in combination with 5-fluorouracil but is considered investigational.

7. The answer is D (2.2.1)

Protonix is the brand name of pantoprazole and, therefore, the correct product to use to fill the prescription. Prilosec (A) is the brand name of omeprazole, and Prevacid (E) is the brand name of lansoprazole, both are proton pump inhibitors like pantoprazole. Zantac (B) is the brand name product of ranitidine, and Pepcid (C) the brand name product of famotidine.

8. The answer is D (1.3.0)

Appropriate treatment of a level 2 emetogen would be with the use of a phenothiazine antiemetic agent such as prochlorperazine. Serotonin antagonist (5-HT$_3$) antiemetic agents, such as ondansetron and granisetron, are not indicated unless patients fail to respond to phenothiazines. Also, serotonin antagonists are much more expensive. Diphenhydramine is not an appropriate agent to treat chemotherapy-induced nausea and vomiting.

9. The answer is B (3.2.1)

The American Cancer Society recommends a screening colonoscopy/sigmoidoscopy for everyone starting at age 50. Because MW is at increased risk due to his family history, he should have had a screening colonoscopy at age 35–40. Patients with a history of genetic syndromes such as Familial Adenomatous Polyposis (FAP) are screened even earlier.

10. The answer is A (3.2.0)

Vicodin is a combination analgesic medication containing hydrocodone (a narcotic) and acetaminophen (a prostaglandin inhibitor). It may be habit-forming, especially with repeated use of high doses. If the medication is not controlling the pain, patients should be instructed to contact their doctor. Narcotic analgesics may cause nausea or upset stomach, and taking Vicodin with food or milk may help to alleviate this side effect. Narcotics can also cause drowsiness or dizziness. Patients should be counseled not to drive or operate machinery until the full effects of the medication are known. Alcohol can potentiate this side effect.

Case 47 Leukemias

1. The answer is C (1.2.1)

Vincristine is an active drug in treating ALL, however, it should never be given intrathecally. An accidental intrathecal injection of vincristine is nearly always fatal within 2 weeks. Methotrexate and cytarabine are suitable agents to be administered intrathecally to BM.

2. The answer is B (1.3.3)

Cyclophosphamide is metabolized to several metabolites, including the active 4-hydroxycyclophosphamide and the inactive metabolite, acrolein. Acrolein irritates the bladder mucosa, resulting in hemorrhagic cystitis. Chloroacetaldehyde is an inactive metabolite of ifosfamide and may cause neurotoxicity. Difluorodeoxyuridine and uracil arabinoside are metabolites of gemcitabine and cytarabine, respectively.

3. The answer is C (1.3.3)

Mesna is a selective urinary tract protectant. It binds directly to the toxic cyclophosphamide metabolite, acrolein, and prevents damage to the bladder.

4. The answer is A (2.2.1)

Adriamycin is doxorubicin. Although idarubicin, daunorubicin, and mitoxantrone are anthracyclines, they are not interchangeable with doxorubicin. Doxil is liposomal doxorubicin and is also not interchangeable with standard doxorubicin. The order would need to specify the liposomal product.

5. The answer is D (3.2.2)

Neutropenic fever is an oncologic emergency and requires immediate evaluation and treatment. Without the protection of neutrophils against bacterial infections, patients can be in septic shock and die within hours. Pseudomonas aeruginosa has a doubling time of approximately 20 minutes in a patient with an ANC <500. Whenever a patient is unsure of his or her white blood cell count and he or she is at risk for low counts, all fevers require that the patient call to alert their medical team. If their ANC is <500 then they should receive empiric antibiotics.

6. The answer is D (1.3.3)

The management of this extravasation should include stopping the infusion and aspirating any drug via the intravenous cannula before it is removed. Cold compresses, as well as DMSO, should be applied to the affected area. A surgeon should be consulted to assess the need for early surgery for minimization of the injury and potential for future skin grafting for serious infiltrations. Sodium thiosulfate is useful in treating cisplatin and mechlorethamine extravasations. Warm compresses and hyaluronidase are local antidotes for extravasations of the vinca alkaloids and epipodophyllotoxins.

7. The answer Is A (2.3.1)

Filtration with a 0.22-μm filter would help to insure a bacteria-free product. A bacteriostatic diluent is not used in intrathecal preparations since it increases the risk of arachnoiditis associated with intrathecal injection of medications. Antineoplastic chemotherapy is always mixed in a class II vertical hood since any chemotherapy aerosolized in a horizontal flow hood would be blown back onto the compounder.

8. The answer is B (1.3.3)

Leucovorin rescue reduces high-dose toxicity. It is a reduced form of folic acid and competes with methotrexate for transport into tissues, including the gastrointestinal tract and the bone marrow. It is metabolized to tetrahydrofolate and thymidylate and DNA synthesis is subsequently resumed, rescuing cells from the toxicity of methotrexate. Levamisole, dexrazoxane, filgrastim, and dolasetron play no role in reducing toxicity in the setting of elevated methotrexate levels.

9. The answer is B (2.1.4)

Sodium bicarbonate contains 1 mEq sodium for each mEq sodium bicarbonate. At 5.7 mg/mEq sodium x 150 mEq = 855 mg sodium in 1L from the sodium bicarbonate. Normal saline has 900 mg/L (i.e., 0.9%). 900 + 855 = 1,755 mg/L or ~1.76% saline in the final solution.

10. The answer is D (2.2.2)

Leucovorin is folinic acid which is already in the reduced form and ready to be utilized by cells. Folic acid must undergo metabolism via dihydrofolate reductase in order to be utilized by cells and this process is blocked by methotrexate so the two agents cannot be substituted. Folic acid is available OTC in 0.4- and 0.8-mg strengths.

Case 48 Lung Cancer

1. The answer is A (2.1.1)

The patient weighs 61.3 kg and is 157.48 cm. The BSA is calculated to be the square root of [(61.3 kg x 157.48 cm)/3600] = 1.638 m². A 50% dose reduction was necessary for this patient, resulting in the dose of 15 mg/m². Thus, the final dose for this patient is 1.638 m² x 15 mg/m² = 25 mg.

2. The answer is C (3.2.1)

Zyban and nicotine patches such as Nicoderm and Habitrol are modalities used alone or in combination for smoking cessation. Zyban is administered for 7–12 weeks at doses of 150 mg po bid. If the patient does not show progress towards quitting, it should be discontinued. Nicoderm and Habitrol patches should be used when a patient has committed to smoking cessation. Patches come in a variety of strengths and should be tapered down at individual time frames. Nicotine gum and counseling may also be used with patients in this population who desire to quit smoking. Niacin has no role in assisting a patient to quit smoking.

3. The answer is B (1.2.2)

Vinorelbine is a vinca alkaloid that acts by inhibiting the polymerization of tubulin.

4. The answer is E (1.3.3)

Grade 3 or 4 nausea and vomiting occurs in 1%–3% of patients receiving vinorelbine; thus, it is low in emetogenicity. Grade 3 or 4 emesis is defined by the Common Toxicity Criteria as no significant intake and requiring intravenous fluids.

5. The answer is A (2.3.1)

To ensure sterility of the final product, aseptic technique should be utilized. It is recommended that chemotherapy be prepared in a class II, type b, or class III biologic safety cabinets, because these cabinets vent the air to the outside. OSHA recommends that small solid spills be cleaned up using wet absorbent gauze.

6. The answer is B (1.3.3)

Grade 3 to 4 neutropenia occurs in 50% of patients who receive vinorelbine; therefore, it is a dose-limiting toxicity. According to the Common Toxicity Criteria, grade 3 neutropenia is defined as a neutrophil/granulocyte count of (0.5 - <1.0 x 10⁹/L) or an absolute neutrophil/granulocyte count of (500 to <1000/mm³). Grade 4 neutropenia is defined as a neutrophil/granulocyte count of <0.5 x 10⁹/L or an absolute neutrophil/granulocyte count <500/mm³. Pulmonary fibrosis, cardiotoxicity, and mucositis are rare. Neuropathy is less common with vinorelbine than with other vinca alkaloids and is rarely dose limiting.

7. The answer is B (1.3.3)

JB received both cisplatin and vinorelbine during this course

Answers

of chemotherapy. Cisplatin is highly emetogenic and induces both acute and delayed chemotherapy-induced emesis. JB now needs to be admitted for hydration and intravenous antiemetics. Of the agents listed only aprepitant plus dexamethasone is considered a standard agent to prevent delayed nausea and vomiting. Other options for the prevention of delayed emesis include dexamethasone with or without metoclopramide. Also prochlorperazine could be added to dexamethasone.

8. The answer is D (2.2.1)

Hydromorphone is the generic name for Dilaudid. Hydrocodone is an antitussive and a narcotic analgesic. It is only available in an oral formulation and in combination with other agents. Hydrocodone is available in many different products, including Hycodan (hydrocodone/homatropine) and Lortab (hydrocodone/acetaminophen). Propoxyphene is only available in an oral formulation and is the generic name for Darvon. Fentanyl is the generic name for Sublimaze (intravenous formulation), Actiq (oral lozenge), and Duragesic (transdermal patch). Acetaminophen is the generic name for Tylenol.

9. The answer is C (2.1.1)

JB has a basal rate of 0.5 mg/h, which totals 12 mg/24 h. She received 11 extra doses of Dilaudid during that time, resulting in an additional 3.3 mg administered. Therefore, her 24-hour total of Dilaudid received is 12 mg + 3.3 mg = 15.3 mg.

10. The answer is E (1.3.5)

Docetaxel 75 mg/m² produces an improvement in quality of life and somewhat prolonged survival when used as second-line therapy in patients with good performance status. Higher doses are generally too toxic. Cytarabine, tamoxifen, carmustine, and vinblastine have no role as second-line therapy against non-small-cell lung cancer.

Case 49 Lymphoma

1. The answer is C (1.1.3)

The staging classification that is currently used for Hodgkin's lymphoma was adopted in 1971 at the Ann Arbor Conference, with some modifications 18 years later from the Cotswolds meeting. Subclassification of stage

Stages I, II, III, and IV adult Hodgkin's lymphoma can be subclassified into A and B categories: B for those with defined general symptoms and A for those without B symptoms. The B designation is given to patients with any of the following symptoms:

Unexplained loss of more than 10% of body weight in the 6 months before diagnosis.

Unexplained fever with temperatures above 38 °C.

Drenching night sweats.

Stage I: Stage I adult Hodgkin's lymphoma is characterized by the involvement of a single lymph node region (I) or localized involvement of a single extralymphatic organ or site (IE).

Stage II: Stage II adult Hodgkin's lymphoma is characterized by the involvement of two or more lymph node regions on the same side of the diaphragm (II) or localized involvement of a single associated extralymphatic organ or site and its regional lymph node(s) with or without involvement of other lymph node regions on the same side of the diaphragm (IIE). Note: The number of lymph node regions involved may be indicated by a subscript. Many investigators divide patients with clinical stage I and II disease into favorable or unfavorable groups based on prognostic factors. The patients in the favorable group are managed with treatment reduction strategies; the patients in the unfavorable group are managed with combined modality therapy. Patients with early-stage disease and favorable prognostic features can undergo radiation therapy without staging laparotomy. These favorable subgroups of patients have an 80% relapse-free survival rate at 5 to 10 years with mantle-field irradiation, alone or in conjunction with para-aortic and splenic irradiation. Favorable features include the following:

Sedimentation rate of <50.

Patient age of 50 or younger.

Lymphocyte predominant or nodular sclerosing histology.

Lack of B symptoms.

Fewer than three sites of involvement.

No bulky adenopathy.

Stage III: Stage III adult Hodgkin's lymphoma is characterized by the involvement of lymph node regions on both sides of the diaphragm (III), which may also be accompanied by localized involvement of an associated extralymphatic organ or site (IIIE), by involvement of the spleen (IIIS), or by involvement of both (IIIE + S). Stage III disease may be subdivided by anatomic distribution of abdominal involvement or by extent of splenic involvement. Stage III(1) indicates involvement that is limited to the upper abdomen above the renal vein. Stage III(2) indicates involvement of pelvic and/or para-aortic nodes. Five or more visible splenic nodules on a cut section constitutes extensive splenic involvement. Zero to 4 nodules is classified as minimal splenic disease.

Stage IV: Stage IV adult Hodgkin's lymphoma is characterized by disseminated (multifocal) involvement of 1 or more extralymphatic organs, with or without associated lymph node involvement, or isolated extralymphatic organ involvement with distant (nonregional) nodal involvement. Massive mediastinal disease has been defined by the Cotswolds meeting as a thoracic ratio of maximum transverse mass diameter <gr than or eq to symbol> >33% of the internal transverse thoracic diameter measured at the T5/6 intervertebral disc level on chest radiography. Some investigators have designated a lymph node mass measuring <gr than or eq to symbol> >10 cm in greatest dimension as massive disease. Other investigators use a measurement of the maximum width of the mediastinal mass divided by the maximum intrathoracic diameter.

KL's Hodgkin's lymphoma is classified as IIB, bulky disease, given the > 2 LN's regions on same side of diaphragm. The "B" refers to the constitutional symptoms that she had been experiencing as outlined above.

2. The answer is C (1.3.1)

Patients who have stage IIB disease with bulky mediastinal involvement should be treated with chemotherapy plus involved-field RT. Whenever possible, the high cervical regions (all patients) and axillae (women) should be excluded from the radiation fields. ABVD is generally still considered the gold standard and is administered for 6–8 cycles. Complete restaging takes place at the completion of chemotherapy. Consolidative irradiation is optimally instituted within 3 weeks (36 Gy to initial sites >5 cm).

CHOP chemotherapy continues to be the gold standard in the treatment of non-Hodgkin's lymphoma.

ABVD therapy for 6 to 8 months is as effective as 12 months of MOPP alternating with ABVD, and both are superior to MOPP alone in terms of failure-free survival. The Intergroup trial comparing ABVD with MOPP/ABV hybrid showed equivalent efficacy in failure-free survival and overall survival, but increased toxic effects in the hybrid arm, especially from second malignancies

Rituximab is an option in selected symptomatic patients who are not candidates for chemotherapy in patients with clinical stage III-IV non-lymphocyte predominant Hodgkin's disease.

3. The answer is D (1.3.2)

Doxorubicin damages cardiac muscle and may result in congestive heart failure. The toxicity increases with increasing total dosage, and this causes most clinicians to limit doxorubicin dosage to about 450 mg/m². A MUGA measures the ejection fraction of the left ventricle. If the ejection fraction falls by ~15% or below 50, clinicians may discontinue use of doxorubicin.

4. The answer is B (1.3.2)

Pulmonary fibrosis is the most common severe toxicity of bleomycin. The incidence increases in: (1) pts > 70 yo, (2) those patients with prior pulmonary radiation, (3) those who have received high concentrations of oxygen post-treatment, (4) those receiving more than a total of 400 units, and (5) those receiving more than 25 units/m² per dose.

Monitoring for lung toxicity: chest auscultation (end inspiratory crackles are indicative of toxicity and the drug discontinuation); pulmonary function test that reveals abnormal carbon monoxide dissuasion capacity if indicative of toxicity.

Lung toxicity prevention: infuse all doses no faster than 1 unit per minute, administer no more than 30 units per dose, avoid administration of high oxygen concentrations, and avoid giving more than 400 units total lifetime dose.

5. The answer is B (1.1.3)

The constitutional symptoms of unexplained fever, drenching night sweats, and unintentional weight loss are present at diagnosis in approximately 30% of patients with Hodgkin's lymphoma. Bulky disease is an important prognostic feature in itself but is not considered one of the three constitutional "B" symptoms.

6. The answer is D (3.1.2)

More than 75% of all newly diagnosed patients with adult Hodgkin's lymphoma can be cured with combination chemotherapy and/or radiation therapy. Careful staging and treatment planning by a multidisciplinary team of cancer specialists is required to determine the optimal treatment for patients with this disease. Hodgkin's lymphoma is the main cause of death over the first 15 years after treatment. By 15 to 20 years after therapy, the cumulative mortality from a second malignancy will exceed the cumulative mortality from Hodgkin's lymphoma. So given this, it is essential that health care providers and patients are educated and aware of the potential long-term sequelae when comparing one regimen to another.

With respect to response rates and cure, ABVD has not been shown to be superior in all clinical trials to date, however, it has demonstrated at least equivalent results or better results in most cases, with significantly less toxicity associated with it. The Intergroup trial comparing ABVD with MOPP/ABV hybrid showed equivalent efficacy in failure-free survival and overall survival, but increased toxic effects in the hybrid arm, especially from second malignancies.

A toxic effect that is primarily related to chemotherapy is infertility, usually after MOPP-containing regimens; ABVD appears to spare long-term testicular and ovarian function.

Acute nonlymphocytic leukemia may occur in patients treated with combined modality therapy or with combination chemotherapy alone. At 10 years following therapy with regimens containing MOPP, the risk of acute myelogenous leukemia is approximately 3%, with the peak incidence occurring 5 to 9 years after therapy. The risk of acute leukemia at 10 years following therapy with ABVD appears to be <1%.

7. The answer is D (1.3.3)

Cold and DMSO are typically used to treat doxorubicin extravasation and prevent development of tissue necrosis. Heat and hyaluronidase are considered the standard of care for vincristine extravasations.

8. The answer is C (1.2.4)

Sulfamethoxazole/trimethoprim would certainly be a reasonable choice, however, KL is allergic to sulfa drugs so it is not an option for her. Fluconazole is an antifungal drug so would not be indicated in a bacterial infection. Ciprofloxacin is the best choice in this situation. Its spectrum of activity consistently covers the identified bacteria while producing high concentrations of drug in the urine. Combination therapy with amoxicillin/clavulanic acid and cipro is overkill and should not

Answers

be utilized with a simple urinary tract infection. Metronidazole is utilized in the treatment of anaerobic infections (bacterial vaginosis).

9. The answer is C (1.1.4)

Though there is uncertainty about the precise etiology of Hodgkin's lymphoma, an association with viral (EBV and mononucleosis), familial factors (same sex siblings= 10x higher risk, monozygotic twin has 99x higher risk of developing HD than a dizygotic twin; single family homes, fewer siblings, early birth order and few playmates), and being exposed to certain chemicals, organic solvents, and herbicides has also been described.

Hodgkin's lymphoma is slightly more predominant in the male gender (1.4: 1) and is characterized by its bimodal distribution: first peak occurs in the mid to late 20's (15–34) and a second rise in incidence occurs after the age of 50.

10. The answer is B (3.2.1)

Dexamethasone may cause fluid retention and weight gain as an adverse event. It does increase appetite in some instances but certainly is not why it was prescribed for KL. Dexamethasone should be given in the morning to reduce sleeplessness and vivid dreams, and it is not uncommon for patients to complain of flu-like syndrome and asthenia when stopping the drug after 5–7 days. In addition, it should be taken with food or milk to help minimize GI intolerance. Being a nurse, she is most likely aware of the potential side effects of steroids so the most helpful information would be gained through direct discussion. Many are somewhat reluctant to take steroids because of known adverse events, so it is important to provide information that helps her to understand the importance of compliance in this situation. Hyperglycemia may occur from corticosteroid use.

Case 50 Prostate Cancer

1. The answer is B (1.1.4)

African American descent is one of the strongest risk factors for prostate cancer. The overall life time risk of developing prostate cancer in African American males is approximately 9.8% compared to 8% in Caucasian males. The risk is lowest in Asian men. Positive smoking history, additional malignancies, alcohol use, and vasectomy are not associated with increased prostate cancer risk.

2. The answer is B (3.2.1)

The American Cancer Society recommends non-African American men and those with a negative family history begin annual PSA screening at age 50. For African American men and those with one or more first-degree relatives with prostate cancer, screening should begin at age 40. Given their positive family history, PN and his brothers should start prostate cancer screening at age 40.

3. The answer is D (1.1.2)

Digital rectal examination and prostate-specific antigen measurement are standard screening tools. The positive predictive value of PSA >4 ng/mL alone is 35% whereas PSA values >4 ng/mL and a positive digital rectal exam is 50%. Ultrasound guided fine needle biopsy is not routinely recommended for screening. However, biopsy should be obtained in men with PSA >4 ng/mL and/or abnormal digital rectal exams suggestive of prostate cancer. Screening based on symptomatology, chemistries, and age are not highly predictive.

4. The answer is A (1.1.2)

A PSA >4 ng/mL generally requires evaluation to rule out malignancy, however, normal range for PSA values will change based on the patient's age.

5. The answer is A (3.2.2)

Nerve-sparing prostatectomies are associated with fewer complications than radical prostatectomies. Common complications of prostatectomies and radiation include local tissue damage, irritation and/or bleeding of surrounding tissues, impotence, and urinary incontinence.

6. The answer is A (1.2.2)

Terazosin is an alpha blocker. Examples of agents belonging to the other pharmacological classes include:

Beta blocker: metoprolol, atenolol

Calcium channel blocker: verapamil, amlodipine

5HT-$_3$ blocker: ondansetron, granisetron

ACE inhibitor: lisinopril

7. The answer is E (2.2.2)

All of the above agents are oral alternatives to PN's alprostadil suppositories.

8. The answer is D (1.2.1)

Dutasteride and finasteride are 5-alpha reductase inhibitors. Finasteride was studied in the Prostate Cancer Prevention Trial. Sildenafil is a phosphodiesterase inhibitor. Gemcitabine is a chemotherapy agent. Tolterodine is an antimuscarinic.

9. The answer is B (1.2.7)

The absorption of Proscar is decreased with food. However, the bioavailability remains unchanged. Therefore, Proscar can be administered without regard to food. The other statements are true.

10. The answer is C (1.2.2)

Aminoglutethimide and bicalutamide are antiandrogens. Goserelin is a LHRH agonist. Estramustine is a chemotherapy agent. Pamidronate is a bisphosphonate.

Case 51 Skin Cancers and Melanomas

1. The answer is C (2.2.5)

The IV and SQ routes can be used to administer interferon alpha-2b. Interferon alpha-2b is not orally bioavailable.

2. The answer is A (3.2.1)

The ABCD rule stands for asymmetry, border irregularity, color variations, and diameter >6 mm. These are the only identified characteristics that help in determining whether a mole is likely to be benign or a melanoma. The other characteristics listed are not a part of this rule.

3. The answer is B (1.2.1)

The approved dose of interferon for the adjuvant treatment of melanoma is 20 million units/m²/day IV x5 days/week x4 weeks, then 10 million units/m² SQ three times weekly x48 weeks. The other dosing regimens, while used for other indications in other disease states, are not the approved doses for the adjuvant treatment of melanoma.

4. The answer is E (3.2.1)

While hypothyroidism is a more common thyroid-related manifestation than hyperthyroidism while receiving interferon alpha-2b therapy, both may be experienced. Patients with pre-existing thyroid dysfunction may have more difficulty with thyroid regulation. Flu-like symptoms are the more common adverse effect from all alpha interferons, including interferon alpha-2b. In some patients, this may be a dose-limiting adverse effect or cause the patient to abandon therapy. Education of the patient is very important to enhance medication adherence. CNS toxicity may be seen with interferon alpha-2b treatment, ranging from depression to somnolence to stupor. Note that virtually all of the side effects from interferon alpha-2b therapy are reversible with discontinuation of therapy.

5. The answer is E (1.2.1)

Capecitabine is an oral prodrug to 5-fluorouracil. Neither have shown activity in melanoma. The other agents have been used for melanoma, whether as standard therapy or on a study protocol, because they have demonstrated efficacy.

6. The answer is D (1.2.3)

The activity of aldesleukin is reduced in the presence of glucocorticoids, even when topically applied. Since aldesleukin acts by stimulating the body's innate immunity to target melanoma, it is not like traditional chemotherapy. As a result, secondary malignancy and neutropenia are not likely. This regimen is given with an approximate 9-day period between cycles.

7. The answer is C (3.2.1)

Acetaminophen (or an NSAID) is recommended as pretreatment for interferon to reduce fever and headache. The other medications listed have little to no impact on either fever or headache in this instance.

8. The answer is E (3.2.2)

All of the characteristics listed are associated with an increased risk of skin cancer.

9. The answer is D (1.1.2)

The only method that is effective for early detection of melanoma lesions is the total body skin examination. While the other tests listed may be useful for identification of a metastatic lesion, they are not used for screening with any type of cancer.

10. The answer is B (1.2.3)

Hepatotoxicity associated with interferon therapy is quite common and can be life-threatening. The most appropriate course of action to take if a patient's LFTs begin to rise is to hold the interferon until the LFTs return to normal, then restart the interferon at half the dose. The benefits of continuing therapy at half the dose rather than completely discontinuing are evident in the survival benefit from this therapy when given to patients such as WW. Therefore, continuing at half the dose is preferable, in terms of the risk-benefit ratio. Continuing interferon (at any dose) in light of an increase in LFTs can be fatal and should not be recommended.

Case 52 Bone and Joint Infections

1. The answer is E (1.1.1)

Elevated temperature and WBC are indicative of acute infectious processes and could be expected to be elevated as in this case. Although relatively nonspecific, the increased ESR and CRP indicate inflammation and are consistent with osteomyelitis. While not very sensitive, the blurred margins presented on the x-ray can be an early sign of osteomyelitis. Finally, the HR and RR of the patient are not elevated significantly, but when considering the physical condition of the patient, these modest compensatory elevations could be a result of an infectious process. Thus, the composite of the s/s presented reveal a likely osteomyelitis.

2. The answer is C (1.1.3)

The most appropriate choice is S. aureus, given the time to presentation postsurgery. The source is most likely skin contamination via surgical wound.

Answers

3. The answer is E (1.3.1)

Necrotic bone, sepsis, and required amputation are all possible sequela from osteomyelitis.

4. The answer is D (3.2.1)

Antibiotics used in the management of acute osteomyelitis should be given in high doses, and, at least initially, should be given intravenously. Patients may be switched later to oral antibiotics to complete therapy if they have a clinical response to parenteral antibiotics. Early antibiotic therapy may reduce the need for surgery because a delay in treatment may allow the development of bone necrosis, thus making it more difficult to eradicate the infection. Finally, ciprofloxacin has inadequate activity against S. aureus to be used for this indication.

5. The answer is D (1.2.6)

Initially, antibiotics used for treating osteomyelitis should be administered IV at high dosages in order to achieve adequate concentrations in the infected bone. Ceftriaxone 2 g IV every 24 hours is the most appropriate choice. Ceftriaxone is not available for oral administration. IM therapy is inappropriate due to the long duration of therapy required, and both the 500-mg and 1-g doses are too low for treatment of osteomyelitis.

6. The answer is C (1.3.3)

Phototoxicity is not a common adverse effect of ceftriaxone. Thrombocytopenia, rash, diarrhea, and nausea all occur more frequently.

7. The answer is C (2.1.4)

To achieve a concentration of 4 mg/mL, the vancomycin 1000 mg dose should be diluted in 250 mL of dextrose 5% in water.

To solve this problem: $4 \text{ mg/mL} = 1000 \text{ mg/X}, X = 250 \text{ mL}$

8. The answer is D (1.3.3)

Linezolid is available in both oral and IV formulations, with the oral tablets approaching 100% bioavailability. Linezolid has mild MAO inhibitor properties and does interact with serotonergic agents, such as fluoxetine, causing a serotonin syndrome when used concomitantly. Finally, myelosuppression, namely thrombocytopenia, has been reported with linezolid therapy.

9. The answer is A (1.3.1)

Initially, all patients with acute osteomyelitis should receive IV antibiotics. However, patients may be able to complete their course of therapy with oral antibiotics if signs of active infection have resolved (i.e., afebrile, reduced WBC count, reduced ESR, and normal CRP), symptoms have improved (i.e., decreased swelling, redness, and pain), and patients have received at least 5 days of parenteral therapy.

10. The answer is C (3.2.1)

Two weeks is not sufficient time for treatment of osteomyelitis. It is advised that 4–6 weeks of adequate antibiotic therapy be administered. In addition, high doses of antibiotics are used in treating osteomyelitis.

Case 53 CNS Infections

1. The answer is A (1.1.3)

Nuchal rigidity is a stiff neck. A petechial rash is a non-raised and non-blanching rash with small red or purple spots resulting from tiny hemorrhages in the skin. A maculopapular rash is described in II. Photophobia is an abnormal sensitivity to light.

2. The answer is C (1.1.4)

Correct interpretation of the CSF findings is critical to the appropriate diagnosis of bacterial meningitis (especially when a pathogen is not cultured). A "clean" tap will have few to no red blood cells present. The presence of red cells suggests a traumatic tap. Since white cells are normally present in the peripheral blood, this can falsely elevate CSF white blood cell counts. This can be reasonably corrected with the equation:

Corrected WBC in CSF= measured WBC in CSF - (WBC in blood x RBC in CSF)/RBC in blood. (Adapted from Bleck TP, Greenlee JE. *Approach to the Patient with Central Nervous System Infection,* in Mandell GL, Bennett JE, Dolin R. *Principles and Practice of Infectious Diseases,* 6th ed., 2005 Churchill Livingstone.)

The hallmark of bacterial meningitis is an elevated CSF protein count (secondary to the compromise of the blood brain barrier), a CSF leukocytic pleocytosis characterized by a polymorphonuclear cell predominance, and a lowered CSF glucose relative to serum glucose secondary to micro-organism consumption.

For an in-depth review of the differences between bacterial, viral, and fungal meningitis, the reader is referred to an excellent review written in the aforementioned chapter of Principles and Practice of Infectious Diseases. The text is also available online through www.mdconsult.com.

3. The answer is C (1.1.0)

Streptococcus pneumoniae and Neisseria meningitidis are the most common causes of atraumatic, community-acquired meningitis. Listeria monocytogenes is an infrequent cause overall, but its frequency is increased in neonates, the elderly, immunocompromised, and patients with comorbid conditions, including alcoholics. Haemophilus influenzae type b meningitis was historically the most common cause of meningitis in neonates, but not in adults, and it is no longer of high prevalence in this country due to effective vaccination programs. Group B Streptococci are common causes of meningitis in the neonate. Staphylococcus aureus, Acinetobacter baumannii, Pseudomonas aeruginosa, and Bacteroides fragilis are not frequently encountered in community-acquired meningitis but may be encountered in the nosocomial setting, particularly in the patient with CNS trauma (injury or surgery).

Answers

4. The answer is B (1.2.1)

Ceftriaxone provides effective coverage for S. pneumoniae and Neisseria. Vancomycin is added for coverage of penicillin-resistant isolates of S. pneumoniae. Gentamicin, azithromycin, and cefazolin (as well as all other first-generation cephalosporins) poorly penetrate the CNS and should be avoided for treatment of meningitis, although gentamicin may be administered intrathecally when infection is caused by a resistant gram-negative aerobe. Daptomycin has not been sufficiently studied clinically at this time and has poor CNS penetration. Metronidazole exhibits a high level of CNS penetration, but activity is limited to anaerobes. As a result, this agent is frequently used when the presence of anaerobic organisms is suspected or confirmed; however, anaerobes are not a frequent cause of community-acquired meningitis. Fluconazole is used exclusively for treatment of fungal infections, which are not common in an immunocompetent individual. Accordingly, choices A, D, and E are not acceptable for the reasons cited above. Choice C is a frequently employed empiric regimen in the patient with hospital-acquired meningitis or the patient with CNS trauma. Ceftazidime is not required in this patient as Pseudomonas aeruginosa coverage is not necessary. Choice B is a preferred treatment regimen for community-acquired meningitis in a young adult patient population. While not pertinent to this case per se, a patient presenting similar to TC with penicillin allergy should receive chloramphenicol for appropriate coverage against S. pneumoniae and Neisseria.

5. The answer is C (1.2.0)

Dexamethasone therapy has been shown to be beneficial in the empiric treatment of adult meningitis. TC, however, has not received any corticosteroids at day 3. Patients who have already received antimicrobial therapy are unlikely to benefit from the anti-inflammatory properties of corticosteroids. Therefore, answers A and B cannot be correct. In addition, some experts believe that benefit is only realized in patients with S. pneumoniae meningitis. While dexamethasone has the theoretical ability to decrease vancomycin concentrations in the CSF, clinical data support its use. However, vancomycin is not useful in the treatment of N. meningitidis. Therefore, answer D cannot be selected. Finally, the absolute stated in answer E, or the presence of a black box warning, does not exist for dexamethasone and leucocytosis. Therefore, the answer is C. Additional information is available for the reader from the IDSA practice guidelines for the management of bacterial meningitis, available at www.idsociety.org.

6. The answer is C (3.2.1)

Prophylaxis is recommended for closed contacts of patients diagnosed with N. meningitidis meningitis. This includes household members, intimate contacts, children in school environments, coworkers in close proximity, and young adults in dormitories. Healthcare workers need not receive prophylaxis unless direct exposure to respiratory secretions exists. The Advisory Committee on Immunization Practices has published guidelines for the proper prophylaxis of N. meningitidis meningitis. These include: rifampin 600 mg q 12 h x 4 doses, ciprofloxacin 500 mg x once, or ceftriaxone 250 mg IM x once. These therapies are recommended secondary to clinical efficacy.

Daptomycin does not cover Neisseria spp. and should not be given PO. Trimethoprim/sulfamethoxazole is active against N. meningitidis, but both the route and duration are excessive for prophylaxis. Vancomycin does not cover gram negative bacilli such as N. meningitidis.

7. The answer is C (1.2.4)

Rifampin is an FDA pregnancy category C, and it has been associated with hemorrhagic disease of the newborn. Studies involving pregnant women are generally supportive that rifampin is not a teratogen; however, its use should be avoided if other alternative agents are feasible. Ciprofloxacin is an FDA pregnancy class C drug, due to animal mutagenicity, and alternates should be used when available. Chloramphenicol has been associated with gray baby syndrome and is an FDA pregnancy category class C drug. It should not be used. SMX/TMP is an FDA pregnancy category class C drug and may interfere with folic acid metabolism. This combination should be avoided, particularly near term due to neonate jaundice, hemolytic anemia, and kernicterus. In addition, it is not a recommended prophylaxis agent. Therefore, ceftriaxone, a recommended agent and an FDA pregnancy category class B drug, should be used.

8. The answer is A (3.2.1)

The meningococcal conjugate vaccine is recommended by the CDC for pre-adolescents (age 11–12) and individuals at high risk such as college freshmen living in dormitories, microbiologists who are routinely exposed to meningococcal bacteria, U.S. military recruits, asplenic individuals, people traveling to countries with meningococcus outbreaks, and those who might have been exposed to meningitis during an outbreak. Therefore, the only age group that is routinely recommended to receive the vaccine is the pre-adolescents through young adults category. Elderly adults should only receive the vaccine if other high-risk situations exist.

9. The answer is E (1.2.7)

Vancomycin is a large glycopeptide molecule (~1500 daltons) that is very irritating to veins and is frequently associated with phlebitis; hence, optimal administration necessitates adequate dilution and slow IV infusion. IM administration may culminate in tissue necrosis, the drug is not systemically absorbed by the oral route, and rapid administration is associated with an infusion reaction commonly referred to as Red Man syndrome. Expert opinion suggests that serum trough levels for vancomycin should be maintained between 15–20 mg/L. Intrathecal use of vancomycin is possible and intraventricular vancomycin can be given in doses of 5–20 mg; however, this use is reserved for patients with an intraventricular shunt or patients unresponsive to therapy.

Answers

10. The answer is E (1.1.3)

Staphylococcus aureus is a gram positive cocci. Neisseria meningitidis is a gram negative cocci. Haemophilus influenzae is a gram negative coccobacilli. Streptococcus pneumonia is a gram positive coccus. Listeria monocytogenes is a gram positive bacillus.

Case 54 Drugs Used to Counter Biological Warfare

1. The answer is D (1.2.1)

Penicillin and doxycycline are approved by the FDA for the treatment of anthrax infection. Penicillin, doxycycline, and ciprofloxacin are FDA approved for postexposure prophylaxis. Other drugs that are usually active in vitro include clindamycin, rifampin, imipenem, aminoglycosides, chloramphenicol, vancomycin, cefazolin, tetracycline, linezolid, and the macrolides. It has been reported that a B anthracis strain was engineered to resist the tetracycline and penicillin classes of antibiotics. With that in mind, antibiotic resistance to penicillin- and tetracycline-class antibiotics should be assumed following a terrorist attack until otherwise demonstrated. Sulfamethoxazole, trimethoprim, cefuroxime, cefotaxime, aztreonam, and ceftazidime should not be used in the treatment or prophylaxis of anthrax infection due to some natural resistance of B anthracis strains that has been seen. The Working Group on Civilian Biodefense has made recommendations based on available evidence, and those recommendations will need to be updated as new information is available.

2. The answer is C (1.2.1)

Penicillin and doxycycline are FDA approved for treatment of anthrax infection, while penicillin, doxycycline, and ciprofloxacin are FDA approved for postexposure prophylaxis.

3. The answer is A (1.1.4)

Early antibiotic administration is essential due to the rapid progression of symptomatic anthrax infection. Because it is difficult to achieve rapid microbiologic diagnosis of anthrax, anyone in a high-risk group who develops fever or evidence of systemic disease should start receiving multiple drug therapy for possible anthrax infection as soon as possible while awaiting the results of laboratory studies. Postal workers, mail room workers, media personnel, politicians and their associates, and microbiology lab personnel are considered high-risk groups. See also the explanation to Question 1.

4. The answer is E (1.3.1)

The 60-day antibiotic course was recommended by the Working Group on Civilian Biodefense because of (1) data showing the potential for prolonged survival of anthrax spores in animals despite antibiotic treatment and (2) data from the acci-

dental release of anthrax from a Soviet bioweapons plant in Sverdlovsk in 1979, showing the potential for delayed development of disease in humans. Illness can develop in 2 days or as late as 6–8 weeks after exposure. In Sverdlovsk, one case developed 46 days after exposure. The risk of recurring disease may persist for a prolonged period because of the possibility of delayed germination of spores. Therefore, it is recommended that antibiotic therapy be continued for at least 60 days postexposure, with oral therapy replacing intravenous therapy when appropriate. It is very important to counsel patients being treated for infection or postexposure prophylaxis about the need to take the antibiotic for the full 60 days.

5. The answer is E (1.1.3)

All of the statements are true.

6. The answer is E (1.1.1)

Early inhalation anthrax symptoms can be similar to those of much more common infections such as influenza. However, a runny nose is a rare feature of anthrax. This means that a person who has a runny nose along with other common influenza-like symptoms is much more likely to have the common cold than to have anthrax.

7. The answer is C (2.1.3)

Ciprofloxacin should be administered over a period of 60 minutes, either by direct IV infusion or through a Y-type IV infusion set, which may already be in place, in order to minimize patient discomfort and reduce the risk of venous irritation. The infusion time should be included on the label information for nursing.

8. The answer is C (1.1.4)

Given the limited experience with inhalation anthrax and the lack of comparative data, it remains unclear whether the use of two or more antibiotics results in a survival advantage; however, combination therapy is a sound therapeutic approach in the face of life-threatening illness.

9. The answer is C (3.2.1)

Out of the 10 patients from the 2001 attack, information on exposure to symptoms was available for only 6. In these 6 patients, the median period from presumed time of exposure to the onset of symptoms was 4 days (range, 4–6 days).

Usually <1 week; may be prolonged for weeks (up to 2 months)

10. The answer is E (3.1.1)

All of the statements are true.

Case 55 Endocarditis

1. The answer is E (1.1.2)

Low-grade fever (80%–90%), heart murmur (85%), dyspnea (40%), and anorexia (25%) are all clinical manifestations commonly associated with patients with infective endocarditis.

2. The answer is D (1.1.1)

Streptococci occurs in 55%–66% of the cases, Staphylococci occurs in 20%–35% of the cases, and Enterococci occurs in 5%–18% of the cases of infective endocarditis.

3. The answer is B (1.1.3)

The two most common pathogens are Streptococci and Staphylococci. Nafcillin will cover both Strep and methicillin (oxacillin) sensitive strains of Staph.

4. The answer is C (1.1.4)

Mitral valve prolapse with regurgitation, IVDA, prosthetic valve, and a previous bacterial endocarditis are all major risk factors for endocarditis. Family history of myocardial infarction is not a risk factor.

5. The answer is C (2.1.1)

20 million units reconstituted with 33 mL of sterile water plus 7 mL displaced by the powder, produces 20 million units per 40 mL, or 500,000 units per mL. 24 million units divided by four equal doses equals 6 million per dose. 6 million units divided by 0.5 million units per mL equals 12 mL per dose.

6. The answer is C (2.3.1)

Typically a horizontal laminar flow hood would provide the appropriate sterile environment to prepare this solution, a vertical laminar flow hood could be used.

7. The answer is E (2.2.5)

Intravenous piggy-back solutions are administered through compatible primary IV solution tubing y-site, non-compatible primary IV solution y-site with primary solution stopped and tube is flushed before and after with saline solution, or through a heparin lock.

8. The answer is A (3.2.1)

Aqueous penicillin G by the intravenous route in high doses (above 10 million units) should be administered slowly because of the adverse effects of electrolyte imbalance from either the potassium or sodium content of the penicillin. Penicillin G potassium contains 1.7 mEq potassium and 0.3 mEq sodium per million units. The patient's renal, cardiac, and vascular status should be evaluated and if impairment of function is suspected or known to exist a reduction in the total dosage should be considered. Frequent evaluation of electrolyte balance, renal and hematopoietic function is recommended during therapy when high doses of intravenous aqueous penicillin G are used.

9. The answer is E (3.2.1)

If an allergic reaction occurs, the drug should be discontinued and the appropriate therapy instituted. Serious anaphylactoid reactions require immediate emergency treatment with epinephrine, oxygen, intravenous steroids, and airway management, including intubation, should also be administered as indicated.

10. The answer is B (3.2.1)

Consider skin testing for a patient with a positive culture for oxacillin-susceptible Staphylococci and questionable history of immediate-type hypersensitivity to penicillin. Cephalosporins should be avoided in patients with anaphylactoid-hypersensitivity to beta-lactams; vancomycin should be used in these cases.

Case 56 Fungal Infections (Invasive)

1. The answer is B (1.1.4)

Risk factors for candidemia include total parenteral nutrition (TPN), central venous catheters, broad-spectrum antibiotic use, immunosuppression, neutropenia, abdominal surgery, mechanical ventilation, and being in the ICU (especially prolonged stays). Hospitalization alone is not a risk; however, as previously mentioned, being in the intensive care unit is a risk. Hypertension is not a risk factor for candidemia. Disseminated candidiasis is being considered in MB because she has had multiple abdominal surgeries, has been on broad-spectrum antibiotics, TPN, has a central venous catheter, and has been in the ICU for 15 days. Also, despite broad-spectrum antimicrobial therapy (vancomycin, meropenem, tobramycin), MB is critically ill. She also has yeast in her urine and sputum. Her blood cultures are negative x 2 days; however, the yield of a positive Candida blood culture is low (<50%). Often, disseminated candidiasis is a diagnosis of exclusion.

2. The answer is D (1.2.1)

In clinical trials in nonneutropenic hosts, fluconazole has shown to be equally effective as amphotericin B for disseminated candidiasis. However, if patients are critically ill/unstable, many clinicians would choose amphotericin over fluconazole. In addition, MB has continued to worsen despite receiving fluconazole for several days. Voriconazole is an option for candidiasis and has a broader spectrum of activity than fluconazole. However, because MB failed fluconazole therapy it may be prudent to avoid the empiric use of voriconazole as the potential for cross-resistance exists. Data demonstrate that voriconazole may not be appropriate therapy in refractory candidiasis in patients previously treated with fluconazole. Ketoconazole is not available IV. Nystatin is not available IV; it is only topical.

3. The answer is B (2.2.3)

Amphotericin is stable in dextrose solutions. Amphotericin B will form a precipitate when mixed with lactated ringers and saline solutions.

Answers

4. The answer is C (1.3.3)

Amphotericin B may cause a reversible, normochromic, normocytic anemia due to decreased erythropoiesis. Nephrotoxicity is the major toxicity associated with amphotericin B occurring in at least 80% of patients. The nephrotoxicity can be glomerular or tubular. Glomerular toxicity manifests as a reduction in glomerular filtration rate and renal blood flow. Tubular toxicity manifests as renal tubular acidosis, hypokalemia, and hypomagnesemia. Infusion-related toxicities may occur in up to 70%–90% of patients and may be characterized by rigors, chills, fever, headache, nausea, and vomiting. Thrombophlebitis may occur; central venous administration minimizes this adverse event.

5. The answer is C (3.2.1)

Nephrotoxicity may be potentiated by sodium depletion and the concurrent administration of other nephrotoxic agents. Diuretics, poor oral intake, and vomiting can induce sodium depletion. Several studies and case reports support the concept of sodium loading. Theoretically, sodium loading may prevent and treat the nephrotoxicity, particularly the reduction in glomerular filtration rate, associated with amphotericin B. It is recommended that 1 L of 0.9% NaCl be given daily to patients receiving amphotericin B. Avoid concomitant use of diuretics, which may cause sodium depletion as well as nephrotoxicity, and other nephrotoxic agents while the patient is receiving amphotericin B.

ACEIs do not provide protection against amphotericin B induced nephrotoxicity.

6. The answer is D (3.2.1)

Infusion-related toxicities include fever, chills, rigors, headache, nausea, and vomiting. Premedication with acetaminophen, ibuprofen, or aspirin may minimize some of these toxicities; however, most patients develop tolerance to these effects. Meperidine reduces rigors associated with amphotericin B administration. Infusion-related toxicities occur during both slow and fast infusions. Faster infusions may be associated with an earlier onset of infusion-related toxicities. Lipid-formulated amphotericin B products may be associated with fewer infusion-related reactions.

7. The answer is C (1.2.0)

Lipid preparations of amphotericin B are associated with reduced rates of nephrotoxicity. These agents are approved for patients who are unresponsive to therapy with amphotericin B deoxycholate or for those patients who are intolerant (secondary to renal toxicity) of amphotericin B deoxycholate. Larger doses of the lipid amphotericin B preparations can be administered. The lipid preparations of amphotericin B and amphotericin B deoxycholate appear to be equally efficacious. The lipid preparations appear to have higher concentrations in some tissues (particularly, liver and spleen) than amphotericin B deoxycholate.

8. The answer is E (1.3.2)

MB should have all of the above laboratory parameters monitored. Amphotericin B induced nephrotoxicity will cause an increase in serum creatinine and blood urea nitrogen. The tubular toxicity associated with amphotericin B manifests as hypokalemia and hypomagnesemia. Wasting of both electrolytes occurs and needs to be monitored closely. Supplementing both potassium and magnesium may be necessary.

9. The answer is B (1.3.3)

Gynecomastia may be seen with Ketoconazole. Hepatotoxicity has been associated with voriconazole as with other azole antifungals. Skin rash occur in <10% of patients, are primarily mild to moderate in nature but, in rare cases, may become severe (e.g. Stevens-Johnson syndrome). Visual disturbances are reported in 20%–45% of patients receiving voriconazole. The disturbances are transient; generally occur 30 minutes after receiving a dose and last ~15–30 minutes. The visual disturbances include photophobia, blurred vision, altered visual acuity, and changes in color vision. Common GI AEs include N/V, and diarrhea.

10. The answer is A (1.2.1)

Fluconazole is not active against Aspergillus sp. of the azole antifungals, only itraconazole and voriconazole are active against Aspergillus sp.

Case 57 Human Immunodeficiency Virus (HIV) and Acquired Immunodeficiency Syndrome (AIDS)

1. The answer is B (1.1.2)

The Centers for Disease Control and Prevention have defined in what clinical circumstances an HIV-infected patient is considered to have AIDS. The criteria are as follows: (1) CD4 count <200/mm³ plus laboratory evidence of HIV-infection or (2) presence of an AIDS-indicator disease (these consist of a number of different opportunistic infections and malignancies) or (3) presence of pulmonary TB, recurrent pneumonia, or invasive cervical cancer in a patient with HIV infection. JJ meets the criteria for AIDS by having a CD4 count <200/mm³ with both serologic and virologic evidence of HIV infection. Flu-like illness, while associated with the acute retroviral syndrome, is not specific to this syndrome and does not contribute to an AIDS diagnosis. A decreased white count with primarily neutrophils is often seen in patients with advanced HIV infection but, again, is not specific to patients with AIDS.

2. The answer is B (1.2.1)

According to the most recent Department of Health and Human Services Guidelines for the Use of Antiretrovirals in Adults and Adolescents, all patients with a diagnosis of AIDS should be treated with antiretrovirals regardless of plasma viral levels. Fatigue and weight loss, while often associated with advanced HIV infection and which often respond to effective antiretroviral therapy, are not of themselves indications for the initiation of antiretroviral therapy.

3. The answer is A (1.2.3)

Delavirdine, amprenavir, and ritonavir are cytochrome P450 3A4 inhibitors and are associated with a number of significant interactions with substrates of this isoenzyme. Nevirapine is a cytochrome P450 3A4 inducer and can cause a significant decrease in activity of other substrates of this isoenzyme. Lamivudine is primarily eliminated unchanged by renal excretion and has not been associated with significant drug interactions.

4. The answer is C (3.2.1)

Adherence to HIV therapy is one of the primary determinants of a successful outcome. In an important adherence trial done in this patient population it was determined that 95% adherence was necessary to achieve the highest likelihood of a successful virologic outcome. Obviously 100% adherence is optimal; however, this is an unrealistic goal and is likely to discourage patients and result in patients giving up on their therapy because they find 100% adherence impossible to achieve. Adherence at the 80% level has been shown to be adequate for other chronic diseases such as hypertension; however, in HIV infection this level of adherence has resulted in suboptimal outcomes. Intracellular pharmacokinetics and pharmacodynamics are the primary determinants of the effect of nucleoside reverse transcriptase inhibitors. There are no data to suggest that administering these agents on a strict time interval has an effect on virologic outcomes.

5. The answer is E (1.2.3)

There are in vitro data to suggest that zidovudine and stavudine are antagonistic. There are no clinical data to indicate a benefit with this combination, and the Department of Health and Human Services (DHHS) Guidelines list this combination on the Not Recommended, Should Not Be Offered list. Obviously, adherence is important, but with a suboptimal regimen, viral resistance may result. Efavirenz containing regimens have been shown to be as efficacious as PI containing regimens, and efavirenz is listed along with protease inhibitors as strongly recommended on the DHHS guidelines. Counseling the patient regarding adverse effects is also very important; however, a change in regimen would be more appropriate in this case. While efavirenz has been associated with central nervous system side effects, there are no data to suggest that St. John's wort offers any benefit, and the potential for St. John's wort to induce cytochrome P450 3A4 precludes its use with antiretrovirals such as efavirenz that are metabolized by this pathway.

6. The answer is C (3.2.2)

Indinavir has been associated with nephrolithiasis due to the crystallization of the drug in the renal tubules. Adequate fluid intake is vital to decrease the incidence of this adverse effect. Dosing indinavir on an empty stomach is not necessary when indinavir is given in conjunction with ritonavir. Ritonavir's inhibition of cytochrome P450 and p-glycoprotein ensure adequate indinavir concentrations for the entire 12-hour dosing interval when administered in either the fed or fasted state. Both St. John's wort and garlic capsules have been associated with significant decreases in protease inhibitor serum concentrations when administered concurrently with a protease inhibitor containing regimen.

7. The answer is D (1.2.4)

Indinavir and ritonavir are both significant inhibitors of cytochrome P450 3A4. All HMG-coA reductase inhibitors except pravastatin have demonstrated significant increases in serum concentrations when administered concurrently with an enzyme inhibitor. Increased concentrations of HMG-coA reductase inhibitors have been associated with rhabdomyolysis.

8. The answer is B (1.1.3)

According to the U.S. Public Health Service/Infectious Disease Society of American Guidelines for the Prevention of Opportunistic Infections in Persons Infected with the Human Immunodeficiency Virus, prophylaxis for Pneumocystis carinii should be initiated in patients with CD4 counts less than 200 cells/mL. Prophylaxis for cytomegalovirus and Mycobacterium avium complex should be initiated when the CD4 count drops below 50 cells/mL.

9. The answer is D (1.3.1)

A decline in viral load to undetectable levels and a significant increase in CD4 counts are the goals of antiretroviral therapy. These are realistic expectations for patients who are adherent to their regimen and have not been extensively treated with other antiretroviral regimens that have failed. It has been demonstrated that most likely due to sanctuary sites to which antiretrovirals fail to penetrate, that viral eradication is unlikely to occur. Maintaining current CD4 count would not be considered an optimal response. Effective antiretroviral therapy would be expected to significantly prolong life, and one would expect a near-normal lifespan for a patient who successfully maintains a response to antiretroviral therapy.

10. The answer is E (1.3.3)

Protease inhibitors have been associated with glucose intolerance, often requiring the addition of medication to assist in glucose control. None of the other agents in JJ's regimen are likely to be associated with glucose intolerance.

Answers

Case 58 Drug Resistance

1. The answer is B (1.2.3)

Ciprofloxacin is generally not a drug of first choice in pediatric patients due to the potential risk of cartilage malformation seen in animal studies. However, there are certain situations when ciprofloxacin would be considered for a pediatric patient with close monitoring, such as when a multidrug resistant pathogen is suspected.

The pharmacokinetic profile of phenytoin (200 mg daily) was essentially unchanged in seven normal subjects following coadministration with ciprofloxacin (500 mg oral twice daily) for 5 days. A separate case report describes a patient who experienced a seizure while on both ciprofloxacin and phenytoin, although no changes in phenytoin serum concentrations were noted. In contrast, one patient in the former study exhibited a significant reduction in the AUC of phenytoin. A number of case reports describe reductions (up to 80%) in serum phenytoin concentrations following the initiation of ciprofloxacin therapy, at times resulting in the occurrence of seizures. Another report describes a ciprofloxacin-receiving patient in whom prescribers struggled to achieve adequate serum phenytoin concentrations on initiation of therapy (loading dose and initiation of maintenance doses). A single case report describes the occurrence of increased phenytoin concentrations during ciprofloxacin therapy.

A mechanism for the increased concentrations of phenytoin in the presence of ciprofloxacin is unclear. It is unlikely related to drug-induced changes in phenytoin metabolism. Animal data indicates that a change in renal phenytoin excretion might occur. It is also important to note the potential of ciprofloxacin alone to cause seizures.

2. The answer is C (1.2.4)

Dosing adjustment in renal impairment: Oral, I.V.: Cl_{cr} 15–30 mL/minute. Administer 50% of recommended dose Cl_{cr} <15 mL/minute. Use is not recommended.

3. The answer is A (1.2.2)

Bacteria such as E. coli and Klebsiella spp most commonly modify DNA gyrase altering the target for quinolone antibiotics.

S. aureus, B. fragilis, and H. influenzae among others, are known to produce a beta lactamase that will hydrolyze the structure of certain penicillins and cephalosporins. This is analogous to drug hydrolysis.

S. pneumoniae will alter the binding the site for penicillin as a means of resistance.

The answer "supernatant production" is incorrect; it is fictitious.

4. The answer is C (1.2.7)

Optimizing drug dosing for age and weight could only have a positive impact on therapy.

5. The answer is C (2.1.1)

Urinary tract infection: Treatment: Oral: 6–12 mg TMP/kg/day in divided doses every 12 hours. 3 mg/kg/dose x 20 kg = 60 mg trimethoprim q12h. Key points to remember is that dosing based on the trimethoprim component, the drug ratio is 5 parts sulfamethoxazole to 1 part trimethoprim, weight based dosing is usually given in mg/kg/day, which must then be divided into the appropriate interval.

6. The answer is D (1.1.4)

Streptococcus pneumoniae is not known to produce a beta lactamase as a means of drug resistance, Streptococcus pneumoniae more commonly alters the binding site of penicillins as a means of resistance.

Common ESBL producing organisms are E. coli, K. pneumoniae, some Enterobacteriaceae, and some Pseudomonas.

7. The answer is A (1.2.2)

Generally, some sort of chromosomal mutation is responsible for bacterial resistance to antibiotics. The genotypic makeup (chromosomal content) of the bacteria will encode for the phenotypic expression (resistance) of the bacteria.

Chromosomal mutation can occur in a number of different ways. A plasmid, or small portion of genetic material, can be transferred from one bacteria to another via a bacteriophage. This plasmid can code for antibiotic resistance in bacteria "A" and transfer it to bacteria "B." Bacteria can incorporate free genetic material in the environment in to their own DNA, creating an antibiotic-resistant bacteria. Finally, DNA itself coding for antibiotic resistance can be directly transferred from one bacteria to another.

Answers II and III are fictitious.

8. The answer is C (3.2.1)

Options I and II will allow more judicious use of antibiotics and allow a better assessment of the patient. Option III is not an approved therapy.

9. The answer is C (3.2.1)

Broad spectrum antibiotics do not necessarily have a higher incidence of renal disease.

10. The answer is E (1.3.5)

I. E. coli are lactose fermenters, this also has no bearing on the questions. II. Quinolones and carbapenems will provide reasonable empirical coverage for a suspected ESBL. III. Glycopeptides will not treat any E. coli. IV. This is not a true statement; ESBL are by definition multi-drug resistant. V. Cefpodoxime or ceftazidime are indicator antibiotics that are strongly correlated to ESBL identification.

<h2>Case 59 Parasitic and Tick-Borne Diseases</h2>

<h3>1. The answer is D (1.1.4)</h3>

Outdoor activities in wooded areas place people at risk for Lyme disease. In the United States, the Centers for Disease Control and Prevention has determined that endemic areas include non-urban communities throughout much of the Northeast (Massachusetts to Maryland), parts of the upper Midwest (Minnesota and Wisconsin) and areas along the West Coast (northern California and Oregon). Lyme disease prevalence has not been shown to differ between gender and age groups.

<h3>2. The answer is E (1.1.3)</h3>

Signs and symptoms found on physical exam include erythema migrans as well as nonspecific symptoms such as low-grade fever, fatigue, malaise, lethargy, stiff neck, myalgia, and arthralgia.

<h3>3. The answer is C (1.1.1)</h3>

Elevated sedimentation rate (ESR) is a nonspecific indicator of inflammation that occurs in 50% of patients with erythema migrans. Platelets are normal in patients with Lyme disease. White blood cell count is normal or mildly elevated in Lyme disease.

<h3>4. The answer is E (1.2.0)</h3>

This patient's Lyme disease is classified as early, uncomplicated Erythema migrans, which is treated using doxycycline 100 mg BID, amoxicillin 500 mg TID or cefuroxime 500 mg PO BID.

<h3>5. The answer is B (1.2.6)</h3>

IDSA guidelines from the CDC recommend a duration of treatment for patients with early, uncomplicated Lyme disease with erythema migrans of 14–21 days.

<h3>6. The answer is B (3.2.1)</h3>

The use of repellents such as DEET (N, N-diethyl-m-toluamide) and picaridin have been shown to prevent Lyme disease. No vaccine is currently available to prevent Lyme disease in humans. Early antibiotic prophylaxis has been used to prevent erythema migrans at the site of a tick bite but not prophylactically prior to exposure.

<h3>7. The answer is D (1.1.2)</h3>

Borrelia burgdorferi belongs to the phylum Spirochaetes. The phylum Spirochaetes contains a single class (Spirochaetes), a single order (Spirochaetales), and three families: Brachyspiraceae, Leptospiraceae, and Spirochaetaceae. The Spirochaetaceae family contains ten genera, including the genus Treponema and the genus Borrelia.

<h3>8. The answer is E (3.2.2)</h3>

Doxycycline can interact with birth control pills, rendering them less effective. Therefore, patients need to use alternative birth control methods. Patients should avoid using antacids concurrently with doxycycline. Doxycycline can increase the sensitivity of the skin to sunlight, requiring the use of a sunscreen.

<h3>9. The answer is C (2.2.5)</h3>

To avoid stomach upset patients should take oral doxycycline with food or a full glass of water. Patients should avoid concurrent alcohol consumption while taking doxycycline and maintain adequate hydration by drinking at least two to three liters of fluid a day. Doxycycline should be stored at a controlled room temperature and protected from light.

<h3>10. The answer is E (2.2.2)</h3>

Doxycycline is available as a tablet, capsule, oral powder for suspension, and syrup.

<h2>Case 60 Sepsis and Septic Shock</h2>

<h3>1. The answer is C (1.3.1)</h3>

In 2003, Critical Care and Infectious Disease experts representing 11 international organizations convened to develop guidelines for severe sepsis and septic shock. They recommended that during the initial (first 6 hours) resuscitation of patients with severe sepsis that therapy should be directed toward specific goals. This was based on a randomized, controlled study, which demonstrated that early goal-directed therapy could reduce the 28-day mortality rate. The goal parameters that were included in the study were the following; central venous pressure of 8–12 mm Hg, mean arterial pressure of equal to or greater than 65 mmHg, urine output of equal to or greater than 0.5 mL/kg/h, and a central venous (superior vena caval) or mixed venous oxygen saturation of equal to or greater than 70%. A temperature of < 39° C was not one of the early goals.

<h3>2. The answer is E (1.2.1)</h3>

High-dose steroids have not been shown to be beneficial in sepsis; indeed, recent meta-analyses have suggested that they may be harmful. JS is currently hypotensive; therefore there is an immediate need to try and elevate her blood pressure. Vasopressors are an option; however, prior to implementing vasopressors, it reasonable to try and maximize the CVP. Current guidelines recommend volume replacement as the initial step in trying to reverse the hypotension. Therefore, administration of IV fluids should continue in order to push the CVP into the range of 8–12 prior to implementing vasopressor therapy. If fluid replacement is unsuccessful in increasing the blood pressure, then vasopressors are the next option.

<h3>3. The answer is A (2.2.5)</h3>

While the initial focus for resuscitation of patients with severe sepsis, should be focused on normalization of hemodynamic

Answers

parameters, quick initiation of appropriate antimicrobial therapy is still an important component for optimal outcomes. The 2003 guidelines suggest that appropriate antimicrobial therapy should be initiated within the first hour of recognition of severe sepsis.

4. The answer is D (1.3.5)

While little published data exists comparing the use of crystalloids to colloids in the treatment of severe sepsis, studies in postsurgical and critical care patients have demonstrated similar outcomes with the use of each. As a result, the 2003 consensus guidelines recommend either strategy as acceptable for fluid resuscitation in patients with severe sepsis. However, one must keep in mind that a greater administration volume is required with the use of crystalloids and, therefore, may result in more edema.

5. The answer is C (1.2.1)

JS's current hemodynamic parameters show an adequate cardiac index (CI) and central venous pressure, but a low mean arterial pressure. Therefore, vasopressor therapy should be directed primarily at improving the blood pressure rather than enhancing inotropic support. The 2003 consensus guidelines list both dopamine and norepinephrine as acceptable options for initiation of vasopressure support in patients with a normal or high cardiac index and a low mean arterial pressure. If JS had a low cardiac output, then inotropic support with the use of dobutamine may have been indicated.

6. The answer is C (2.1.3)

The infusion rate for dopamine for JS should be based on her dry weight or her weight on admission and not on her weight after receiving massive amounts of fluid in surgery. To calculate the infusion rate: Wt. = 185 lb = 84.1 Kg.

Dose = 5 µ/kg/min x 84.1 kg = 420.5 µ/min.

Dopamine 400 mg/500 mL = 0.8 mg/mL or 800 µ/mL.

420.5 µ/min / 800 µ/mL = 0.526 mL/min.

0.526 mL/min x 60 min/h = 32 mL/h

7. The answer is E (1.3.2)

The response to IV dopamine should be evaluated using blood pressure, hemodynamic parameters, and clinical outcome measures that demonstrate adequate tissue perfusion. A MAP of equal to or greater than 65 mmHg is generally necessary to prevent symptomatic hypotension and maintain organ perfusion. Ideally, a goal for hemodynamic parameters of CI, CVP, and SVR is to titrate the dopamine to obtain normal or near-normal values. PCWP should be maximized, while preventing the development of pulmonary edema, which generally occurs at values > 18 mmHg.

8. The answer is A (3.2.1)

In order to answer specific questions about a published clinical trial, it is often necessary to pull the primary source of the information. While you may find reviews or abstracts regarding clinical trials in secondary reference sources, it may take months for these references to be included.

9. The answer is B (1.2.6)

Because of the location, JS's infection is most likely polymicrobial, including the possibility of gram positive organisms, gram negative Enterobacteriaceae, and anaerobes. As a result, target gentamicin peak levels should generally be 6–8 µg/mL with trough levels <2 µg/mL. In order to obtain peaks and troughs within these ranges with conventional dosing, it will be necessary to both increase the dose and extend the dosing interval.

10. The answer is D (3.2.1)

Both Trissel's *Handbook on Injectable Drugs* and Micromedex can be useful references for IV admixture incompatibility.

Case 61 Sexually Transmitted Diseases

1. The answer is C (1.1.2)

Neisseria gonorrhea is the only gram-negative diplococci listed. Chlamydia trachomatis and T. pallidum do not stain on Gram stain, while B. fragilis is a gram-negative anaerobe. Candida albicans is a yeast.

2. The answer is C (1.2.1)

According to the 2002 CDC STD treatment guidelines, individuals infected with gonococci are often coinfected with C. trachomatis. Hence, optimal antimicrobial therapy requires coverage for both organisms.

3. The answer is B (2.1.1)

The patient and her partner should be treated for both N. gonorrhea and C. trachomatis.

A single 400-mg dose of cefixime or single 500-mg dose of ciprofloxacin effectively treats N. gonorrhea, but not C. trachomatis. A single 1-g dose of azithromycin or 7-day course of doxycycline 100 mg po bid effectively eradicates C. trachomatis, but not N. gonorrhea.

Accordingly, ciprofloxacin 500 mg #2 tablets plus azithromycin 250 mg #8 tablets would be required to adequately treat RC and her partner.

The cefixime and doxycycline regimen contains enough cefixime to treat both individuals for N. gonorrhea, but only enough doxycycline to adequately treat one individual for C. trachomatis.

Cefixime monotherapy covers only N. gonorrhea, but not C. trachomatis.

Additionally, cefixime 400-mg tablets are currently unavailable.

4. The answer is E (3.2.2)

Photosensitivity reactions are commonly observed in patients on tetracycline antibiotics. While these reactions may occur with other antibiotics as well, particularly some quinolones, the incidence of this reaction is most prevalent with tetracyclines.

5. The answer is B (1.3.0)

To minimize transmission, a patient with gonorrhea and chlamydia should abstain from sex for 7 days following single-dose treatment or until a 7-day treatment regimen is completed and is asymptomatic.

6. The answer is A (2.3.1)

IM injections of cephalosporins can be quite irritating, so dilution in a 1% lidocaine solution is often recommended to minimize discomfort. The volume for a single IM injection generally should not exceed 2.5 mL. When IM injections of drugs of greater than 2.5 mL are necessary, multiple IM injections are required to deliver the total concentration of agent.

7. The answer is D (1.2.4)

The rate of fluoroquinolone-resistant N. gonorrhea is high in Asia, the Pacific Islands, Hawaii, and California. The use of a fluoroquinolone, like ciprofloxacin, for the treatment of gonorrhea is not recommended for residents in these areas nor for individuals with recent travel history to these locations.

8. The answer is E (3.2.0)

Ciprofloxacin is best absorbed on an empty stomach spaced from divalent cations such as calcium, iron, magnesium, and aluminum, which are also present in food, milk, antacids, and multivitamins. Divalent cations bind ciprofloxacin in the GI tract and significantly reduce its absorption.

9. The answer is C (1.2.1)

According to the CDC guidelines (2002), the following regimens are recommended for a recurrent episode of genital HSV: acyclovir 400 mg po tid, 200 mg po 5x/day or 800 mg po bid, famciclovir 125 mg po bid, or valacyclovir 500 mg po bid or 1 g po q day for a duration of 5 days. Valganciclovir is not recommended for the treatment of genital HSV. IV acyclovir is recommended in severe disease. A duration of 7–10 days is recommended for the treatment of the first episode of genital HSV. Famciclovir 250 mg po tid and valacyclovir 1 g po bid are regimens recommended for treatment of a first episode.

10. The answer is E (2.2.1)

Valtrex is the brand name of valacyclovir. Famvir is the brand name of famciclovir. Zovirax is the brand name of acyclovir. Valcyte is the brand name of valganciclovir. Cytovene is the brand name of ganciclovir.

Case 62 Skin and Soft Tissue Infections

1. The answer is A (1.2.1)

Prior to the late 1990s virtually all infections associated with MRSA were health care related. Recently, widespread cases of CA-MRSA have been reported. Infections caused by CA-MRSA usually involve superficial skin infections like boils or furuncles, but more complicated infections can occur. Risk factors for infections caused by CA-MRSA are different than health care related MRSA. Common CA-MRSA risk factors include: age (common in pediatrics), steam baths, close skin contact such as participation in contact sports, crowded living conditions such as prisons or military barracks, or poor hygiene. Unlike health care acquired MRSA, community acquired MRSA generally remains susceptible to most non-beta lactam based antibiotics. Many of these antibiotics have been used successfully to treat skin infections caused by CA-MRSA. Vancomycin is not absorbed from the gastrointestinal tract, and must be administered intravenously. Oral vancomycin should only be used to treat infections in the gastrointestinal tract such as Clostridium difficile associated diarrhea. While clindamycin can be used to treat CA-MRSA infections, an inducible mechanism of resistance has been reported. Occasionally, therapeutic failures are encountered. Microbiology labs test for inducible clindamycin resistance and reports such isolates as resistant. However, if clindamycin is to be used empirically to treat presumed CA-MRSA infections, confirmation of clindamycin sensitivity and appropriate follow-up may be warranted.

2. The answer is C (1.2.3)

Linezolid has demonstrated mild, reversible inhibitor of monoamine oxidase-A (MAO-AI) activity. MAO-A deaminates noradrenaline, adrenaline, and 5-hydroxtryptamine (serotonin), which may mediate untoward reactions through increased adrenergic tone. Because of the MAO-I properties of linezolid, the potential exists for drug interactions with serotonergic or noradrenergic properties, as well as tyramine, which is capable of releasing stored catecholamines. Patients should be advised to avoid foods rich in tyramine such as aged, smoked, pickled, or fermented foods or beverages while on linezolid. However, the average amount of tyramine in most servings of red wine, smoked meats, etc., are in the range of 1–15 mg per serving. Transient increases in systolic and diastolic blood pressure have occurred when linezolid is administered concurrently with pseudoephedrine, phenylpropanolamine, dopamine, or other pressor agents. When given concurrently with the selective serotonin reuptake inhibitors, there have been case reports of serotonin syndrome, and prescribers should be aware of this possible interaction.

3. The answer is C (1.1.0)

While a variety of organisms occasionally cause cellulitis, Streptococcus pyogenes and occasionally Staphylococcus aureus are the first organisms that should be considered in non-diabetic (i.e., uncomplicated) cellulitis infections. Other organisms that

Answers

should be on the differential include Group C and G Streptococcus and Haemophilus influenzae in children. Group B strep infections can be seen in newborns. E. coli is rarely associated with uncomplicated cellulitis in immunocompetent patients.

4. The answer is B (1.1.3)

Cellulitis associated with carbuncles, furuncles, and abscesses is generally caused by Staphylococcus aureus, whereas cellulitis that is diffuse in presentation or does not appear to have an established portal of entry is generally caused by Streptococcus species. E. coli is rarely associated with uncomplicated cellulitis.

5. The answer is A (1.1.1)

Puncture wounds through a tennis shoe can result in Pseudomonas spp. Infection from this pathogen can also occur after hot-tub use or after swimming in underchlorinated swimming pools. Pseudomonas is highly resistant and should be treated with an antipseudomonal fluoroquinolone (ciprofloxacin or levofloxacin), IV piperacillin, or piperacillin/tazobactam, IV ceftazidime, or IV cefepime. The newer fluoroquinolones (moxifloxacin and gatifloxacin) do not provide reliable Pseudomonas aeruginosa coverage. Vancomycin has activity only against gram-positive organisms and would not be effective treatment for Shigella or Salmonella, which are Gram-negative bacteria. Wounds of this kind can also cause deep tissue abscess, fever, and leukocytosis. Treatment should continue for at least 2 weeks.

6. The answer is D (1.2.6)

The goal trough vancomycin level for skin and soft tissue infections is 5–15 mg/dL. The dose should not be decreased; his current trough level is below goal. A 50% increase in dose to 1500 mg every 12 hours will result in a 50% increase in trough, which will not be sufficient to achieve adequate troughs. Decreasing the interval to every 8 hours will result in increased trough concentrations and is the best choice.

7. The answer is D (3.2.1)

Cellulitis involves infection of the dermis, whereas impetigo involves infection of the epidermis. The former generally involves treatment with systemic antibiotics, whereas the latter generally can be treated with topical antimicrobials such as mupirocin. Impetigo can also successfully be treated with oral antibiotics as well. The treatment for furuncles (boils) usually involves moist heat and or surgical drainage. As furuncles are caused by Staphylococcus aureus, patients with recurrent disease may benefit from nasal decolonization of Staphylococcus aureus with mupirocin placed in each nare for 5 days.

8. The answer is D (1.3.3)

Red-man syndrome is an infusion-related toxicity related to vancomycin. When infused too quickly (> 15 mg/min), it can cause flushing, hypotension, urticaria, and pruritus. Nephrotoxicity may be a dose-related side effect of vancomycin, but data supporting specific "toxic levels" are scant. Most studies

that have attempted to link elevated serum concentrations with renal damage were retrospective, had variable renal endpoints, and in many cases vancomycin levels were measured after serum creatinine increased, making causality difficult to determine. In prospective randomized controlled trials where vancomycin is used as a comparator drug, the incidence of nephrotoxicity is similar. Nephrotoxicity rarely occurs when used as monotherapy. Administration with other nephrotoxins (i.e., aminoglycosides) greatly increases the nephrotoxic potential of vancomycin. Aplastic anemia and grey-baby syndrome are classic side effects of chloramphenicol.

9. The answer is D (1.1.1)

Dicloxacillin is semi-synthetic penicillinase resistant penicillin with good activity against methicillin sensitive Staphylococcus aureus (MSSA) like nafcillin. The MIC for cephalosporins are generally higher. Cephalexin possesses fair activity, but the MIC are relatively high for MSSA. Ampicillin is poorly absorbed. Both ampicillin and penicillin would be hydrolyzed by Staph beta-lactamases. Amoxicillin/clavulanate would also be a good empiric choice. If the doctor has reason to suspect MRSA infection, patients should be treated with linezolid, clindamycin, sulfamethoxazole/trimethoprim, or minocycline.

10. The answer is E (3.2.1)

MRSA is considered to be a resistant pathogen and most health care facilities have infection control policies that direct preventative measures to decrease patient-to-patient transmission. Staphylococcus aureus, including MRSA, generally colonizes a host's nares prior to causing infection. The primary mode of transmission of MRSA in hospital environments is via health care workers' hands. This can occur when a health care worker touches an infected patient or comes into contact with contaminated environmental surfaces. The health care worker then spreads the bacteria to other patients if preventative measures are not taken. All answers are correct. All health care workers should wash their hands prior to and after coming into contact with each patient, including DH. DH should be placed in a private room, and visitors should wear a gown and gloves when touching the patient or their close environment.

Case 63 Tuberculosis

1. The answer is E (1.1.1)

The PPD skin test (Mantoux test) is used to detect MTB infections in individuals with subclinical disease (latent infection). Infection can lead to positive PPD reactions within 6–8 weeks of exposure. Those individuals with a history of significant exposure to a known case of active TB should be screened for infection using the PPD skin test. In this case, since MB's husband, grown daughter, and grandchildren all have significant exposure, they all should be screened with the PPD skin test.

2. The answer is C (1.1.2)

A reaction of >5 mm to 5 TU Mantoux test after 48 hours is considered positive for those patients with recent close contact with infectious TB cases and also for patients who are HIV positive, persons with fibrotic changes consistent with old healed TB, patients with organ transplants, and other immunosuppressed patients. A reaction of >10 mm is positive for patients who are recent arrivals from high-prevalence countries, intravenous drug users, residents or employees of high-risk congregate settings, mycobacteriology lab personnel, persons with clinical conditions that place them at risk, children <4 years old, and adolescents exposed to adults in the high-risk category. A reaction of >15 mm is positive for patients with no TB risk factors. The area of induration measures a patient with a positive TB reaction. Erythema is not considered.

3. The answer is A (1.2.0)

Various conditions may result in a false-negative TB skin test. One of these is the use of immunosuppressive drugs, such as corticosteroids, HIV infection, or anything that might overwhelm TB. Therefore, many patients may have active TB but not a positive PPD skin test. In these patients, Candida and mumps are used to determine whether the patient is able to mount an immune response. If the patient reacts to the controls (mumps and Candida) and not to the TB, he or she is assumed to have a competent immune system and to be without TB disease. If a patient does not react to the Candida and/or mumps or PPD, he or she is considered anergic and still may have active TB disease. While the CDC does not recommend the routine use of anergy panels when skin testing for TB, in persons in whom anergy is suspected, it can be evaluated by giving at least two delayed-type hypersensitivity antigens along with the TB antigen test (mumps and Candida). Mumps and Candida do not increase the potency of the TB antigen. Mumps and Candida do not boost the immune response to the TB antigen.

4. The answer is A (1.1.3)

The short course or 6-month regimen is preferred for therapy of TB. This consists of 2 months of isoniazid, rifampin, and pyrazinamide followed by 4 months of isoniazid and rifampin. Ethambutol or streptomycin should be included in the initial regimen if drug resistance is suspected or until drug susceptibility results are known. TB should be treated with at least two agents to which the organism is susceptible to prevent the emergence of resistance. The 6-month course is the shortest duration of effective therapy.

5. The answer is D (1.3.3)

Many clinicians consider adding daily doses of pyridoxine (25–50 mg) in patients who are treated with isoniazid (INH) to offset potential neurological side effects of INH therapy. While MB's hematocrit is borderline low, there is no evidence she is iron deficient. Likewise, although MB is postmenopausal, there is no evidence she has osteoporosis requiring alendronate treatment. While the use of vitamin E and vitamin C is commonplace today, there is no specific reason MB should be started on these agents.

6. The answer is D (3.2.2)

Rifampin therapy can lead to orange-red discoloration of body fluids. Ethanol consumption can increase the risk of INH-induced hepatotoxicity, so abstinence is recommended during therapy. Pyrazinamide does not cause optic neuritis, but ethambutol does.

7. The answer is A (1.3.3)

In the presence of symptoms, elevation of LFTs to three times normal range may warrant discontinuation of drug at least temporarily. If no symptoms are present, continuation of medications until the LFTs are over five times the normal range may be reasonable.

8. The answer is A (1.1.3)

"Prophylaxis" (treatment of latent TB infection, LTBI) with INH is recommended for those individuals who have a new conversion of a PPD and no other clinical manifestations of TB. The dose of INH shown is correct. Moxifloxacin should not be used in pediatric patients. Rifampin can be used as an alternative to INH, but the dose shown is incorrect. Ethambutol has not been used as a single agent for TB prophylaxis.

9. The answer is C (1.3.3)

Pyrazinamide may cause elevation of uric acid concentrations. Acute episodes of gout may occur but are uncommon. Rifampin does not cause cartilage destruction. Isoniazid does not cause arthritis. Pain in the large toe without any other history of trauma is an unlikely presentation of osteomyelitis. Tuberculous osteomyelitis presents as a single lesion, usually in the long bones, ribs, pelvis, skull, mastoid, or mandible.

10. The answer is E (3.1.0)

The local chapter of the American Lung Association has numerous educational resources and counselors available to assist with patient/family information needs. While the local library may have some resources, they are not focused on providing this information. The Infectious Diseases Society of America focuses on the needs of ID physicians and clinicians and not on patient-specific education. The other agencies do not generally address tuberculosis.

Case 64 Upper and Lower Respiratory Tract Infections

1. The answer is B (1.1.0)

Streptococcus pneumoniae is the most common cause of community-acquired pneumonia. It is also implicated in early on-

Answers

set nosocomial pneumonias. However, late onset nosocomial pneumonias are more likely to be caused by gram-negative bacteria (Pseudomonas, Enterobacter, or Klebsiella) and Staphylococcus aureus. AS has been intubated and hospitalized for 13 days; therefore, Streptococcus pneumoniae is the least likely pathogen to be causing nosocomial pneumonia. For additional information on nosocomial pneumonia, refer to the "Guidelines for the Management of Adults with Hospital-Acquired, Ventilator-Associated, and Healthcare-Associated Pneumonia."

2. The answer is E (1.3.2)

A reduction in WBC and temperature are positive responses to therapy and an indication that the infection is resolving. An improvement in oxygenation (a reduction in supplemental oxygen) also shows that the pneumonia is resolving. Oxygenation can be monitored via oxygen saturation or the amount of supplemental oxygen a patient is receiving (e.g., via mechanical ventilation, nasal cannula, and oxygen mask).

3. The answer is D (1.2.0)

Piperacillin/tazobactam plus gentamicin is the most appropriate choice for AS. He has a nosocomial pneumonia; therefore, nosocomial gram-negative pathogens (e.g., Pseudomonas, Enterobacter, and Klebsiella) must be covered. He is currently on ampicillin/sulbactam for his perforated ulcer. Ampicillin/sulbactam does not provide adequate coverage against nosocomial gram-negative pathogens. However, AS does need anaerobic coverage for his perforated ulcer: piperacillin/tazobactam will provide this coverage as well. The addition of an aminoglycoside (gentamicin) to piperacillin/tazobactam is usually recommended for the treatment of Pseudomonas. The combination of an antipseudomonal beta-lactam plus an aminoglycoside provides synergy against Pseudomonas.

Vancomycin is not appropriate in AS because his gram stain showed gram-negative bacilli. Vancomycin covers only gram-positive organisms.

Ceftriaxone does not provide coverage against Pseudomonas or anaerobic bacteria. Levofloxacin plus metronidazole does not provide coverage against Pseudomonas. Pseudomonas must be empirically covered in AS because his sputum gram stain shows gram-negative bacilli.

4. The answer is E (3.2.1)

Prior antimicrobial agent use may lead to increasing colonization and potential infection with resistant organisms. Prior antimicrobial agent use may have exerted selective pressure that may have induced resistance as well. Prolonged hospitalization leads to increasing colonization and infection with resistant organisms. Underdosage of antimicrobial agents leads to the emergence of resistant pathogens.

5. The answer is C (1.3.0)

On the basis of culture and susceptibility data, meropenem is the most appropriate agent based on MIC data. It is the most susceptible agent listed with an MIC of 0.5 and a breakpoint of 8; the MIC is four dilutions away from the breakpoint, whereas ceftazidime is only two dilutions away from the breakpoint and, therefore, resistance may emerge. Piperacillin is not an appropriate choice as the Pseudomonas is resistant to the drug. Pseudomonas infections are generally recommended to be treated with two drugs for synergy. Synergy occurs with a beta-lactam and an aminoglycoside. Therefore, adding gentamicin to the meropenem is the most appropriate choice as meropenem also provides anaerobic coverage for his perforated ulcer. Ciprofloxacin plus gentamicin is probably only additive; however, some believe that the combination is synergistic. Ciprofloxacin with or without gentamicin or ceftazidime plus gentamicin will not provide anaerobic coverage for his perforated ulcer.

6. The answer is D (1.3.2)

AS's CrCl has decreased from 56 to 28 mL/min (based on Cockcroft Gault equation). As aminoglycosides can cause nephrotoxicity, it is reasonable to recommend that the gentamicin be discontinued. Meropenem is renally eliminated, and the manufacturer recommends a dosage adjustment at CrCl of 26–50 mL/min to 1 g q 12 h. Failure to dose adjust may increase the risk of adverse effects, including seizures. Imipenem/cilastatin has a higher risk of seizures than meropenem: however, a risk exists with meropenem.

On the basis of susceptibilities, the Pseudomonas is resistant to the piperacillin, and tobramycin is an aminoglycoside, which may also worsen AS's renal function. It would not be a reasonable option to change therapy to piperacillin plus tobramycin.

7. The answer is A (1.3.0)

Enterobacter spp. may contain inducible beta-lactamase genes that in the presence of ceftazidime (a third-generation cephalosporin) may be induced. Both Klebsiella and Enterobacter spp may contain extended spectrum beta-lactamases (ESBLs). In these cases, the carbapenems appear to be first-line therapy. Therefore, what shows to be susceptible in the lab is not actually susceptible in vivo. Beta-lactam agents are cell wall active agents and, therefore, alterations in the DNA gyrase of organisms will not affect their activity against an organism. Quinolones act on DNA gyrase. Although underdosing may promote the emergence of resistant organisms, ceftazidime at a dose of 2 g q 8 h is not underdosed.

8. The answer is D (1.3.5)

On the basis of culture and susceptibility data, ciprofloxacin is the only listed agent that is active against the Pseudomonas aeruginosa. Meropenem does not come as an oral agent. Cefuroxime, amoxicillin/clavulanate, and moxifloxacin do not have activity against Pseudomonas aeruginosa.

9. The answer is C (1.3.0)

Ciprofloxacin may cause theophylline levels to increase; therefore, the patient should be counseled on his theophylline and what to expect if the levels increase (tachycardia, nervousness, tremors, nausea, vomiting, and abdominal pain). Ciprofloxacin and glyburide interact and may lead to hypoglycemia. It is important that the patient know the signs and symptoms of hypoglycemia. AS should closely monitor his blood glucose. Ciprofloxacin may be taken with or without food.

10. The answer is D (3.2.3)

Quinolone absorption is significantly reduced if taken with multivalent cations (magnesium, calcium, zinc, iron, and aluminum). Therefore, antacids, vitamins, iron, zinc, calcium, and enteral products should be taken at least 2 hours before or 2 hours after taking an oral dose of a quinolone. Warfarin will not affect the absorption of a quinolone. However, quinolones will increase the activity of warfarin, increasing the PT/INR.

Case 65 Viral Infections

1. The answer is D (2.2.1)

The brand name for acyclovir is Zovirax. The other brand name-generic name matches are Famvir-famciclovir, Cytovene-ganciclovir, Valtrex-valacyclovir, and Foscavir-foscarnet.

2. The answer is B (1.2.1)

Valacyclovir may be used for and is FDA-approved for treatment of HSV infections. Oseltamivir is an oral neuraminidase inhibitor antiviral used for influenza treatment and prophylaxis. Foscarnet may be used for treatment of HSV infections but is not available in an oral dosage form.

3. The answer is B (1.3.1)

Acyclovir treatment of recurrent genital HSV infections does not eradicate the virus. The role of acyclovir treatment in this setting is for control of HSV-induced symptoms through inhibition of ongoing viral replication. Periodic short courses of acyclovir are unlikely to prevent herpes zoster infection. While bacterial superinfection may be a complication of HSV infection, treatment with acyclovir would not manage bacterial superinfection, nor would acyclovir prevent acquisition of other STDs.

4. The answer is E (1.2.1)

Each of the therapies would be appropriate to use as chronic suppressive therapy of genital HSV in patients experiencing at least six recurrent episodes per year.

5. The answer is C (1.2.5)

The active moiety of the prodrug valacyclovir is acyclovir. Famciclovir is a prodrug for penciclovir. Zanamivir is an antiviral agent used for treatment of influenza. Atazanavir is an antiretroviral agent used as a component of combination therapy for HIV infection.

6. The answer is E (1.2.6)

Acyclovir is primarily eliminated in the urine, and dosage reduction is necessary in a patient with renal dysfunction. Therefore, the dose should be reduced from 400 mg po tid. Answer E is the only response that provides a daily dose lower than the current dose of 1200 mg per day.

7. The answer is B (1.2.1)

Parenteral antiviral therapy is indicated in HIV-infected patients with severe or disseminated HSV infection. The parenteral form of acyclovir would be indicated in this setting. Ganciclovir IV and foscarnet IV have activity against HSV but are typically reserved for CMV treatment and are not preferred therapies for HSV infection. Oral dosage forms of both acyclovir and ganciclovir are relatively poorly absorbed and would not be expected to provide high enough systemic concentrations to effectively treat severe or disseminated HSV in immunocompromised hosts.

8. The answer is A (3.2.1)

Sexual partners of patients with documented STDs should be referred to their physician for evaluation and possible treatment of that particular STD. TJ's partner should not take some of TJ's prescription, as both individuals would ultimately end up receiving suboptimal treatment courses of acyclovir. The chickenpox vaccine is utilized to prevent primary varicella zoster virus infection and not HSV. Immune globulin is not routinely indicated for postexposure prophylaxis of HSV, particularly in patients who are not immunosuppressed.

9. The answer is D (3.2.1)

HIV and syphilis testing is recommended for all patients with documented STDs. HIV and other STDs commonly coexist, and STDs can increase risk of HIV transmission. Hepatitis A is not considered to be a STD and routine screening for this infection in immunocompetent hosts is not indicated.

10. The answer is E (3.2.1)

Nonadherence with acyclovir therapy can lead to subtherapeutic drug exposure, which can, in turn, lead to both an extended duration of symptoms and increased symptom intensity. Due to resultant subtherapeutic acyclovir concentrations induced by nonadherence, the possibility of development of resistance to this medication must be considered.

Case 66 Neonatal Therapy

1. The answer is B (1.1.1)

A neonate is defined as age 0–30 days. An infant is defined as age 1 month to 1 year. A toddler is defined as age 1–3 years. A child is defined as age 3–12 years. An adolescent is defined as age 12–18 years.

2. The answer is A (1.1.1)

Answers

Normal AST, ALT, and Alkaline Phosphate levels for a neonate are 25–75 U/L, 13–45 U/L, and 150–420 U/L, respectively. Potassium levels in a newborn range from 3.7–5.9 mEq/L. Chloride levels in a newborn range from 98–113 mEq/L. BG Hill's hepatic enzymes, potassium, and chloride levels are normal.

3. The answer is B (1.1.1)

Group B streptococcus is a gram-positive cocci organism in pairs or chains. Listeria monocytogenes is a gram-positive bacilli organism. Escherichia coli is a gram-negative rod organism. Group B Streptococcus, Escherichia coli, Haemophilus influenzae, Klebsiella sp., Enterobacter sp., and Listeria monocytogenes are common causes of early-onset sepsis, which is usually acquired from the mother.

4. The answer is E (2.1.1)

BG Hill is being administered 200 mg/kg/day of ampicillin divided every 12 hours. The standard dose for rule out sepsis in a neonate is 200 mg/kg/day; 200 mg x 1.747 kg = 349 mg/day. This equals 175 mg twice daily.

5. The answer is C (1.2.6)

The goal trough is less than 2 mcg/mL. A peak of 4–8 mcg/mL is goal. No change is needed for the current dose.

6. The answer is C (1.3.1)

Antibiotics may be discontinued if the patient shows no signs of illness, is feeding well, and if the cultures are negative for 48 hours. Ninety-five percent of neonates with a GBS infection will show signs and symptoms of illness within the first 24 hours.

7. The answer is B (2.1.3)

During the first and second day of life, newborns require 60–80 mL/kg/day, and 60–80 mL x 1.474 kg /day = 104–140 mL/day. Then divide by 24 hours. This calculates to be approximately 4–6 mL/hr.

8. The answer is C (1.1.1)

The APGAR score is a quick and easy way to assess whether a newborn needs resuscitation immediately after birth. It is calculated based on color, heart rate, respiratory rate, muscle tone, and reflex irritability. Each category is rated from 0–2 and added to a maximum score of 10. The APGAR score is calculated at 1, 5, and 10 minutes after birth. An initial low score does not predict mortality or developmental concerns, but it may signify that the newborn needs assistance.

9. The answer is C (1.2.2)

Gentamicin is an aminoglycoside antibiotic and binds to the 30S and 50S ribosomal subunit. This causes an inhibition of protein synthesis and results in a faulty cell wall membrane. Ampicillin is a penicillin antibiotic and causes cell death by binding to penicillin-binding proteins and affecting the cell wall.

10. The answer is A (2.2.2)

Ampicillin sodium is the only intravenous formulation. Ampicillin trihydrate is available as a capsule and powder for suspension. There is no sulfate formulation available.

Case 67 Pediatric Infectious Diseases

1. The answer is C (1.1.4)

In children older than 5 years of age, streptococcus pneumoniae (C) and Neisseria meningitides are the most common causes of bacterial meningitis. Group B strep (A), E. coli (B), and Listeria monocytogenes (E) are common causes of bacterial meningitis in the newborn age. Streptococcus pneumoniae, Neisseria meningitides, and Haemophilis influenzae type b (Hib) are common causes of bacterial meningitis in infants and children less than 5 years of age.

2. The answer is D (1.2.2)

The incidence of hearing loss in children with documented bacterial meningitis is still unacceptably high, despite appropriate antimicrobial therapy. Dexamethasone along with ceftriaxone for patients with meningitis caused by Haemophilus influenzae (Hib) has been proven to reduce the incidence of hearing loss and neurologic sequelae. Less benefit was seen with dexamethasone in pneumococcal meningitis. The greatest benefit seen is when dexamethasone is administered with or shortly before the first dose of parenteral antibiotics. Current recommendations support the use of dexamethasone in Hib meningitis and for it to be considered in pneumococcal meningitis. Corticosteroids have not demonstrated anti-infective properties. They are reported to cause immunosuppression. Decreased inflammation leading to decreased penetration is correct; however, it is not a benefit in treating meningitis. Data does not support the use of dexamethasone in GB.

3. The answer is B (2.1.1)

GB's correctly prescribed dose is 250,000 units/kg/d, which equals 8 million units divided by 6 equals 1.33 million units/dose and then divide by 50,000 units/ mL = 26.7 mL/dose; thus, the other answers are incorrect.

4. The answer is A (1.2.2)

Penicillin does bind to several enzymes in the cytoplasmic membrane that are involved in cell wall synthesis. (B) describes the mechanism of action of tetracyclines and (C) describes the mechanism of action of bacitracin. (D) is not the mechanism of any currently available antibiotic. (E) is the mechanism of action for sulfa-type antibiotics.

5. The answer is C (3.2.1)

Currently, the CDC recommends universal vaccinations for H. flu type b (Hib) and Streptococcus pneumoniae. A vaccine to

E. coli does not exist. Meningitis due to Hib has drastically decreased by 99% since the mid-1980s when the conjugate vaccine was recommended to be administered to all infants and children. Invasive disease, including meningitis, due to streptococcus has decreased by more than 90% after implementation of the pneumococcal vaccine in 2000 for infants and children. A vaccine for Neisseria meningitis has been available since 1982; however, a conjugate vaccine was approved in 2005. With the approval of the new conjugate, the vaccine is now recommended to be administered to all children ages 11–12 years and those with risk factors. It is anticipated that vaccine implementation will reduce the incidence of meningococcal meningitis due to the serotype A, C, Y, and W-135, which are the serotypes in the vaccine. However, type b is a common cause of meningitis but is not included in the vaccine due to poor immunogenicity. Data from England, where a serogroup C vaccine was introduced in 1999, has shown an 81% decrease in serogroup C disease. It would have been appropriate to offer GB the meningococcal vaccine prior to camp due to his risk factor of attending a camp where the kids would live in a dorm setting.

6. The answer is A (1.1.3)

Fever, headache, increased white count with a left shift, or increased number of immature white cells are common signs of meningitis in children and adults. Pulmonary infiltrates are not common in meningitis but are common in pneumonia and other pulmonary diseases. Nuchal rigidity, photophobia, and a positive Kernig's sign are present at diagnosis in many children. A positive Kernig's sign means the patient will resist leg extension after the knee is brought to the chest while lying supine. Kernig originally performed the test while the patient was seated. Brudzinski's sign most commonly cited is the "nape of the neck sign," in which the patient's hips and knees flex on flexion of the neck. Other common signs of meningitis in children are mostly nonspecific and include changes in activity level, somnolence, confusion, and lethargy. Infants may develop irritability, altered sleep patterns, vomiting, high-pitched crying, decreased oral intake, and seizures.

7. The answer is E (3.2.1)

Chemoprophylaxis for meningococcal meningitis is recommended for the following individuals: 1) All household contacts, 2) childcare/nursery school contact during 7 days before the onset of illness, 3) direct exposure to the index case's secretions during 7 days before the onset of illness, 4) healthcare workers who performed unprotected mouth-to-mouth resuscitation, intubation, or suction, 5) frequently slept or ate in same dwelling as index case during 7 days before onset of illness. Anyone who meets the criteria above should receive chemoprophylaxis because of contact with GB.

8. The answer is B (3.2.1)

The most appropriate thing to do is to determine whether home care is possible. If the home environment and caregivers are conducive to providing good care, it may be considered.

Although parenteral penicillin could be continued at home, it is administered so frequently that adherence may become an issue. Pen G is standard of care for PCN-sensitive N. meningitidis meningitis, but ceftriaxone is a reasonable alternative for treatment. Ceftriaxone offers an acceptable choice for GB at home. Once-daily therapy with 80–100 mg/kg provides serum levels many-fold higher than the MIC of the common organisms. The serum level remains high enough at the end of the 24-hour dosing interval to be efficacious. Some studies have documented that the large single-daily dose may saturate protein binding and lead to increased free ceftriaxone. The free concentration is able to cross into CNS and eradicate the infecting organism. Many physicians may treat with ceftriaxone empirically in this patient, which is appropriate as well.

9. The answer is C (2.2.2)

Pediatric physicians often become very comfortable with mg/kg calculations but fail to recognize that the child does not need more than the adult dose. In this example, 600 mg qd divided into 300 mg doses is easily dispensed and recommended. Compounding a suspension to make the dose 640 mg q day increases costs and may decrease adherence if the patient does not tolerate the taste of the suspension. Rifampin dosing for Neisseria meningitidis is recommended at 10 mg/kg po once daily for 2 days.

10. The answer is A (3.2.1)

Many people, including health care professionals, are reluctant to use appropriate medications in appropriate doses for pain relief, especially in children. Children and infants experience pain and need relief. Literature has documented improved healing when pain is controlled, both psychologically and physically. Catecholamine levels can be measured, and they correlate with pain or pain relief. Increased levels may indicate, among other things, inadequate pain relief. Thus, effective treatment of GB requires trying to relieve his pain. Once antibiotics have been started and clinical symptoms abate, morphine may be switched to a less potent agent, such as acetaminophen with codeine. Many studies have demonstrated the safety and efficacy of opioids and nonopioids in neonates and children. Our healthcare providers need to use them more often.

Case 68 Pediatric Nutrition

1. The answer is D (2.1.0)

Utilizing the Holiday-Segar formula for calculating fluid requirements involves the following: 0–10 kg: 100 mL/kg/day; 10–20 kg: 1000 mL + 50 mL/kg for each kg > 10 kg; > 20 kg: 1500 mL + 20 mL/kg for each kg > 20 kg.

Since very low birthweight (VLBW) infants often require greater than maintenance, their daily volume is often 25%–75% greater than their actual maintenance fluids. It is often difficult to fully assess all of the infant's fluid requirements, so utilizing

Answers

weight gain/loss and laboratory parameters is essential. Some practitioners would use 150 mL/kg for VLBW infants as maintenance, which also yields 165 mL/day for this patient.

2. The answer is C (2.1.2)

Since baby Jones is a pre-term infant, it is common to slowly increase the parenteral feedings in order to avoid causing side effects (hyperglycemia, hypertriglyceridemia, and prerenal azotemia). Starting low and increasing to goal requirements is the preferred practice for carbohydrates and fats. Current studies suggest that starting on the first day of life with 2–3 grams/kg of protein may minimize protein catabolism, and it may improve overall weight gain. Slowly increasing the fat emulsion and liberalizing the glucose infusion rate can be accomplished on subsequent days of therapy.

3. The answer is D (2.1.2)

Premature infants on PN will often meet their goal macronutrients within 5–7 days after initiating therapy. An infant this size would require approximately 3–3.5 g/kg/day of protein. She would require approximately 3–4 g/kg/day of intravenous fat emulsion as tolerated by serum triglycerides. She would require 8–12 mg/kg/min of glucose.

4. The answer is D (2.1.2)

Since premature infants do not obtain their full supply of nutrients from their mother prior to birth, they are at risk for growth failure and failure to thrive. It is important to provide a balanced supply of calories. The usual parenteral intake of calories for premature infants is between 80 and 100 kcal/kg/day. Enteral intake typically ranges from 100–130 kcal/kg/day for premature infants.

5. The answer is C (1.3.2)

Monitoring serum triglycerides is the most useful test to aid in adjusting the intravenous fat emulsion. It responds more quickly to intake and metabolism. Cholesterol is a measure of long-term fat metabolism and will most likely not be useful while on PN. HDL will not indicate the patient's ability to utilize the lipid emulsion. Alkaline phosphate may be monitored, but more for appropriate calcium, phosphate, and vitamin D intake. Alpha-1 anti-trypsin is not related to fat metabolism.

6. The answer is C (1.3.2)

In patients with metabolic bone disease associated with long-term PN usage, the alkaline phosphatase usually increases significantly. Patients usually develop metabolic bone disease and calcium and phosphate deficiency. The bones will re-distribute calcium and phosphorus, so it appears that the serum levels are normal. Some infants may have metabolic bone disease due to poor absorption or poor intake of vitamin D, although less commonly. Appropriate monitoring would include alkaline phosphatase. If a patient's alkaline phosphatase increases, the patient's calcium and phosphate intake should be maximized.

If the alkaline phosphatase does not decrease, or continues to increase, additional vitamin D may be warranted. The ability to measure vitamin D serum levels is not common. Alpha-1 antitrypsin is not related to bone homeostasis.

7. The answer is E (1.3.3)

As mentioned in Question 6, osteopenia or metabolic bone disease occurs frequently in neonates on long-term PN. Cholestasis occurs, less frequently in the same population. An inability to metabolize amino acids may be the cause. The incidence of cholestasis decreased dramatically following the use of neonatal parenteral amino acid solutions. These solutions ensure that all essential amino acids are provided to the neonate and reduce the likelihood that metabolic immaturity will lead to toxic levels of other amino acids. Selenium deficiency has been documented in patients of all ages on long-term PN. The trace element solutions for pediatric and adult patients contain selenium; as yet, neonatal trace elements do not. However, it may be prudent to supplement with low dose selenium. Consider that 1 µg/kg/day will prevent deficiency and also not lead to toxicity. Serum levels will be low but safe until enteral nutrition, which contains selenium, is started.

8. The answer is D (1.1.4)

Infants receive most of their calcium and phosphorus stores in utero during the third trimester. During pregnancy, the infant acquires calcium and phosphorus at a consistent rate of 2 mg of calcium for every 1 mg of phosphorus. The range is between 1.5 and 2.1. Keep in mind that 1 mmol of phosphorus is equivalent to 30 mg of phosphorus. Calcium can be ordered in units of the salt, milliequivalents, or in mg of elemental calcium. Be sure to choose the correct conversion when making this comparison.

9. The answer is E (2.3.3)

Many factors play a role in calcium phosphate solubility in PN solutions. Most important and easiest to monitor are the dose of each in the solution. A role of pharmacy in neonatal PN management is to maximize the calcium and phosphate intake. This is often challenging as the doses of each needed to prevent osteopenia and promote adequate bone growth are very difficult and sometimes impossible to provide in PN solutions. Many graphs and formulas are available (from amino acid solution manufacturers, for example) to help determine the calcium phosphate solubility in the specific PN solution being prepared.

The pH is one other important factor. The more acidic the PN, the greater the calcium phosphate solubility. Dextrose itself is acidic at high concentrations, so not only do neonates receive a large portion of calories in PN from dextrose concentrations of 12.5%–20%, the more dextrose the solution contains, the more calcium phosphate it can simultaneously accommodate. Amino acid solution, like the word "acid" implies, has an acidic pH. Also, cysteine is routinely added by the pharmacy department when compounding TPN solutions.

Cysteine has a pH of 1.0 and, thus, further acidifies the PN and increases calcium phosphate solubility. Temperature increases negatively impact calcium phosphate solubility. It is not uncommon for a solution to be clear and free of precipitate when sent to the neonatal unit. However, many neonates are under warmers to help maintain body temperature and sometimes near windows or other light sources to treat or prevent hyperbilirubinemia. These increases in environmental temperature can decrease the calcium phosphate solubility in a PN solution to the point of precipitation.

10. The answer is C (1.3.3)

Both manganese and copper are excreted in the bile. Since patients with cholestatic liver disease do not eliminate bile effectively, there is a possible benefit of holding manganese and copper from their PN solution. Patients will require supplementation of these trace elements periodically or they may develop a deficiency. Chromium, selenium, and zinc are all eliminated renally, and they may need to be adjusted in cases of severe renal impairment.

Case 69 Pediatric ICU

1. The answer is E (1.2.3)

Daunorubicin is an anthracycline agent indicated for the treatment of acute non-lymphocytic leukemia in adults and for the treatment of acute lymphocytic leukemia in adults and children. Daunorubicin, as with any chemotherapeutic agent, is associated with myelosuppression at therapeutic doses. The drug is also associated with cardiac toxicity, manifested as potentially fatal congestive heart failure. Cardiac toxicity associated with daunorubicin therapy appears to be dose related, most commonly occurring when the total cumulative dosage exceeds 400–550 mg/m^2 in adults, 300 mg/m^2 in children > 2 years of age, or 10 mg/kg in children < 2 years of age. Daunorubicin-induced cardiac toxicity may occur during therapy or several months to years after completion of therapy. It is difficult to predict which patients may be at highest risk for cardiac toxicity associated with daunorubicin therapy, so baseline ejection fraction, obtained by echocardiogram, as well as an ECG are appropriate in all patients. Daunorubicin is extensively metabolized by the liver and dosage reductions are recommended for patients with hepatic insufficiency.

2. The answer is B (2.2.5)

Vincristine is fatal if given intrathecally.

3. The answer is C (1.3.5)

Pneumocystis carinii pneumonia is an opportunistic infection that occurs in immunosuppressed populations, particularly HIV-infected patients and those patients receiving aggressive therapy for leukemia, lymphoma, or transplant. The drug of choice for PCP prophylaxis is IV or PO trimethoprim/ sulfamethoxazole. Dapsone and aerosolized pentamidine are acceptable alternatives to trimethoprim/sulfamethoxazole for this indication. Daptomycin is an IV antibiotic indicated for resistant gram-positive and complicated skin and skin structure infections. It is not indicated for pneumonia.

4. The answer is D (3.2.1)

Hyperuricemia usually develops 2–3 days after initiation of treatment for leukemia. Rapidly growing tumor cells carry a large nucleic acid burden, due to their high cellular activity and turnover. Once chemotherapy is begun, tumor cells are lysed into purine nucleic acids, which are further broken down into hypoxanthine. Hypoxanthine is then converted into uric acid by the enzyme xanthine oxidase. A number of measures may be implemented to prevent and manage uric acid levels in newly diagnosed leukemic patients. Adequate fluid hydration is recommended in order to reduce serum concentrations of uric acid. Hydration should be aggressive in those patients who are not fluid restricted and should begin at least 1–2 days prior to chemotherapy, continuing until 2–3 days after chemotherapy is administered. Urinary alkalinization with sodium bicarbonate (usually diluted in D$_5$W or 0.45% NaCl) increases the solubility of uric acid and its renal excretion. The goal of urinary alkalinization is to raise the pH of urine to > 7.0. Allopurinol is a competitive inhibitor of xanthine oxidase, acting to prevent the formation of uric acid. Rasburicase, a recombinant form of urate oxidase, acts to increase the solubility and renal excretion of uric acid by catalyzing the oxidation of uric acid to allantoin. Apresoline is considered a "look-alike, sound-alike" drug to allopurinol. Apresoline is the trade name for hydralazine, which is a peripheral vasodilator.

5. The answer is D (1.3.3)

The major goals of managing hyperkalemia include intracellular shift of potassium, cardiac membrane stabilization, and reduction of total potassium levels. Sodium polystyrene sulfate is a resin that exchanges sodium ions for potassium ions in the intestine before the resin is eliminated. The drug, commercially available as a suspension, may be administered either orally or as a rectal enema. Calcium gluconate is administered to patients with hyperkalemia to prevent cardiac arrhythmias through stabilization of the cardiac membrane. Regular insulin, administered IV, promotes the intracellular shift of potassium. Insulin is given in combination with concentrated dextrose to prevent hypoglycemia. Sodium bicarbonate also promotes the intracellular shift of potassium. Magnesium does not alter potassium levels.

6. The answer is A (2.2.5)

Calcium chloride is 27% elemental calcium; calcium gluconate is 9% elemental calcium. Thus, calcium chloride has three times more calcium than calcium gluconate. Oral absorption of calcium varies depending on the form. Calcium carbonate is only available in an oral form but does provide the most elemental calcium, 40%.

Answers

7. The answer is C (1.2.6)

Due to the renal elimination of cefepime, dosage adjustments are recommended for patients with creatinine clearance < 60 mL/min. Accumulation of allopurinol, as well as its metabolite oxypurinol, may occur in renal failure. Dosage adjustments are not necessary for dexamethasone in renal failure.

8. The answer is D (1.3.5)

As with all medications, hypersensitivity to the agent, including anaphylaxis, is a contraindication to use. Rasburicase may continue to break down uric acid following blood sample collections for uric acid. By placing the blood sample on ice immediately after collection, this drug-lab interaction may be avoided. A by-product of the conversion of uric acid to allantoin is hydrogen peroxide. Patients with G6PD deficiency may be unable to appropriately metabolize hydrogen peroxide, leading to an increased risk of hemolytic anemia or methemoglobinemia. Rasburicase does not require dosage adjustment in renal insufficiency.

9. The answer is B (1.2.2)

Urate oxidase catalyzes the oxidation of uric acid to allantoin, which is five to ten times more water soluble than uric acid. The increased solubility of allantoin facilitates the urinary excretion of uric acid. This enzyme, although present in most mammals, is not expressed in humans due to a genetic mutation. Rasburicase is a recombinant form of urate oxidase. Allopurinol inhibits the conversion of hypoxanthine to xanthine, as well as the conversion of xanthine to uric acid, by inhibiting the enzyme xanthine oxidase.

10. The answer is A (2.1.1)

The recommended dose of rasburicase is 0.15 - 0.2 mg/kg/dose given once daily for up to 5 days. The effect of rasburicase on uric acid levels is dramatic; often, just one dose of rasburicase will be sufficient to bring uric acid levels to within normal limits. Due to the significant cost of rasburicase, it is not uncommon for institutions to round the dose to the nearest full 1.5-mg vial to avoid waste.

Case 70 Acne

1. The answer is E (1.2.2)

Keratinolytic compounds break down keratin, the hard, fibrous protein in skin cells. This process helps break up the stratum corneum, the outermost skin layer composed of dead, enucleated, keratinized cells, and allows the cells to be shed more easily. Preventing keratinocyte clumping helps prevent the clogged pores that lead to acne. All three compounds listed have keratinolytic properties. Benzoyl peroxide is the most effective against acne because it also has anti-bacterial and thus anti-inflammatory properties. Salicylic acid can help maintain clear skin in mild acne cases, but is not as effective. Lactic acid is

not used in acne; instead, products such as Lac-Hydrin feature this agent in oily bases to reduce lichenification, thereby softening skin and aiding topical medication penetration in conditions such as psoriasis. However, the oily product formulations would be counterproductive in acne.

2. The answer is A (1.2.4)

Minocycline has a higher incidence than the other two of adverse CNS effects, such as vertigo, skin discoloration, and lupus-like syndrome (A). Minocycline is considered by some to be even more effective than doxycycline or tetracycline, and is often used when one of the other two has failed (B). It can be dosed bid or even qd so it does not require more frequent dosing (D). It is better absorbed than tetracycline and does not have a larger number of drug interactions than the other two (C, E).

3. The answer is B (3.2.3)

Tea tree oil is widely used as a topical anti-infective or antiseptic. Some research suggests it could be beneficial in acne (B) as well as in fungal skin and nail infections.

Grape seed extract (A) has been promoted for treating diabetic complications and hastening wound healing, but with little evidence. Arnica (C) has been used topically for bruises, sprains, aches, and dandruff, but little research is available. Neither has been promoted or studied for acne.

Flaxseed oil (D) has been used as a cooking oil, topically as a moisturizer, and orally as a dietary supplement for uses ranging from relieving arthritis or constipation to lowering cholesterol and triglycerides. It has not been promoted for acne. It is a dietary source of a;-linolenic acid. Though research continues into possible cardiovascular benefits, no strong evidence supports any of its therapeutic uses.

Feverfew (E) has been taken orally for migraines, allergies, asthma, and arthritis, and used topically for dental pain or as an antiseptic. It has not been studied or promoted for acne, but some evidence suggests it may be useful for migraines.

4. The answer is E (1.3.5)

Although any single agent may be effective in a given patient, studies reveal that Accutane (isotretinoin) is the best for severe, recalcitrant acne. It is the only agent with mechanisms of action against all four of the causative factors behind acne: 1) normalization of keratinization of cells lining the sebaceous glands; 2) reduction of excessive sebum production; 3) anti-bacterial effects; 4) anti-inflammatory effects. Patients often experience "cure" of their acne or at least months to years of total or near-total remission.

5. The answer is D (3.2.2)

Although patients with acne are sometimes told not to use any makeup, careful use of non-comedogenic (non-pore-clogging) cosmetics is acceptable (D) in all but the most severe cases (e.g., broken skin, superinfection). Makeup should be applied over topical acne medications and removed every night using a mild, oil-free cleanser. Like all makeup users, patients with acne should periodically wash brushes and other application tools and replace old, potentially contaminated products. Dietary oils do not affect sebum production, and no dietary changes are recommended for acne (A). Although some patients report that sun exposure improves their acne, the effect is not reliable, and in any case sunbathing cannot be recommended in light of the long-term benefit-to-risk ratio (B). In addition, patients using benzoyl peroxide or tetracycline are advised to use sunscreen. Acne is not caused by dirt, so neither harsh nor frequent (more than once or twice daily) cleansing is called for (C). Benzoyl peroxide or other keratinolytic agents provide appropriate exfoliation, while popular "exfoliating scrubs" containing abrasives only scratch the skin and irritate it further. Patients should not pick at or pop their own pimples (E); any comedo extraction should be performed at the dermatologist's office.

6. The answer is E (1.3.2)

Because oral isotretinoin is known to be extremely teratogenic and can elevate liver function tests, cholesterol, and triglycerides, as well as lower HDL, all three of the above lab tests are performed at baseline (in fact, two negative pregnancy tests are required before therapy begins) and monthly during therapy. Additionally, the same schedule of tests applies to blood glucose and CBC. Hyperglycemia has been observed in patients on isotretinoin. Decreases in hematocrit, hemoglobin concentration, red blood cell counts, and white blood cell counts occur in significant numbers of patients, as well as increases in platelet counts; serious hematologic abnormalities have been reported. It is also important to monitor the patient's mood for signs of depression, aggression, or other changes.

7. The answer is C (2.2.5)

The iPLEDGE program has replaced the SMART program for Accutane and the similar programs for generic isotretinoin products. The FDA hopes the iPLEDGE program will simplify isotretinoin dispensing by consolidating the various programs, and will be even more effective than the earlier programs at preventing unintended pregnancies in patients on isotretinoin. The iPLEDGE program requires registration of all parties involved in the chain of distribution: not only prescribers and patients but also pharmacies and drug wholesalers (I). In general, the new program is similar to the old ones. Patients have to sign consent forms to take isotretinoin, and female patients of child-bearing age who have not had bilateral oophorectomies or a hysterectomy must commit to two reliable methods of birth control or complete sexual abstinence for a month before, during, and for a month after therapy. As before, prescriptions may be for no more than 30 days' supply and cannot have any refills (II). Prescriptions still must be filled within 7 days of the date they were written. However, the yellow sticker requirement is gone (III), so prescribers are free to phone or fax isotretinoin prescriptions. The dispensing pharmacist must call in to the iPLEDGE database and get authorization before each fill. A prescriber may only write the month's prescription

for a female patient of child-bearing age after the patient has had another negative pregnancy test; the prescriber calls this result in to the iPLEDGE database so that the prescription fill will be authorized. Not just the prescriber but the female patient of child-bearing age must call in to the iPLEDGE database or contact it through the internet every month. All patients, male or female, must not donate blood during or for a month after isotretinoin therapy.

8. The answer is A (1.2.1)

Hormonal contraceptives may improve, aggravate, or not affect acne. The tendency to improve acne comes from estrogens and from estrogenic effects of the progestins. The tendency to aggravate acne comes from the androgenic effects of progestins. Only Ortho Tri-Cyclen has received FDA approval for treating acne. It contains ethinyl estradiol and a progestin with high estrogenic activity, norgestimate. However, patients may notice acne improvement when they begin any estrogen/progestin combined contraceptive, or when they switch from one to another with a more estrogenic progestin. Note that when SJ is on Accutane with its multiple mechanisms of action, she will no longer need to take oral antibiotics, so concerns about oral contraceptive efficacy in patients taking antibiotics will not be an issue. Available data suggest that tetracycline does not actually impair the efficacy of oral contraceptives, but many pharmacists still mention the theoretical interaction to patients based on medicolegal fears.

9. The answer is B (1.2.7)

Ery-Tabs are enteric coated, meaning they will not release medication in the very low pH environment of the stomach. Erythromycin base is susceptible to degradation by stomach acid, so enteric coating improves bioavailability and allows for administration with food. However, Ery-Tabs are not designed for sustained-release qualities; they dissolve completely and immediately release all medication once they are in the less acidic environment of the intestines.

10. The answer is C (2.1.1)

SJ weighs 160 lb, or divided by 2.2 lb/kg, about 73 kg. Since she should get 0.5–1 mg/kg/d, her ideal daily dose would range from 36.5–73 mg/d. Dosing regimens of 20 mg po bid (40 mg/d) and 30 mg po bid (60 mg/d) are within this range. Answers D and E are eliminated.

Her cumulative dose should be about 120 mg/kg x 73 kg = 8760 mg. If taking 20 mg po bid (40 mg/d), she would need 8760 mg divided by 40 mg/d, or 219 days, to finish. 219 days divided by 7 days/week = 31.3 weeks. Therefore, neither of the regimens in answer A or B is long enough.

If taking 30 mg po bid (60 mg/d), she would need 8760 mg divided by 60 mg/d, or 146 days, to finish. 146 days divided by 7 days/week = 20.8 weeks. Answer C looks close. To check, multiply 21 weeks x 7 days/week = 147 days, just one extra day of therapy.

Answers

Case 71 Photosensitivity and Burns

1. The answer is D (3.2.1)

Blanching, or turning white, when pressure is applied to a burn is not a dire sign; this is a characteristic of superficial and superficial partial-thickness burns (I). However, burns caused by electricity or chemicals, as well as inhalation burns, should be seen by a physician immediately (II). White, painless burns are deep partial-thickness or full-thickness burns. The whiteness, which may develop in the hours following the burn, indicates loss of blood supply and the painlessness indicates the destruction of nerve endings. These most severe burns require emergency care (III).

2. The answer is D (3.2.1)

Weeping of serous fluid is an expected stage in the healing of vesicles and bullae (D). New pain, warmth, redness, or swelling could indicate bacterial infection. Pus, streaking, or systemic symptoms (e.g., fever, malaise) are further, more serious indicators.

3. The answer is C (1.1.3)

Superficial burns, once called first-degree burns, involve only the epidermis and are usually only indicated by erythema and slight swelling. Nerve endings in the dermis are not affected, so pain and tactile sensation remain (A). The old category of second-degree burns has been broken down into superficial partial-thickness and deep partial-thickness burns. These burns extend through the epidermis and part of the dermis. Superficial partial thickness burns do not affect nerve endings in the dermis and so are also painful and sensitive (B); these burns are characterized by erythema and blistering. However, some areas of a deep partial thickness burn have dermis sufficiently damaged to destroy nerve endings. These areas become white and lose sensation (C). Full-thickness burns, once called third-degree burns, involve the destruction of the entire epidermis and dermis.

4. The answer is B (1.1.3)

See the answer to Question 3 for a full description of burn categorization.

5. The answer is E (1.2.2)

Counterirritants, such as menthol (E) and camphor, reduce itch and minor pain perception by irritating nerve endings to supply competing, less noxious nerve stimulation. They are not usually the best choice to treat burns because they further irritate the sensitive, damaged skin.

Pramoxine (A) and lidocaine (C) are topical anesthetics that work by disrupting the neural transmission of pain signals and reducing sensation. Though topical anesthetics provide relief for less than an hour (except for lidocaine patches),

patients should not apply them more often than qid to avoid systemic absorption and hypersensitization.

Topical diphenhydramine (B) is an antihistamine. Allantoin (D) is a keratinolytic agent.

6. The answer is C (1.2.5)

The patient needs to use a skin protectant to prevent the irritation and pruritus that can result from a dried-out wound and to promote fast healing. Bacitracin ointment is the best of the alternatives provided because the petrolatum base will keep the skin protected and moist and prevent sticking of bandages (C). Though the bacitracin may modestly reduce the chances of secondary bacterial infection, the skin protectant vehicle provides most of the product's benefit. Note that ointments are not appropriate on a blistering burn acutely; they trap heat and exudate.

Benadryl (diphenhydramine) Gel is a poor choice because the gel vehicle will dry out the lesion and topical diphenhydramine can be very sensitizing (A). Creams can be more neutral in terms of moisturizing vs. drying out lesions. However, the erosion is an area of broken skin so systemic absorption should be taken into account. Hydrocortisone cream offers less skin protection than the bacitracin ointment and might make it easier for the burn to become infected (B). Gold Bond Cream contains menthol, a counterirritant that is counterproductive in painful, sensitized skin (D). Lanacane Cream contains benzocaine, a topical anesthetic that only provides short-lived relief and causes hypersensitivity reactions in many patients (E). Its inactive ingredients do not provide as much skin protection as the petrolatum found in the ointment.

7. The answer is B (3.2.1)

Alcohol-containing preparations should be avoided because they cause drying and severe pain (B). The initial management of minor burns includes cleansing with water and mild soap (A) and use of a nonadherent dressing (C). Hydrophobic skin protectants such as cocoa butter (D) or white petrolatum (E) can be helpful unless the burn is hot, blistered, or weeping.

8. The answer is E (1.1.3)

Extensive burns disrupt the integrity of the skin over a critically large area, compromising the skin's ability to serve as a barrier against infection and body water loss. Dehydration can lead to inadequate blood pressure, inadequate kidney perfusion, and shock. Massive amounts of hemoglobin and other substances released from widespread muscle tissue destruction can overwhelm kidney filtration and result in rhabdomyolysis.

9. The answer is D (1.2.1)

Ice should not be applied to burns acutely or later in the healing process (I). The ice may be left on the skin too long and can even make the burn more painful. Also, once past the warm, blistering phase, MJ's burn will get dried out by repeated wetting and evaporation from ice.

Although there isn't clear-cut evidence that aloe helps burns heal, its topical use is not associated with any toxicity. There is no need to discourage MJ from using aloe in an appropriate vehicle (II). She also has no contraindications to the use of ibuprofen to relieve pain (III).

10. The answer is C (1.3.1)

Superficial partial thickness burns usually heal within 2–3 weeks and leave minimal to no scarring (C). Superficial burns may heal within 4 days, but MJ's will take longer (A, B). It should not, however, take 6 weeks (D, E). Deep partial thickness and full thickness burns heal over months and leave significant scarring.

Case 72 Cold and Flu

1. The answer is C (1.1.2)

A cough can be present in both influenza and rhinovirus infections, which doesn't help differentiate from which condition MH is suffering. A person suffering from an influenza infection usually has a fever 100°F and experiences chills and myalgias. A person suffering from a rhinovirus will not usually experience a fever > 100°F or chills and myalgias with their other symptoms.

2. The answer is B (1.1.2)

Nasal congestion and the lack of a fever are common to both rhinovirus infections and allergies. A fever > 100°F is usually only present in influenza infections. A patient suffering from allergies will likely have paroxysmal sneezing and/or watery or itchy eyes, nose and throat.

3. The answer is C (1.1.3)

A systemic decongestant will provide relief for the patient's stuffy nose, and possibly help relieve his headache, which sounds like it might be due to sinus congestion. An expectorant is no longer recommended as a first-line treatment for cough or chest congestion according to guidelines published in 2006 by the American College of Chest Physicians, although the patient should be encouraged to drink plenty of liquids to help loosen chest secretions. An analgesic will help relieve his headache and mild myalgias.

4. The answer is D (1.2.0)

Systemic decongestants (sympathomimetics) can increase blood pressure, which can cause problems in hypertension and benign prostatic hyperplasia. They can also cause urinary retention, which is also a problem with BPH. The patient's physician should determine if the use of a decongestant is appropriate with the status of their disease state. Decongestants don't propose a problem with gastroesophageal reflux disease.

5. The answer is B (1.2.1)

Mucinex contains guaifenesin, which is the only available expectorant ingredient. Delsym is dextromethorphan, which is a cough suppressant. Actifed is pseudoephedrine and triprolidine, a decongestant and antihistamine.

6. The answer is D (3.1.1)

MicroMedex/DrugDex is a software program that lists the trade/generic names for drug inquiries. Facts and Comparisons is a loose-leaf resource that contains drugs grouped by category and ingredients for ease of comparison. It is indexed by brand and generic names, making it useful to cross reference products and their ingredients. Medline is a medical research database that locates journal articles on specific topics, which would not be useful in this instance.

7. The answer is A (2.2.1)

Mucinex is a long-acting (12 hour formulation) guaifenesin product. Robitussin is available OTC, but is not long acting (4–6 hour formulation). Tussionex is a CIII medication requiring a prescription.

8. The answer is C (3.2.5)

Humidifiers and vaporizers provide moisture in the air, which acts as an expectorant to soften and loosen mucous, to relieve congestion. A sitz bath is used to soak the hips and/or buttocks to ease pain associated with recent surgery, hemorrhoids, or other pelvic related conditions.

9. The answer is E (1.2.0)

Because topical decongestants can increase blood pressure, raise heart rates and cause urinary retention as possible side effects, it is not recommended for use by people with disease states that can be affected by those effects, unless under the supervision of a physician. Oxymetazoline is the longest acting topical decongestant, used every 10 to 12 hours. Phenylephrine is the shortest acting topical decongestant, used every 4 to 6 hours. Xylometazoline is an intermediate acting topical decongestant, used every 8 to 10 hours. Topical decongestants should not be used for a duration longer than 3 days, because it can worsen symptoms by causing rebound congestion.

10. The answer is B (1.2.4)

With the use of NSAIDs, the risk of severe GI events (GI bleeding and/or ulceration) is increased by the history of peptic ulcer disease and/or GI bleeding. From the PMH, we know the patient experienced a peptic ulcer associated with GI bleeding 7 years ago, precluding him from the use of NSAIDs. Acetaminophen is not associated with these risks, and can be safely taken by patients with a history of peptic ulcers and/or GI bleeding.

Answers

Case 73 Ophthalmic Disorders and Contact Lenses

1. The answer is E (1.1.0)

All three instances could be indicative of conditions too severe to be treated with over the counter medications. Although watery discharge is likely due to allergies, mucous or thick, discolored discharge is likely due to infection, which can't be treated with over the counter remedies. Recent trauma to the eye, or contact with foreign matter should be addressed by a physician, to ensure there is no damage to the eye.

2. The answer is E (1.1.3)

Pheniramine and Antazoline are ophthalmic antihistamines that will relieve watery, itchy eyes. Methylcellulose is used in lubricants to help relieve dry eye symptoms by preventing tear evaporation through tear film stabilization (excessive tearing, paradoxically, is often one of the signs, at least initially, of dry eyes).

3. The answer is D (2.2.1)

Vasocon-A, Visine-A, Opcon-A and Naphcon-A all have either pheniramine or antazoline as the active antihistamine ingredient, which are available without a prescription. Patanol contains olopatadine, which does require a prescription.

4. The answer is C (1.2.4)

Olopatadine would be therapeutic duplication if she used it at the same time as an OTC ophthalmic antihistamine. Phenazopyridine can discolor her soft contact lenses because it discolors bodily fluids, including tears. Although lubricants will help alleviate her dry eye symptoms at night by preventing tear evaporation, it will not alleviate her itchy, watery eyes because they do not block histamine.

5. The answer is E (3.3.2)

Ointments are retained in the eye for longer periods of time, increasing their ocular contact time, because of their greater viscosity. The greater viscosity and retention time in the eye enhances the integrity of the tear film to alleviate symptoms of dry eye. Because ointments tend to blur vision for some time after use, it is best administered at bedtime, so the blurred vision will not be present during waking hours.

6. The answer is C (3.2.3)

The eye requires time for the first drop to be absorbed, or the first drop is likely to be flushed out by the second drop, and overflow out of the eye. Preservatives are not effective after the stated expiration date and once the bottle is open for an extended period, which can lead to contamination. Drops should be administered BEFORE ointments, otherwise the ointment will act as a barrier to the aqueous drops.

7. The answer is D (1.2.4)

All are eye preparation preservatives, except for boric acid, which is an antiseptic.

8. The answer is D (3.3.2)

Lid scrubs will not help prevent dry eye, as they are intended to remove excess oils, debris and desquamated skin that is associated with inflamed eyelids. Protecting soft contact lenses from drying out from exposure to extreme winds and temperatures can help prevent dry eye symptoms. Allegra is a systemic antihistamine with potential anticholinergic properties that can dry out the eyes.

9. The answer is B (1.3.1)

An ophthalmic antihistamine can be expected to resolve allergic conjunctivitis symptoms after 2 to 3 days of use. After 2 to 3 hours, they may notice some relief, but possibly not complete resolution of symptoms. If there is no relief after weeks or months, their condition needs to be reevaluated by their physician. And a patient should always be educated on self monitoring tips and to contact their doctor if they are not feeling better, as physicians are often too busy to follow up on all of their patients.

10. The answer is C (3.2.3)

Never recommend inserting any solution into the eye, while wearing contact lenses, unless the product is specifically formulated for contact lens use, like rewetting drops. I and II are considered proper administration techniques to successfully placing the medication in the eye, without additional contamination of the eye.

Case 74 Vaginal Preparations

1. The answer is C (1.1.3)

Insufficient vaginal lubrication can be caused from a variety of factors, which include: low estrogen concentrations (menopause, oophorectomy or postpartum), Sjogren's syndrome, diabetes mellitus, systemic lupus erythematosus, stress, fatigue, strenuous exercise, endometriosis, and medications.

2. The answer is D (1.2.1)

A douche is generally used for vaginal hygiene and would be inappropriate for improving vaginal dryness.

3. The answer is A (1.2.6)

Vaginal lubricants can be used as often as needed for the patient. The patient should, also, use the quantity that is needed to keep them comfortable.

4. The answer is D (1.3.5)

The patient could try a different vaginal lubricant to see if symptoms improve. If changing products does not work, then the patient should be referred. If the patient chooses to see a physician, a vaginal estrogen product would be the next step. HRT rather than ERT would be recommended orally since the patient's uterus is intact.

5. The answer is B (1.1.4)

Regular sexual activity will help maintain the vaginal lining so that it is more capable of producing adequate vaginal lubrication during sexual arousal. Both baths and sitz baths can flush lubrication from the vaginal area. Petroleum jelly is not recommended as a lubricant, and regular exercise has not been proven to increase lubrication.

6. The answer is D (2.2.3)

Glycerin is safe for use with latex condoms. All of the other choices are unsafe and will harm the integrity of the latex condom.

7. The answer is E (3.2.4)

All of the options would be appropriate. The sponge might require additional lubrication, but would be an appropriate alternative.

8. The answer Is D (3.2.4)

The onset of action of the sponge is immediate upon insertion; therefore, 15 minutes lead time is not needed prior to use. All of the other answers are correct counseling points regarding use of a contraceptive sponge.

9. The answer is E (2.2.3)

Astroglide is a lubricant and does not contain any spermicide. The other options all contain nonoxynol-9 as a spermicide.

10. The answer is B (3.2.4)

The female condom should only be used once. It should be discarded after use. Combination of a male and female condom can increase friction and cause displacement of the female condom.

Case 75 Skin Disorders and Sunscreens

1. The answer is C (1.1.4)

Since DD's fever blister developed while on vacation, excessive sun exposure is the most likely cause.

2. The answer is E (1.2.1)

Any of the treatment options would be appropriate. Abreva will be less effective in reducing healing time since the scab has already appeared, but it would still be considered an appropriate treatment option.

3. The answer is D (3.2.4)

Docosanol should be applied five times daily while awake for up to 10 days. Therapy should begin at the first sign of a fever blister.

4. The answer is E (3.2.2)

All of the statements are appropriate recommendations to make for the patient to prevent future recurrences induced by sun.

5. The answer is C (3.2.4)

Lip balms should have a minimum of 15 SPF in order to ensure adequate protection for the lips.

6. The answer is D (3.2.4)

A topical application of a triple antibiotic ointment/cream should be started. If no improvement or worsening, then the patient should be referred to a physician. The patient should be instructed to not remove the scab.

7. The answer is E (1.1.3)

The patient has plaque psoriasis. The lesions begin as small papules that will grow until they are joined together. The lesions range in color from pink to red to maroon. The lesions will have a scaly layer over them.

8. The answer is E (3.2.4)

Depending on the severity of the patient's symptoms, all of the recommendations would be appropriate.

9. The answer is E (1.2.1)

All of these ingredients may be found in various OTC preparations to treat psoriasis.

10. The answer is E (1.3.1)

After 7 days of unresponsive treatment with over-the-counter products, it would be best to refer the patient. Psoriasis is often unresponsive to self-treatment, and prescription products are required.

Answers
Federal Law
Review

1. The answer is C (1.02)

Under the PDMA, federal legend drug samples may be distributed by manufacturer's representatives only when a prescriber requests the samples in writing. Community pharmacies are not allowed to have any samples of federal legend drugs. Hospital pharmacies are allowed to possess samples but only when they are requested to do so by a prescriber.

2. The answer is C (1.04)

All of the listed individuals must obtain a DEA registration number to prescribe controlled substances except a medical resident who is employed by a teaching or research hospital. The resident uses the hospital's DEA registration number when prescribing controlled substances.

3. The answer is B (1.01)

The term "pharmacist-in-charge" is used most frequently to indicate which individual pharmacist can be held legally responsible for complying with the applicable laws. A few states do not use this term and, instead, elect to hold any "pharmacist on duty" responsible for legal compliance. The other terms are usually used in conjunction with employment status.

4. The answer is C (2.02)

Drug product interchange (generic selection or generic substitution), monitoring drug therapy, counseling patients, and interpreting prescriptions are all activities associated with core pharmacy practice. Making a physical assessment of a patient for the purpose of diagnosis is considered the practice of medicine and is generally outside the legal scope of pharmacy practice in the vast majority of practice settings.

5. The answer is D (1.04)

With the exception of a pharmacist who owns a pharmacy solely in his or her own name (a "sole practitioner"), pharmacists do not register with the DEA as a predicate to handling or dispensing controlled substances. Most, but not all, states issue a separate controlled substances license to pharmacists and other practitioners who handle these drugs. Physicians, hospitals, pharmacies, and nursing homes that dispense or otherwise handle controlled substances do need to obtain a DEA registration.

6. The answer is B (1.04)

The issue of who is allowed to prescribe which drugs is determined by state law. Most state laws make these determinations by defining the scope of practice of the practitioner. In the vast majority of cases podiatry is limited to the treatment of feet and nails (including fingernails). Prescribing contraceptive drugs is outside the scope of the practice of podiatry.

7. The answer is C (1.05)

Originally, OBRA-90 mandated that state law require pharmacists or their agents to offer to counsel in certain situations. That counseling requirement has been expanded to include new prescriptions for all patients. The laws are specific that while others may make the offer to counsel, only a pharmacist (or perhaps a pharmacist intern under the supervision of a pharmacist) may actually provide the counseling. Under the concept of professional discretion or judgment, a pharmacist may advise any patient at any time about the use of OTC and prescription-only medication.

8. The answer is D (2.02)

CMS administers Medicare and Medicaid programs. JCAHO only certifies institutions as complying with its standards of practice. DHHS is the federal administrative agency that oversees the FDA. The FDA does not license or register pharmacies even though, to a limited extent, it does have regulatory authority over some pharmacy activities. The states, through the Board of Pharmacy or an equivalent body, actually grant a pharmacy authority to operate and the DEA registers pharmacies to handle and dispense controlled substances.

9. The answer is A (3.02)

Controlled substances are placed into one of five schedules by the DEA. Federal legend drugs are those designated by the FDA as available only on the prescription of a licensed prescriber. INDs are drugs authorized for research uses by the FDA. A sample drug is one designated by a manufacturer or wholesaler as available for distribution without charge. A generic drug is one that is made by more than one manufacturer.

10. The answer is A (3.01)

Federal law requires pharmacies to keep controlled substances prescriptions at least 2 years after the date most recently dispensed. Having dispensed a refill on July 1, 2007, First Community must keep it on file until at least June 30, 2009.

11. The answer is C (3.01)

Using the same rule explained in the previous question, because ABC last dispensed the controlled substance on November 1, 2007, it must keep the prescription on file until at least October 31, 2009.

12. The answer is B (3.02)

Federal law limits refills on Schedule 3 and 4 drugs to five times within a 6-month period from the date the prescription is issued. This five refill limit applies even though a physician indicates, as in this case, that more than five refills are authorized. Here, because the patient has already obtained five refills, the pharmacy must refuse to dispense any additional medication. Likewise, no other pharmacy could dispense any other refills on the authority of this prescription. In any event the prescription could not be transferred back to the original pharmacy or any other pharmacy because DEA regulations limit the transfer of controlled substances prescriptions to one time only between unrelated pharmacies. Although not listed as a possible answer, the pharmacist could call the physician to obtain a new prescription authorization.

13. The answer is A (2.03)

DEA regulations allow a hospital pharmacy to supply a limited number of doses of controlled substances drugs to the emergency room if the drugs are stored in a locked cabinet. Procedures must be established under an approved protocol for stocking, restocking, and logging out all drugs stored in the cabinet. The pharmacy director must approve the protocol.

14. The answer is E (3.02)

Most states issue controlled substances licenses, in addition to other kinds of licenses, to pharmacists, pharmacies, physicians, and other authorized prescribers. The Board of Pharmacy or an equivalent agency usually issues the licenses.

15. The answer is A (3.01)

The FDA makes the determination that drugs are safe and effective for intended purposes when it approves an NDA for an individual drug. The DEA determines if FDA approved drugs should be controlled and how they should be scheduled. DHHS is the parent agency of the FDA but does not make determinations about drugs directly. CMS administers Medicare and Medicaid and, at least in part, pays suppliers for those drugs used by beneficiaries of those programs. The BNDD is the predecessor to the DEA and no longer exists.

16. The answer is B (3.01)

As explained in the answer to question 15, the DEA determines which drugs should be designated as controlled substances.

17. The answer is D (3.01)

Both the federal and individual state governments have authority to regulate controlled substances. The World Trade Federation is not a government agency. Local municipalities usually do not have direct authority to regulate controlled substances.

18. The answer is C (3.02)

Authority to designate which schedule a controlled substance will be placed in is vested in the United States Attorney General under federal statute. This cabinet-level presidential appointee is in charge of the Department of Justice, which is the parent agency of the DEA.

19. The answer is A (2.02)

Pharmacists and pharmacy interns are not required to register with the DEA before handling controlled substances. Neither police officers nor employees of manufacturers of controlled substances are required to obtain DEA registration. Pharmacies, however, must register with the DEA if controlled substances are handled.

20. The answer is C (1.04)

The federal "transfer warning," ("Federal law prohibits the transfer of this drug to any person other that the patient for whom it was prescribed"), must appear on the pharmacy label of dispensed controlled substances listed in Schedules II, III, and IV. The warning is not required for Schedule V controlled substances.

21. The answer is E (2.03)

DEA regulations allow pharmacies to either stock controlled substances in a locked cabinet in the pharmacy or disperse these medications throughout the other drug inventory. A combination of both methods is also permissible. For example, many pharmacies lock up Schedule 2 controlled substances while dispersing Schedule 3, 4, and 5 drugs with the rest of the pharmacy inventory.

22. The answer is A (1.04)

The term "purported prescription" is used in DEA regulation 21 CFR 1306.04 to describe an order for a controlled substance that may originate from a physician and appear to be a prescription in all other regards but is not deemed to be a prescription because it was issued for a non-legitimate reason. For example, a prescription that is sold to a patient by a physician outside of a normal patient-physician relationship for purposes of diversion, is a purported prescription. Note that even though a pharmacist might verify that an authorized prescriber issued a prescription, it is no less an unlawful purported prescription if issued for a reason that is not a legitimate medical purpose.

23. The answer is D (1.04)

Unlike the limits on refills of Schedule 3 and 4 controlled substances (five times in 6 months), Schedule 5 prescriptions may be refilled as many times as authorized by the prescriber or allowed by state law (usually 1 year from the date of issuance).

24. The answer is D (1.06)

Federal law limits the transfer of controlled substance prescriptions to one time between unrelated pharmacies. For purposes of this rule, "unrelated" means not under common ownership. For example, an independently owned pharmacy and a chainstore pharmacy corporation are unrelated.

25. The answer is D (1.04)

Two chain-store pharmacies owned by the same corporation are related and may transfer controlled substances prescriptions as often as refills are authorized but only if the two pharmacies are linked by a real-time online network. Chain pharmacies, even though owned by one corporation, are limited to the one-time transfer rule if they are not linked by a real-time online computer network.

26. The answer is B (1.06)

Schedule 2 controlled substances may be distributed (i.e., transferred) between DEA registrants only by use of DEA Form

Answers

222. Schedule 2 drugs cannot be dispensed by a pharmacy to a prescriber by use of a prescription that indicates the drugs will be used for the prescriber's office. Form 106 is used to report stolen or missing controlled substances.

27. The answer is D (1.02)

In contrast to the procedure for transferring Schedule 2 controlled substances between DEA registrants, Schedule 3 and 4 drugs are to be distributed using an invoice that is to be filed with other Schedule 3 and 4 records.

28. The answer is C (1.07)

Federal law requires pharmacies to complete a controlled substance inventory every 2 years. Note that many states require inventories to be taken more frequently. A 1-year period is common.

29. The answer is B (1.07)

Federal law requires pharmacies to maintain records of controlled substances prescriptions, invoices, and transfer records as well as inventories for at least 2 years. Note that many states have requirements that at least some of these records be kept for a longer period. For example, some states require that all prescriptions be kept a minimum of 5 years.

30. The answer is E (3.02)

Penalties for willful or knowing violations of the controlled substances laws may include criminal and civil sanctions as well as administrative actions against the pharmacy's DEA registration. Therefore, all of the answers are correct.

Compounding

Powders

1. The answer is A (3.2.3)

As listed in the directions for the patient, "bid" is the Latin abbreviation for two times daily or twice daily.

2. The answer is C (2.1.1)

By subtracting the ingredients, excluding corn starch, from the total amount to be dispensed, you obtain the required quantity of corn starch. Therefore, for 20 g:

Tolnaftate	1% w/w	= 0.2 g
Zinc oxide	5% w/w	= 1.0 g
Talc	20% w/w	= 4 g
Total ingredients	5.2 g	

20 g - 5.2 g = 14.8 g corn starch

3. The answer is A (2.1.1)

By subtracting the ingredients, excluding corn starch, from the total amount to be dispensed, this gives the required quantity of corn starch. Therefore, for 30 g:

Tolnaftate	1% w/w	= 0.3 g
Zinc Oxide	5% w/w	= 1.5 g
Talc	20% w/w	= 6 g
	7.8 g total ingredients	

30g - 7.8 g = 22.2 g corn starch

4. The answer is B (2.1.1)

1% tolnaftate = (1 g tolnaftate/100 g total) x 30 g total= 0.3 tolnaftate

5. The answer is B (2.1.1)

(0.2 g tolnaftate/20 g total)=1:100::tolnaftate:total

6. The answer is B (3.2.3)

Since this preparation is in powder form and will be administered to the feet, the only auxiliary label required is "not to be taken by mouth."

7. The answer is E (2.1.4)

0.0014 g/10 g x 300 g = 0.042 g

8. The answer is B (2.1.4)

1.4 mg/10 g x 10 g = 1.4 mg = 0.0014 g

9. The answer is D (2.1.4)

0.0014 g/10 g x 100 g = 0.014%

10. The answer is C (3.2.3)

The Latin abbreviation "au" in the patient instructions is translated as administration in both ears.

11. The answer is A (3.2.3)

The Latin abbreviation "tid" in the patient instructions is translated to mean administration of the drug product three times daily.

12. The answer is E (2.1.1)

2% = (2 g/100 g) x 100 g = 2 g Miconazole

13. The answer is D (2.1.1)

Since 2 grams of the total 100-gram preparation are made up of miconazole, the remaining 98 grams (100 g - 2 g) will be boric acid powder.

14. The answer is E (3.2.3)

Based on the patient instructions and on the formulation type, the auxiliary labels include "for external use only" and "for the ear."

15. The answer is E (2.1.1)

(400 µg/15 g) x (1 mg/1000 µg) x 30 g = 0.8 mg

16. The answer is A (2.1.1)

Since 0.8 mg is required for a 30-gram preparation, twice that, or 1.6 mg would be required for the 60-gram preparation. 1.6 mg or 0.0016 g.

17. The answer is C (2.1.1)

30 g x (15.432 gr/1 gr) = 462.96 gr

18. The answer is D (2.1.1)

30 g x (1 mL/1.3 g)=23.1 mL

19. The answer is A (3.2.3)

The Latin abbreviation for powder is "pulv."

20. The answer is B (2.1.1)

Since misoprostol and polyethylene oxide are in a ratio of 0.4 mg:200 mg, dividing 200 mg by 0.4 reduces the ratio.

21. The answer is D (2.1.1)

(0.0004 g misoprostol/15 g total) x 100=0.0027% w/w

Capsules

1. The answer is E (2.1.1)

Assuming that there is no overage, the total six capsules will contain 60 mg pseudoephedrine and 12 mg chlorpheniramine, both of which are below SAW of the balance.

2. The answer is B (2.1.1)

8 capsules x (160 acetaminophen/1 capsule) x (1 g/1000 mg) x (15.432 gr/1 g) = 19.8 gr

3. The answer is A (2.1.1)

10 capsules x (10 mg pseudoephedrine/1 capsule) x (1 g/1000 mg) x (15.432 gr/1 g) = 1.54 gr

4. The answer is A (2.1.1)

(350 mg/1 capsule) x 6 capsules = 2100 mg or 2.1 g

5. The answer is C (2.1.1)

350 mg - 10 mg - 2 mg - 160 mg = 178 mg lactose

6. The answer is A (2.1.1)

(160 mg acetaminophen/350 mg total) x 100 = 45.7%

7. The answer is C (3.2.3)

The Latin abbreviations "tid" and "prn" are translated as three times daily as needed.

8. The answer is E (3.2.3)

None of the auxiliary labels listed there are required for this type of formulation.

9. The answer is C (3.2.3)

The Latin abbreviation "qid" is translated as four times daily.

10. The answer is B (2.1.1)

(50 mg dehydroepiandosterone/350 mg total) x 100 = 14.3%

11. The answer is A (2.1.1)

350 mg - 50 mg = 300 mg/capsule of lactose

10 capsules x (300 mg/1 capsule) = 3000 mg or 3 g

12. The answer is C (2.1.1)

50 mg x 12 = 600 mg or 0.6 g dehydroepiandrosterone

13. The answer is C (2.1.1)

Since 300 mg lactose are required for each capsule, 10 capsules would require three grams of lactose

3 g x (15.432 gr/1 g) = 46.296 gr

14. The answer is B (2.1.1)

300 mg lactose/50 mg dehydroepiandrosterone = 6; therefore, there is 1 part dehydroepiandrosterone per 6 parts lactose.

15. The answer is C (2.1.1)

(280 - 1 - 8 - 1 - 150) x 100 = 12,000 mg or 12 g

16. The answer is C (2.1.1)

8 mg/280 mg x 100 mg = 2.857% w/w

17. The answer is C (2.1.1)

60 capsules x 150 mg/capsule = 9000 mg or 9 g

Answers

Tablets

1. The answer is B (2.1.1)

150 mg x 200 tablets = 30 g

30 g + 0.01 (30 g) = 30.3 g

2. The answer is C (3.2.3)

The Latin abbreviation "tid prn" in the patient instructions is translated as three times daily as needed.

3. The answer is B (2.1.1)

(15 mg pseudoephedrine/150 mg total) x 100 = 10% w/w

4. The answer is A (2.1.1)

15 mg pseudoephedrine x 200 tablets = 3000 mg or 3 g

3 g + 0.01(3 g) = 3.03 g

3.03 g x (15.432 gr/1 g) = 46.75 gr

5. The answer is A (2.1.1)

10 mg loratadine x 200 tablets = 2000 mg or 2 g

2 g + 0.01 (2 g) = 2.02 g

6. The answer is B (2.1.1)

150 mg total/10 mg loratadine = 1.5; so, 1 part loratadine per 1.5 parts total or 1:1.5

Troches and Lozenges

1. The answer is B (3.2.3)

The Latin abbreviation "bid" in the patient instructions is translated as twice daily.

2. The answer is B (2.1.1)

50 mg sodium fluoride x 10 lozenges = 500 mg or 0.5 g

0.5 g + 0.2 (0.5 g) = 0.60 g

3. The answer is A (2.1.1)

(2 g/mold) x (1 mL/0.98 g) = 2.04 mL/mold

4. The answer is B (2.1.1)

10 lozenges x (2 g/lozenge) = 20 g

20 g - (10 x 0.05 g sodium fluoride) = 19.5 g sorbitol

5. The answer is A (2.1.1)

(50 mg sodium fluoride/2000 mg total) x 100 = 2.5% w/w

Solutions

1. The answer is C (2.1.1)

Since one fluid ounce is 30 mL, the amount dispensed will be 60 mL (2 x 30 mL).

(Q.27 in CBT)

2. The answer is B (2.1.1)

(20 mg phenobarbital/5 mL) x 60 mL = 240 mg phenobarbital

240 mg x (1 mL/25 mg) = 9.6 mL stock solution

3. The answer is C (2.1.1)

60 mL total x (10 mL simple syrup/100 mL total) x (1.3 g simple syrup/1 mL simple syrup) = 7.8 g simple syrup

4. The answer is C (2.1.1)

Since each teaspoon is 5 mL and the instructions call for two teaspoons per dose, the total dose in milliliters is 10 mL.

5. The answer is C (3.2.3)

The Latin abbreviation "tid" in the patient instructions is translated as three times daily.

6. The answer is B (2.1.1)

(20 mg phenobarbital/5 mL) x 60 mL = 240 mg phenobarbital

7. The answer is A (2.1.1)

60 mL total x (10 mL simple syrup/100 mL total) = 6 mL

8. The answer is A (2.1.1)

(0.1 g methylparaben/100 mL) x 5 mL = 0.005 g or 5 mg methylparaben

20 mg phenobarbital/5 mg methylparaben = 4

9. The answer is B (2.1.1)

2.5 g/100 mL = 2.5% w/v

10. The answer is A (2.1.1)

(2.5 g/100 mL) x 15 mL = 0.375 g or 375 mg meperidine

11. The answer is D (2.1.1)

(200 mg/100 mL) x 15 mL = 30 mg

12. The answer is B (3.2.3)

The Latin abbreviation "qid prn" in the patient instructions translates to four times daily as needed.

13. The answer is D (3.2.3)

The preparation should not be taken by mouth and is intended for use in the nose.

Answers

Suspensions

1. The answer is A (2.1.1)
(0.9 g/100 mL) x 100 mL = 0.9 g

2. The answer is A (2.1.1)
(0.24 g/250 mL) x 100 = 0.096% w/v

3. The answer is A (2.1.1)
(0.24 g/250 mL) x 150 mL = 0.144 g
0.144 g x (15.432 gr/1 g) = 2.2 gr

4. The answer is B (3.2.3)
The Latin abbreviation "bid" in the patient instructions translates to twice daily.

5. The answer is C (2.1.1)
(0.24 g/250 mL) x 100 mL = 0.096 g or 96 mg

6. The answer is B (2.1.1)
10.5 lb x (1 kg/2.2 lb) x (0.5 mg/1 kg) x 250 mL/240 mg) = 2.48 mL

7. The answer is A (3.2.3)
Since the preparation is a suspension, the required auxiliary label is "Shake Well."

8. The answer is C (2.1.1)
Each fluid ounce is 30 mL, so two fluid ounces is 60 mL.

9. The answer is A (2.1.1)
(5 mL/100 mL) x 60 mL = 3 mL 2N sodium hydroxide
3 mL x (1.2 g/1 mL) = 3.6 g

10. The answer is A

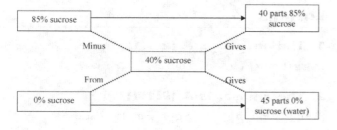

The parts given in the above allegation can be reduced to 4:4.5 (2.1.1)

11. The answer is B (2.1.1)
3/4 tsp x (5 mL/1 tsp)=3.75 mL

12. The answer is A (3.2.3)
The Latin abbreviation "qd" given in the patient instructions is translated to once daily

13. The answer is B (2.1.1)
(5 mL/100 mL) x 60 mL=3 mL 2N sodium hydroxide

14. The answer is A (2.1.1)
(0.02 g/100 mL) x 60 mL=0.012 g or 12 mg sodium lauryl sulfate

12 mg x (100 mL/1000 mg)=1.2 mL stock solution

Sterile Solutions

1. The answer is B (2.1.1)
(1 mg/1 mL) x 2 mL = 2 mg albuterol per dose

2. The answer is C (3.2.3)
According to the patient instructions, the Latin abbreviation tqid prn is translated as "three to four times daily as needed."

3. The answer is A (2.1.1)
(0.01 g/100 mL) x 20 mL = 2 mg benzalkonium chloride

4. The answer is B (2.1.1)
(0.01 g/100 mL) x 20 mL = 2 mg benzalkonium chloride

2 mg x (100 mL/100 mg) = 2 mL stock solution

Ointments

1. The answer is A (2.1.1)
(0.5 g/100 g) x 10 g = 0.05 g hydrocortisone

2. The answer is A (2.1.1)
10 g x (1 mL/1.1 g) = 9.09 mL

3. The answer is A (2.1.1)
Hydrocortisone 0.5% w/w = 0.05 g

Methylparaben 0.1% w/w = 0.01 g

Propylparaben 0.01% w/w = 0.001 g

0.05 g + 0.01 g + 0.001 g = 0.06 g

So, the total amount of white petrolatum needed is 10 g - 0.06 g = 9.94 g

4. The answer is B (2.1.1)
(0.1 g/100 g) x 10 g = 0.01 g methylparaben

5. The answer is D (3.2.3)
According to the patient instructions, the Latin abbreviation "qod" is translated as "every other day."

6. The answer is D (3.2.3)
The Latin abbreviation "ung" is translated as ointment.

Answers

7. The answer is E (3.2.3)

Ointments are for external use only and should not be taken by mouth. There is no need to shake semisolid dosage forms.

8. The answer is C (3.2.3)

The Latin abbreviation "q2–3h prn" in the patient instructions are translated as "every 2–3 hours as needed."

9. The answer is C (2.1.1)

$(10 g/100 g) \times 15 g = 1.5 g$ anhydrous lanolin

10. The answer is B (2.1.1)

$(18 g/100 g) \times 15 g = 2.7 g$ cetyl esters wax

11. The answer is E (2.1.1)

$(30 g/100 g) \times 15 g = 4.5 g$ yellow wax

12. The answer is C (2.1.1)

$(42 g/100 g) \times 15 g = 6.3 g$ liquid petrolatum

13. The answer is B (2.1.1)

$(42 g/100 g) \times 15 g = 6.3 g$ liquid petrolatum

$6.3 g \times (1 mL/0.89 g) = 7.08 mL$

14. The answer is C (2.1.1)

42% liquid petrolatum/18% cetyl esters wax = 2.33
Therefore, there is 1 part cetyl esters wax per 2.33 parts liquid petrolatum

15. The answer is E (3.2.3)

Ointments are for external use only and should not be taken by mouth. There is no need to shake semisolid dosage forms.

Pastes

1. The answer is B (2.1.1)

$(53 g/100 g) \times 30 g = 15.9$ zinc oxide ointment

2. The answer is A (2.1.1)

$(17 g/100 g) \times 30 g = 5.1 g$ white petrolatum

Plus

$((100 g - (20 g$ zinc oxide $+ 15 g$ mineral oil$))/100 g) \times (53 g/100 g) \times 30 g = 10.34 g$ white petrolatum (zinc oxide ointment)
So, $10.34 + 5.1 = 15.44 g$ total white petrolatum

3. The answer is D (2.1.1)

$(17 g/100 g) \times 30 g = 5.1 g$ white petrolatum

4. The answer is C (2.1.1)

$(25 g/100 g) \times 30 g = 7.5 g$ mineral oil

$7.5 g (1 mL/0.89 g) = 8.4 mL$

5. The answer is C (2.1.1)

$(5 g/100 g) \times 30 g = 1.5 g$ white wax

6. The answer is B (2.1.1)

53 g zinc oxide ointment/5 g white wax = 10.6
Therefore, there is 1 part white wax per 10.6 parts zinc oxide ointment.

Creams

1. The answer is C (2.1.1)

$15 g \times (1 mL/1.1 g) = 13.6 mL$

2. The answer is B (2.1.1)

$(5 g/1000 g) \times 15 g = 0.075 g$ or 75 mg boric acid

$75 mg \times (100 mL/5000 mg) = 1.5 mL$ stock solution

3. The answer is E (3.2.3)

The Latin abbreviation "q2–3 h prn" in the patient instructions is translated "every 2–3 hours as needed."

4. The answer is A (2.1.1)

$(125 g/1000 g) \times 15 g = 1.875 g$ cetyl esters wax

5. The answer is C (2.1.1)

$(125 g/1000 g) \times 100 = 12.5\%$ cetyl esters wax

6. The answer is C (2.1.1)

$(560 g/1000 g) \times 15 g = 8.4 g$ mineral oil

$8.4 g \times (1 mL/0.89 g) = 9.4 mL$

7. The answer is B (2.1.1)

100% cream/12.5% cetyl esters wax = 8
Therefore, there is 1 part cetyl esters wax per 8 parts cream

Lotions

1. The answer is A (2.1.1)

$15 g \times (1 mL/1.2 g) = 12.5 mL$

2. The answer is A (2.1.1)

$(0.5 g/100 g) \times 15 g = 0.075 g$ or 75 mg lactic acid

$75 mg \times (1 mL/25 mg) = 3 mL$ stock solution

3. The answer is B (2.1.1)

Since 0.5 g are contained in 100 g of the total preparation, the concentration of lactic acid is 0.5% w/w.

4. The answer is D (2.1.1)

0.5 g lactic acid/0.1 g methylparaben = 5
Therefore, there is 1 part methylparaben per 5 parts lactic acid.

5. The answer is C (2.1.1)

(6 g/100 g) x 15 g = 0.9 g mineral oil

0.9 g x (1 mL/0.89 g) = 1.01 mL

Gels

1. The answer is B (2.1.1)

(0.02 g/15 g) x 100 = 0.133% capsaicin

2. The answer is C (2.1.1)

50 mg x (100 mL/1250 mg) = 4 mL stock solution

3. The answer is D (2.1.1)

Dissolving 100 mg capsaicin in 10 mL ethanol will form a 10-mg/mL solution; 2 mL will contain the correct amount of capsaicin for the preparation.

4. The answer is B (2.1.1)

5 drops x (1 mL/20 drops) = 0.25 mL TEA

5. The answer is B (3.2.3)

According to the patient instructions, the Latin abbreviation qod prn is translated "every other day as needed."

6. The answer is C (2.1.1)

(0.3 g/100 mL) x 0.3 mL = 0.9 mg scopolamine HBr

7. The answer is A (2.1.1)

0.1 mL x (1.2 g/1 mL) = 0.12 g

8. The answer is A (2.1.1)

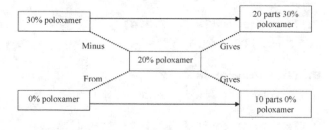

The ratio of 10 parts water to 20 parts 30% poloxamer can be reduced to 1:2.

9. The answer is D (2.1.1)

(0.1 g/100 mL) x 0.3 mL = 0.3 mg methylparaben

10. The answer is C (3.2.3)

The Latin abbreviation ud is translated "as directed."

Aqueous Nasal Sprays

1. The answer is A (2.1.1)

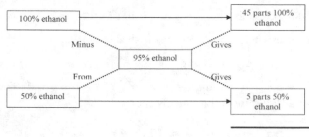

(5 parts 50% ethanol/50 parts total) x 1000 mL = 100 mL 50% ethanol

2. The answer is A (2.1.1)

(0.2 g/100 mL) x 30 mL = 0.06 g or 60 mg methylparaben
60 mg x (100 mL/3000 mg) = 2 mL stock solution

3. The answer is C (2.1.1)

(0.25 g/100 mL) x 100 = 0.25% dihydroergotamine mesylate

4. The answer is A (2.1.1)

(5 mL/100 mL) x 30 mL = 1.5 mL glycerin

1.5 mL x (0.92 g/1 mL) = 1.38 g

5. The answer is E (2.1.1)

(250 mg/10 sprays) x (1 mL/1000 mg) = 0.025 mL

6. The answer is E (2.1.1)

(0.25 g/100 mL) x (0.025 mL/spray) = 0.0625 mg

7. The answer is B (2.1.1)

(30 g - 28.4 g)/10 sprays x (1 mL/1 g) = 0.16 mL/spray

2 mg Morphine Sulfate/mL x 0.16 mL/spray = 0.32 mg/actuation or 320 mcg/actuation

8. The answer is A (2.1.1)

(30 g - 29.1 g)/10 sprays x 1 mL/0.8 g = 0.1125 mL/spray

0.02 mg naltrexone/mL x 0.1125 mL/spray = 0.00225 mg/actuation or 2.25 mcg/actuation

9. The answer is B (2.1.1)

0.115 mL x 2 mg/mL x 12 actuations/day = 2.76 mg

Rectal suppositories

1. The answer is B (3.2.3)

According to the patient instructions listed on the prescription order, the Latin abbreviation q 8 h prn can be translated "every 8 hours as needed."

Answers

2. The answer is A (2.1.1)

(10 mg/1 suppository) x 6 suppositories = 60 mg

If balance SAW is 100 mg, needs an aliquot

100 mg/60 mg = 200 mg/120 mg

So, weigh out 100 mg resorcin, dilute to 200 mg with zinc oxide and remove 120 mg of that mixture.

3. The answer is A (2.1.1)

3 mL x (1.1 g/1 mL) = 3.3 g for each suppository

3.3 g x 6 suppositories = 19.8 g total

19800 mg - 6 (50 mg + 20 mg + 10 mg + 300 mg) =

17520 mg or 17.52 g

4. The answer is B (2.1.1)

(50 mg/1 suppository) x 4 suppositories = 200 mg

5. The answer is A (2.1.1)

2 g x 4 suppositories = 8 g total

8000 mg - 4 (50 mg + 20 mg + 10 mg + 300 mg) = 6480 mg or 6.48 g

Vaginal suppositories

1. The answer is C (2.1.1)

2 g x 4 suppositories = 8 g total

2. The answer is D (3.2.3)

According to the patient instructions listed on the prescription drug order, the Latin abbreviation qhs is translated "before bedtime."

3. The answer is A (2.1.1)

2 g x 4 suppositories = 8 g total

8000 mg - 4[40 mg + ((5 g/100 g) x 2000 mg)] = 7440 mg or 7.44 g

4. The answer is C (2.1.1)

(5 g/100 g) x 2 g = 0.1 g or 0.1 mL water

Solutions

1. The answer is B (2.1.1)

0.2 g/100 mL = 0.2% w/v

2. The answer is C (2.1.1)

100 mL - (200 mg x 1 mL/50 mg) - (25 mg x 1 mL/25 mg) = 95 mL of saline required, such that 5 mL of saline must be removed from the 100 mL bag.

3. The answer is C (2.1.1)

0.025 mg/100 mL = 0.025%

4. The answer is A (2.1.1)

0.9 g/100 mL x 90 mL = 0.81 g NaCl

0.81 g/100 mL = 0.81% w/v

Calculations

Basic Principles of Pharmaceutical Calculations

1. The answer is E (2.1.4)

1.45 mg x $(1 \times 10^9$ pg/1 mg) = 1.45×10^9 picograms

2. The answer is C (2.1.4)

5 quarts x (32 fluid ounces/1 quart) = 160 fluid ounces

3. The answer is A (2.1.4)

3 lb x (1 kg/2.2 lb) x (1000 g/1 kg) x (15.432 gr/1 g) = 2.1×10^4 gr

4. The answer is C (2.1.4)

110 lb x (1 kg/2.2 lb) x (2.5 mg/1 kg) = 125 mg

5. The answer is D (2.1.4)

94 g/100 mL = 0.94 g/mL

6. The answer is E (2.1.4)

2 g x (1 mL/0.976 g) = 2.05 mL

7. The answer is C (2.1.4)

2 g x (1 mL/1.02 g) = 1.96 mL

8. The answer is A (2.1.4)

Specific volume = (1/specific gravity) = (1/0.956) = 1.05

9. The answer is A (2.1.1)

1.5 kg x (1000 g/1 kg) x (15.432 gr/1 g)=23148 gr

10. The answer is A (2.1.1)

Specific Gravity = 6.5 g/30 mL = 0.22

11. The answer is B (2.1.4)

1 mL/6.5 g x 9 g = 1.38 mL

Basic Pharmaceutical Calculations

1. The answer is C (2.1.4)

$20 \text{ g}/1000 \text{ mL} = 5 \text{ g}/X$

$x = 250 \text{ mL}$

2. The answer is C (2.1.4)

Only C is correct because the answer for B requires measurement below the SAW for the balance.

3. The answer is B (2.1.4)

Dissolving 90 mg methylparaben in 12 mL forms a 7.5 mg/mL solution, which 2 mL will contain 15 mg.

4. The answer is A (2.1.4)

$(50 \text{ mg}/1 \text{ mL}) \times (1000 \text{ µg}/1 \text{ mg}) \times (1000 \text{ mL}/1 \text{ L}) = 5 \times 10^7 \text{ µg}/\text{mL}$

5. The answer is C (2.1.1)

$(750 \text{ mL}/5 \text{ hr}) = (150 \text{ mL}/\text{hr})$

$(150 \text{ mL}/\text{hr}) \times (1 \text{ hr}/60 \text{ min}) = (2.5 \text{ mL}/\text{min})$

6. The answer is D (2.1.1)

$(700 \text{ drops}/\text{hr}) \times 8 \text{ hr} = 5600 \text{ drops}$

$(5600 \text{ drops}/1000 \text{ mL}) = 5.6 \text{ drops}/\text{mL}$

Dosage Calculations

1. The answer is A (2.1.4)

Using Fried's Rule for infants,
$(3 \text{ months}/150 \text{ months}) \times 500 \text{ mg} = 10 \text{ mg}$

2. The answer is E (2.1.4)

Using Clark's Rule,
$15 \text{ kg} \times (2.2 \text{ lb}/1 \text{ kg}) = 33 \text{ lb}$

$(33 \text{ lb}/150) \times 65 \text{ mg} = 14.3 \text{ mg}$

3. The answer is A (2.1.4)

$200 \text{ lb} \times (1 \text{ kg}/2.2 \text{ lb}) \times (2 \text{ mg}/1 \text{ kg}) = 182 \text{ mg}$

4. The answer is C (2.1.4)

Drawing a line from the 300-lb mark to the 71-inch mark on the nomogram for body surface area, the surface area of this patient is 2.5 m²

$(2.5 \text{ m}^2/1.73 \text{ m}^2) \times 300 \text{ mg} = 434 \text{ mg}$

5. The answer is A (2.1.4)

Since each teaspoon is 5 mL, 30 mL is 6 teaspoons.

6. The answer is B (2.1.4)

$(2 \text{ tablespoons}/1 \text{ day}) \times (15 \text{ mL}/1 \text{ tablespoon}) \times 30 \text{ days} = 900 \text{ mL}$

7. The answer is B (2.1.4)

$(30 \text{ drops}/5 \text{ mL}) = 6 \text{ drops}/\text{mL}$

8. The answer is A (2.1.4)

$1.2 \text{ mL} \times (5 \text{ drops}/1 \text{ mL}) = 6 \text{ drops}$

9. The answer is B (2.1.4)

$30 \text{ mL} \times (5 \text{ drops}/1 \text{ mL}) \times (1 \text{ dose}/15 \text{ drops}) = 10 \text{ doses}$

10. The answer is A (2.1.4)

$1.5 \text{ mg} \times (1 \text{ g}/1000 \text{ mg}) \times (1000 \text{ mL}/1 \text{ g}) = 1.5 \text{ mL}$

11. The answer is B (2.1.4)

$0.8 \text{ mg} \times (1000 \text{ mcg}/1 \text{ mg}) \times (2 \text{ mL}/500 \text{ mcg}) = 3.2 \text{ mL}$

Concentration

1. The answer is C (2.1.4)

$(0.05 \text{ g}/500 \text{ mL}) \times 100 \text{ mL} = 0.01\% \text{ w/v}$

2. The answer is B (2.1.4)

$20 \text{ g ZnO}/100 \text{ g mixture} = 20\% \text{ w/w}$

3. The answer is A (2.1.4)

50% w/v is a ratio of 50 g of substance to 100 mL solution, so the ratio can be reduced to 1:2.

4. The answer is C (2.1.4)

Since the lidocaine HCl solution is diluted in half, the resulting concentration is 0.5%, or:

$1(250) = x(500)$, where $x = 0.5$

5. The answer is C (2.1.4)

$90(500 \text{ mL}) = 50(X \text{ mL})$ where $X = 900 \text{ mL}$ total solution

However, since 500 mL of the final solution is taken from the ethanol, only 400 mL of water are needed.

6. The answer is B (2.1.4)

5 x 300	1500
2 x 400	800
8 x 250	2000
7.5 x 400	3000
1350	7300

$7300 \div (1350 \text{ mL}) = 5.4\%$

7. The answer is E (2.1.4)

$5\% = 5 \text{ g}/100 \text{ mL} = 50 \text{ mg}/\text{mL}$

$200 \text{ mL} \times (50 \text{ mg}/1 \text{ mL}) = 10,000 \text{ mg}$

$(10,000 \text{ mg} \times 1)/74.5 = 134.23 \text{ mEq}$

Answers

8. The answer is A (2.1.4)

5% = (5 g/100 mL) x 1000 mL = 50 g/L

((50 g/L)/74.5 g) x 2 species x 1000 = 1342 mOsm/L

9. The answer is A (2.1.4)

0.9% sodium chloride solution is considered to be isotonic.

10. The answer is A (2.1.4)

0.9 g/100 mL x 100 mL = 0.9 g

0.9 g - 0.01 x 0.16 = 0.8984 g = 898.4 mg

11. The answer is D (2.1.4)

2.5 mL x 20 mEq/5 mL = 10 mEq

10 mEq/1000 mL = 0.01 mEq/mL

12. The answer is B (2.1.4)

25 drops/min x 1 mL/15 drops = 1.67 mL/min

1.67 mL/min x 22.5 mEq/1000 mL x 60 min/1 hr = 2.25 mEq/hr

13. The answer is B (2.1.4)

0.8 g/100 mL x 50 mL/hr = 0.4 g/hr = 400 mg/hr

Calculations For Sterile Products

1. The answer is C (2.1.4)

0.8 mg x 1 mL/0.4 mg = 2 mL

2. The answer is A (2.1.4)

50 units x 1 mL/100 units = 0.5 mL

3. The answer is A (2.1.4)

1000 mL/4 hr x 1 hr/60 min x 8 drops/mL=33.3 drops/min

4. The answer is E (2.1.4)

500 mL x 1 hr/55 mL = 9 hr

5. The answer is D (2.1.4)

450 mL/100 min x 10 drops/mL = 45 drops/min

6. The answer is B (2.1.4)

25 mL/hr x 0.5 hr = 12.5 mL

7. The answer is A (2.1.4)

The powder has 2 mL of volume

10 mL/12 mL x 400,000 Units/mL=333,333 Units/mL

8. The answer is A (2.1.4)

1000 Units/hr x 4 hr = 4000 units

9. The answer is C (2.1.4)

500 mg/4 mL = 125 mg/mL

10. The answer is A (2.1.4)

450 mL x 5 g/100 mL = 22.5 g

11. The answer is C (2.1.4)

Flow Rate = 240 mg/hr x 1000 mL/4000 mg = 60 mL/hr

12. The answer is A (2.1.4)

2500 Units/2 hr x 0.5 hr = 625 Units

13. The answer is C (2.1.4)

0.015 g x 1000 mL/10 g = 1.5 mL

14. The answer is D (2.1.4)

0.45 g x 10 mL/0.5 g = 9 mL

15. The answer is B (2.1.4)

(900 mg x 1)/58 = 15.5 mEq

16. The answer is E (2.1.4)

500 mL/1000 mg x 60 mg/hr = 30 mL/hr

17. The answer is E (2.1.4)

30 mL x 10 g/100 mL = 3 g

18. The answer is A (2.1.4)

500 mL/3 hr x 1 hr/60 min x 8 drops/mL = 22 drops/min

19. The answer is D (2.1.4)

6 %w/v = 6 g/100 mL or 60 g/L

20. The answer is C (2.1.4)

4 mL/500 mL x 350 mg/1 mL = 2.8 mg/mL

21. The answer is B (2.1.4)

30 mL x 1 g/10,000 mL = 0.003 = 3 mg